SpringerWienNewYork

H. Parvez, P. Riederer (eds.)

Oxidative Stress and Neuroprotection

Journal of Neural Transmission
Supplement 71

SpringerWienNewYork

Prof. Dr. H. Parvez
Institute Alfred Fessard de Neurosciences, CNRS,
Gif Yvette, France

Prof. Dr. P. Riederer
Klinik und Poliklinik für Psychiatrie und Psychotherapie
Würzburg, Germany

Printed in Austria

SpringerWienNewYork is part of Springer Science+Business Media
springer.com

Typesetting: Thomson Press India Ltd., New Dehli
Printing: Druckerei Theiss GmbH, 9431 St. Stefan im Lavanttal, Austria

Printed on acid-free and chlorine-free bleached paper

SPIN: 11733454

Library of Congress Control Number: 2006932707

With 72 Figures

ISSN 0303-6995
ISBN-10 3-211-33327-4 SpringerWienNewYork
ISBN-13 978-3-211-33327-3 SpringerWienNewYork

J Neural Transm (2006) [Suppl] 71: V–IX

Journal of Neural Transmission
Printed in Austria

My love with monoamine oxidase, iron and Parkinson's disease

M. B. H. Youdim

Technion-Rappaport Family Faculty of Medicine, Eve Topf and US National Parkinson Foundation, Centers of Excellence for Neurodegenerative Diseases Research and Teaching and Department of Pharmacology, Haifa, Israel

I had intended to go to medical school and was accepted to McGill University, Montreal (1959). During my preclinical B.Sc (1961) degree, the courses of biochemistry and neurochemistry were to influence me so much that I gave up the idea of medicine and decided to take a Ph.D in neurochemistry-neuropharmacology and was directed to Theodore L. Sourkes, at the Allan Memorial Institute (McGill University Department of Psychiatry), who was working on monoamine oxidase (MAO), MAO inhibitors, serotonin, depression, dopamine and Parkinson's disease. Ted, as he is affectionately known to all his colleagues, accepted me for an Msc. and Ph.D where I started to work on serotonin metabolism and MAO. In my M.Sc thesis I provided one of the first physico-chemical and pharmacological evidence for two forms of MAO in rat liver and brain mitochondria, which have now been shown to be two separate proteins (MAO A and MAO B). I presented these data at FASEB meeting in Atlantic City (1963), where I met Menek Goldstein and Toshi Nagatsu who remained my close friends ever since and the chairman was Albert Zeller, the discoverer of first MAO inhibitor, iproniazid. For my PhD I decided to purify MAO. After two years we eventually were able to solubilize and purify MAO. We showed that the purified enzyme still exhibited two forms of MAO with different inhibitor sensitivities. In 1966 I went back to England to continue my work on MAO and its multiple forms with Merton Sandler, where I remained until 1972 as a Welcome Research Fellow. These were to be some of my formidable years. It was while with Merton Sandler that I met Keith Tipton with whom I forged a friendship and collaboration that remain until today. With Merton Sandler, in a series of papers published in Nature, we described the multiple forms of MAO in rat and human brains and showed that human basal ganglia contains mostly MAO B. This finding was to have a major impact later on in the treatment of Parkinson's disease with MAO B inhibitor l-deprenyl (selegiline). We also showed for the first time the effect of selective MAO A (clorgyline) and non selective MAO inhibitors (tranylcypromine, isocarboxazide) on MAO and amine metabolism in human brains, obtained at autopsy from geriatric subjects with terminal diseases treated with MAO inhibitor antidepressants. In the Nature paper (Youdim et al. 1972) we predicted the future development of selective MAO inhibitors directed at each enzyme form as antidepressants, but devoid of their major side effect, namely potentiation of sympathomimetic action of indirectly acting amines (tyramine), known as the "cheese reaction" (which eventually led to the development of reversible MAO A inhibitor antidepressants such as moclobemide and brofaromin. In 1972 Jacques Glowinski invited me to spend a year at College de France in Paris as Welcome Trust Fellow, and with Michel Hamon we purified tryptophan hydroxylase and during which time I met Hasan Parvez as consequence being his Ph.D examiner. While in Paris David Grahame-Smith offered me a position at the MRC Unit and Department of Clinical Pharmacology at Oxford.

The four years (1973–1977) I spent at Oxford was to profoundly change my carrier. The department consisted of a dynamic group of young individuals (A. R. Green, F. Woods and J. Aronson, and David Boulin) with different talents who wanted to succeed badly. Thanks to Grahame-Smith, the department and its members achieved world

Correspondence: Moussa B. H. Youdim, PhD, Technion-Rappaport Family Faculty of Medicine, Eve Topf and US National Parkinson Foundation, Centers of Excellence for Neurodegenerative Diseases Research and Teaching and Department of Pharmacology, Haifa, Israel prominence. Here I continued to study the physiological roles of MAO A and B. Specially MOA-B, with highest encouragement from High Blaschko, who was at the department of pharmacology. Blaschko, never failed to support me and was responsible for me to come to Oxford. Within the first year at Oxford I meet two individuals who influenced me so much, that if I had not met them, my carrier would certainly have taken a different turn. The first was the hematologist Dr. Shiela Calendar, Reader in the Department of Medicine at Oxford. She had read an earlier paper of mine on iron and MAO from my years with Ted Sourkes and thought why I had not continued my studies on brain iron metabolism and neurotransmitter metabolism. The reason being that nutritional iron deficiency was the major nutritional deficiency in the world affecting 4–600 million individuals and iron deficient children have abnormal behavior and cognitive defect. Iron is a cofactor of the major enzymes of the mitochondrial electron transport system and for synthetic and metabolic aminergic neurotransmitter enzymes (tyrosine hydroxylase, tryptophan hydroxylase and monoamine oxidase). An abnormality in serotonin, dopamine and noradrenaline might explain the altered behavior in the iron deficient children. Practically there were no published works on brain iron distribution, regulation, metabolism had been done. I set up a rat model of nutritional iron deficiency with Richard Green and showed it resulted in reduction of brain iron metabolism and diminution of aminergic (serotonin and dopamine) neurotransmission and behavioral responses. In retrospect we were among the first to suggest that dopamine sensitive adenylate cyclase was not the dopamine receptor, since in iron deficiency this enzyme and its response to dopamine was not changed in the striatum. Yet the behavioral response of iron deficient rats to amphetamine and apomorphine were almost completely diminished. We suggested that either dopamine sensitive adenylate cyclase is not the receptor or that iron deficiency affects some component after adenylate cyclase. Indeed when the radio ligand (haloperidol and spiperone) were identified by S. H. Snyder to bind to dopamine D2 receptor, we examined these receptors in the striatum of iron deficient rats and showed that they are decreased which explained the dopaminergic subsensitivity and the reduction in apomorphine behavioral responses (Ben Shachar et al.). These studies have continued to receive world wide recognition from WHO, pediatritions, nutritionists and neurologists.

The second individual, who was to have the greatest impact on my carrier was meeting Peter Riederer for the fist time in Nov./Dec. 1973 in London and again in Vienna in early 1974. Another influencial person was Alfred Pletscher who believed in MAO inhibitors as therapeutic agents and invited me to my first CINP Congress in Paris. The association with Peter has been one of the most fruitful and productive period that is still on going. He was a member of Prof. Walther Birkmayer's, Neurology Department at Lainz Geriatric Hospital, Vienna. Peter wanted to know whether there was any new MAO inhibitors without "cheese reaction" he could use in Parkinson's disease as adjuvant to L-dopa. Some years earlier (1961) Birkmayer and Oleh Hornykiewicz had employed iproniazid, nardil and nialamide with L-dopa in parkinsonian subjects. Although the beneficial effects of L-dopa were potentiated, severe side effects were observed. Peter and I decided that MAO-B inhibitor l-deprenyl was the choice since it did not produce a cheese reaction as reported by Knoll and Magyar and dopamine was equally well metabolized by both MAO-A and B in vivo). On a visit to meet Joseph Knoll in October of 1974. I was able to get 5 gm of l-deprenyl and a study in 47 Parkinsonian patients by Walther Birkmayer in Vienna could be immediately related. Its success was reported at 5th Congress of Parkinson's Disease in Vienna (1975). Eventually other neurologists became aware of l-deprenyl and among the first was Melvin Yahr and l-deprenyl became one of the major innovative antiParkinson drugs. The other reason why L-deprenyl received such prominence was the description of our data in 1983 and 1985 pointing to its possible ability to slow down the degeneration of nigrostriatal dopamine neurons in Parkinsonian subjects. This was the first time the concept of "neuroprotection" and retarding the neurodegeneration of nigrostriatal dopamine neurons was discussed. L-deprenyl and MAO-B inhibition received further prominence as consequence of the discovery of the human inducing parkinsonism by the synthetic neurotoxin MPTP (N-methyl-4-phenyl-1,2,3,6-tetrahydropyridine) resulting from the observation that MPTP was a substrate of MAO-B and l-deprenyl pretreatment prevented its neurotoxicity in vivo and cell culture. This led to a floury of pharmaceutical companies developing MAO-A and MAO-B inhibitors, the presumption being that Parkinson's Disease is consequence of an environmental or endogenous factor similar to MPTP. Non of these MAO inhibitors survived into the clinic, except moclobemide (reversible MAO-A antidepressant) and rasagiline (to be discussed later). By this time l-deprenyl was in European clinics and did not reach USA until 1989, some fifteen years later from our first publication, named selegiline.

At Oxford together with Gretel Holzbauer, Hasan Parvez and Simmone Parvez we extended the work started by Margaret Southgate and Merton Sandler on hormonal regulation of MAO-A and B and the profound effect oestrous cycle has on brain MAO activity, specially in the hypothalamus and striatum.

It was in on the occasion of International Neurochemistry Society meeting in Copenhagen (1978) that Peter and I came up with the concept of "iron, radical oxygen species and oxidative stress roles" in neurodegenerative aspect of Parkinson's disease. The basis of it was laid down in a paper I presented at the Iron Symposium, which I had organized with Alan Jacobs (Professor of Hematology at Cardiff University) in 1976 at Ciba Foundation in London. I had reviewed the human and animal brain iron metabolism in relation to work with Richard Green on the effect of nutritional iron deficiency on aminergic neurotransmission. I came across several papers from 1920's by Spatz that distribution of iron was uneven in the brain, with the highest being in globus pallidus, substantia nigra, red nucleus, detate gyrus and thalamus, with most of brain iron being found in extrapyramidal regions. What puzzled me are papers by Lehermitte et al. (1924) and Earle (1968) that iron is increased in substantia nigra of Parkinsonian brains as compared with matched controls. With Peter we decided to re-examine brain iron in Parkinsonian brains subjects and its implication for oxidative stress induced neurodegeneration. Peter had analysed iron and other elements in a pilotstudy in controls and PD brain areas already in 1976 and 1977 based on work published by Ule and his group in 1972 and 1974 on the age-dependent distribution of iron in the "normal" brain. These date were presented at the 75th birthday symposium for Walther Birkmayer in 1985 and published in the thereof proceedings. In 1989 we published our work on a summary of iron and oxidative stress related parameters in J. Neurochem. and showed that iron was increased, GSH and ascorbate were decreased in substantia nigra, the implication being that iron induced oxidative stress may have a pivotal role in dopaminergic neurodegeneration with confirmation coming from other laboratories. We went on to show that indeed iron was increased in those melanin containing dopamine neurons of substantia nigra that selectively die. Furthermore similar events occur with 6-hyroxydopamine and MPTP. I demonstrated for the first time that iron chelators (desferal and Vk-28) can prevent the neurotoxicity of these neurotoxins. This led to suggest brain permeable iron chelators as therapeutic approach to PD a concept confirmed by other groups and chelation therapy is now considered one approach to neuroprotection.

With Margaret Thatcher coming to power and the lack of available university position in UK, I decided to leave Oxford (1977) and was offered to set up the Department of Pharmacology in the newly opened Medical School at Technion in Israel. During the time at Oxford one of the great scientific pleasure was to visit Hugh Blaschko, when ever opportunity arose. We discussed many aspect of MAO-A and B functions. He was fascinated by our findings on the antiParkinson action of l-deprenyl. He advised me to concentrate on studying MAO-B many times, including the time I went to bid him good bye, before leaving UK. I clearly remembered that among the MAO inhibitors which we received, while with Sandler, were two compounds (AGN1133 and AGN1135) with similar structures to l-deprenyl. l-Deprenyl was the only MAO inhibitor known that did not give cheese reaction. The intriguing question was whether l-deprenyl had a specific pharmacological action that prevented the cheese reaction (as suggested by Knoll and Magyar) or that any MAO B inhibitor would do the same thing. By the time John Finberg joined my department in Haifa we had identified that AGN1135 was the second selective MAO B inhibitor and went on to show that it had pharmacological actions identical to l-deprenyl and that it did not produce a cheese reaction in animal and pharmacological preparations at its selective MAO-B inhibitory dosage. Further more unlike l-deprenyl it was devoid of sympathomimetic activity. Indeed it was John Finberg and Meir Tenne who established that the cheese reaction is the property of MAO-A inhibition within the adrenergic neurons and that when MAO-B is inhibited selectively, no cheese reaction would occur. As a consequence we were among the first to suggest development of MAO-A inhibitors with out the cheese reaction as antidepressant that led to my long association with Alfred Pletscher, William Haefely and Moshe Da Prada at Roche and led to the discovery of the first reversible MAO-A inhibitor, moclobemide, without the cheese reaction by Moshe Da Prada and others followed. These findings were the imputes for the development of other MAO-B inhibitors as antiParkinson drugs and reversible MAO-A inhibitors as antidepressant by some of the major pharmaceutical companies. It is ironical that non of those newly developed found their way into the clinic (except eventually moclobemide and rasagiline). Because AGN1135, unlike l-deprenyl, did not have sympathomimetic activity or be metabolized to amphetamine and was a potent MAO-B inhibitor, we suggested its development as anti PD drug. Eventually it was co-developed with Teva Pharmarmaceutical Co. and rasagiline (Azilect) has been approved for Europe and Israel and letters of approval have been received from FDA. This would not have been achieved with if it were not for the unflinching efforts of my colleague and friend Dr. Ruth Levy of Teva, who one day in came to my office back in 1987 saying they are interested to develop AGN1135 as antiParkinson drug. Together with Makato Naoi, Wakako Maruyama and members of our Center (Tamar Amit, Silvia Mandel, Ori Bar Am, Orly Weinreb and Yotam Sagi) we elucidated the molecular mechanism of rasagiline's neuroprotective activity and showed that it was not dependent on its MAO inhibitory activity, but rather on the propargyl moiety, since the S-optical isomer of rasagiline, TVP 1022 and propargylamine are poor inhibitors of MAO, yet have the same molecular neuroprotective property with similar potency. The mechanism of these propargylamines results from interaction of Bcl-2 family protein with PKC-dependent MAPkinase pathway.

The conventional neurochemistry, genomic and proteomic profiling studies were demonstrating that neurodegeneration is associated with a cascade of events and failure of several neurotransmitter systems. The concept of targeting multiple disease etiologies that lead to neurodegenerative disorders (such as Alzheimer's disease, Parkinson's disease amyotrophic lateral sclerosis and stroke), is challenging the widely held assumption that "silver bullet" agents are superior to "dirty drugs" in drug therapy. Accumulating evidence in the literature suggests that a drug with two or more mechanisms of action targeted at multiple etiologies of the same disease, may offer more therapeutic benefit in certain disorders than a drug that targets one disease etiology only. In addition, such multiple mechanism/multifunctional drugs may exhibit a more favorable side-effect profile than a polypharmacology combination of several drugs that individually target the same disease etiologies than those identified for a single multifunctional drug. In the last few years in collaboration with Marta Weinstock (the developer of the antiAlzheimer drug, rivastigmine) we designed and developed several novel cholinesterase- brain selective monoamine oxidase AB inhibitor compounds (TV3326 and TV3279). These compounds were developed from the pharmacophore of rasagiline, its S-isomer and carbamate cholinesterase inhibitor moiety in order to possess the neuroprotective and MAO and cholinesterase inhibitory activities for treatment of AD subjects having co-morbidity with depression and Parkinson's disease. Ladostigil (TV3326) is a unique brain selective MAO-AB-cholinesterase inhibitor that in animal studies shows antiAlzheimer, antiParkinson and antidepressant activities, besides being neuroprotective and the ability to process amyloid precursor protein implicated in Alzheimer's disease. Ladostigil (Teva Pharmaceutical Co. Israel) is finishing its Phase II clinical studies. Another example of multifunctional neuroprotective drug that we recently designed and are under development are the iron chelator-brain selective MAO-AB inhibitors, M30 and HLA-20. In these drugs we have introduced a propargyl MAO inhibitory moiety at different sites in our brain permeable neuroprotective iron chelator, VK-28 which Avraham Warshawsky (deceased) and I developed in 1989 and Mati Fridkin took over the project successfully with our Ph.D student Hailin Zheng. Unlike l-deprenyl and rasagiline, which do not increase brain levels of dopamine, ladostigil and M30 does so, as consequence their ability to inhibit MAO-AB. Thus, they may represent more effective as drugs for PD. We have shown that these multifunctional propargylamine drugs have neuroprotective activity in vitro neuronal cell cultures, and in vivo models of Parkinson's disease, Alzheimer's disease and Huntington disease similar to rasagiline. An added bonus for the iron chelator-MAO inhibitor, M30, is its ability to prevent the neurotoxicity resulting from dysregulation of iron in MPTP, 6-hydroxy-dopamine and kainate treated animals and which has also been established at brain sites in the neurodegenerative disorders models, where neurons die. Our present efforts now are directed at determining the brain selectivity of ladostigil and M30 for brain MAO inhibition, which may allow us to synthesize further similar drugs.

More recently I have ventured back to studies on depressive illness specially in Parkinson's disease and mechanism of action of different classes of antidepressants including MAO inhibitors employing the technique of gene expression with cDNA microarray and proteomic profiling, the first group to do so. With this system we have identified how complex the mechanisms of antidepressant actions are and have identified a homology of 37 gene expressions with 5 different classes of antidepressants that may explain their common final pathway as antidepressants. The down stream gene pathways identified may lead to novel new drugs away from the classical MAO and amine up take inhibitors presently in the clinic.

In 2006 The British Pharmacology Society decided to celebrate its 75th Anniversary of the founding of Society, and the 60th Anniversary of the first issue of its Journal, BJP, the British Journal of Pharmacology. To commemorate these important anniversaries, BJP decided to publish a special supplement, comprising a series of articles by distinguished scientists who have been actively involved in areas of the subject in which British pharmacologists have made a contributions and major pharmacological discoveries of the past half-century. I was honoured and delighted that they chose the subject of monoamine oxidase and its inhibitors by including my contribution to the field (Youdim and Bakhle, 2006).

I wish to express my gratitude and thanks to all who a have contributed to this publication, which I consider an honour, since there is no substitute to be recognized by ones colleagues. Special thanks to Peter Riederer and Hasan Parvez for organizing this volume and allowing me to give a biography of my 40 years love affair with MAO. Special appreciation and thanks to Keith Tipton for the long association, who never failed to support any suggestion I had and more recently for collaborating on the new MAO review, 40 years on to appear in Nature Review Neuroscience (Youdim et al., 2006) I have been lucky to have worked and collaborated with some of the finest scientific colleagues, with out whose collaboration, insights, efforts and patience I would not have achieved some of the goals I set for myself. As a consequence of space I have left out the names of many other colleagues and students who worked with me in other projects. Special thanks to them.

References

Youdim MB, Bakhle YS (2006) Monoamine oxidase: isoforms and inhibitors in Parkinson's disease and depressive illness. Br J Pharmacol 147 [Suppl 1]: S287–S296

Youdim MBH, Edmondson D, Tipton KF (2006) Therapeutic potentials of monoamine oxidase inhibitors. Nat Rev Neurosci 7: 295–309

J Neural Transm (2006) [Suppl] 71: XI–XII

Journal of Neural Transmission
Printed in Austria

Preface
Moussa Youdim – an appreciation

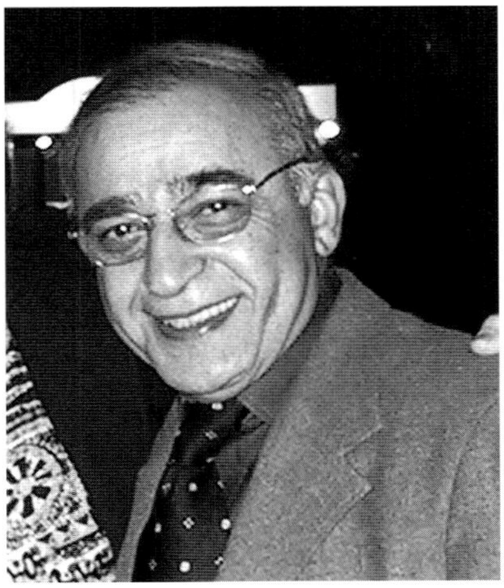

It would be possible to write at considerable length about Moussa and still not do him full justice on his 65th birthday. Indeed, within the constraints of this brief appreciation, many things that might be said about the numerous awards he has won, his contribution as an editor of many journals, the books that he has edited etc., will have to be left out. Nonetheless, a brief resume of his career is important to illustrate his unique personality and achievements.

Born in what was formally known as Persia, and educated in England, he is reported to have said that during his studies he accepted the "European lifestyle" and never moved back. His career as a research scientist began in the Laboratory of Ted Sourkes at McGill University in Canada, where he gained his PhD in Biochemistry. There could have been few better places to absorb a passion for research allied with a rigorous and critical approach than in Ted's laboratory. It was there that he developed his dual interests in monoamine oxidases and the roles of iron in the brain, both of which were to play central roles in much of his subsequent research. He then relocated to England in order to work in the laboratory of Merton Sandler in Queen Charlotte's Hospital London where his interests in monoamine oxidase fitted in well with those of Merton's group. This, as well as the time he spent at Oxford where he developed collaborations with many other laboratories in the UK, notably that of David Graham-Smith and Richard Green in Oxford, proved to be a most productive period for him. He also spent an all-too-brief period working in my laboratory in Cambridge looking at MAO in the adrenal medulla-in addition to having a lot of fun. Whilst there he developed friendships with a scholar of ancient Persian Literature as well as with Sir Rudolph Peters, who among many other accomplishments, developed the concept of lethal synthesis and founded the journal Biochemical Pharmacology. More notably, he developed collaborations with Walther Birkmayer and one of us (P.R.) in Vienna, which led to the demonstration of the effectiveness of *l*-deprenyl (Selegiline) in the treatment of Parkinson's disease. This work attracted worldwide attention and led to an explosion of research and publications on deprenyl as a 'neuroprotective' drug and the revival of MAO inhibitors as antidepressants. His continuing collaboration with Peter Riederer also resulted in the further development of fundamental ideas about defects of iron homeostasis being an important contributing factor in the aetiology of neurodegenerative diseases.

In 1977 he was invited to set up a department of Pharmacology at the Technion Institute in Haifa. Although one does not normally find much good to say for the baleful bureaucrats who run many of our institutions, this was however, an admittedly inspired move on their part. Certainly England's loss was Israel's gain. In addition to getting the department organised, he continued his own research at an ever increasing pace with the able assistance of our collaborator John Finberg. At the same time he was extremely active at promoting Technion around the world and obtaining funding for its activities. He subsequently moved from the department to set up his own research centre within the Technion institute; a centre for neurodegenerative diseases research which now bears such a long name that it would exceed the allowable word count were I to give it in full here. That notwithstanding, it is recognized as a Center of Excellence by the National Parkinson Foundation (USA).

He formed a collaboration with the gifted chemist Asher Kali, resulting in the synthesis of a range of novel monoamine oxidase inhibitors, including anti Parkinson's drug Rasagiline, which appears to have several advantages over Selegiline. It is not necessary to discuss the drugs merits here, since it has been the subject of many scientific and clinical publications, including the present volume of our Journal. It appears very likely that we will hear much more about Rasagiline and its efficacy in treating neurodegenerative diseases in the future.

His interest in bifunctional drugs that developed around this time resulted in his collaboration with Marta Weinstock. Their collaboration brought forth the synthesis of a compound, which contains monoamine oxidase and amine reuptake inhibitory functions in a single molecule and is indicated for the treatment of Alzheimer's disease. Although this compound was less effective than might have been hoped, the same approach resulted in the development of a series of drugs including combined iron chelator-monoamine oxidase inhibitor drugs and the cholinesterase-monoamine oxidase inhibitor, ladostigil. Both classes of bifunctional drugs show considerable promise and the outcomes of further studies are eagerly awaited.

Translational research is a popular buzzword in the biological sciences at the moment and granting agencies appear to believe that is what we should all be doing. It seems that the policy makers have discovered something that Moussa has been doing for much of his career: He has typified the "from-the-laboratory-to-the-patient" approach in the areas of monoamine oxidases and brain iron metabolism by developing them to their full extent in order to determine their physiological roles in the central nervous system, and then, by further pursuing them in the clinic. His continuing relationship with the pharmaceutical company Teva has been a key element in ensuring the success of these developments.

It is not the intention of this preface to reference Moussas' curriculum in detail. Indeed, it would be impossible in this short format to reference the seventy two pages of his CV and publications list. However, we would like to point to his incredible working capacity resulting in more than 450 original publications, some 220 full papers published in international symposia proceedings, the over 40 books and 96 invited articles, reviews, book chapters and commentaries – not to forget the 97 international patents awarded. As impressive as his scientific work is, and the list of awards, prizes and honours which he has received from around the world, perhaps most prestigious are the two Honorary Doctorate Degrees from the Universities in Budapest (1997) and Pisa (1998). Moussa is a member of 17 international scientific and professional associations and holds a current appointment on 19 editorial boards for international journals.

The list of graduate students and post-doctoral fellows is equally as impressive as that of the postdoctoral research associates that have worked with him. Together, they are creating "Moussa's school of medicine".

Finally, we would like to mention Moussa's talent of organizing and co-organizing international meetings and his extraordinary ability as invited plenary speaker.

Moussa is always fun to be with, spinning off ideas at a great rate and is seemingly able to carry on several detailed conversations simultaneously. Perhaps his inventive humour is best captured by naming the most successful amine oxidase workshop, which he organised in Haifa in 1996, "MAO: the mother of all amine oxidases". However, all of this is far from being meant as a valediction, and perhaps one day we will say that we "shall not look upon his like again" – and that will be true: Unless of course he invents an anti-death drug! But for now we can be glad that we have Moussa around and can be certain that he will continue to surprise and excite us with new developments and concepts.

"We are thankful, Moussa, for your friendship and open discussions. And we think that this collection of scientific work is a tribute which reflects your brilliant personality".

Keith Tipton, Dublin
Hasan Parvez, Gif Sur Yvette
Peter Franz Riederer, Würzburg, March 2007

Contents

Listed in Current Contents/Life Sciences

J Neural Transm (2006) [Suppl] 71: 1–15

Journal of Neural Transmission
Printed in Austria

Levodopa in the treatment of Parkinson's disease

S. Fahn

Columbia University, New York, U.S.A.

Summary Levodopa is the most efficacious drug to treat the symptoms of Parkinson's disease (PD) and is widely considered the "gold standard" by which to compare other therapies, including surgical therapy. Response to levodopa is one of the criteria for the clinical diagnosis of PD. A major limiting factor in levodopa therapy is the development of motor complications, namely dyskinesias and motor fluctuations. The ELLDOPA study was designed to determine if levodopa affected the progression of PD. This double-blind randomized study showed that the subjects treated with levodopa for 40 weeks had less severe parkinsonism than the placebo treated subjects even after a 2-week washout of medications, with the highest dose group showing the greatest benefit. Thus, levodopa may actually have neuroprotective value, but the result was not conclusive of slowing disease progression, because the same result could have arisen from a very long-lasting symptomatic benefit of levodopa.

Introduction

Parkinson's disease (PD) was first described in 1817 with the publication by James Parkinson of a book entitled "An Essay on the Shaking Palsy" (Parkinson, 1817). In it, he described six individuals with the clinical features that have come to be recognized as a disease entity. One of the people was followed in detail over a long period of time; the other five consisted of brief descriptions, including two whom he had met walking in the street, and another whom he had observed at a distance. Such distant observations without a medical examination demonstrates how readily distinguishable the conditions. The physical appearance of flexed posture, resting tremor, and shuffling gait are readily recognizable. Parkinson's opening description has the key essentials: "Involuntary tremulous motion, with lessened muscular power, in parts not in action and even when supported; with a propensity to bend the trunk forward, and to pass from a walking to a running pace: the senses and intellects being uninjured." In the small monograph, Parkinson provided a detailed description of the symptoms and also discussed the progressive worsening of the disorder, which he called "the shaking palsy" and its Latin term "paralysis agitans."

After the publication of Parkinson's book, the disease was widely accepted in the medical community. It took 70 years for the name of the disorder to be referred to as "Parkinson's disease," as recommended by the French neurologist Charcot who argued against the term "paralysis agitans" (see Goetz, 1987, for English translation). Charcot argued that there is no true paralysis, but rather the "lessened muscular power" is what is today called akinesia, hypokinesia or bradykinesia; all three terms often being used interchangeably. These terms represent a paucity of movement not due to weakness or paralysis. Similarly, Charcot emphasized that tremor need not be present in the disorder, so "agitans" and "shaking" are not appropriate as part of the name of the disorder.

Parkinson's disease (PD) vs. parkinsonism

The syndrome of parkinsonism must be understood before one can understand what is PD. Parkinsonism is defined by any combination of six specific, non-overlapping, motoric features, so-called cardinal features: tremor-at-rest, bradykinesia, rigidity, loss of postural reflexes, flexed posture and the "freezing" phenomenon (where the feet are transiently "glued" to the ground) (Fahn and Przedborski, 2005). Not all six of these cardinal features need be present, but at least two should be before the diagnosis of parkinsonism is made, with at least one of them being tremor-at-rest or bradykinesia. Parkinsonism is divided into four categories (Table 1). PD or primary parkinsonism will be the principal focus of this chapter; not only is it the one that is most commonly encountered by the general clinician, it is also the one in which levodopa is particularly

Correspondence: Stanley Fahn, MD, Neurological Institute, 710 West 168th Street, New York, NY 10032, U.S.A.
e-mail: fahn@neuro.columbia.edu

Table 1. *Classification of the parkinsonian states*

I. Primary parkinsonism (Parkinson's disease)
- Sporadic
- Known genetic etiologies (see Table 2)

II. Secondary parkinsonism (environmental etiology)
- A. Drugs
  - 1. Dopamine receptor blockers (most commonly antipsychotic medications)
  - 2. Dopamine storage depletors (reserpine)
- B. Postencephalitic
- C. Toxins – Mn, CO, MPTP, cyanide
- D. Vascular
- E. Brain tumors
- F. Head trauma
- G. Normal pressure hydrocephalus

III. Parkinsonism-Plus Syndromes
- A. Progressive supranuclear palsy
- B. Multiple system atrophy
- C. Cortical-basal ganglionic degeneration
- D. Parkinson-dementia-ALS complex of Guam
- E. Progressive pallidal atrophy
- F. Diffuse Lewy body disease (DLBD)

IV. Heredodegenerative disorders
- A. Alzheimer disease
- B. Wilson disease
- C. Huntington disease
- D. Frontotemporal dementia on chromosome 17q21
- E. X-linked dystonia-parkinsonism (in Filipino men; known as lubag)

effective in ameliorating. Three of the most helpful clues that one is likely to be dealing with PD rather than another category of parkinsonism are 1) an asymmetrical onset of symptoms (PD often begins on one side of the body), 2) the presence of rest tremor (although rest tremor may be absent in patients with PD, it is almost always absent in Parkinson-plus syndromes), and 3) substantial clinical response to adequate levodopa therapy (usually, Parkinson-plus syndromes do not respond to levodopa therapy).

The great majority of cases of primary parkinsonism are sporadic, but in the last few years several gene mutations have been discovered to cause PD (Table 2). Whether genetic or idiopathic in etiology, the common denominator is that it is not caused by known insults to the brain (the main feature of secondary parkinsonism) and is not associated with other motoric neurologic features (the main feature of Parkinson-plus syndromes). The uncovering of genetic causes of primary parkinsonism has shed light on probable pathogenetic mechanisms that may be a factor in even the more common sporadic cases of PD.

Clinical description of Parkinson's disease

Although non-motor symptoms (e.g., constipation, aching shoulder, hypo-osmia, depression) may begin before the motor features of PD, these non-motor symptoms are too common in the general population to lead to a diagnosis of PD on their own. The motor symptoms of PD begin insidiously and gradually worsen. Symptoms, such as rest tremor, can be intermittent at the onset being present only in stressful situations. Symptoms tend to worsen on one side of the body before spreading to involve the other side. Rest tremor, because it is so obvious, is often the first symptom recognized by the patient. But the illness sometimes begins with bradykinesia, and in some patients, tremor may never develop. Bradykinesia manifests as slowness and small amplitude of movement, such as slower and smaller handwriting, decreased arm swing and leg stride when walking, decreased facial expression, and decreased amplitude of voice.

There is a steady worsening of symptoms over time, which, if untreated, leads to disability with severe immobility and falling. The early symptoms and signs of PD – rest tremor, bradykinesia and rigidity – are related to progressive loss of nigrostriatal dopamine and are usually correctable by treatment with levodopa and dopamine (DA) agonists. As PD progresses over time, symptoms that do not respond to levodopa develop, such as flexed posture, the freezing phenomenon and loss of postural reflexes appear; these are often referred to as non DA-related features of PD. Moreover, bradykinesia that responded to levodopa in the early stage of PD increases as the disease worsens and no longer fully responds to levodopa. It is particularly these intractable motoric symptoms that lead to the disability of increasing immobility and balance difficulties.

While it may be difficult to distinguish between PD and Parkinson-plus syndromes in the early stages of the illness, with disease progression over time, the clinical distinctions of the Parkinson-plus disorders become more apparent with the development of other neurological findings, such as cerebellar ataxia, loss of downward ocular movements, and autonomic dysfunction (e.g., postural hypotension, loss of bladder control, and impotence).

There are no practical diagnostic laboratory tests for PD, and the diagnosis rests on the clinical features or by excluding some of the other causes of parkinsonism. The research tool of fluorodopa positron emission tomography (PET) measures levodopa uptake into dopamine nerve terminals, and this shows a decline of about 5% per year of the striatal uptake. A similar result is seen using ligands for the dopamine transporter, either by PET or by single photon emission computed tomography (SPECT); these ligands also label the dopamine nerve terminals. All these neuroimaging techniques reveal decreased dopaminergic nerve terminals in the striatum in both PD and the Parkinson-plus syndromes, and do not distinguish between them. A

Table 2. *Genetic linkage and gene identification in Parkinson's disease*

Name and locus	Gene or protein	Mode of inheritance; pathological and clinical features	Protein function	Where found	Pathogenic mutations
PARK1 4q21.3	alpha-synuclein	autosomal dominant; Lewy bodies; young onset; dementia occurs	possibly synaptic vesicle trafficking; elevated in bird song learning	families in Germany, Italy-U.S. (Contoursi kindred), Greece, Spain	A53T and A30P, may promote aggregation; Lewy body and Alzhemer plaque component; protofibrils (toxic) accumulation
PARK2 6q25.2–q27	parkin	autosomal recessive; (also dominant?); often juvenile onset w/o Lewy bodies; slowly progressive	ubiquitin E3 ligase, attaches short ubiquitin peptide chains to a range of proteins, likely to mark degradation	ubiquitous, originally in Japan, very common in juvenile onset	Over 70 mutations identified; mostly likely loss of function mutations
PARK3 2p13	unknown	autosomal dominant; Lewy bodies, indistinguishable from idiopathic PD		4 families in southern Denmark and northern Germany, probable common ancestor	
PARK4 4q13–q22	multiple copies of wild-type alpha-synuclein	autosomal dominant; wide range of symptoms from idiopathic PD to dementia with Lewy bodies	See PARK1	"Spellman-Muenter" and the "Waters-Miller" families with common ancestor in the United States, European families	Duplications/triplications of chromosomal region that contains wild-type alpha-synuclein gene
PARK5 4p14	ubiquitin-C-terminal hydrolase L1	possibly autosomal dominant	removes polyubiquitin	1 family in Germany	
PARK6 1p35–p36	PINK-1	autosomal recessive; juvenile onset	mitochondrial protein; provides protection against multiple stress factors	1 family in Sicily	
PARK7 1p36	DJ-1	autosomal recessive; early onset	sumoylation pathway	families in Holland, Italy, Uruguay	L166P, M261, and a variety of other candidates
PARK8 12p11.2–q13.1	dardarin (leucine rich repeat kinase 2, LRRK2)	autosomal dominant; nigral degeneration, Lewy bodies; onset at 65; tremor, benign; responds to low doses of L-dopa.	Probably a cytoplasmic kinase	First family in Japan; many now around the world. Gene identified in 4 families in Basque (Spain) and 1 in England	
PARK9 1p36	unknown	autosomal recessive; Kufor-Rakeb syndrome, a Parkinson-plus disorder		1 family in Jordan	
PARK10 1p32	unknown	autosomal recessive; typical late-onset		Families in Iceland	
PARK11 2q36–q37	unknown	autosomal dominant		Families in the U.S.	

substantial response to levodopa is most helpful in the differential diagnosis, indicating presynaptic dopamine deficiency with intact postsynaptic dopamine receptors, features typical for PD.

Dementia is a common late complication of PD. Following patients over an 8-year period, Aarsland et al., (2003) found the prevalence of dementia to affect more than 75% of patients with PD. The development of dementia in a patient with parkinsonism remains a difficult differential diagnosis. If the patient's parkinsonian features did not respond to levodopa, the diagnosis is likely to be Alzheimer disease, which can occasionally present with parkinsonism. If the presenting parkinsonism responded to levodopa, and the patient developed dementia over time, the diagnosis is usually called PD-Dementia (PDD) and also diffuse Lewy body disease (DLBD), also called Dementia with Lewy Bodies (DLB).

If hallucinations occur with or without levodopa therapy, DLBD is the most likely diagnosis. DLBD is a condition where Lewy bodies are present in the cerebral cortex as well as in the brainstem nuclei. The heredodegenerative disease, known as frontotemporal dementia, is an autosomal dominant disorder due to mutations of the tau gene on chromosime 17; the full syndrome presents with dementia, loss of inhibition, parkinsonism, and sometimes muscle wasting.

Some adults may develop a more benign form of PD, in which the symptoms respond to very low dosage levodopa, and the disease does not worsen severely with time. This form is usually due to the autosomal dominant disorder known as dopa-responsive dystonia, which typically begins in childhood as a dystonia. But when it starts in adult life, it can present with parkinsonism. There is no neuronal degeneration. The pathogenesis is due to a biochemical deficiency involving dopamine synthesis. The gene defect is for an enzyme (GTP cyclohydrolase I) required to synthesize the cofactor for tyrosine hydroxylase activity, the crucial rate-limiting first step in the synthesis of dopamine and norepinephrine. Infantile parkinsonism is due to the autosomal recessive deficiency of tyrosine hydroxylase, another cause of a biochemical dopamine deficiency disorder.

Epidemiology of Parkinson's disease

Although PD can develop at any age, it begins most common in older adults, with a peak age at onset around 60 years. The likelihood of developing PD increases with age (Fig. 1), with a lifetime risk of about 2% (Elbaz et al., 2002).

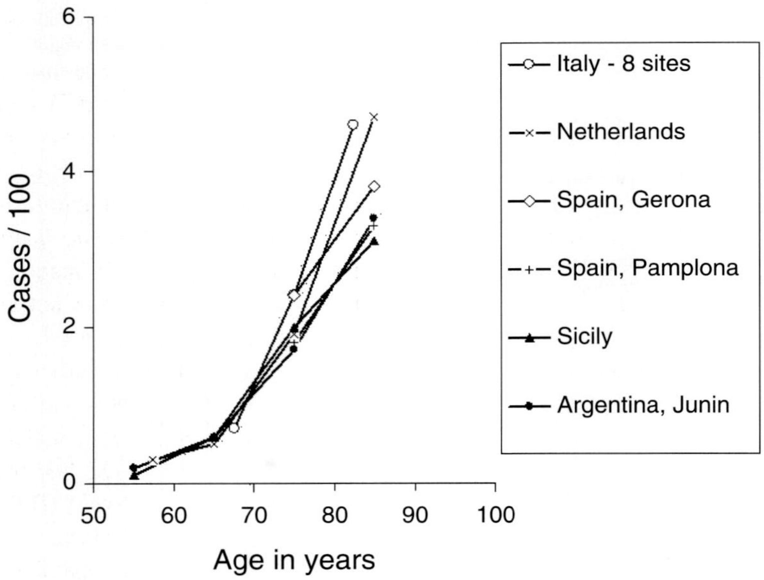

Fig. 1. Age-specific prevalence rates of PD in different countries. This figure is a modification of a figure in de Rijk et al. (1997), provided by W. A. Rocca, personal communication, along with permission to reproduce

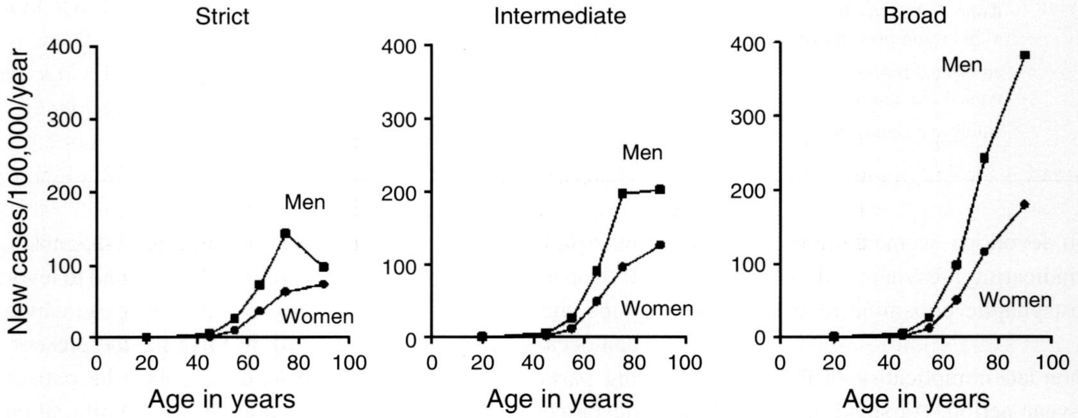

Fig. 2. Age- and sex-specific incidence rates of Parkinson disease based on strict, intermediate or broad definitions of the disease. Data from Rochester, MN from 1975 to 1990. From Bower et al. (2000) with permission from the Movement Disorder Society

A positive family history doubles the risk of developing PD to about 4%. Twin studies indicate that PD with an onset under the age of 50 years is more likely to have a genetic relationship than for patients with an older age at onset (Tanner et al., 1999). Males have higher prevalence (male-to-female ratio of 3:2) and incident rates than females (Fig. 2). The prevalence of PD is approximately 160 per 100,000, and the incidence is about 20 per 100,000/yr. Prevalence and incidence increase with age. At age 70, the prevalence is approximately 550 per 100,000, and the incidence is 120 per 100,000/yr. At the present time, approximately 850,000 individuals in the U.S. have PD, with the number expected to grow as the population ages.

In the pre-levodopa era, excess mortality was reported to be 3-fold greater in patients with PD (Hoehn and Yahr, 1967). The excess mortality rate was reduced to 1.6-fold greater than age-matched non-PD individuals after the introduction of levodopa (Yahr, 1976; Elbaz et al., 2003). Today, patients with PD can live 20 or more years, depending on the age at onset. Death in PD is usually due to some concurrent unrelated illness or due to the effects of decreased mobility, aspiration, or increased falling with subsequent physical injury. The Parkinson-plus syndromes typically progress at a faster rate and often cause death within nine years. Thus, the diagnosis of PD is of prognostic importance, as well as of therapeutic significance because it almost always responds to at least a moderate degree to levodopa therapy, whereas the Parkinson-plus disorders do not.

Pathology and biochemical pathology of Parkinson's disease

It was many years after Parkinson's original description before the basal ganglia were recognized by Meynert in 1871 as being involved in disorders of abnormal movements. And it was not until 1895 that the substantia nigra was suggested to be affected in Parkinson disease. Brissaud (1895) suggested this on the basis of a report by Blocq and Marinesco (1893) of a tuberculoma in that site that was associated with hemiparkinsonian tremor. These authors were careful to point out that the pyramidal tract and the brachium conjuctivum above and below the level of the lesion contained no degenerating fibers. The importance of the substantia nigra was emphasized by Tretiakoff in 1919 who studied the substantia nigra in nine cases of Parkinson disease, one case of hemiparkinsonism, and three cases of postencephalitic parkinsonism, finding lesions in this nucleus in all cases. With the hemiparkinsonian case Tretiakoff found a lesion in the nigra on the opposite side, concluding that the nucleus served the motor activity on the contralateral side of the body. The substantia nigra, so named because of its normal content of neuromelanin pigment, was noted to show depigmentation, loss of nerve cells, and gliosis. These findings remain the histopathologic features of the disease. In his study, Tretiakoff also confirmed the earlier observation of Lewy (1914) who had discovered the presence of cytoplasmic inclusions in Parkinson disease, now widely recognized as the major pathologic hallmark of the disorder, and referred to as Lewy bodies.

Foix and Nicolesco made a detailed study of the pathology of Parkinson disease in 1925 and found that the most constant and severe lesions are in the substantia nigra. Since then many workers, including Hassler (1938) and Greenfield and Bosanquet (1953), have confirmed these findings and added other observations, including involvement of other brainstem nuclei such as the locus ceruleus.

PD and the Parkinson-plus syndromes have in common a degeneration of substantia nigra pars compacta dopaminergic neurons, with a resulting deficiency of striatal dopamine due to loss of the nigrostriatal neurons. Accompanying this neuronal loss is an increase in glial cells in the nigra and a loss of the neuromelanin normally contained in the dopaminergic neurons. In PD, intracytoplasmic inclusions, called Lewy bodies, are usually present in many of the surviving neurons. It is recognized today, that not all patients with PD have Lewy bodies, for those with the a homozygous mutation in the PARK2 gene, mainly young-onset PD patients, have nigral neuronal degeneration without Lewy bodies. Lewy bodies contain many proteins, including the fibrillar form of α-synuclein, discovered because PARK1's mutations involve the gene for this protein. There are no Lewy bodies in the Parkinson-plus syndromes.

With the progressive loss of the nigrostriatal dopaminergic neurons, there is a corresponding decrease of dopamine content in both the nigra and the striatum, which accounts particularly for bradykinesia and rigidity in PD. There are compensatory changes, such as supersensitivity of dopamine receptors, so that symptoms of PD are first encountered only when there is about an 80% reduction of dopamine concentration in the putamen (or a loss of 60% of nigral dopaminergic neurons) (Bernheimer et al., 1973). With further loss of dopamine concentration, parkinsonian bradykinesia becomes more severe (Table 3). The progressive loss of the dopaminergic nigrostriatal pathway can be detected during life using PET and SPECT scanning; these show a continuing reduction of FDOPA and dopamine transporter ligand binding in the striatum (Snow et al., 1994; Seibyl et al., 1995; Eidelberg et al., 1995; Morrish et al., 1996; Benamer et al., 2000).

Table 3. *Dopamine concentration in striatum is associated with severity of bradykinesia*

Severity of bradykinesia	Caudate nucleus	Putamen
Mild	0.58 (13)	0.44 (12)
Marked	0.44 (9)	0.05 (9)
Normal Controls	2.64 (28)	3.44 (28)

Data from Bernheimer et al. (1973). Results are means in µg/g fresh tissue. Numbers in parentheses are the number of cases studied

The consequence of nigrostriatal loss is an altered physiology downstream from the striatum. The striatum contains D1 and D2 receptors. Current thinking is that dopamine is excitatory at the D1 receptor and inhibitor at the D2 receptor. Deficiency of dopamine at these receptors results in alteration at the downstream nuclei: excessive activity of the subthalamic nucleus and globus pallidus interna, and increased inhibition in the thalamus and cerebral cortex (Penney and Young, 1986; Miller and DeLong, 1988; Mitchell et al., 1989). These altered physiology patterns are restored towards normal with treatment with levodopa.

Although the etiology and pathogenesis of PD remain unkown (except for the gene-specific defects listed in Table 2), there are many clues to factors that can lead to degeneration of the dopamine neurons.(see review by Fahn and Sulzer, 2004). Oxidative stress due to excessive cytosolic dopamine, mitochondrial dysfunction, and toxic protein accumulation are some of the leading suspects, and these factors can interact with each other. This topic is too huge to be considered here.

Levodopa therapy for Parkinson's disease

Historical introduction

Following the discovery of striatal dopamine deficiency in PD (Ehringer and Hornykiewicz, 1960; Bernheimer et al., 1973), Birkmayer and Hornykiewicz (1961) injected small doses of levodopa (up to 150 mg) intravenously and reported a transient reversal of akinesia. Levodopa was previously shown by Carlsson and colleagues (1957) to reverse reserpine-induced parkinsonism in rabbits. Barbeau and his colleagues (1962) also reported benefit with small oral doses of levodopa (200 mg). Subsequently, many other investigators using small oral or intravenous doses reported similar results in very brief communications (Friedhoff et al., 1964; Umbach and Bauman, 1964; Hirschmann and Mayer, 1964; Fazzagli and Amaducci, 1966; Bruno and Bruno, 1966). However, not every investigator reported benefit from such small doses of levodopa. Greer and Williams (1963) failed to find benefit in two patients after 1 gm of D,L-dopa orally. Aebert (1967) saw no benefit after 70 to 100 mg L-dopa intravenously, nor did Rinaldi and colleagues (1965) even with inhibition of monoamine oxidase. Double-blind trials with low dosage levodopa also failed to provide benefit (Fehling, 1966; Rinne and Sonninen, 1968) using up to 1.5 mg/kg of intravenous levodopa. McGeer and Zeldowicz in 1964 were the first to use high doses of D,L-dopa that were later found to be successful by Cotzias et al. in 1967. They used up to 5 gm per day in ten patients for several days, and in one patient, 3 gm daily for 2 years, but only two patients showed any objective improvement.

The breakthrough in establishing levodopa as a therapeutically useful drug was the report of Cotzias et al. (1967). They treated 16 patients with doses of D,L-dopa of 3–16 gm per day, building the dosage up slowly to avoid anorexia, nausea and vomiting, which had been dose-limiting complications with previous investigators. They reported marked improvement in eight patients and less improvement in two others. Of the eight who received 12 g/or more per day, seven showed marked benefit. Granulocytopenia was seen in four patients, and bone marrow examination revealed vacuoles in the myeloid cells in four of the 12 patients who had bone marrow examinations.

Because of the hematologic problems and because D-dopa in not metabolized to form dopamine, Cotzias and his colleagues subsequently used L-dopa (1969), and these problems were no longer encountered. The first double-blind study with high dosage levodopa was carried out by Yahr and his colleagues (1969). Many subsequent reports showed significant improvement in approximately 75% of patients with parkinsonism. Although a complete remission is rarely obtained, the benefit in akinesia and rigidity were generally most benefited, and many who had been unable to turn in bed or arise from a chair became able to do so. Tremor has a more variable response; sometimes it is eliminated by levodopa, and in other patients, the tremor is resistant. A number of other symptoms, including postural instability and speech disturbance, are typically unaffected by levodopa therapy, suggesting these symptoms are not solely due to dopamine deficiency. The introduction of levodopa therapy by Cotzias was a revolutionary treatment for PD, not just an evolutionary one.

The development of inhibitors of L-aromatic amino acid decarboxylase that do not cross the blood-brain barrier was the next major step. Carbidopa and benserazide are such peripheral decarboxylase inhibitors. When given with levodopa, they allow for a 4-fold increase in the effectiveness of a given dose because peripheral metabolism to dopamine was blocked. More importantly, these agents block the gastrointestinal side effects, which were due to peripheral dopamine acting upon the vomiting center of the area postrema, which is not protected by the blood-brain barrier. The combination of levodopa with carbidopa was commercially marketed under the trade name of Sinemet, to indicate without ("sine") emesis. Sinemet (carbidopa/levodopa) is sold in 10/100, 25/100 and 25/250 mg strengths. Many patients require at least 50–75 mg of carbidopa a day to have adequate inhibition of peripheral dopa decarboxylase. If the dose of levodopa is less than 300 mg per day, then one should use the 25/100 mg strength tablets and not the 10/100 mg tablets. In some patients even 75 mg per day of carbidopa is inadequate, and nausea, anorexia or vomiting still occur. In such patients, one needs to use higher doses of carbidopa, which are available under the trade name of Lodosyn. The combination of benserazide and levodopa is marketed under the brand name of Madopar.

The other enzyme that metabolizes levodopa is catechol-O-methyltransferase (COMT), and two inhibitors of this enzyme have also become available, namely tolcapone and entacapone. These COMT inhibitors delay the peripheral decay of levodopa plasma levels, allowing a slightly longer half-life. An enzyme that metabolizes dopamine centrally and peripherally is monoamine oxidase (MAO), which comes in two genetically distinct forms, known as MAO-A and MAO-B. Inhibition of the A-type makes patients susceptible to dietary tyramine, and can trigger hyper- and hypotensive episodes if levodopa is taken with MAO-A inhibitors. But inhibition of MAO-B alone does not create this hazard, commonly known as the cheese-effect because of the presence of high levels of tyramine in some fermenting cheeses. Inhibitors of MAO-B can be taken safely with levodopa, which potentiate the symptomatic benefit of levodopa by about one-third. Two such MAO-B inhibitors are now commercially available, selegiline (formerly called deprenyl) and rasagiline.

Drugs that act directly on the dopamine receptor have also been developed. None are as powerful as levodopa, except possibly apomorphine, which is administered parenterally, and which easily induces nausea and vomiting, and which has a very short half-life. However, a number of orally active dopamine agonists have received considerable use in the treatment of PD, because their side effect profile is different from that of levodopa's.

To provide a longer plasma half-life of levodopa, delayed release formulations have been developed. One product is Sinement CR (for continuous release); another is Madopar HBS. As seen in the early days of levodopa therapy, this drug is now known not to have an immediate antiparkinsonian effect. It takes several days to weeks of high dosage therapy to achieve the desired degree of benefit. Once a patient has been primed, though, then restarting levodopa after a withdrawal period brings on the benefit almost immediately.

Clinical benefit from levodopa therapy

Levodopa remains today the most powerful drug available to treat PD. In fact, the absence of a robust response to high-dose levodopa essentially excludes the diagnosis of PD and suggests there must be another explanation for the parkinsonian symptoms. In contrast, a marked and sustained response strongly supports the diagnosis of PD (Marsden and Fahn, 1982). Although numerous other treatment options are available in early PD when the disease is mild, virtually all patients will eventually require levodopa therapy as the disease worsens.

However, as mentioned above, not all symptoms of PD are equally responsive to levodopa. Bradykinesia and rigidity generally show the most dramatic improvement with dopaminergic therapy. In fact, the presence of residual rigidity is a good means by which to determine if a patient would further improve by increasing the dose. Tremor has a more variable (and often incomplete) response to levodopa. A number of other symptoms, including postural instability, micrographia and speech disturbance, are typically poorly responsive to dopaminergic therapy, suggesting they are likely due to deficits in other neurotransmitter systems. Recognition of the differential responsiveness of these symptoms to levodopa is critical for setting realistic treatment goals.

Early in the course of disease, levodopa provides a long-duration response that can last several days even if levodopa is discontinued. This continuous response occurs in the presence of a short plasma half-life of a little more than 30 minutes (Muenter and Tyce, 1971; Tolosa et al., 1975).

Problems with levodopa therapy

As PD worsens (or with long-term usage of levodopa), more serious and persistent complications, such as "wearing off" fluctuations and dyskinesias (abnormal involuntary movements) emerge; these motor complications affect 75% of patients after 6 years of levodopa therapy (Fahn, 1992). These problems markedly impair the quality of life and functional status of affected patients, and prove challenging not only for the patient, but also for the treating physician. Today, these motor complications, especially clinical fluctuations and abnormal involuntary movements (dyskinesias), have limited the usefulness of levodopa.

The initial paper by Cotzias and his colleagues (1967) describing the successful use of high dosage D,L-dopa in patients with PD did not mention motor complications. Adverse effects that were mentioned were predominantly anorexia, nausea, vomiting, faintness and hematologic changes. Cotzias et al. (1969) then substituted levodopa for D,L-dopa, which eliminated the hematologic adverse effects. This paper also presents the first report of levodopa-induced dyskinesias, as well as mental symptoms of irritability, anger, hostility, paranoia, insomnia, and an awakening effect. The dyskinesias described were chorea, myoclonus, hemiballism (ipsilateral to the side of a prior thalamotomy), and dystonia. These investigators noted that the adverse effects would subside with a lowering of the dosage of levodopa. They also reported that the appearance of dyskinesias is not an early occurrence after initiating levodopa therapy. Dyskinesias were not seen during the first three weeks of treatment, but occurred later on.

The next paper reporting on the use of levodopa was by Yahr and his colleagues (1969). In their 60 patients, gastrointestinal adverse effects were encountered in 51, dyskinesias in 37, hypotension in 14, cardiac abnormalities in 13, and psychiatric symptoms in 10. By 1970 McDowell and colleagues and Schwarz and Fahn were reporting that dyskinesias were as common as gastrointestinal side effects. They noted that the gastrointestinal effects could often be avoided by building up the dose of levodopa very slowly, and that often patients build up tolerance, with the result that few patents would have persistent gastrointestinal difficulties. On the other hand, dyskinesias, although occurring later, would persist, and would increase and become more prominent with continuing treatment. By 1971 dyskinesias were noted to be the most common dose-limiting adverse effect (Calne et al., 1971). The abnormal movements were seen in all parts of the body, and most often were choreic in nature.

The first review article on levodopa-induced dyskinesias was presented by Duvoisin (1974a, b), based on an analysis of levodopa therapy in 116 patients with PD. He found that by 6 months of treatment, 53% of patients had developed dyskinesias; by 12 months, 81% had. Although described earlier by Cotzias, myoclonic jerking in patients with PD, especially as a toxic reaction to levodopa, was further elaborated by Klawans et al. (1975).

Besides dyskinesias, the treating physician began to become more aware of motor fluctuations, especially as the return of parkinsonian symptoms during these episodes were more prominent due to the underlying worsening of the disease. Various terms were coined to label these fluctuations. "On–off" was coined in 1974 to describe a sudden loss of levodopa's benefit and replacing it with the parkinsonian state (the "off" state) (Sweet and McDowell, 1974; Duvoisin, 1974a, b; Yahr, 1974; Fahn, 1974). The speed of this change was likened to that of a light switch turning on and off. The "on" state was equated with the time when the patient was having a good response from levodopa; the reemergence of the "on" state was sometimes sudden, without even the benefit of another dose of levodopa. But often the "on" state would not appear until another dose of levodopa was ingested. The more common gradual development of the "off" state, taking many minutes to develop and appearing as the plasma levels of levodopa had fallen, was labeled in 1976 as the "wearing-off" phenomenon (Fahn, 1976) and also the "end-of-dose deterioration (Marsden and Parkes, 1976). Both of these terms refer to the identical clinical situation and have been used interchangeably since.

A new dyskinetic state related to the timing of levodopa dosing was described in 1977. Up to this point, all dyskinesias were considered to occur at the peak effect of the levodopa dose. Muenter and his colleagues (1977) described dyskinesias appearing at the beginning and at the end of the dose, which they called "D-I-D" for dystonia (dyskinesia)-improvement-dystonia (dyskinesia). These workers contrasted this to the much more common peak-dose dyskinesia, labeled by Muenter as "I-D-I." Subsequently, the D-I-D phenomena have been labeled diphasic dyskinesias (Marsden et al., 1982; Fahn, 1982).

Not all dyskinesias appear at the peak, the beginning or the end of the dose. Melamed (1979) described painful dystonia occurring in the foot early in the morning, when the effect of the previous night's dose of levodopa has completely worn off. This is a dyskinesia, appearing as a dystonia, that occurs during the "off" state, a time when bradykinesia and other signs of the parkinsonian state would be manifest. Instead, the "off" state dystonia is seen in place of parkinsonism. Early morning dystonia is the most common type of "off" dystonia, but these tight, cramped muscles can appear at other times of the day when the medication wears off.

In addition to the motor offs, a phenomenon known as "sensory offs" or equivalently "behavioral offs" are now recognized. These sensory and behavioral phenomena may accompany a motor (parkinsonian) "off" or be present as an "off" in the absence of much parkinsonian signs. Sensory "offs" can consist of pain, akathisia, depression, anxiety, dysphoria, or panic, and usually a mixture of more than one of these. Sensory "offs," like dystonic "offs" are extremely poorly tolerated. It is often the presence of one of these sensory and behavioral phenomena – more so than

Table 4. *Major fluctuations and dyskinesias as complications of levodopa*

Fluctuations ("Offs")	Dyskinesias
Slow "wearing-off"	Peak-dose chorea, ballism and dystonia
Sudden "off"	Diphasic chorea and dystonia
Random "off"	"Off" dystonia
Yo–yo-ing	Myoclonus
Episodic failure to respond	Simultaneous dyskinesia and parkinsonism
Delayed "on"	
Weak response at end of day	
Response varies in relationship to meals	
Sudden transient freezing	
Sensory and Behavioral "Offs"	
Pain	
Akathisia	
Depression	
Anxiety	
Dysphoria	
Panic	

parkinsonian or dystonic "offs" – which drives the patient to take more and more levodopa, turning them into "levodopa junkies."

Levodopa-related motor and sensory complications can be subdivided according to the clinical phenomena that occur (Table 4). They can also be classified according to their temporal relationship with levodopa dosing. The latter approach is useful when discussing the treatment of motor complications (see below).

There is usually a pattern of progressively worsening response fluctuations in patients who are on chronic levodopa therapy (Table 5). Response fluctuations usually begin as mild wearing-off (end-of-dose failure). Wearing-off can be defined to be present when an adequate dosage of levodopa does not last at least 4 hours. Typically, in the first couple of years of treatment, there is a long-duration response (Muenter and Tyce, 1971). As the disease progresses or as levodopa treatment continues, the long-duration response fades, and the short-duration response is becomes predominant, leading to the wearing-off effect.

The "offs" tend to be mild at first, but over time often become deeper with more severe parkinsonism; simultaneously, the duration of the "on" response becomes shorter. Eventually, many patients develop sudden "offs" in which the deep state of parkinsonism develops over minutes rather than tens of minutes, and they are less predictable in terms of timing with the dosings of levodopa. Many patients who develop response fluctuations also develop abnormal involuntary movements, i.e., dyskinesias.

A number of investigators have found that the major risk factors for motor complications are the duration (Horstink et al., 1990; Roos et al., 1990) or dosage (Poewe et al., 1986; Parkinson Study Group, 2004b) of levodopa therapy. Several studies have also shown that using dopamine agonists are much less likely to induce these motor complications, and therefore using them initially to treat PD symptoms, rather than levodopa, can delay the start of the "wearing off" and dyskinesia effects (Montastruc et al., 1994; Przuntek et al., 1996; Rinne et al., 1998). In a double-blind direct comparison of starting with levodopa or the dopamine agonists, pramipexole and ropinirole, the CALM-PD and 056 trials, respectively, also showed that levodopa was statistically more likely than these agonists to induce both motor fluctuations and dyskinesias (Parkinson Study Group, 2000, 2004a; Rascol et al., 2000).

Table 5. *Temporal development of response fluctuations and dyskinesias*

Dyskinesias
1. Peak-dose dyskinesias
2. Diphasic dyskinesias
3. Chorea → dystonia
4. Yo–yo-ing

Fluctuations
1. Mild wearing-off
2. Deeper wearing-off; shorter time "on"
3. Delayed "ons"
4. Dose failures
5. Sudden, unpredictable "offs" (on–offs)
6. Early morning dystonia
7. Off dystonia during day

Somatotopic response
e.g. dyskinetic in neck, bradykinetic in legs

Freezing phenomenon
1. Freezing when "off"
2. Freezing when "on"

Alertness
1. Drowsy from a dose of levodopa
2. Reverse sleep–wake cycle

Myoclonus
1. Myoclonic jerks during sleep
2. Myoclonic jerks while awake

Behavioral and cognitive
1. Vivid dreams
2. Benign hallucinations
3. Malignant hallucinations
4. Delusions
5. Paranoia
6. Confusion
7. Dementia

Sensory offs
1. Pain
2. Akathisia
3. Depression
4. Anxiety
5. Dysphoria
6. Panic

The mechanism by which levodopa induces these motor complications is not understood. A current hypothesis is that these may be a function of the higher potency and shorter half-life of levodopa as compared with dopamine agonists. Since the development of motor complications relates, in part, to the dose (Parkinson Study Group, 2004b), it is probably best to use the lowest dose of levodopa possible to achieve adequate clinical benefit. In light of concerns that pulsatile administration of levodopa may contribute to the development of motor complications (Mouradian et al., 1990; Chase, 1998; Zappia et al., 2000), there is some rationale for the initial use of extended-release levodopa preparations or catechol-O-methyltransferase (COMT) inhibitors to extend the half-life of levodopa. Unfortunately, clinical trials of early use of regular (Sinemet) vs. long-acting (Sinemet CR) carbidopa/levodopa failed to show differences in the rate of development of motor fluctuations in the two treatment groups (Block et al., 1997; Capildeo, 1998; Wasielewski and Koller, 1998; Koller et al., 1999). There are as yet no clinical trials to determine whether the early use of COMT inhibitors will delay motor complications.

Is levodopa neurotoxic or neuroprotective?

One of the most controversial questions regarding the treatment of PD is whether levodopa is neurotoxic. The results of many *in vitro* studies have suggested that levodopa may be injurious to dopaminergic neurons (see reviews by Fahn, 1996, 1997). These findings have raised concerns that chronic levodopa exposure might hasten disease progression in PD patients. Accordingly, some physicians and patients have opted to defer the use of levodopa for as long as possible (Fahn, 1999). Others physicians have continued to use levodopa as first-line therapy, arguing that it is inappropriate to withhold the most potent symptomatic treatment for PD in the absence of clinical evidence of toxicity (Agid, 1998; Weiner, 1999; Factor, 2000).

Until very recently, there was little clinical data to support or refute the possibility of levodopa toxicity. In 2002, however, two studies were published in which functional neuroimaging techniques had been used to compare patients initially treated with pramipexole vs. levodopa (CALM-PD) and ropinirole vs. levodopa (REAL-PET), respectively. The CALM-PD trial used single photon emission computerized tomography (SPECT) to look at striatal

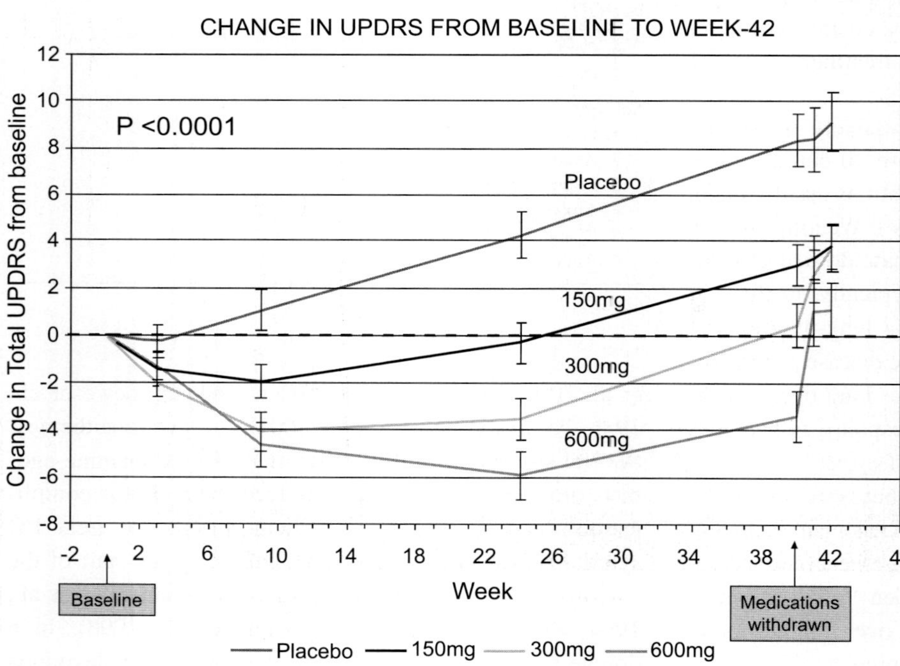

Fig. 3. Changes in Unified Parkinson's disease Rating Scale (UPDRS) from baseline to Week-42. The changes in subjects treated with levodopa at different dosages or with placebo were determined on the basis of the total score of UPDRS. The scores were obtained by the blinded treating investigator who performed the evaluations before the morning dose of the daily dose of the study drug. The points on the curves represent mean changes from baseline in the total scores at each visit. Improvement in parkinsonism is represented by lower scores, and worsening by higher scores. Negative scores on the curves indicate improvement from baseline. The bars indicate standard error. Figure from Parkinson Study Group, 2004b. Reproduced with permission from the New England Journal of Medicine.

dopamine transporter (DAT) activity (β-CIT uptake) as a marker for intact terminals of nigrostriatal dopaminergic neurons. This four-year trial showed a more rapid rate of decline of β-CIT uptake in the group assigned to early levodopa compared with early pramipexole treatment (Parkinson Study Group, 2002). A similar result was found in the REAL-PET trial, which used positron emission tomography (PET) to look at putaminal ^{18}F accumulation (due to ^{18}F-DOPA uptake and decarboxylation) as a marker for functional dopaminergic terminals. This two-year study showed a more rapid rate of reduction of ^{18}F accumulation in patients who were initially treated with levodopa versus ropinirole (Whone et al., 2003). Since there was no placebo group in either study, the findings of the two studies could be interpreted to show that dopamine agonists slow the progression of PD, levodopa hastens the progression of PD, or both. They also raise the question of whether levodopa or dopamine agonists have direct pharmacological effects on DAT or L-aromatic amino acid (dopa) decarboxylase that might confound the interpretation of these results. Thus, caution must be used in interpreting these and other studies that use imaging markers to document "neuroprotection" (Morrish et al., 1996; Marek et al., 2002; Albin and Frey, 2003).

Because of ongoing controversy about whether levodopa is toxic, a large, multicenter, randomized controlled clinical trial comparing three different doses of levodopa with placebo treatment in patients with early PD (the ELLDOPA study) was designed to answer this question (Parkinson Study Group, 2004b). This was a double-blind, placebo-controlled, parallel group, multicenter trial of patients with early PD who had not been previously treated with symptomatic therapy. A total of 361 patients were enrolled, and were randomized to receive treatment with either low- (150 mg/day), middle- (300 mg/day), or high- (600 mg/day) dosage levodopa, or placebo. After forty weeks of treatment, the patients underwent a three-day taper of their medications, followed by a two-week washout period during which they received no treatment for their PD. The primary outcome measure was the change in the total Unified Parkinson's disease Rating Scale (UPDRS) score between baseline and after the washout

SPECT SCAN RESULTS IN ELLDOPA
Subjects with Low Putamen < 3.25 (n=116)

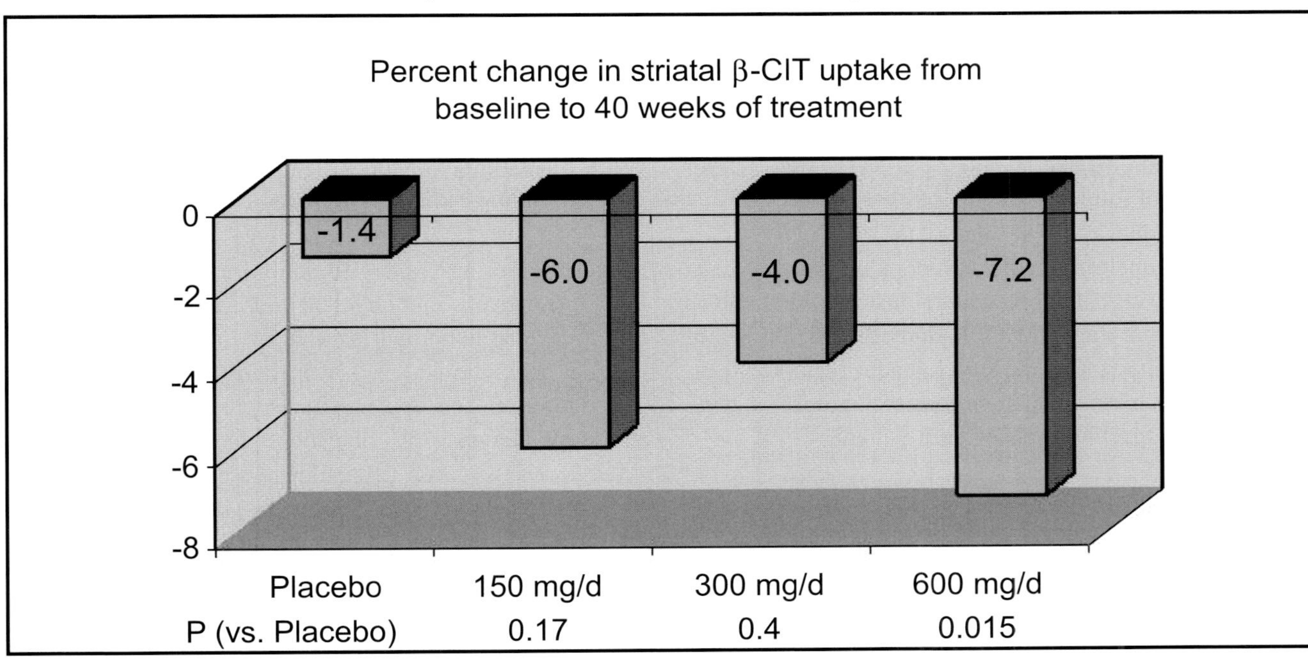

P (dose-response) = 0.036

Fig. 4. Percent changes in striatal binding of β-CIT binding using SPECT from baseline to Week-40 in 116 subjects with low putamen binding (<3.25) at baseline. The bar graphs reveal the percent reduction in β-CIT binding from baseline to Week-40 when subjects were taking the highest assigned dosage of study drug. Data from Parkinson Study Group (2004b) period at Week-42. The goal of the study was to determine whether levodopa treatment affects the rate of progression of PD.

At the end of the two-week washout period, the UPDRS scores of patients treated with all three doses of levodopa were lower (better) than those of the placebo-treated group, in a dose-response pattern (Fig. 3). These findings suggest that levodopa is not neurotoxic, and may even be neuroprotective, though the possibility that patients were experiencing a longer duration of symptomatic response to levodopa that had extended beyond the two-week wash-out period could not be excluded. The highest dosage of levodopa was, however, associated with a higher incidence of motor complications, including dyskinesias and a trend to develop the "wearing off" phenomenon. The ELLDOPA study publication provides a listing of the different adverse events from different dosages of levodopa as well as from placebo.

In addition to the clinical data, a subset of patients in the ELLDOPA trial was also evaluated with β-CIT SPECT imaging, which (as in the CALM-PD trial) was used as a marker for intact nigrostriatal dopaminergic neurons by labeling the dopamine transporter (DAT). These neuroimaging studies showed that there was a larger decrease in striatal DAT binding in patients treated with levodopa, in a dose-response pattern (Fig. 4). Thus, in contrast with the clinical data, the imaging findings suggested that levodopa may hasten the progression of PD. As with other neuroimaging studies, however, it is possible that the observed changes in the levels of uptake of this marker reflected a pharmacological effect of levodopa on DAT activity, rather than evidence of injury to dopaminergic neurons.

Thus, intriguing as the results of the ELLDOPA study are, it remains unclear whether levodopa may (either positively or negatively) affect the natural history of PD. Given the evidence from the ELLDOPA study that the dosage of levodopa is important in the development of motor complications, it is reasonable to customize the dose of levodopa to fit the specific needs of each patient.

Levodopa in patients with a history of melanoma

Levodopa is an intermediary metabolite in the synthesis of melanin. For this reason, there has been longstanding concern that this medication might potentially promote the growth of melanoma. While melanoma obviously occurs in patients on levodopa therapy, there is no evidence that the incidence differs from that in the general population (Skibba et al., 1972; Przybilla et al., 1985; Rampen, 1985; Fiala et al., 2003), other than that there seems to be a higher risk for melanoma in patients with PD even without levodopa treatment (Olsen et al., 2004). In studies of patients with melanoma, levodopa exposure is rare (Sober and Wick, 1978). Thus, although package inserts warn that levodopa should not be used patients with melanoma or suspicious skin lesions (Sinemet, Madopar, Madopar HBS and Stalevo package inserts), there is no clinical evidence to support this admonition (Weiner et al., 1993; Woofter and Manyam, 1994; Pfutzner and Przybilla, 1997; Siple et al., 2000). Nonetheless, in patients with PD and a history of melanoma, it would seem prudent both to defer levodopa therapy until other medications prove inadequate, and to monitor closely for recurrent melanoma.

Summary of clinical phases of levodopa therapy

One can usually discern four clinical phases of PD in relation to treatment with levodopa.

Phase 1 – Honeymoon period

When levodopa is first introduced, there is a "long-duration response" from each dose, with few motoric complications. This is the initial period of maximum benefit without adverse motor effects. The duration of this phase varies, but usually lasts 2–3 years.

Phase 2 – Motoric complication period

With continuing treatment the duration of beneficial response gradually shortens in almost all patients (Muenter and Tyce, 1971), who then need to take levodopa more frequently during the day to minimize the duration of the "off" (relatively immobile) periods; in addition, patients often develop abnormal involuntary movements (dyskinesias) at peak plasma levels of levodopa that are parallel to the timing of their doses. After approximately 5 years of levodopa therapy, 75% of patients have either developed *troublesome* response fluctuations ('wearing-off' and 'on–off' phenomena) or *troublesome* dyskinesias (Fahn, 1992). During the 'wearing-off', dose-failures, and 'on–off' states (which can total 50% or more of the waking day), there is disability with pronounced parkinsonian symptoms and signs, leaving patients immobile or akinetic for hours at a time, sometimes with painful sustained contractions, known as 'off' dystonia. Dyskinesias are usually choreic in nature, and classically show a temporal correlation with peak plasma levodopa levels (peak-dose dyskinesias). Peak-dose dyskinesias may also be dystonic ('on' dystonia).

Some patients, particularly younger ones, may alternate between states of dyskinesia and 'off', with little normal periods in between, a state referred to as 'yo–yo-ing' (Marsden et al., 1982; Fahn, 1982). Sometimes, diphasic dyskinesias develop when the plasma levels of levodopa are low (Muenter et al., 1977); the mechanism of this complication remains unknown.

Whether the motor complications seen with chronic levodopa therapy in patients with PD are actually caused by long-term levodopa therapy or simply reflect the progression of the disease is unknown and widely debated (de Jong et al., 1987; Quinn et al., 1987; Blin et al., 1988; Roos et al., 1990; Caraceni et al., 1991; Cedarbaum et al., 1991). The ELLDOPA study showed that dyskinesias are more common with higher doses of levodopa (Parkinson Study Group, 2004b).

Phase 3 – Period of progression and drug-resistant parkinsonism

Also, after 2–3 years of levodopa therapy, the degree of benefit begins to fade, and the signs and symptoms of parkinsonism increasingly recur. By 5 years of levodopa treatment, the clinical severity of PD, even while on levodopa, has been shown to reach the level it was prior to initiating levodopa, and the severity steadily continues to increase further with time (Yahr, 1976; Markham and Diamond, 1986; Parkinson Study Group, 2000). Thus, levodopa therapy can be considered to set back the signs and symptoms by about 5 years. Beyond this time period, there is development of new symptoms that are resistant to treatment: loss of postural reflexes, falling, freezing, dysphonia, dysarthria, and flexed posture.

Phase 4 – Dementia period

The development of dementia in patients with PD is a most ominous sign, for there is no satisfactory reversal of this feature. Besides causing great physical and emotional stress for the caregivers, the presence of dementia often leads to nursing home placement. The leading cause for patients with PD to be admitted to nursing homes is the presence of hallucinations (Goetz and Stebbins, 1993), which occurs commonly in demented PD patients receiving anti-PD medications. The presence of dementia greatly limits the amount of levodopa the patient can tolerate, because confusion and hallucinations are easily induced as the dosage of levodopa is increased. Atypical antipsychotics, such as clozapine and quetiapine, can ease the hallucinations.

References

Aarsland D, Andersen K, Larsen JP, Lolk A, Kragh-Sorensen P (2003) Prevalence and characteristics of dementia in Parkinson disease – An 8-year prospective study. Arch Neurol 60: 387–392

Aebert K (1967) Was leistet L-DOPA bei der Behandlung der Parkinson-Akinese? Deutsch Med Wschr 92: 483–487

Agid Y (1998) Levodopa: is toxicity a myth? Neurology 50: 858–863

Albin RL, Frey KA (2003) Initial agonist treatment of Parkinson disease: a critique. Neurology 60: 390–394

Barbeau A, Sourkes TL, Murphy GF (1962) Les catecholamines dans la maladie de Parkinson. In: de Ajuriaguerra J (eds) Symposium Sur les Monoamines et Systeme Nerveux Central. Georg & Cie, Geneve: pp 247–262

Benamer HTS, Patterson J, Wyper DJ, Hadley DM, Macphee GJA, Grosset DG (2000) Correlation of Parkinson's disease severity and duration with I-123- FP-CIT SPECT striatal uptake. Mov Disord 15: 692–698

Bernheimer H, Birkmayer W, Hornykiewicz O, Jellinger K, Seitelberger F (1973) Brain dopamine and the syndromes of Parkinson and Huntington. J Neurol Sci 20: 415–455

Birkmayer W, Hornykiewicz O (1961) Der L-3,4-Dioxyphenylalanin (DOPA)-Effekt bei der Parkinson-Akinese. Wien Klin Wochenschr 73: 787–788

Blin J, Bonnet A-M, Agid Y (1988) Does levodopa aggravate Parkinson's disease? Neurology 38: 1410–1416

Block G, Liss C, Reines S, et al. (1997) Comparison of immediate-release and controlled release carbidopa/levodopa in Parkinson's disease. A multicenter 5-year study. The CR First Study Group. Eur Neurol 37: 23–27

Blocq P, Marinesco G (1893) Sur un cas de tremblement Parkinsonien hemiplegique, symptomatique d'une tumeur de peduncule cerebral. C R Soc Biol Paris 5: 105–111

Bower JH, Maraganore DM, McDonnell SK, Rocca WA (2000) Influence of strict, intermediate, and broad diagnostic criteria on the age- and sex-specific incidence of Parkinson's disease. Mov Disord 15: 819–825

Brissaud E (1895) Lecons sur les Maladies Nerveuses. Masson et Cie, Paris

Bruno A, Bruno SC (1966) Effetti dell L-2,4-dihydossifenilalanina (l-Dopa) nei pazienti parkinsoniani. Riv Sper Freniat 90: 39

Calne DB, Reid JL, Vakil SD, Pallis C (1971) Problems with L-dopa therapy. Clin Med 78: 21–23

Capildeo R (1998) Implications of the 5-year CR FIRST trial. Sinemet CR Five-Year International Response Fluctuation Study. Neurology 50 [Suppl 6]: 15–17; discussion 44–18

Caraceni T, Scigliano G, Musicco M (1991) The occurrence of motor fluctuations in parkinsonian patients treated long term with levodopa: role of early treatment and disease progression. Neurology 41: 380–384

Carlsson A, Lindqvist M, Magnusson T (1957) 3,4-Dihydroxyphenylalanine and 5-hydroxytryptophan as reserpine antagonists. Nature 180: 1200

Cedarbaum JM, Gandy SE, McDowell FH (1991) Early initiation of levodopa treatment does not promote the development of motor response fluctuations, dyskinesias, or dementia in Parkinson's disease. Neurology 41: 622–629

Chase TN (1998) The significance of continuous dopaminergic stimulation in the treatment of Parkinson's disease. Drugs 55 [Suppl 1]: 1–9

Cotzias GC, Papavasiliou PS, Gellene R (1969) Modification of parkinsonism – chronic treatment with L-dopa. N Engl J Med 280: 337–345

Cotzias GC, Van Woert MH, Schiffer LM (1967) Aromatic amino acids and modification of parkinsonism. N Engl J Med 276: 374–379

de Jong GJ, Meerwaldt JD, Schmitz PIM (1987) Factors that influence the occurrence of response variations in Parkinson's disease. Ann Neurol 22: 4–7

de Rijk MC, Tzourio C, Breteler MM, Dartigues JF, Amaducci L, Lopez-Pousa S, et al. (1997) Prevalence of parkinsonism and Parkinson's disease in Europe: the EUROPARKINSON Collaborative Study. European Community Concerted Action on the Epidemiology of Parkinson's disease. J Neurol Neurosurg Psychiatry 62: 10–15

Duvoisin RC (1974a) Hyperkinetic reactions with L-DOPA. In: Yahr MD (ed) Current Concepts in the Treatment of Parkinsonism. Raven Press, New York: 203–210

Duvoisin RC (1974b) Variations in the "on–off" phenomenon. Adv Neurol 5: 339–340

Duyckaerts C (2000) Images. Les corps et prolongements de Lewy. Rev Neurol (Paris) 156: 800–801

Ehringer H, Hornykiewicz O (1960) Verteilung von Noradrenalin und Dopamin (3-Hydroxytyramin) im Gehirn des Menschen und ihr Verhalten bei Erkrankungen der extrapyramidalen Systems. Klin Wochenschr 38: 1236–1239

Eidelberg D, Moeller JR, Isikawa T, Dhawan V, Spetsieris P, Chaly T, Robeson W, Dahl JR, Margouleff D (1995) Assessment of disease severity in parkinsonism with fluorine-18- fluorodeoxyglucose and PET. J Nucl Med 36: 378–383

Elbaz A, Bower JH, Maraganore DM, McDonnell SK, Peterson BJ, Ahlskog JE, Schaid DJ, Rocca WA (2002) Risk tables for parkinsonism and Parkinson's disease. J Clin Epidemiol 55: 25–31

Elbaz A, Bower JH, Peterson BJ, Maraganore DM, McDonnell SK, Ahlskog JE, Schaid DJ, Rocca WA (2003) Survival study of Parkinson disease in Olmsted county, Minnesota. Arch Neurol 60: 91–96

Factor SA (2000) The initial treatment of Parkinson's disease. Mov Disord 15: 360–361

Fahn S (1974) "On–off" phenomenon with levodopa therapy in parkinsonism: Clinical and pharmacologic correlations and the effect of intramuscular pyridoxine. Neurology 24: 431–441

Fahn S (1976) Medical treatment of movement disorders. In: Davis FA (ed) Neurological Reviews 1976. Minneapolis; American Academy of Neurology: 72–106

Fahn S (1982) Fluctuations of disability in Parkinson's disease: pathophysiological aspects. In: Marsden CD, Fahn S (eds) Movement Disorders. London, Butterworth Scientific, pp 123–145

Fahn S (1992) Adverse effects of levodopa. In: Olanow CW, Lieberman AN (eds) The Scientific Basis for the Treatment of Parkinson's disease. Carnforth, England; Parthenon Publishing Group: 89–112

Fahn S (1996) Is levodopa toxic? Neurology 47: 184–195

Fahn S (1997) Levodopa-induced neurotoxicity: Does it represent a problem for the treatment of Parkinson's disease? CNS Drugs 8: 376–393

Fahn S (1999) Parkinson disease, the effect of levodopa, and the ELLDOPA trial. Arch Neurol 56: 529–535

Fahn S, Przedborski S (2005) Parkinsonism. In: Rowland LP (ed) Merritt's neurology, 10th ed. Lippincott Williams & Wilkins, Philadelphia, pp 828–846

Fahn S, Sulzer D (2004) Neurodegeneration and neuroprotection in Parkinson disease. NeuroRx 1: 139–154

Fazzagli A, Amaducci L (1966) La Sperimentazione clinica del Dopa nelle sindromi parkinsoniane. Riv Neurobiol 12: 138–145

Fehling C (1966) Treatment of Parkinson's syndrome with L-DOPA, a double-blind study. Acta Neurol Scand 42: 367–372

Fiala KH, Whetteckey J, Manyam BV (2003) Malignant melanoma and levodopa in Parkinson's disease: causality or coincidence? Parkinsonism Relat Disord 9(6): 321–327

Foix C, Nicolesco I (1925) Anatomie Cerebrale; Les Noyeux Gris Centraux et la Region Mesencephalo-Sous-Opitique, Suive d'un Appendice sur l'Anatomie Pathologique de la Maladie de Parkinson. Masson et Cie, Paris

Friedhoff AJ, Hekiman L, Alpert M, Tobach E (1963) Dihydroxyphenylalanine in extrapyramidal disease. JAMA 184: 285–286

Goetz CG (1987) Charcot, the Clinician: The Tuesday Lessons. Excerpts from Nine Case Presentations on General Neurology Delivered at the Salpetriere Hospital in 1887–88 By Jean-Martin Charcot. Translated with Commentary. Raven Press, New York: 123–124

Goetz CG, Stebbins GT (1993) Risk factors for nursing home placement in advanced Parkinson's disease. Neurology 43: 2227–2229

Greenfield JG, Bosanquet FD (1953) The brain-stem lesions in parkinsonism. J Neurol Neurosurg Psychiatry 16: 213–226

Greer M, Williams CM (1963) Dopamine metabolism in Parkinson's disease. Neurology 13: 73–76

Hassler R (1938) Zur Pathologie der Paralysis Agitans und des postenzephalitischen Parkinsonismus. J Psychol Neurol 48: 387–476

Hirschmann J, Mayer K (1964) Zur Beeinflussung von L-Dopa (L-Dihydroxyphenylananin) Deutsch Med Wschr 89: 1877–1880

Hoehn MM, Yahr MD (1967) Parkinsonism: Onset, progression and mortality. Neurology 17: 427–442

Horstink MW, Zijlmans JC, Pasman JW, et al. (1990) Which risk factors predict the levodopa response in fluctuating Parkinson's disease? Ann Neurol 27: 537–543

Klawans HL, Goetz C, Bergen D (1975) Levodopa-induced myoclonus. Arch Neurol 32: 331–334

Koller WC, Hutton JT, Tolosa E, et al. (1999) Immediate-release and controlled-release carbidopa/levodopa in PD: a 5-year randomized multicenter study. Carbidopa/Levodopa Study Group. Neurology 53: 1012–1019

Lewy FH (1914) Zur pathologischen Anatomie der Paralysis agitans. Dtsch Z Nervenheilk 1: 50–55

Madopar HBS (2002) [summary of product characteristics]. Wellwyn Garden City, Hertfordshire: Roche Products, Ltd

Marek K, Jennings D, Seibyl J (2002) Do dopamine agonists or levodopa modify Parkinson's disease progression? Eur J Neurol 9[Suppl 3]: 15–22

Markham CH, Diamond SG (1986) Long-term follow up of early dopa treatment in Parkinson's disease. Ann Neurol 19: 365–372

Marsden CD, Fahn S (1982) Problems in Parkinson's disease. In: Marsden CD, Fahn S (eds) Movement Disorders. Butterworth Scientific, London, pp 1–7

Marsden CD, Parkes JD (1976) 'On–off' effects in patients with Parkinson's disease on chronic levodopa therapy. Lancet 1: 292–295

Marsden CD, Parkes JD, Quinn N (1982) Fluctuations of disability in Parkinson's disease – clinical aspects. In: Marsden CD, Fahn S (eds) Movement Disorders. Butterworth Scientific, London, pp 96–122

McDowell F, Lee JE, Swift T, Sweet RD, Ogsbury JS, Kessler JT (1970) Treatment of Parkinson's syndrome with dihydroxyphenylalanine (levodopa). Ann Int Med 72: 29–35

McGeer PL, Zeldowicz LR (1964) Administration of dihydroxyphenylalanine to parkinsonian patients. Canad Med Assn J 90: 463–466

Melamed E (1979) Early-morning dystonia: A late side effect of long-term levodopa therapy in Parkinson's disease. Arch Neurol 36: 308–310

Meynert T (1871) über Beiträge zur differential Diagnose der paralytischen Irrsinns. Wiener Med Presse 11: 645–647

Miller WC, DeLong MR (1988) Parkinsonian symptomatology: an anatomical and physiological analysis. Ann NY Acad Sci 515: 287–302

Mitchell IJ, Clarke CE, Boyce S, Robertson RG, Peggs D, Sambrook MA, Crossman AR (1989) Neural mechanisms underlying parkinsonian symptoms based upon regional uptake of 2-deoxyglucose in monkeys exposed to 1-methyl-4-phenyl-1,2,3,6-tetrahydropyridine. Neuroscience 32: 213–226

Montastruc JL, Rascol O, Senard JM, et al. (1994) A randomised controlled study comparing bromocriptine to which levodopa was later added, with levodopa alone in previously untreated patients with Parkinson's disease: a five year follow up. J Neurol Neurosurg Psychiatry 57: 1034–1038

Morrish PK (2002) Brain imaging to assess the effects of dopamine agonists on progression of Parkinson disease. JAMA 288: 312; author reply 312–313

Morrish PK, Sawle GV, Brooks DJ (1996) An [F-18]dopa-PET and clinical study of the rate of progression in Parkinson's disease. Brain 119: 585–591

Mouradian MM, Heuser IJE, Baronti F, Chase TN (1990) Modification of central dopaminergic mechanisms by continuous levodopa therapy for advanced Parkinson's disease. Ann Neurol 27: 18–23
Muenter MD, Sharpless NS, Tyce GM, Darley FL (1977) Patterns of dystonia ('I-D-I' and 'D-I-D') in response to L-dopa therapy of Parkinson's disease. Mayo Clin Proc 52: 163–174
Muenter MD, Tyce GM (1971) L-dopa therapy of Parkinson's disease: Plasma L-dopa concentration, therapeutic response, and side effects. Mayo Clin Proc 46: 231–239
Olsen JH, Frils S, Frederiksen K, McLaughlin JK, Mellemkjaer L, Moller H (2004) Atypical cancer pattern in patients with Parkinson's disease. Br J Cancer: 1–5
Parkinson J (1817) An Essay on the Shaking Palsy, Sherwood, Neely, and Jones, London
Parkinson Study Group (2000) Pramipexole versus levodopa as the initial treatment for Parkinson's disease: a randomized controlled trial. JAMA 284: 1931–1938
Parkinson Study Group (2002) Dopamine transporter brain imaging to assess the effects of pramipexole vs levodopa on Parkinson disease progression. JAMA 287: 1653–1661
Parkinson Study Group (2004a) Pramipexole vs levodopa as initial treatment for Parkinson disease – A 4-year randomized controlled trial. Arch Neurol 61: 1044–1053
Parkinson Study Group (2004b) Levodopa and the progression of Parkinson's disease. N Engl J Med. 351: 2498–2508
Penney JB Jr, Young AB (1986) Striatal inhomogeneities and basal ganglia function. Mov Disord 1: 3–14
Pfutzner W, Przybilla B (1997) Malignant melanoma and levodopa: is there a relationship? Two new cases and a review of the literature. J Am Acad Dermatol 37: 332–336
Poewe WH, Lees AJ, Stern GM (1986) Low-dose L-dopa therapy in Parkinson's disease: a 6-year follow-up study. Neurology 36: 1528–1530
Przuntek H, Welzel D, Gerlach M, et al. (1996) Early institution of bromocriptine in Parkinson's disease inhibits the emergence of levodopa-associated motor side effects. Long-term results of the PRADO study. J Neural Transm Gen Sect 103: 699–715
Przybilla B, Schwab U, Landthaler M, et al. (1985) Development of two malignant melanomas during administration of levodopa. Acta Derm Venereol 65: 556–557
Quinn N, Critchley P, Marsden CD (1987) Young onset Parkinson's disease. Mov Disord 2: 73–91
Rampen FH (1985) Levodopa and melanoma: three cases and review of literature. J Neurol Neurosurg Psychiatry 48: 585–588
Rascol O, Brooks DJ, Korczyn AD, et al. (2000) A five-year study of the incidence of dyskinesia in patients with early Parkinson's disease who were treated with ropinirole or levodopa. 056 Study Group. N Engl J Med 342: 1484–1491
Rinaldi F, Marghertia G, De Divitus E (1965) Effetti della somministrazione de DOPA a pazienti parkinsoniani pretrattati con inhibitore delle monoaminossidasi. Ann Fren Scienze Affini 78: 105–113
Rinne UK, Bracco F, Chouza C, et al. (1998) Early treatment of Parkinson's disease with cabergoline delays the onset of motor complications. Results of a double-blind levodopa controlled trial. The PKDS009 Study Group. Drugs 55[Suppl 1]: 23–30
Rinne UK, Sonninen V (1968) A double-blind study of L-dopa treatment in Parkinson's disease. Europ Neurol 1: 180–191
Roos RAC, Vredevoogd CB, van der Velde EA (1990) Response fluctuations in Parkinson's disease. Neurology 40: 1344–1346
Schwarz GA, Fahn S (1970) Newer medical treatments in parkinsonism. Med Clin No Am 54: 773–785
Seibyl JP, Marek KL, Quinlan D, Sheff K, Zoghbi S, Zea-Ponce Y, Baldwin RM, Fussell B, Smith BS, Charney DS, Hoffer PB, Innis RB (1995) Decreased single-photon emission computed tomographic [(123)]I beta-CIT striatal uptake correlates with symptom severity in Parkinson's disease. Ann Neurol 38: 589–598
Sinemet CR (2002) [package insert]. Bristol-Myers Squibb Co, Princeton, NJ
Siple JF, Schneider DC, Wanlass WA, et al. (2000) Levodopa therapy and the risk of malignant melanoma. Ann Pharmacother 34: 382–385
Skibba JL, Pinckley J, Gilbert EF, et al. (1972) Multiple primary melanoma following administration of levodopa. Arch Pathol 93: 556–561
Snow BJ, Lee CS, Schulzer M, Mak E, Calne DB (1994) Longitudinal fluorodopa positron emission tomographic studies of the evolution of idiopathic Parkinsonism. Ann Neurol 36: 759–764
Sober AJ, Wick MM (1978) Levodopa therapy and malignant melanoma. JAMA 240: 554–555
Stalevo (2003) [package insert]. Novartis Pharmaceuticals Corp, East Hanover, NJ
Sweet RD, McDowell FH (1974) The "on–off" response to chronic L-DOPA treatment of parkinsonism. Adv Neurol 5: 331–338
Tanner CM, Ottman R, Goldman SM, Ellenberg J, Chan P, Mayeux R, Langston JW (1999) Parkinson disease in twins – An etiologic study. JAMA 281: 341–346
Tolosa ES, Martin WE, Cohen HP, Jacobson RL (1975) Patterns of clinical response and plasma dopa levels in Parkinson's disease. Neurology 25: 177–183
Tretiakoff C (1919) Contribution a l'etude de l'anatomie pathologique du locus niger de Soemmering avec quelques dedutions relatives a la pathogenie des troubles du tonus musculaire et de la maladie de Parkinson. These de Paris
Umbach W, Bauman D (1964) Die Wirksamkeit von L-Dopa bei Parkinson-Patienten mit und ohne sterotaktischen Herneingriff. Arch Psychiat Nervenkr 205: 281–292
Wasielewski PG, Koller WC (1998) Quality of life and Parkinson's disease: the CR FIRST Study. J Neurol 245[Suppl 1]: 28–30
Weiner WJ (1999) The initial treatment of Parkinson's disease should begin with levodopa. Mov Disord 14: 716–724
Weiner WJ, Singer C, Sanchez-Ramos JR, et al. (1993) Levodopa, melanoma, and Parkinson's disease. Neurology 43: 674–677
Whone AL, Watts RL, Stoessl AJ, et al. (2003) Slower progression of Parkinson's disease with ropinirole versus levodopa: The REAL-PET study. Ann Neurol 54: 93–101
Woofter MJ, Manyam BV (1994) Safety of long-term levodopa therapy in malignant melanoma. Clin Neuropharmacol 17: 315–319
Yahr MD (1974) Variations in the "on–off" effect. Adv Neurol 5: 397–399
Yahr MD (1976) Evaluation of long-term therapy in Parkinson's disease: Mortality and therapeutic efficacy. In: Birkmayer W, Hornykiewicz O (eds) Advances in Parkinsonism. Basle, Editiones Roche: 444–455
Yahr MD, Duvoisin RC, Schear MJ, Barrett RE, Hoehn MM (1969) Treatment of parkinsonism with levodopa. Arch Neurol 21: 343–354
Zappia M, Oliveri RL, Bosco D, et al. (2000) The long-duration response to L-dopa in the treatment of early PD. Neurology 54: 1910–1915

J Neural Transm (2006) [Suppl] 71: 17–25

Journal of
Neural
Transmission
Printed in Austria

Changing dopamine agonist treatment in Parkinson's disease: experiences with switching to pramipexole

H. Reichmann[1], **P. Odin**[2], **H. M. Brecht**[3], **J. Köster**[3], **P. H. Kraus**[4]

[1] Department of Neurology, Technical University of Dresden, Dresden, Germany
[2] Central Hospital Bremerhaven, Department of Neurology, Germany
[3] Boehringer Ingelheim Pharma GmbH & Co. KG, Division Medicine, Germany
[4] Department of Neurology, St. Josef-Hospital, Ruhr-University Bochum, Germany

Summary 1202 patients suffering from Parkinson's disease switched from other dopamine agonists to pramipexole under open conditions either abruptly or in an overlapping, gradual manner. Mostly insufficient effectiveness motivated the switch. The investigators gave equal preference to either an abrupt or an overlapping switch to pramipexole in this observational study. There was a tendency in favour of the overlapping switch procedure in those patients who were on a relatively higher dose of a dopamine agonist before the switch. The switch was performed because the investigators expected the effect of pramipexole on tremor, motor functions and depression/anhedonia to be better compared with previous dopamine agonists. The main reasons for switching to pramipexole (anti-tremor effect, anti-depressive/anti-anhedonic effect) as given by the physicians at baseline came up to expectations.

The switch to pramipexole mostly yielded further improvements irrespective of the mode of switching.

Introduction

Dopamine agonists are a mainstay in the pharmacotherapy of Parkinson's disease. They are currently favoured as monotherapy or adjunct to levodopa over levodopa monotherapy as first treatment option in early disease (Olanow et al., 2001; American Academy of Neurology, 2002; Agency for Healthcare Research and Quality, 2003; German Society of Neurology, 2003), because of indications that they delay the onset of motor complications in comparison to levodopa and their supposed neuroprotective properties. In Germany, seven dopamine agonists are available for oral use, two of them are second generation nonergot derivatives (pramipexole and ropinirole) and five of them (bromocriptine, cabergoline, alpha-dihydroergocryptine, lisuride, pergolide) are ergot derivatives.

Correspondence: H. Reichmann, Department of Neurology, Technical University of Dresden, Fetscherstr. 74, 01307 Dresden, Germany
e-mail: heinz.reichmann@mailbox.tu-dresden.de

Dopamine agonists not only differ from each other with respect to their chemical structure but also with respect to their binding affinities to the different dopamine receptor subtypes D_1–D_5, contraindications, pharmacokinetics, dosage regimen, duration of the titration period and to their side effect profiles (Brecht, 2001).

Concerning tolerability and side effects meta-analyses suggest that ropinirole may be associated with a higher risk of hypotension and somnolence compared to pramipexole, which seems to be associated with a higher risk of hallucinations than ropinirole (Etminan et al., 2003).

Ergot-type dopamine agonists seem to be associated with an increased risk of cardiovascular adverse events and of pleural, pericardial and retroperitoneal effusions and fibroses (Müller and Fritze, 2003) as well as valvular heart disease (VHD) involving one or more valves (Rascol et al., 2004; Horvath et al., 2004; van Camp et al., 2004; Basemann et al., 2004), while these risks appear to be low or non-existing under pramipexole. The ergot dopamine agonist pergolide is currently under special scrutiny because of VHD (Flowers et al., 2003). Thus, in patients with valvular heart disease a switching from an ergot-type dopamine agonist to a non-ergot agonist may be indicated.

Moreover, there are several other reasons for switching: insufficient or declining effectiveness, side effects, pharmacokinetic interactions or concomitant diseases. The reasons why patients can profit from a switch in terms of effectiveness are still poorly understood. Therefore, switching strategies are worth being investigated for all dopamine agonists, which may also include switches from nonergot-type dopamine agonists to ergot-type ones. In principle, switching may be achieved by gradually up-titrating of the new dopamine agonist while in parallel tapering-off the other one or, alternatively, by abruptly substituting the dopamine agonist by an equivalent dose of the new one from one day to the other. Theoretically, abrupt switching may induce increasing motor impairment or even an akinetic crisis if the dosage is too small – or dyskinesias and hallucinations in case of overdose. The same holds true for the gradual overlapping switch as dose equivalents are still not well established. Nevertheless, there is evidence from at least one systematic although small trial that tolerability of immediate switching is superior to tapering (Goetz et al., 1999). Therefore, abrupt switching is currently recommended (Grosset et al., 2004).

The present post-marketing surveillance (PMS) study focused on the effectiveness and tolerability of overlapping versus abrupt switching to pramipexole from other dopamine agonists. Moreover, additional information on the reasons for switching as well as for preferring the non-ergot pramipexole over the other options could be collected. A PMS study may be expected to increase insight in which dosage of the various dopamine agonists might be equivalent to that of pramipexole.

Material and methods

This was an open post-marketing surveillance study. Data on 1216 patients were collected from 487 centres including 26 in-patients from 9 centres. Neurologists were supplied with recommendations for dosing (average daily dose) and titration (increase of dose per week and time to reach the average daily dose) of the following dopamine agonists: Alpha-dihydroergocryptine (alpha-DHEC), bromocriptine, cabergoline, lisuride, pergolide, ropinirole according to the respective Summaries of Product Characteristics (SPCs); the choice between overlapping versus abrupt switching to pramipexole, however, was left to the neurologist.

Clinical assessments were performed at screening as well as four to eight weeks later, providing a 4 week treatment period after the switching was completed. Assessments included demographic data, previous type and dosage of antiparkinsonian drugs, reasons for discontinuation of the dopamine agonist and selection of pramipexole, and type of switching to pramipexole. Motor functioning and psychopathology were assessed by the Short Parkinson's Disease Evaluation Scale (SPES) (Rabey et al., 1997, Marinus et al., 2004). Additionally, tremor was assessed by the spiral drawing test (Bain, 1993) and the scanned drawings were computer analysed (Kraus, in preparation). Mood and drive were assessed by self-rating using seven visual analogue scales (VAS) for the dimensions mood, anxiety/restlessness, drive, somatic fitness, general wellbeing, happiness, pleasure, respectively. Finally a global clinical assessment of effectiveness and tolerability of pramipexole as well as a comparison to the previous dopamine agonist were performed by the investigator. All spontaneously reported adverse drug reactions were documented. All patients receiving at least a single dose of pramipexole were included into the safety analyses.

Statistical analyses were performed descriptively and exploratively.

Dose comparisons between previous dopamine agonist and pramipexole were calculated in those patients only, in whom the investigator considered the switch to be completed, the concurrent antiparkinsonian therapy had not been changed and the Global Clinical Assessment of effectiveness was rated equal or even superior in comparison to the previous dopamine agonist. The proportion of patients with equal effectiveness was too small (15%) to estimate the equivalent dosage for the various dopamine agonists.

All pramipexole doses mentioned in this paper refer to the pramipexole salt. For conversion into the pramipexole base dose the milligrams have to be multiplied by 0.7, i.e. 1.5 mg salt corresponds to 1.05 mg base.

Results

Subjects

For safety analyses 1202 out of 1216 patients were included, as $n = 14$ patients provided only baseline data. Further $n = 113$ patients had an "incorrect" switch (no previous dopamine agonist treatment or previous treatment with 2 dopamine agonists, where only one was substituted by pramipexole), leaving $n = 1089$ for effectiveness analysis and comparison of the switching procedure.

The 1202 patients comprised 58% males, 41% female patients with a mean age of 69.2 years and a median duration of PD 4.2 years.

Previous PD therapy

87% were simultaneously treated with levodopa (plus a dopa-decarboxylase inhibitor, DCI) and 43% with other antiparkinsonian drugs, essentially the NMDA-antagonist amantadine (66%), followed by MAO-inhibitors (23%), COMT-inhibitors (19%) and anticholinergics (11%). Table 1 presents the number of patients treated with the various antiparkinsonian drugs as well as the daily dosages (where applicable).

Reason for withdrawal of the previous dopamine agonist

Among the reasons for withdrawal of the previous dopamine agonist insufficient effectiveness on motor functions

Table 1. *Antiparkinsonian drug treatment before switching*

Parkinson therapy	Number of patients *n*	%	Daily dose (mg) (median)
Dopamine agonists	1089	100	
Cabergoline	300	27	2.0
Bromocriptine	197	18	10.0
Alpha-Dihydroergocryptine	179	16	40.0
Pergolide	175	16	1.5
Lisuride	154	14	0.6
Ropinirole	98	9	6.0
levodopa (+DCI)	944	87	300.0*
Other antiparkinsonian drugs	470	43	–

*Dose calculated for levodopa

Table 2. *Reasons for withdrawal of previous dopamine agonist*

	Total	
	*n**	%
Number of patients	1089	100.0
Insufficient effectiveness on tremor	741	68.0
Insufficient effectiveness on motor function	513	47.1
Insufficient effectiveness on depression/anhedonia	485	44.5
Insufficient gastrointestinal tolerability	223	20.5
Insufficient cardiovascular tolerability	143	13.1
Effusions/fibroses	4	0.4
Other reasons	86	7.9

*Multiple naming allowed

especially on tremor predominated, followed by anhedonia and depression (Table 2).

Reason for switching to pramipexole

The neurologists' leading reason for choosing the switch to pramipexole was the anticipation of an improved anti-tremor (70%), antidepressant (56%), and neuroprotective (27%) effect as well as a low interaction potential (25%) and favourable pharmacokinetic profile (17%) (Table 3).

Switching procedure

From the protocol no preference was given for the switching procedure and no reason was requested for the specific choice from the investigator. A nominally observation period of 4 to 8 weeks was foreseen to allow an assessment after a maintenance period of 4 weeks following the end of the switching period. The median observational period lasted 50 days (direct switch) respectively 51 days (overlapping switch).

Table 3. *Reasons for the choice of pramipexole*

	Total	
	*n**	%
Number of patients	1089	100.0
Better anti-tremor effect	767	70.4
Better antidepressant/anti-anhedonic effect	614	56.4
Neuroprotective effect, especially in younger patients	294	26.2
Lower potential for interactions	275	27.0
Favourable pharmacokinetics	205	18.1
Daily therapy costs	118	10.8
Other reasons	87	7.9
Concomitant disease RLS	27	2.5
Impaired liver function	13	1.2
Missing	9	0.8

*Multiple naming allowed

Table 4. *Switching procedure*

		Direct switching		Overlapping switching
Number of patients		553		536
Gender (male)	%	61		58
Age (years)	mean	69		69
Duration of PD (years)	median	4.1		5.0
SPES motor function	median	15.0		16.0
SPES psychopath disturbance	median	2.0		2.0
Previous dopamine agonist	*n*	median daily dose (mg)	*n*	median daily dose (mg)
Cabergoline	151	2.0	148	2.0
Bromocriptine	108	7.5	87	10.0
Alpha-DHEC	83	40.0	93	40.0
Pergolide	83	1.5	91	1.5
Lisuride	79	0.6	74	0.8
Ropinirole	52	3.0	46	6.0

The two modes of switching were equally distributed 51%:49%, and no clinically relevant difference could be observed with respect to gender, age or previous dopamine agonist, although there was a trend that duration of Parkinson disease and relatively higher daily doses of the previous dopamine agonist (bromocriptine, lisuride and ropinirole) favoured the overlapping switch procedure (Table 4). In addition the reasons for switching to pramipexole had no influence on choosing one or the other mode of switching (not shown in Table 4).

Effectiveness of switching to pramipexole compared to the previous DA in the total population

Effectiveness of pramipexole after 4–8 weeks was comparable between the two groups established by the switching procedure; therefore results are presented for the total group only.

Global clinical effectiveness of pramipexole

The global clinical effectiveness of pramipexole in direct comparison to the previous DA was rated by the investigator to be superior to the previous DA (84.3%), equal (14.7%) and worse in 1 patient from the direct switch group (Fig. 1).

Motor function (SPES)

The median sum score of motor function improved from 15.0 on the respective previous DA to 9.0 on pramipexole ($n = 1089$, signed rank test, $p < 0.0001$).

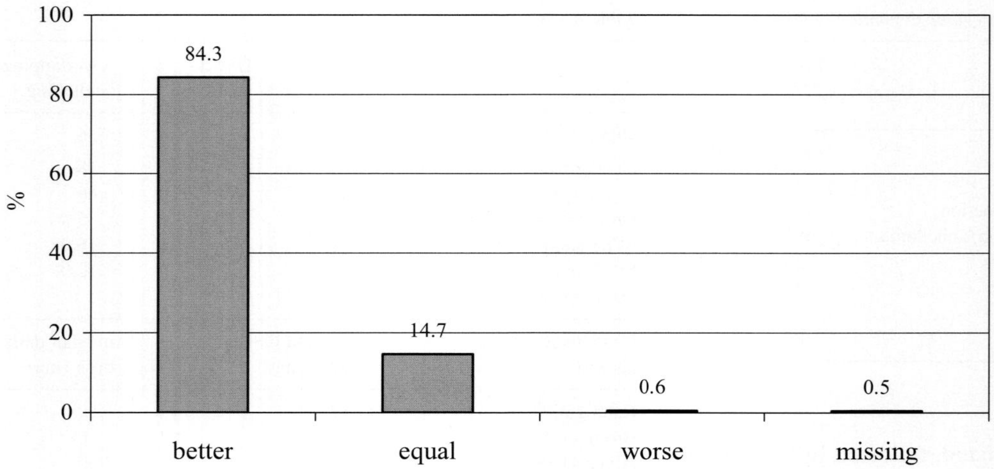

Fig. 1. Global clinical effectiveness of pramipexole in comparison to the previous dopamine agonist

Psychopathological disturbances (SPES)

The median sum score of psychopathological disturbances improved from 2.0 on the respective previous DA to 1.0 on pramipexole ($n = 1088$, signed rank test, $p < 0.0001$).

Kinetic tremor (Spiralometry)

The median kinetic tremor amplitude was improved from 11.0 on the respective previous DA to 9.3 on pramipexole ($n = 885$, signed rank test, $p < 0.0001$) for the tremor dominant hand (possible amplitude range between 0 and 30).

Mood and drive (Visual analogue scales)

Mood and drive as measured by 7 visual analogue scales (10 cm) significantly ($n = 1016$–1041, paired t-tests, $p < 0.001$) improved on pramipexole.

Effectiveness of switching to pramipexole in subgroups

To investigate whether the expectations of investigator and patient were fulfilled by the switching to pramipexole, three subgroups were analysed:

1. Anti-tremor effect of pramipexole in those patients where the anti-tremor effect of the previous DA was insufficient ($n = 741$, see Table 2) and post pramipexole data were available ($n = 721$).
   a) Resting tremor estimated by the SPES (max. score 12).
      A median resting tremor of 4 on previous DA was reduced to 2 on pramipexole ($n = 707$, signed rank test, $p < 0.0001$).
   b) Postural tremor estimated by the SPES (max. score 6).
      A median resting tremor of 2 on previous DA was reduced to 1 on pramipexole ($n = 706$, signed rank test, $p < 0.0001$).

In categories 'change from previous DA to pramipexole' the results are shown in Figs. 2, 3.

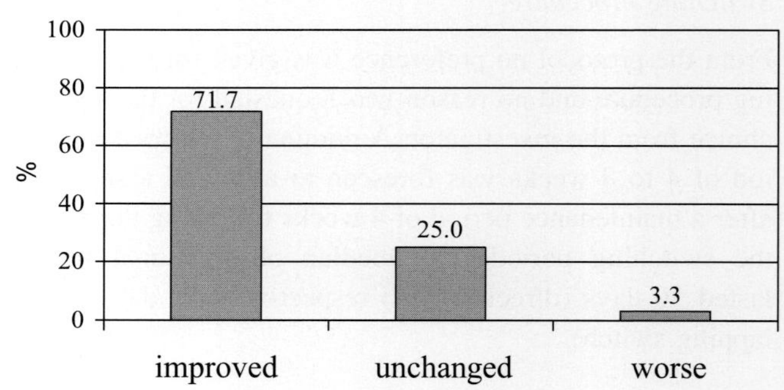

Fig. 2. Categorised change of the sum of *resting tremor* items between previous DA and 4–8 weeks on pramipexole (n = 707)

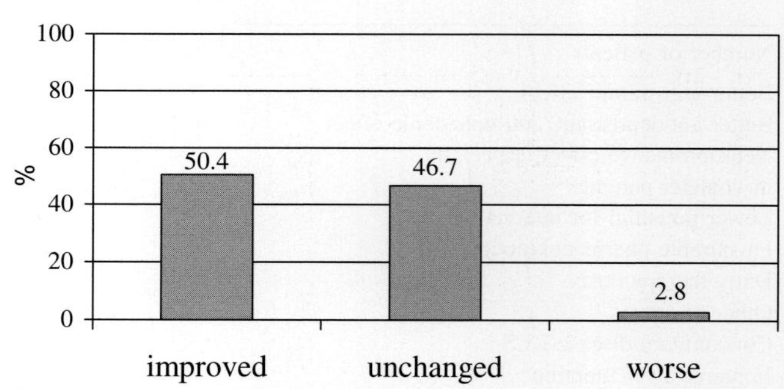

Fig. 3. Categorised change of the sum of *postural tremor* items between previous DA and 4–8 weeks on pramipexole (n = 706)

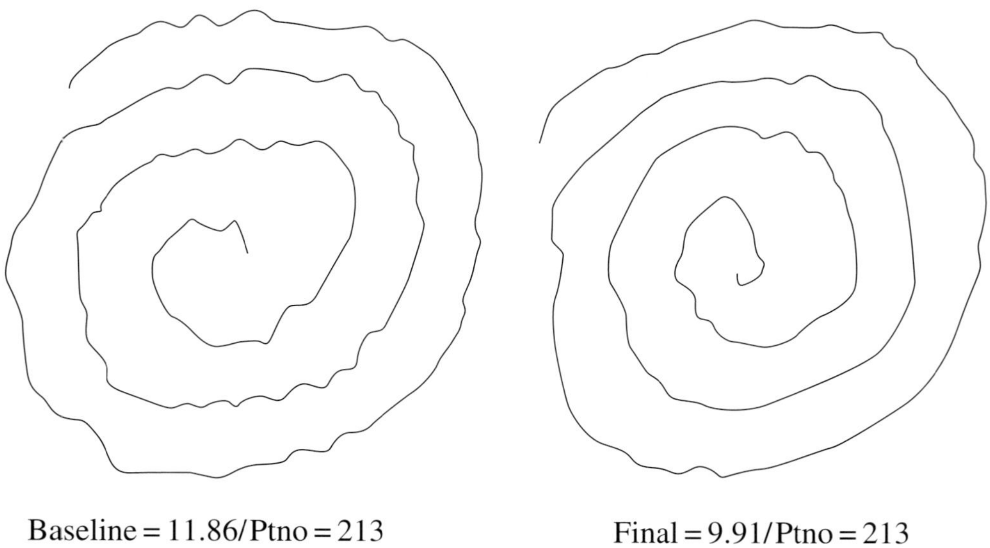

Fig. 4. Example for an improvement of 1.8/1.9 points in kinetic tremor in two patients on the previous DA and after 4–8 weeks on pramipexole

c) Kinetic tremor as estimated by the computerized evaluation of the spiral drawing test (maximal amplitude about 30).

The median of kinetic tremor improved from 11.0 on previous DA to 9.3 at the final visit (signed rank test, $p < 0.0001$) for the tremor dominant hand (Fig. 4).

2. Anti-depressive/anti-anhedonic effect of pramipexole in those patients ($n = 485$) where the anti-depressive/anti-anhedonic effect of the previous DA was insufficient (see Table 2).

a) Anti-depressive/anti-anhedonic effect estimated by SPES item 'Depression' For 384 patients SPES depression data were available. In categories of change from previous dopamine agonist 49.1% patients improved, 50.2% remained unchanged and 0.6% worsened after 4–8 weeks pramipexole treatment. The rating of the depression item is displayed below (Fig. 5).

b) Anti-depressive/anti-anhedonic effect estimated by visual analogue scales (VAS).

Mood and drive as measured by seven VASs (10 cm) significantly improved ($n = 446$–458, paired t-test, $p < 0.001$) from previous DA to the final visit (Fig. 6).

3. Cabergoline pre-treated patients.

Patients previously treated with cabergoline ($n = 300$) constituted the largest subgroup (Table 1) thus allowing a separate analysis.

Both switching procedures were equally represented (Table 4). At the end of the observational period the

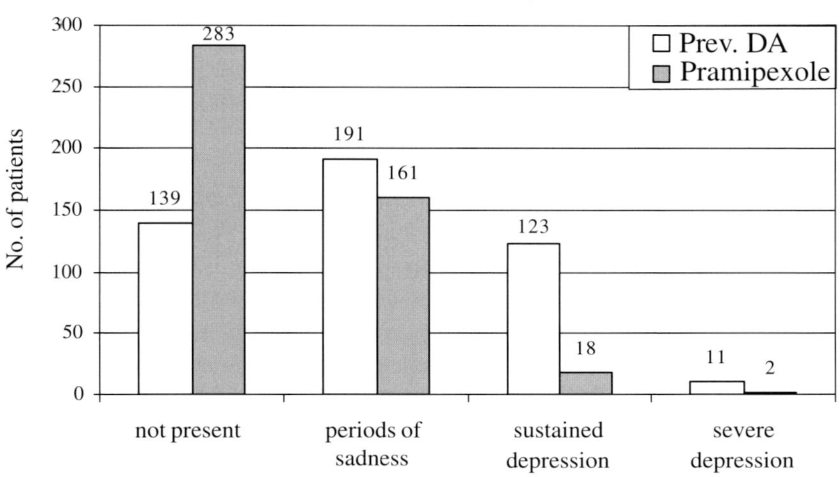

Fig. 5. Change in the distribution of the depression item (SPES) on previous DA to 4–8 weeks on pramipexole

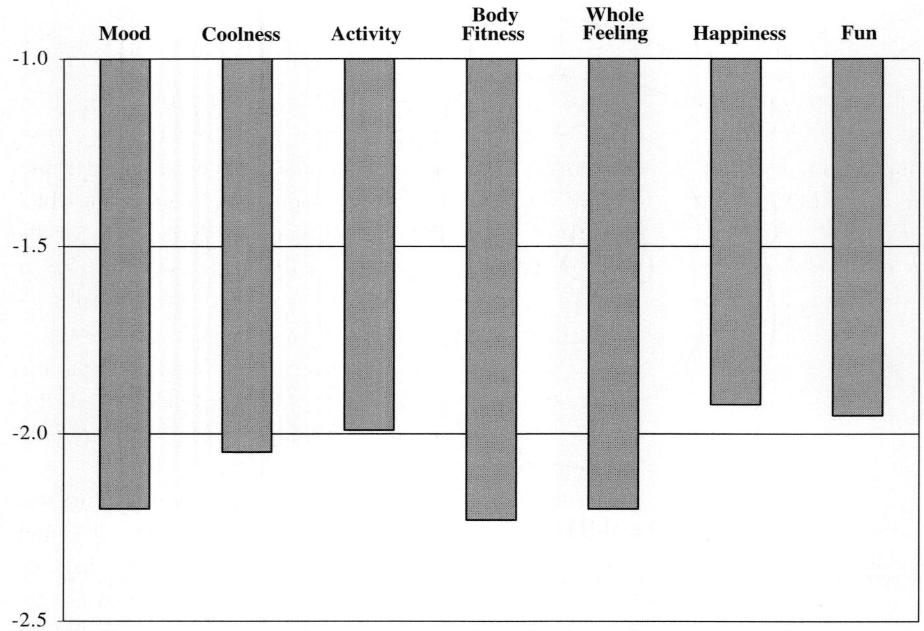

Fig. 6. Mean change in the 7 dimensions of mood and drive self rated by VASs between previous DA and 4–8 weeks on pramipexole

global clinical assessment of effectiveness was rated. Pramipexole with a median daily dose of 1.5 mg was preferred over cabergoline with a median daily dose of 2.0 mg in 82% after direct switch and 86% after overlapping switch and equal in 18% and 13% respectively. Only in one patient (direct switch) the pramipexole treatment was rated worse than cabergoline.

Four patients in the direct switch group experienced Adverse Drug Reactions (dizziness, nausea, headache, fatigue and/or confusion, hallucination) and one patient in the overlapping switch group reported nausea.

Final pramipexole maintenance dose

A median daily dose of 1.5 mg was found at the end of the treatment phase in both switching groups (Table 5).

Table 5. *Median daily doses of previous dopamine agonists and of pramipexole after 4–8 weeks*

Dopamine agonist	Number of patients (*n*)	Daily dose of previous DA (mg)	Daily dose after 4–8 weeks on pramipexole (mg)
Alpha-DHEC	109	40.0	1.5
Bromocriptine	118	9.4	0.7
Cabergoline	184	2.0	1.5
Lisuride	89	0.6	1.5
Pergolide	102	1.5	1.5
Ropinirole	53	6.0	1.5

Table 6. *Final pramipexole dose in comparison to the dose of the previous dopamine agonists stratified by switching procedure*

Final pramipexole dose (mg)	Direct switch (%)	Overlapping switch (%)
≤0.7	34	20
>0.7–1.5	42	44
>1.5–4.5	24	35

The final maintenance daily doses of pramipexole do not represent the equivalent doses of the previous DA, especially as the treatment outcome was favourable for pramipexole.

The decision to perform a direct or overlapping switch was projected into the final pramipexole maintenance dose. Therefore higher doses of pramipexole were seen more frequently in the overlapping switch group (Table 6).

Tolerability of pramipexole

The data of all 1216 patients were included in the safety analysis. Adverse drug reactions (ADRs) under pramipexole were reported by 40 patients (3.3%). The MedDRA system organ classes with more than 1.0% of cases were gastrointestinal disorders (1.3%), with nausea, constipation reported by more than 1 patient, general disorders and administration site conditions (1.1%) mainly fatigue, and the nervous system disorders (1.0%), dizziness (excl. vertigo) and somnolence reported by more than 1 patient. One patient reported sudden onset of sleep. There were no serious adverse drug reactions.

The neurologists rated the tolerability of pramipexole mostly as good (39.6%) to even very good (54.8%). Tolerability of pramipexole was rated as equal or superior to the previous dopamine agonist for 43.1% and 52.8% of the patients, respectively.

Pramipexole was discontinued in a total of 37 patients (3.0% of the total sample). In most cases, discontinuation occurred at the patients' own request ($n = 24$, 2.0%), followed by insufficient tolerability ($n = 16$, 1.3%) and insufficient effect ($n = 8$, 0.7%).

Tolerability of switching procedure

In the direct switch group, the number of patients with ADRs was slightly higher compared with the overlapping switch group (20 patients (3.6%) vs. 14 patients (2.6%)).

Discussion

With the change of the clinical importance of dopamine agonists during the last decade, the question of switching from one dopamine agonist to another is an important issue in routine daily practice.

This observational study was aimed to document the reasons of the treating physician to switch a patient from another dopamine agonist to pramipexole, to find out whether the physicians handled the switch in an overlapping manner or abruptly, to investigate the effect of the switch to pramipexole on motor functions, psychopathological disturbances and mood, to determine the equivalent doses at the end of the switch and to investigate the tolerability of both switch procedures to pramipexole in ambulatory patients suffering from idiopathic Parkinson's disease under routine conditions of daily practice.

Pramipexole, a non-ergot dopamine agonist of the second generation, has been shown to bind selectively and specifically to the D2-dopamine receptor family with high affinity and preference for the D3 receptor subtype (Mierau et al., 1995). As a result of these specificities, it demonstrated special anti-tremor (Pogarell et al., 2002), anti-anhedonic and antidepressant properties (Corrigan et al., 2000; Rektorova et al., 2003; Lemke et al., 2005).

Most physicians undertook the switch because of an insufficient effect of the previous dopamine agonist on tremor (68%), followed by an insufficient effect of the previous dopamine agonist on motor function (47%) and on depression/anhedonia (45%). Surprisingly gastrointestinal (20%) as well as cardiovascular safety aspects (13%) were only minor reasons for withdrawal of the previous dopamine agonist.

Most physicians decided to switch to pramipexole because of its anticipated better effects on tremor (70%), depression/anhedonia (56%), and supposed neuroprotection (26%). When analysing subgroups of patients in which the reason for withdrawal was insufficient effect of the previous dopamine agonist on tremor, motor function or depression/anhedonia, the switching to pramipexole led in all subgroups to a clinically significant improvement.

However, uncertainty concerning adequate dopamine agonist dosages before switching to pramipexole and physicians' expectations of a subsequent improvement may limit the interpretation of those results.

In total no preference for either switching procedure was found: 51% patients underwent a direct or abrupt switch and 49% patients an overlapping switch to pramipexole. The demographics and disease characteristics such as gender, age, age of onset, duration of the Parkinson' disease, and dose of levodopa had no influence on the physicians' choice of the switching procedure.

A tendency in favour of the overlapping switch procedure was observed in those patients who were on a relatively high dose of their previous dopamine agonist, which also resulted in higher doses of pramipexole in these patients, compared to the patients with an abrupt switch procedure.

A median daily dose of 1.5 mg was found at the end of the maintenance treatment phase in both switching groups. This median maintenance daily dose of pramipexole stands in agreement with the median daily maintenance dose derived from another prospective observational study in 657 patients with advanced Parkinson disease (Reichmann et al., 2000).

L-Dopa dose at the final visit had remained unchanged in about 89.6% of the patients in both groups. It was reduced in about 6.8% and increased in about 3.6% of the patients.

The finding that the anti-tremor effect of pramipexole is more marked on the tremor at rest is in accordance with the results of a double blind, randomised, placebo controlled clinical trial (Pogarell et al., 2002).

For the first time a positive effect of pramipexole on kinetic tremor could be demonstrated using a computerised analysis of spiral drawings, which allowed a more objective assessment in comparison to the visual rating according to Bain (1993).

A number of trials have been performed in order to establish equivalent doses between pramipexole and other dopamine agonists (Goetz et al., 1999; Tetrud et al., 2000; Hanna et al., 2001; Linazasoro, 2004; Grosset et al., 2004).

They all lack appropriate methodological design elements such as randomization, double-blindness, both directions of switching, appropriate number of patients, constant conditions (no change in co-medication, UPDRS scores, and tolerability). In all published studies as well as in the present observational study after conversion from bromocriptine, cabergoline, pergolide or ropinirole to pramipexole the Parkinson symptoms have significantly improved, so no equivalent doses could be derived under constant conditions.

A total number of 40 out of 1216 patients (3.3%) of the safety population reported adverse drug reactions. All adverse drug reactions reported according to MedDRA preferred terms occurred with an incidence of $\leq$1.0%. The more common reported adverse drug reactions were nausea, vomiting, dyspepsia (13 patients) and fatigue, somnolence, tiredness (12 patients). All ADRs reported in this PMS study were listed in the SPC for pramipexole.

When compared with their previous dopamine agonist most patients tolerated pramipexole better or equally well (53.4 and 43.5% of the patients, respectively).

The tolerability and safety of both switch procedures were comparable in the present study even though there was a slight but clinically irrelevant difference in the incidence of known and non-serious adverse events: 3.6% in the abrupt switch group and 2.6% in the overlapping switch group. The abrupt switch from bromocriptine, cabergoline, pergolide and or ropinirole to pramipexole has already been reported to be safe and well tolerated (Goetz et al., 1999; Tetrud et al., 2000; Linazasoro, 2004; Grosset et al., 2004). The slow overlapping switch procedure from either bromocriptine or pergolide to pramipexole has been described to be not as safe as a rapid conversion in Parkinson patients with advanced disease (Goetz et al., 1999). Another switch study using an overlapping conversion over a one month period from pergolide to pramipexole resulted in no relevant safety problems (Hanna et al., 2001).

No advantage of abrupt over overlapping switching could be detected. This does not exclude the possibility of such an advantage, because this observational study has the limitations of an open design without randomisation and control, but the large number of patients included in this PMS reduces this deficit. Moreover, there was only one assessment at the end of the switching process.

Interestingly in the subgroup of 300 patients, who were switched from cabergoline to pramipexole, no preference was given to the overlapping switching as theoretically could be expected due to the long half-life of cabergoline. In the abrupt switching group, however, four patients reported adverse drug reactions, one of them confusion and auditory hallucination.

In this PMS study, the excellent efficacy of pramipexole on tremor, motor functions and psychopathological disturbances in patients with idiopathic Parkinson's disease was again confirmed by the positive results obtained on the SPES, VASs, kinetic tremor (spiralometry) and the assessment of the global clinical effect of pramipexole. In addition, its good tolerability could be demonstrated in view of the low number of ADRs reported.

Dopamine agonists can be safely substituted by pramipexole in an abrupt or overlapping mode. The switch to pramipexole may yield further improvement in motor function, tremor, depression and anhedonia, respectively.

In general the overlapping switch procedure should be recommended for those patients who are supposed to be switched from a relatively high dose of a dopamine agonist. The major part of patients, who are treated with low to medium daily dopamine doses can be switched safely from one day to another.

In summary this study clearly demonstrates that switching from other dopamine agonists to pramipexole can be performed safely and effectively. To better support physicians in the choice of the most efficient dopamine agonists, controlled clinical trials directly comparing the maximal effects of different dopamine agonists on different parts of the parkinson symptomatology would be of high value.

References

American Academy of Neurology, Miyasaki JM, Martin W, Suchowersky O, Weiner WJ, Lang AE (2002) Practice parameter: Initiation of treatment for Parkinson's disease: An evidence based review. Neurology 58: 11–17

Agency for Healthcare Research and Quality (2003) Diagnosis and Treatment of Parkinson's Disease: A Systematic Review of the Literature. Summary, Evidence Report/Technology Assessment: Number 57. AHRQ Publication Number 03-E039. Rockville, MD

Bain P (1993) A combined clinical and neurophysiological approach to the study of patients with tremor. J Neurol Neurosurg Psychiatry 56: 839–844

Baseman DG, O'Suilleabhain PE, Reimold SC, Laskar SR, Baseman JG, Dewey Jr RB (2004) Pergolide use in Parkinson's disease is associated with cardiac valve regurgitation. Neurology 63: 301–304

Brecht HM (2001) Dopaminagonisten im Vergleich. In: Riederer P, Laux G, Pöldinger W (eds) Neuro-Psychopharmaka 5: 226–237

Van Camp G, Flamez A, Cosyns B, Weytjens C, Muyldermans L, van Zandijcke M, de Sutter J, Santens P, Decoodt P, Moerman Ch Schoors D (2004) Treatment of Parkinson's disease with pergolide and relation to restrictive valvular disease. The Lancet 363: 1179–1183

Canesi M, Antonini A, Mariani CB, Tesei S, Zecchinelli AL, Barichella M, Pezzoli G (1999) An overnight switch to ropinirole therapy in patients with Parkinson's disease. Short communication. J Neural Transm 106: 925–929

Corrigan MH, Denahan AQ, Wright CE, Ragual RJ, Evans D (2000) Comparison of pramipexole, fluoxetine, and placebo in patients with major depression. Depression Anxiety 11: 58–65

Etminan M, Sudeep G, Samii A (2003) Comparison of the risk of adverse events with pramipexole and ropinirole in patients with Parkinson's disease. A Meta-Analysis. Drug Safety 26: 439–444

Flowers CM, Racoosin JA, Lu SL, Beitz JG (2003) The US Food and Drug Administration's registry of patients with pergolide-associated valvular heart disease. Mayo Clin Proc 78: 730–731

German Society of Neurology (2003) Leitlinien für Diagnostik und Therapie in der Neurologie; 2. revised and enlarged edition, Thieme, Stuttgart, New York

Gimenez-Roldan S, Esteban EM, Mateo D (2001) Switching from bromocriptine to ropinirole in patients with advanced Parkinson's disease: open label pilot responses to three different dose-ratios. Clin Neuropharmacol 24: 346–351

Goetz CG, Blasucci L, Stebbins GT (1999) Switching dopamine agonists in advanced Parkinson's disease: is rapid titration preferable to slow? Neurology 52: 1227–1229

Grosset K, Needleman F, Macphee G, Grosset D (2004) Switching from ergot to nonergot dopamine agonists in Parkinson's disease: A clinical series and five-drug dose conversion table. Mov Disord 19: 1370–1374

Hanna PA, Ratkos L, Ondo WG, Jankovic J (2001) Switching from pergolide to pramipexole in patients with Parkinson's disease. J Neural Transm 108: 63–70

Horvath J, Fross RD, Kleiner-Fisman G, Lerch R, Stalder H, Liaudat S, Raskoff WJ, Flachsbart KD, Rakowski H, Pache JC, Burkhard PR, Lang AE (2004) Severe multivalvular heart disease: a new complication of the ergot derivative dopamine agonists. Mov Disord 19: 656–662

Kraus P, Hoffmann A (2006) (in preparation) Spiralometry: A new technique for a computer based evaluation of paper-pencil spirals

Lemke MR, Brecht HM, Koester J, Kraus PH, Reichmann H (2005) Anhedonia, Depression and Motor Functioning in Parkinson's Disease during treatment with Pramipexole. J Neuropsychiatry Clin Neurosci 17: 214–220

Linazasoro G (2004) Spanish Dopamine Agonists Study Group: conversion from dopamine agonists to pramipexole. An open-label trial in 227 patients with advanced Parkinson's disease. J Neurol 251: 335–339

Marinus J, Visser M, Stiggelbout AM, Rabey JM, Martínez-Martín P, Bonuccelli U, Kraus PH, van Hilten JJ (2004) A short scale for the assessment of motor impairments and disabilities in Parkinson's disease: the SPES/SCOPA. J Neurol Neurosurg Psychiatry 75: 388–395

Mierau J, Schneider FJ, Ensinger HA, Chio CL, Lajines ME, Huff RM (1995) Pramipexole binding and activation of cloned and expressed dopamine D_2, D_3 and D_4 receptors. Eur J Pharmacol 290: 29–36

Müller Th, Fritze J (2003) Fibrosis associated with dopamine agonist therapy in Parkinson's disease. Clinical Neuropharmacol 26: 109–111

Olanow CW, Watts RL, Koller WC (2001) An algorithm (decision tree) for the management of Parkinson's disease: treatment guidelines. Neurology 56 [Suppl 5]: S1–S88

Pogarell O, Gasser T, Van Hilten JJ, Spieker S, Pollentier S, Meier D, Oertel WH (2002) Pramipexole in patients with Parkinson's disease and marked drug resistant tremor: a randomised, double blind, placebo controlled multicentre study. J Neurol Neurosurg Psychiatry 72: 713–720

Rabey JM, Bass H, Bonucelli U, Brooks D, Klotz P, Korczyn AD, Kraus P, Martinez-Martin P, Morrish P, van Sauten W, van Hilten B (1997) Evaluation of the short Parkinson's Evaluation Scale: a new friendly scale for the evaluation of Parkinson's disease in clinical drug trials. Clin Neuropharmacol 20: 322–337

Rascol O, Pathak A, Bagheri H, Montastruc JL (2004) New concerns about old drugs: Valvular heart disease on ergot derivative dopamine agonists as an exemplary situation of pharmacovigilance. Mov Disord 19: 611–613

Reichmann H, Brecht HM, Köster J, Kraus PH (2003) Pramipexole in routine clinical practice. CNS Drugs 17: 965–973

Reichmann H, Herting B, Miller A, Sommer U (2003) Switching and combining dopamine agonists. J Neural Transm 110: 1393–1400

Reichmann H, Sommer U, Fuchs G, Hefter H, Mark G, Muller T, Thumler R, Ulm G, Vieregge P (2000) Workshop IV: drug treatment guidelines for the long-term management of parkinson's disease. J Neurol 247 [Suppl 4]: 40–41

Rektorova I, Rektor I, Bares M, Dostál V, Ehler E, Fanfrdiovà Z, Fiedler J, Klaiblova H, Kulisták P, Ressner P, Svátová J, Urbánek K, Velísková J (2003) Depression in Parkinson's disease: an eight-month, randomised, open-label, national multi-centre comparative study of pramipexole and pergolide. Eur J Neurol 10: 399–406

Stewart D, Morgan E, Burn D, Grosset D, Chaudhuri KR, MacMahon D, Needleman F, Macphee G, Heywood P (2004) Dopamine agonist switching in Parkinson's disease. Hosp Med 65: 215–219

Tan EK, Ratnagopal P, Han SY, Wong MC (2003) Piribedil and bromocriptine in Parkinson's disease: a single-blind crossover study. Acta Neurol Scand 107: 202–206

Tetrud JW, Zhang J, Gomez-Mancilla B, Greenfield JC (2000) Abrupt conversion of Parkinson's disease patients to pramipexole from bromocriptine or pergolide: Safety, tolerance, and optimal conversion ratio. Neurology 54 [Suppl 3]: 279–280

J Neural Transm (2006) [Suppl] 71: 27–30

Journal of Neural Transmission
Printed in Austria

The DONPAD-study – Treatment of dementia in patients with Parkinson's disease with donepezil

T. Müller[1], J. Welnic[1], G. Fuchs[3], H. Baas[4], G. Ebersbach[5], H. Reichmann[2]

[1] Department of Neurology, St. Josef Hospital, Ruhr University Bochum, Bochum, Germany
[2] Department of Neurology, Medical Faculty of the Technical University, Dresden, Germany
[3] Parkinson – Clinic, Wolfach, Germany
[4] Department of Neurology, City Hospital Hanau, Germany
[5] Movement Disorder Clinic, Beelitz – Heilstätten, Germany

Summary Inhibition of acetylcholinesterase improves symptoms of dementia in patients with Parkinson's disease (PD). Dementia in PD has a cumulative incidence of up to 80% and is mainly caused by a distinct cholinergic deficit. Objectives of this investigator initiated multicenter open label trial were to confirm the efficacy of donepezil in the treatment of dementia in PD patients and to investigate the tolerability and safety of donepezil. The Mini Mental State Examination (MMSE)-score significantly increased in patients, who finished the trial. A detailed analysis of the various items of the MMSE revealed, that only task performance of orientation and recall significantly improved. Scores of the short syndrome test and the Clinical Global Impression Scale improved, motor impairment did not increase. Only 14 out of 24 PD patients finished the trial due to predominant onset of vomiting, nausea, dizziness and confusion. This may result from the titration regime of donepezil, that allows only 5 and 10 mg dosages. Participants with premature study termination had a significant longer duration of PD, less motivation and sleep disturbances at night. Treatment with donepezil was only effective in PD patients with dementia, who experience nearly no side effects from the drug.

Introduction

There is increasing evidence, that inhibitors of acetylcholinesterase also improve symptoms of dementia in patients with Parkinson's disease (PD) and allied conditions (Emre, 2004). Clinical symptoms of dementia are deficits of attention, cognitive slowing and impairment of executive, visualspatial and memory function with a cumulative incidence of up to 80% particularly in PD patients of older age (Aarsland et al., 1996). A distinct cholinergic deficit in PD patients is looked upon as the main cause for this non-dopaminergic feature of the disease in particular from the neurochemical point of view (Tiraboschi et al., 2000). Accordingly, predominant open label smaller trials with donepezil and rivastigmine demonstrated an improvement of cognitive function in various kinds of patients with impairment of motor and cognitive function (Werber and Rabey, 2001; Giladi et al., 2003; Leroi et al., 2004). Then the multicenter EXPRESS study compared the efficacy of rivastigmine, an inhibitor of both acetylcholinesterase and butyrylcholinesterase, with placebo. In this trial, rivastigmine produced a moderate but significant improvement in global ratings of dementia, cognition with measurements of executive functions and attention, and neuropsychiatric behavioural symptoms among patients with dementia associated with PD. The mean rivastigmine dosage was 8.6 mg at the end of the dose-escalation phase and remained stable throughout the maintenance phase. Predominant cholinergic adverse effects, i.e. nausea or vomiting, occurred. The rivastigmine treated participants mostly characterised these side effects as mild to moderate and accordingly the rate of premature withdrawal was relatively low (Emre et al., 2004). In contrast to rivastigmine with its selective inhibition of the G 1 cholinesterase isoform in predominant cortical and hippocampal regions is donepezil less selective (Weinstock, 1999). Whereas rivastigmine administration allows a slow, more complex, but individually adapted titration within a dose range between 3 and 12 mg according to the patient's tolerability of the drug, is the treatment with donepezil more simple with the administration of a 5 mg or a 10 mg oral dosage. However this drug regimen may hypothetically result in a higher incidence of the onset typical adverse effects of central acetylcholinesterase inhi-

Correspondence: T. Müller, MD, Department of Neurology, St. Josef Hospital, Ruhr University Bochum, Gudrunstrasse 56, 44791 Bochum, Germany
e-mail: thomas.mueller@ruhr-uni-bochum.de

Table 1. *Clinical characteristics at baseline*

	All participants	Regular finish	Drop out
age	71.08 ± 6.1; 57–79	71.14 ± 7.41	71.00 ± 3.97
size (cm)	168.5 ± 8.87; 143–183	170.14 ± 8.60	166.20 ± 9.16
weight (kg)	71.48 ± 11.17; 53–98	73.86 ± 11.23	68.15 ± 10.74
duration of PD (years)	5.06 ± 3.92; 0.5–16	3.29 ± 2.03	7.55 ± 4.65***
duration of dementia (years)	1.19 ± 1.18	1.11 ± 1.1	1.30 ± 1.34
levodopa dosage (mg)	423.33 ± 227.84	394.64 ± 178.18	463.50 ± 289.37
UPDRS I, item 4 (motivation)	1.17 ± 1.03	1.57 ± 1.02	0.56 ± 0.73*
SKT item 1 (naming of objects)	1.82 ± 1.22	2.21 ± 1.12	1.13 ± 1.13*
NOS item 4 (disturbed behaviour at night)	3.68 ± 1.21	4.14 ± 0.95	2.88 ± 1.25*
NOS item 5 (interest)	2.17 ± 0.98	2.50 ± 1.02	1.67 ± 0.71*
NOS item 14 (clean and tidy)	1.39 ± 0.50	1.21 ± 0.43	1.67 ± 0.50*

CGI clinical global impression scale of severity respectively improvement, *UPDRS* unified Parkinson's disease rating scale, *NOS* nurses observation scale for geriatric patients, Version II, *SKT* short syndrome test, *MMSE* mini mental state examination; $^{+}p<0.05$, $^{++}p<0.01$, $^{+++}p<0.001$; comparisons versus baseline in the post hoc analysis $^{*}p<0.05$, $^{**}p<0.01$, $^{***}p<0.001$

bition. Therefore we conducted an investigator initiated multicenter open label trial in Germany with the objectives to confirm the efficacy of donepezil in the treatment of dementia in PD patients and to investigate the tolerability and safety of donepezil.

Methods

Patients

We enrolled men or women with a diagnosis of PD according to the clinical diagnostic criteria of the United Kingdom Parkinson's Disease Society Brain Bank (Hughes et al., 1992) and a diagnosis of dementia according to the fourth edition of the Diagnostic and Statistical manual of mental Disorders (ICD 294.1) (for clinical characteristics see Table 1). Further inclusion criteria were a score within the range of 10 to 26 in the Mini Mental State Examination (MMSE) with an onset of symptoms occurring at least two years after the diagnosis of PD and a regular contact with a caregiver. Exclusion criteria were a history of major depressive episodes, presence of any other primary neurodegenerative disorders or other causes of dementia, seizures, prior long term intake of anticholinergic compounds. The patients had to be on a stable dopaminergic drug regime ($N=2$, bromocriptine [5 mg t.i.d., 5,5,7.5 mg]; $N=3$, cabergoline [6 mg o.i.d., 4 mg o.i.d., 5 mg o.i.d.]; $N=1$, dihydroergocriptine [20 mg o.i.d.]; $N=4$, pergolide [0.5 mg o.i.d., 0.5 mg o.i.d., 0.75 mg t.i.d., 0.75 mg t.i.d.]; $N=3$, pramipexole [0.18 mg t.i.d., 0.7 mg t.i.d., 0.7 mg t.i.d. + 0.35 mg]; $N=1$, selegiline [5, 2.5 mg]; $N=5$, amantadine [150 mg o.i.d., 100 mg o.i.d., 300 mg daily dosage {d.d.}, 200 mg d.d., 450 mg d.d.] for at least four weeks before study participation. The inclusion criteria allowed change of the antiparkinsonian drug regime in case of increase of motor symptoms and intake of atypical neuroleptics in low dosages on a regular basis. Institutional ethical boards at each center reviewed the protocol, the informed-consent form and other all information provided to patients and caregivers. Both, participants (or the legally authorised representative) and the caregiver gave written informed consent. We conducted all procedures in accordance with the ethical standards of the responsible committee on human experimentation and with the Helsinki Declaration of 1983.

Design

This was a 12-week open label out patient trial. Treatment started with 5 mg Donepezil once daily, an increase of dosage to 10 mg was performed after the second visit. Assessments were performed at baseline (I), after six weeks (II) and after 12 weeks (III). There were standardised visits via phone with the patients respectively their caregivers one week after I and II in order to check compliance of the patients, onset of side effects, change of concomitant medication and tolerability of the drug. The Clinical Global Impression Scale of severity respectively improvement (CGI), MMSE (Koch et al., 2005), Unified Parkinson's Disease Rating Scale (UPDRS) (Goetz et al., 2003) and Nurses Observation scale for geriatric patients, Version II (NOS) (Wahle et al., 1996) were performed at visits I, II, III, the Short Syndrome Test (SKT) (Overall and Schaltenbrand, 1992) only at visits I and III. Investigators were trained for diagnostic and rating procedures under standardized conditions.

Safety measures

At each visit, patients and caregivers were asked for adverse events in an interview with open questions. Efficacy ratings, adverse events, concomitant treatments and drug accountability (pill counting) were assessed, detailed physical examinations, clinical laboratory and vital signs were performed at visits I, II, III.

Study medications

Donepezil was provided by EISAI®, Germany.

Statistics

Data showed a normal distribution according to the Kolmogorow-Smirnow test. We used ANOVA with repeated measures design and as post hoc test the Tukeys HSD test for comparisons against baseline. Comparisons between baseline data of patients, who finished the trial, and those, who did not, was performed with the *t*-test of independent samples.

Results

Efficacy of donepezil

The MMSE-score significantly increased in patients, who finished the trial. The detailed analysis of the various items of the MMSE revealed, that only the performance of the tasks orientation and recall significantly improved. The SKT and the CGI significantly reduced. The UPDRS nearly remained unchanged, the daily levodopa dosage was not

Table 2. *Clinical outcomes*

	I	II	III	F
MMSE	21.57 ± 4.43	$25.57 \pm 4.18^{***}$	$24.71 \pm 5.05^{***}$	18.25^{+++}
orientation	7.5 ± 2.50	$8.79 \pm 1.76^{**}$	$8.71 \pm 1.73^{**}$	9.18^{+++}
memory	3	3	3	n.s.
attention	2.43 ± 1.16	3.36 ± 1.69	3 ± 1.88	2.36
recall	1.14 ± 0.95	$2.21 \pm 0.89^{**}$	$2.07 \pm 1^{**}$	8.89^{++}
speech	7.5 ± 1.29	8.21 ± 0.97	7.93 ± 1.14	2.66
SKT	14.27 ± 6.65		12.27 ± 6.15	5.83^{+}
CGI	4.29 ± 0.92	$3.14 \pm 0.77^{**}$	$3.21 \pm 0.80^{*}$	7.27^{+++}
NOS	92.86 ± 8.46	87.93 ± 16.18	90.86 ± 8.83	1.59
UPDRS total	34.79 ± 10.18	32.29 ± 12.24	34 ± 12.69	1.17
UPDRS I	4.79 ± 2.42	4.07 ± 2.59	4.43 ± 2.31	0.82
UPDRS II	13.64 ± 5.54	12.36 ± 5.47	12.79 ± 5.92	0.94
UPDRS III	15.43 ± 5.27	14.93 ± 6.38	15.29 ± 5.98	0.16
UPDRS IV	0.93 ± 1.27	1.07 ± 1.14	0.79 ± 0.70	0.61

CGI Clinical global impression score, *MMSE* mini mental state examination, *SKT* short syndrome test, *I, II, III* Visits 1, 2, 3; *F* F-value of ANOVA, $^{+}p<0.05$, $^{++}p<0.01$, $^{+++}p<0.001$; comparisons versus baseline in the post hoc analysis $^{*}p<0.05$, $^{**}p<0.01$, $^{***}p<0.001$

significantly altered (results not shown). There was no effect on the outcomes of the NOS (see Table 2).

Drop out rate

Only 14 out of 24 PD patients finished the trial. Causes for premature withdrawals and early study termination were nausea and dizziness ($N=3$, before visit II), hallucinations, anxiety and panic attacks ($N=1$, before visit II), confusion ($N=3$, before visit II), increase of bradykinesia ($N=1$, before visit II), onset of pankreatitis ($N=1$, before visit II), withdrawal of consent ($N=1$, before visit II). This relative high rate of early study terminations allows a comparison of baseline characteristics of both patient groups. Participants with premature withdrawal from the study had a longer duration of PD, a higher score of UPDRS I item 4, which indicates increasing loss of initiative and a deteriorated performance of the SKT task of naming of objects. Patients, who finished the trial, showed a better sleep behaviour at night, were more clean and tidy and had more interest in their daily surroundings according to the corresponding items of the NOS (see Table 1). There was no change of the concomitant drug regime of participants, who finished the trial. The analysis of the concomitantly applied drugs did not reveal, that a specific kind of agent predisposed for early study termination.

Discussion

We show, that donepezil administration provided a moderate but significant improvement of cognition only in patients with PD associated with dementia, who tolerated treatment with donepezil. In particular, orientation and word recall became significant better in the MMSE, which reflects brain function and short term memory. The magnitude of the effect is similar to the one observed in patients with Alzheimer's disease in placebo controlled trials. There was no significant change of daily levodopa intake in our study participants during the trial (results not shown) and their UPDRS-scores, respectively the various subscores, did not significantly worsen. This is of interest, since there is a controversial debate on onset or aggravation of extrapyramidal symptoms during cholinesterase inhibition in AD patients or patients with parkinsonism in dementia with lewy bodies (Richard et al., 2002; Heinze et al., 2002; Hegerl et al., 2003; Di Lazzaro et al., 2004). In particular, there are reports on deterioration of fine motor behaviour during treatment with cholinesterase inhibitors, but concomitant application of typical and atypical neuroleptics may have confounded study outcomes or case reports in AD- or PD patients with dementia (Werber et al., 2001; Richard et al., 2002; Heinze et al., 2002; Bohnen et al., 2004). We show, that PD patients do not experience an essential impairment of motor function due to additional intake of donepezil. States of confusion, nausea, dizziness and vomiting were the main common causes for premature study withdrawal. This drop out rate with 10 out of 24 participants was relative high compared to other trials with rivastigmine (Emre et al., 2004). This may result from the titration regimen, that allows only 5 and 10 mg dosages in the case of donepezil. In contrast, rivastigmine with its oral treatment dosage range between 3 to 12 mg may be titrated in a more slow, continuous and smooth fashion. A further, still hypothetical reason may be an increased affinity of donepezil to the area postrema, which may result in onset of cholinergic side effects, i.e. nausea and vomiting, in contrast to rivastigmine with its more selective place of action in cortical and hippocampal regions (Weinstock, 1999; Poirier, 2002; Edwards et al., 2004).

The comparisons of baseline characteristics between patients with early and normal study termination revealed, that mostly PD patients with longer duration of PD, sleep disturbances and motivation deficits dropped out. We suggest that open label trials are better suitable for this kind of analysis, since the drop out rate is not biased by study participants, who realised their treatment with placebo. This may cause disappointment and a lack of motivation for further study participation. Nevertheless in view of the size and the design of this open label trial, our results only allow a cautious preliminary interpretation. On the one hand these outcomes may indicate, that treatment with cholinesterase inhibitors is efficient and best tolerated in preponderant early stages of PD associated with dementia. On the other hand we also hypothesise, that study participants with motivational deficits and sleep disturbances are not the best candidates for these kind of studies.

In conclusion we show, that treatment with donepezil is effective on symptoms of dementia in PD patients, when it is tolerated. Particularly, this is the case in patients with a shorter duration of PD and without severe sleep disturbances. 10 out of 24 participants dropped out of the study due to onset of side effects. This may suggest a slower more careful titration regime of donepezil in future trials.

References

Aarsland D, Tandberg E, Larsen JP, Cummings JL (1996) Frequency of dementia in Parkinson disease. Arch Neurol 53: 538–542

Bohnen N, Kaufer D, Hendrickson R, Ivanco L, Moore R, DeKosky S (2004) Effects of donepezil on motor function in patients with Alzheimer disease. J Clin Psychopharmacol 24: 354–356

Di Lazzaro, V, Oliviero A, Pilato F, Saturno E, Dileone M, Marra C, Daniele A, Ghirlanda S, Gainotti G, Tonali PA (2004) Motor cortex hyperexcitability to transcranial magnetic stimulation in Alzheimer's disease. J Neurol Neurosurg Psychiatry 75: 555–559

Edwards K, Therriault OJ, Gorman C (2004) Switching from donepezil or rivastigmine to galantamine in clinical practice. J Am Geriatr Soc 52: 1965

Emre M (2004) Dementia in Parkinson's disease: cause and treatment. Curr Opin Neurol 17: 399–404

Emre M, Aarsland D, Albanese A, Byrne EJ, Deuschl G, De Deyn PP, Durif F, Kulisevsky J, van Laar T, Lees A, Poewe W, Robillard A, Rosa MM, Wolters E, Quarg P, Tekin S, Lane R (2004) Rivastigmine for dementia associated with Parkinson's disease. N Engl J Med 351: 2509–2518

Giladi N, Shabtai H, Gurevich T, Benbunan B, Anca M, Korczyn AD (2003) Rivastigmine (Exelon) for dementia in patients with Parkinson's disease. Acta Neurol Scand 108: 368–373

Goetz CG, LeWitt PA, Weidenman M (2003) Standardized training tools for the UPDRS activities of daily living scale: newly available teaching program. Mov Disord 18: 1455–1458

Hegerl U, Mergl R, Henkel V, Gallinat J, Kotter G, Muller-Siecheneder F, Pogarell O, Juckel G, Schroter A, Bahra R, Emir B, Laux G, Moller HJ (2003) Kinematic analysis of the effects of donepezil hydrochloride on hand motor function in patients with Alzheimer dementia. J Clin Psychopharmacol 23: 214–216

Heinze M, Andreae D, Grohmann R (2002) Rivastigmin and impaired motor function. Pharmacopsychiatry 35: 79–80

Hughes AJ, Daniel SE, Kilford L, Lees AJ (1992) Accuracy of clinical diagnosis of idiopathic Parkinson's disease: a clinico-pathological study of 100 cases. J Neurol Neurosurg Psychiatry 55: 181–184

Koch HJ, Gurtler K, Szecsey A (2005) Correlation of Mini-Mental-State-Examination (MMSE), Syndrom-Kurztest (SKT) and Clock test (CT) scores in patients with cognitive impairment assessed by means of multiple regression and response surface analysis. Arch Gerontol Geriatr 40: 7–14

Leroi I, Brandt J, Reich SG, Lyketsos CG, Grill S, Thompson R, Marsh L (2004) Randomized placebo-controlled trial of donepezil in cognitive impairment in Parkinson's disease. Int J Geriatr Psychiatry 19: 1–8

Overall JE, Schaltenbrand R (1992) The SKT neuropsychological test battery. J Geriatr Psychiatry Neurol 5: 220–227

Poirier J (2002) Evidence that the clinical effects of cholinesterase inhibitors are related to potency and targeting of action. Int J Clin Pract Suppl: 6–19

Richard IH, Justus AW, Greig NH, Marshall F, Kurlan R (2002) Worsening of motor function and mood in a patient with Parkinson's disease after pharmacologic challenge with oral rivastigmine. Clin Neuropharmacol 25: 296–299

Tiraboschi P, Hansen LA, Alford M, Sabbagh MN, Schoos B, Masliah E, Thal LJ, Corey-Bloom J (2000) Cholinergic dysfunction in diseases with Lewy bodies. Neurology 54: 407–411

Wahle M, Haller S, Spiegel R (1996) Validation of the NOSGER (Nurse's Observation Scale for Geriatric Patients): reliability and validity of a caregiver rating instrument. Int Psychogeriatr 8: 525–547

Weinstock M (1999) Selectivity of cholinesterase inhibition – Clinical implications for the treatment of Alzheimer's disease. CNS Drugs 12: 307–323

Werber EA, Rabey JM (2001) The beneficial effect of cholinesterase inhibitors on patients suffering from Parkinson's disease and dementia. J Neural Transm 108: 1319–1325

J Neural Transm (2006) [Suppl] 71: 31–37

Journal of
Neural
Transmission
Printed in Austria

PD-related psychosis: pathophysiology with therapeutical strategies

E. Ch. Wolters

Department of Neurology, Research Institute Neurosciences Vrije Universiteit, VU University Medical Center, Amsterdam, The Netherlands

Summary Parkinson's disease (PD) is a chronic, neurodegenerative disease with degeneration of the central dopaminergic neurons in the substantia nigra, leading to a depletion of dopamine (DA) in the striatum. This depletion causes the clinical hallmarks of this disease: bradykinesia, hypokinesia, rigidity, tremor and postural instability. Besides these well known motor symptoms, non-motor symptoms may develop, such as hyposmia, sleep disorders, autonomic disturbances, depression, cognitive impairment and psychosis. Pathophysiological mechanisms underlying these symptoms not only comprise Lewy body pathology in the central dopaminergic system, but also in the noradrenergic, serotinergic and cholinergic transmittersystems. Indeed, in Parkinson's disease, about 30–40% of the patients suffers fluctuating psychotic symptoms, mainly paranoid delusions and/or visual or acoustic hallucinations, symptoms considered to represent major contributors to patient and caregiver distress and nursing home placement.

Endogenous (related to the disease process itself) as well as exogenous (related to therapeutical interventions) psychotogenic factors may contribute to the development of psychotic symptoms in PD. Therapeutical strategies, therefore, are aimed to reduce both endogenous and exogenous factors. To reduce endogenous psychotogenic factors, cholinesterase inhibitors, suggested to reduce cognitive deterioration, now seem to be the drugs of choice. In exogenously induced psychotic symptoms, atypical antipsychotics are considered the most effective. However, as psychotic symptoms in PD are often influenced by both endogenous and exogenous factors, a combination of both strategies may be preferred.

Introduction

Parkinson's disease (PD) is a chronic neurodegenerative disease, characterized by the presence of bradykinesia, hypokinesia, rigidity, tremor and other signs and symptoms of motor parkinsonism, caused by Lewy body pathology in the nigral substance with consequent striatal dopamine deficiency, allowing the diagnosis in this disease. However, these clinical hallmarks of the disease may be accompanied by other Lewy body pathology-induced symptoms, due to degenerative changes in the ascending central noradrenergic, serotonergic and cholinergic transmitter systems. At a given time, depending on the actual localisation and progression of this pathological process, many if not all PD patients will suffer hyposmia, sleep disorders, autonomic disturbances, depression, dementia and/or psychosis, sometimes preceding the first appearance of motor signs in PD patients (Wolters and Braak, 2006). Especially in dementing PD patients, due to a loss of reality testing, psychotic symptoms constitute important predictors of the patient's quality of life, caregiver distress and nursing home placement (Aarsland et al., 1999a, 2000; Goetz and Stebbins, 1993; Karlsen et al., 1998).

In psychosis, hallucinations, mainly visual, are the most frequent symptom, often preceded by sleep disturbances and vivid dreaming. These are mostly non-threatening and consist often of vivid, colourful and sometimes fragmented figures of beloved (deceased) familiar persons and/or animals, described in detail (Poewe, 2003). Auditory hallucinations may accompany the visual hallucinations but are not common in isolation. As a rule, insight is retained in the majority of occasions, but with reality testing deteriorating; in time, the hallucinations may change and become more frightening, possibly inducing anxiety and panic attacks (Wolters, 2001). Delusions (false beliefs based on incorrect inference about external reality) are less common than hallucinations and are mainly of the paranoid type, dealing with persecution, spousal infidelity or jealousy (Wolters and Francot, 1998). Hallucinations and/or delusions with complete loss of reality testing and insight are rare, they occur particularly in demented elderly PD patients.

The pathophysiology of delusions and hallucinations is still poorly understood. Psychotogenic factors include both exogenous (related to therapeutical interventions) as well as endogenous (related to the disease process itself) factors. As a matter of fact, most of these symptoms will probably

Correspondence: Prof. Dr. E. Ch. Wolters, Department of neurology, Vrije Universiteit Medical Center, De Boelelaan 1117, 1081 HV Amsterdam, The Netherlands
e-mail: e.wolters@vumc.nl

be evoked by a combination of such factors. Antiparkinsonian treatment, with dopaminomimetics and/or anticholinergics (Saint Cyr et al., 1993), is considered the major risk factor, although several observations suggest that the role of antiparkinsonian treatment is not exclusive and that other factors might also provoke psychotic symptoms. Psychotic symptoms were already described before the use of levodopa in a number of PD-patients (Rondot, 1984), although in these earlier studies patients with postencephalitic parkinsonism, dementia with Lewy bodies or premorbid psychiatric illness might have been included. Moreover, psychotic symptoms are also not directly related to the dose or duration of dopaminomimetic treatment (Wolters, 2001) and may even occur in the absence of antiparkinsonian therapy (for instance in patients suffering dementia with Lewy bodies (DLB). Other well identified and even more significant risk factors include cognitive impairment and dementia (Holroyd, 2001): compared to non-demented PD-patients, psychosis is much more common in demented PD patients, suffering PDD (PD with dementia) or DLB (McKeith et al., 1996).

In fact, fluctuating cognitive function, attentional deficits, visual hallucinations and parkinsonism are the clinical hallmarks in both, DLB and PDD. Clinically, PDD and DLB are often difficult to distinguish other than by the temporary onset of dementia and psychosis in relation to motor parkinsonism. In both conditions, Lewy body pathology is present in the brainstem as well as the cortex and it may be impossible to pathologically distinguish the two conditions (Harding and Halliday, 2001; Wolters and Braak, 2006). Both conditions might thus be part of the same disease spectrum: pending the relative contribution of the various endogenous and exogenous psychotogenic factors, a continuum might be seen ranging from psychotic symptoms purely induced by exogenous factors to pure endogenous psychotic symptoms, with in between combinations thereof. At the one end, DLB serves as an example of an endogenous, purely acetylcholine and dopamine deficiency-induced psychosis (with cognitive deficits and confusion), even in the absence of dopaminomimetic or anticholinergic therapy (McKeith et al., 1996). At the other end, dopaminomimetics in cognitively unaffected mainly dopamine deficient PD-patients may provoke exogenous psychotic symptoms in the presence of a clear sensorium. In between, increasing (endogenous) choline deficiency renders cognitive impaired PD-patients vulnerable to develop psychotic symptoms due to dopaminomimetic and anticholinergic therapy. However, as a rule, each PD patient, to some extent will be exposed to both endogenous and exogenous psychotogenic factors. Treatment of psychotic symptoms will be based on the preponderance of one of them (Wolters and Francot, 1998).

Endogenous psychotogenic factors

Identified risk factors for psychotic symptoms related to the disease process itself include age, duration and severity of PD, depression, sleep disturbances and above all, as stated before, cognitive impairment. The cholinergic and the dopaminergic neurotransmitter systems, both are essential in cognitive functioning and their disintegration strongly correlates with cognitive impairment.

The cholinergic system

Not only in normal aging (Perry et al., 1992) and in Alzheimer's disease (AD) (Davies and Maloney, 1976), also in PDD and DLB, the central cholinergic deficit correlates strongly with sleep disturbances and cognitive impairment. In comparison to AD, Lewy body pathology induces a more pronounced degeneration of both, the nucleus basalis of Meynert (Perry et al., 1985, 1991) and pedunculopontine nucleus (PPN) (Zweig et al., 1989) in combination with frontal cortical denervation due to disintegration of the ascending cholinergic transmitter system.

Meynert's nucleus, mainly projecting to the amygdala and neocortex, is thought to play an essential role in higher cortical functions by modulating detection, selection, discrimination and processing of sensory stimuli. Due to confusion and fluctuating attention, degeneration of this nucleus may result in defective processing of sensory stimuli (Perry et al., 1999) with delusions and hallucinations.

Through reciprocal thalamic connections, the cholinergic PPN is thought to play a major role in the control of locomotion and posture as well as in sleep, especially REM sleep (Perry et al., 1999). Interestingly, many PD-patients suffer from REM sleep disturbances and/or REM sleep behavioural disorders (Comella et al., 1993; Pappert et al., 1999) and, as a matter of fact, recently, a temporal relationship between REM sleep intrusions and hallucinations in daytime has been established (Arnulf et al., 2000). The cholinergic system is also suggested to be linked with visual hallucinations by the cholinergic inactivity with hypometabolism in the higher visual temporal association cortices in hallucinating DLB-patients (Perry et al., 1991; Shimomuro et al., 1998). Further evidence in support of cholinergic involvement in psychosis comes from pharmacological studies with antimuscarinic compounds such as atropine or scopolamine, which were found to induce visual hallucinations very similar to the hallucinations seen in PD and DLB (Perry et al., 1995). The most striking clinical evidence in agreement with the suggestions above is the beneficial effect of cholinesterase inhibitors on psychotic symptoms not only in AD but also in DLB as well as PDD, especially by applying dual inhibition of acetylcholinesterase (AChE) and butyrylcholinesterase (BuChE) (Bartorelli et al., 2005).

The dopaminergic system

Due to the disintegration of the dopaminergic nigrostriatal projections, caudate dopamine depletion leads to striato-prefrontal disconnection (Alexander et al., 1986), whereas disintegration of the mesocorticolimbic projections will lead to prefrontal dopaminergic denervation (Paulus and Jellinger, 1991). The prefrontal cortex is thought to play an essential role in executive function. Executive function is a broad term used to describe a range of cognitive functions under the control of the frontal lobes, such as (selective) attention, inhibition, task management, planning, monitoring and encoding. Indeed, already in early PD-patients, disturbances in executive function resembling those found in patients with frontal lobe damage, are often found (Dubois and Pillon, 1997).

Dopamine is suggested to improve the physiological signal-to-noise ratio in the prefrontal cortex during tasks relying on the executive functions and thus plays a major role in the regulation of cognition and attention. Therefore, cortical dopaminergic denervation will reduce selective attention and may predispose PD-patients to psychotic symptoms. In that case, concomitant degeneration of other, especially cholinergic, ascending projections will reduce further the threshold for these symptoms to emerge (Stam et al., 1993).

Exogenous psychotogenic factors

Together with non specific psychotogenic factors (dehydration, fever, infections, alcohol or drug withdrawal, social isolation or social overexposure), exogenous factors, related to extern interventions in PD, such as dopaminomimetic or anticholinergic therapy might also induce psychotic symptoms. Dopaminomimetics are often associated with non-threatening hallucinations in the absence of confusion or delirium, whereas anticholinergics are more likely to produce more frightening hallucinations in combination with a confusional state (Goetz et al., 1982; Wolters, 2001), especially in patients with an endogenous cholinergic cortical denervation, as previously described. However, it should not be forgotten that other antiparkinsonian drugs (Saint-Cyr et al., 1993) as well and several selective serotonin reuptake inhibitors (SSRI's) may induce psychotic symptoms (Lauterbach, 1991).

The pathophysiology of dopaminomimetic psychosis is still poorly understood. As the specific mechanism of action of most antipsychotic agents is based on serotonergic and dopaminergic receptor blockade, both dopaminergic and/or serotonergic mechanisms have been implicated. Early in the disease, DA deficiency-induced hypersensitivity of striatal dopaminergic receptors might contribute to the manifestation of the psychotic symptoms (Moskovitz et al., 1978). Later on, chronic dopaminomimetic treatment-induced mesocorticolimbic DA receptor hypersensitivity (Klawans et al., 1977) or mesocorticolimbic 5HT serotoninergic overstimulation (induced by the transformation of DA neuronal loss-related excess of levodopa into serotonin) (Melamed et al., 1996), might play a more important facilitating role. This does not explain, though, the higher propensity of dopamine agonists to induce psychotic symptoms as compared to levodopa. Trying to explain this phenomenon, (Graham et al., 1997) in this respect suggests that specific dopamine receptors might be involved or, alternatively, that mesocorticolimbic projections in hallucinating patients degenerate faster (and thus induce higher compensatory DA-receptor densities) than nigrostriatal projections.

Management of psychosis

Identification of the specificly involved endogenous and/or exogenous psychotogenic factors is essential to install proper treatment. In the case of a pure endogenous psychosis (for instance in drug-naïve PD patients with dementia) cholinomimetic therapy seems the proper treatment option, whereas in the treatment of a pure exogenous psychosis (such as induced by the first gift of dopaminomimetics in de-novo PD patients without cognitive impairment) atypical antipsychotics will prevail. One has to keep in mind, though, that most psychoses in PD patients are induced by a combination of endogenous and exogenous factors. Therefore, in psychotic PD patients, first of all, infections, metabolic disturbances or other physical illnesses should be excluded as cause of the psychotic symptoms and anticholinergic drugs, amantadine and selegiline should be discontinued.

PD patients with cognitive dysfunction

In PD patients with cognitive dysfunction, as is the case in DLB and PDD, endogenous deterioration of the cholinergic system is suggested to be the major psychotogenic factor.

Therefore, it seems reasonable to treat these patients with AChE and/or BuChE inhibitors to compensate for this deficit. These inhibitors promote cholinergic transmission by slowing down the acetylcholine break down in the synaptic clefts.

Cholinesterase inhibitors

As cholinesterase inhibitors were found to induce some beneficial effects on cognition in Alzheimer's disease (Bullock, 2004; Cummings et al., 1998; Gabelli, 2003; Kaduskiewicz et al., 2005; Takeda et al., 2006), due to the greater presynaptic cholinergic deficit and the relative sparing of the cortex, its efficacy in DLB and PD was expected to be superior (Perry et al., 1993). Indeed, in patients suffering these conditions, so far several studies established a fair clinical effect of these molecules, such as tacrine, galantamine, donepezil and rivastigmine.

The AChE inhibitors tacrine (removed from the marked because of hepatoxicity), galantamine (which also stimulates the nicotinic receptor) and donezepil were also reported to improve psychotic behaviour (Aarsland et al., 1999b, 2003; Fergusson and Howard, 2000; Shea et al., 1998; Fabbrini et al., 2002; Kaufer et al., 1998; Hutchinson and Fazzine, 1996; Bergman and Lerner, 2002) in DLB and/or PDD patients.

In open label and also in randomized controlled studies, similar results were found for rivastigmine, a dual AChE and BuChE inhibitor (Bullock and Cameron, 2002; Grace et al., 2001; McKeith, 2000; McKeith et al., 2000; Reading et al., 2001; Wesnes et al., 2005). In these studies, again, not only cognitive functions but also psychotic behaviour improved and sleep disturbances were found to be decreased (McKeith, 2000; McKeith et al., 2000; Reading et al., 2001). Although donepezil has been described to increase extrapyramidal symptoms in some patients (Shea et al., 1998; Fabrini et al., 2002), studies with rivastigmine unexpectedly established a tendency to improve motor parkinsonism (McKeith et al., 2000; Reading et al., 2001). The increased tremor as found in a large double-blind study with this molecule (Emre et al., 2004; Poewe et al., 2006), in this respect also may be explained as an improvement of motor behaviour, as tremor is found to become more overt when rigidity decreases (Winogrodzka et al., 2001). Frequently reported side effects in cholinesterase inhibitors are nausea, vomiting and anorexia, sometimes interfering with drug titration (up to the maximum dose of 6 mg two times a day). Therefore, these drugs should be started at low dose with a gradual increase to the maximum tolerated dose. About 70% of AD patients, deteriorating during treatment with selective AChE inhibitor treatment, benefits from switching these selective drugs into the dual AChE-BuChE inhibitor rivastigmine, in terms of stabilization of disease, improvement in cognitive function and reduction of the burden of concomitant psychoactive treatment (Bartorelli et al., 2005). A possible explanation might be a more powerful effect on cholinergic transmission of dual cholinesterase inhibitors as compared to selective inhibitors. It should be noted that cholinesterase inhibitors, but not atypical antipsychotics, take several weeks (usually 10–12) before showing any antipsychotic effect. Unfortunately, cholinesterase inhibitors still await approval for treatment of dementia and psychosis in PD and DLB.

PD patients with relatively unaffected cognition

In PD patients with relatively unaffected cognition, exogenous factors usually play a major role. Here, dopaminomimetics might be reduced, though at the risk of aggravation of extrapyramidal symptoms. Usually, however, this strategy takes several days to weeks to reach its goals and is often not sufficient to alleviate psychosis. When psychotic behaviour starts to interfere with daily life activities of the patient, a more active strategy is needed. In those cases, benzodiazepines in combination with a reinforcing, structuring program to improve reality testing and/or a night-light for better nocturnal orientation initially may be very helpful. When this strategy fails, or when psychotic behaviour may harm the patient and/or his environment, active treatment with antipsychotics must be initiated.

Atypical antipsychotics

The exact mechanism of action of atypical antipsychotic agents remains to be resolved. One hypothesis is the combination of high affinity for the serotonergic $5HT_{2A}$-receptor and weak affinity for the dopaminergic D2-receptor of atypical agents compared to the relative selective D2-receptor antagonism of typicals (Meltzer et al., 1989). The antipsychotic effect of $5HT_{2A}$-receptor activity might be explained by its modulation of dopaminergic activity in different regions of the brain. In this respect, also $5HT_{1A}$-receptors (inducing the opposite action compared to the $5HT_{2A}$-receptor), and other 5HT-receptors ($5HT_{2C}$, $5HT_3$, and $5HT_{6/7}$) have been implicated in the mechanism of atypical antipsychotics, but further research is needed to clarify their role (Meltzer et al., 2003). Others, however, emphasize the importance of D2-receptor antagonism even in the absence of $5HT_{2A}$ receptor blockade. They suggest that transient D2 occupancy with fast dissociation from the receptor explains the antipsychotic effect in the absence of extrapyramidal side effects of atypical agents, the so called 'fast off' theory (Seeman, 2002).

Atypical antipsychotics also, to some extent, block the histaminergic, (nor)adrenergic and muscarinic (cholinergic) receptors. In most PD-patients, as mentioned before, these neurotransmitter systems are already endogenously compromised. Therefore, these patients are highly vulnerable to the development of specific transmitter deficiency-related side-effects of these drugs, a phenomenon known as neuroleptic sensitivity (McKeith et al., 1992). A rare, but possibly lethal complication associated with this neuroleptic hypersensitivity is the neuroleptic malignant syndrome (Friedman and Wagner, 1987). This syndrome comes with hyperthermia, autonomic disturbances, rigidity and disturbances of consciousness, in up to 20% of the cases in combination with fatal respiratory or renal failure, cardiac arrhythmia or cardiovascular insufficiency. This syndrome, associated with the withdrawal of dopaminomimetics and the use of typical antipsychotics, is hypothesized to be the consequence of striatal D2-receptor blockade (Keyser and Rodnitzky, 1991), but cases have also been reported during treatment with some atypical antipsychotics (Ballard et al., 1998). To avoid neuroleptic hypersensitivity, antipsychotic drugs should always be started at low doses with a gradual increase to a dose with clinically relevant effect.

Atypical antipsychotics best studied are clozapine, quetiapine, olanzapine and risperidone. Clozapine, a dibenzodiazepine derivate, displays not only antagonistic action at the serotonergic ($5HT_{2A}$) and dopaminergic (D2) receptors but also at muscarinic, adrenergic and histaminergic receptors (therefore inducing 'side-effects' such as sedation, confusion, orthostatic hypotension, hypersalivation and tachycardia). Clozapine was proven very effective in alleviating psychotic symptoms without a decline in motor function (The Parkinson Study Group, 1999; The French Clozapine Parkinson Study Group, 1999). However, it also has an idiosyncratic potential of 1–2% for inducing agranulocytosis, which potential could be reduced to 0.38% by mandatory white blood cell testing (weekly), which sofar is not reported in comparable drugs such as quetiapine. Interestingly, in PD patients, clozapine may reduce tremor, improve sleep quality (increase of REM sleep) and relieve anxiety, depression and hypersexuality. Though lacking affinity to muscarinic receptors, and therefore without risk of inducing confusion, quetiapine is structurally similar to clozapine and displays more or less the same antipsychotic effects and the same side-effects with a low propensity for extrapyramidal symptoms (Fernandez et al., 2003). In order to change patients from clozapine and or olanzapine into quetiapine, a more gradual switch is advised to avoid an increase of psychotic behaviour (Fernandez et al., 2000). Olanzapine is also structurally similar to clozapine. Although first reports were encouraging (Wolters et al., 1996), double blind, placebo-controlled trials later showed worsening of motor function in the absence of a statistically beneficial effect on psychotic symptoms in PD patients (Ondo et al., 2002; Breier et al., 2002). Significant extrapyramidal side-effects are also reported in clinical studies with risperidone in psychotic PD and DLB patients (Ellis et al., 2000; Knable et al., 1997; Rich et al., 1995; McKeith et al., 1995). Therefore, olanzapine and risperidone are not considered first-choice treatment in PD-related psychosis.

Conclusions

Psychotic symptoms are relatively common in PD. Most prominent symptoms are visual hallucinations, sometimes accompanied by auditory hallucinations, and paranoid delusions. Especially when insight is lost, these symptoms can be very distressing to patient and caregiver, and often results in nursing home placement.

Psychotic symptoms in PD might be caused by a combination of endogenous and exogenous psychotogenic factors. Important endogenous psychotogenic factors comprise PD-related dopamine and choline deficiency-induced cortical hypoactivity as well as choline deficiency-induced REM sleep disturbances. Significant exogenous factors are dopaminomimetic and/or anticholinergic drug therapy, as well as age, dehydration, infections, alcohol or drug withdrawal, fever, social isolation or social overexposure. Pending the preponderance of either one of them, a treatment strategy can be chosen.

In pure exogenous, dopaminomimetic-induced psychosis, atypical antipsychotics are considered the treatment of choice. In the case of endogenous psychosis due to progressive attentional and cognitive deficits, however, cholinesterase inhibitors seem to be preferred. By alleviating cognitive defects, especially attention, these drugs make those patients less vulnerable to the development of psychosis. It might be wise, however, to treat psychotic PD patients with a combination of atypical antipsychotics and cholinesterase inhibitors, as in most cases, endogenous as well as exogenous psychotogenic factors will be involved.

Although cholinesterase inhibitors are considered to be safe and without serious adverse effects, atypical antipsychotics should be used with caution, as in psychotic PD patients those drugs easily induce neuroleptic hypersensitivity as well as noradrenergic, serotonergic and/or cholinergic deficiency-related side effects. Of the available atypical antipsychotics, clozapine is still the preferred drug in the treatment of dopaminomimetic psychosis in PD, despite the need for weekly control of blood cell counts. It has been most extensively studied and displays excellent antipsychotic properties without exacerbating extrapyramidal symptoms. Quetiapine is the next alternative. Its antipsychotic properties are less established compared to clozapine, but it lacks the side effect of agranulocytosis, making administration much easier. Because of extrapyramidal side-effects, olanzapine and risperidone are not first-choice drugs in the treatment of drug-induced psychosis in PD patients.

References

Aarsland D, Larsen JP, Karlsen K, Lim NG, Tandberg E (1999a) Mental symptoms in Parkinson's disease are important contributors to caregiver distress. Int J Geriatr Psychiatry 14: 866–874

Aarsland D, Bronnick K, Karlsen K (1999b) Donepezil for dementia with Lewy bodies: a case study. Int J Geriatr Psychiatry 14: 69–72

Aarsland D, Larsen JP, Tandberg E, Laake K (2000) Predictors of nursing home placement in Parkinson's disease: a population-based, prospective study. J Am Geriatr Soc 48: 938–942

Aarsland D, Hutchinson M, Larsen JP (2003) Cognitive, psychiatric and motor response to galantamine in Parkinson's disease with dementia. Int J Geriatr Psychiatry 18: 937–941

Alexander GE, Delong MR, Strick PL (1986) Parallel organization of functionally segregated circuits linking basal ganglia and cortex. Annu Rev Neurosci 9: 357–381

Arnulf I, Bonnet AM, Damier P, Bejjani BP, Seilhaen D, Derenne JP, Agid Y (2000) Hallucinations, REM sleep, and Parkinson's disease: a medical hypothesis. Neurology 55: 281–288

Ballard C, Grace J, McKeith I, Holmes C (1998) Neuroleptic sensitivity in dementia with Lewy bodies and Alzheimer's disease. Lancet 351: 1032–1033

Bartorelli L, Giraldi C, Saccardo M, Cammarata S, Bottini G, Fasarano AM, Trequattrini A (2005) Effects of switching from an AChE inhibitor to a dual AChE-BuChE inhibitor in patients with Alzheimer's disease. Curr Med Res Opin 21: 1809–1818

Bergman J, Lerner V (2002) Successful use of donepezil for the treatment of psychotic symptoms in patients with Parkinson's disease. Clin Neuropharmacol 25: 107–110

Breier A, Sutton VK, Feldman PD, Kadam DL, Ferchland I, Wright P, Friedman JH (2002) Olanzapine in the treatment of dopamimetic-induced psychosis in patients with Parkinson's disease. Biol Psychiatry 52: 438–445

Bullock R, Cameron A (2002) Rivastigmine for the treatment of dementia and visual hallucinations associated with Parkinson's disease: a case series. Curr Med Res Opin 18: 258–264

Bullock R (2004) Galantamine: use in Alzheimer's disease and related disorders. Expert Rev Neurother 4: 153–163

Comella CL, Tanner CM, Ristanovic RK (1993) Polysomnographic sleep measures in Parkinson's disease patients with treatment-induced hallucinations. Ann Neurol 34: 710–714

Cummings JL, Cyrus PA, Bieber F, Mas J, Orazem J, Gulanski B (1998) Metrifonate treatment of the cognitive deficits of Alzheimer's disease. Metrifonate Study Group. Neurology 50: 1214–1221

Davies P, Maloney AJF (1976) Selective loss of central cholinergic neurons in Alzheimer's disease. Lancet 2: 1403

Dubois B, Pillon B (1997) Cognitive deficits in Parkinson's disease. J Neurol 244: 2–8

Ellis T, Cudkowicz ME, Sexton PM, Growdon JH (2000) Clozapine and risperidone treatment of psychosis in Parkinson's disease. J Neuropsychiatry Clin Neurosci 12: 364–369

Emre M, Aarsland D, Albanese A, Byrne EJ, Deuschl G, De Deyn PP, Durif F, Kulisevski J, van Laar T, Lees A, Poewe W, Robillard A, Rosa MM, Wolters E, Quarg P, Tekin S, Lane R (2004) Rivastigmine for the dementia associated with Parkinson's disease. N Engl J Med 351: 2509–2518

Fabbrini G, Barbanti P, Aurilia C, Pauletti C, Lenzi GL, Meco G (2002) Donepezil in the treatment of hallucinations and delusions in Parkinson's disease. Neurol Sci 23: 41–43

Fergusson E, Howard R (2000) Donepezil for the treatment of psychosis in dementia with Lewy bodies. Int J Geriatr Psychiatry 15: 280–281

Fernandez HH, Lannon MC, Friedman JH, Abbott BP (2000) Clozapine replacement by quetiapine for the treatment of drug-induced psychosis in Parkinson's disease. Mov Disord 15: 579–581

Fernandez HH, Trieschmann ME, Burke MA, Jacques C, Friedman JH (2003) Long-term outcome of quetiapine use for psychosis among Parkinsonian patients. Mov Disord 18: 510–514

Friedman JH, Wagner RL (1987) Symptoms of neuroleptic malignant syndrome. Am J Psychiatry 144: 1105–1106

Gabelli C (2003) Rivastigmine: an update on therapeutic efficacy in Alzheimer's disease and other conditions. Curr Med Res Opin 19: 69–82

Goetz CG, Tanner CM, Klawans HL (1982) Pharmacology of hallucinations induced by long-term drug therapy. Am J Psychiatry 139: 494–497

Goetz CG, Stebbins GT (1993) Risk factors for nursing home placement in advanced Parkinson's disease. Neurology 43: 2227–2229

Grace J, Daniel S, Stevens T, Shankar KK, Walker Z, Byrne EJ, Butter S, Wilkinson D, Wodford J, Waite J, McKeith IG (2001) Long-term use of rivastigmine in patients with dementia with Lewy bodies: an open-label trial. Int Psychogeriatr 13: 199–205

Graham JM, Grunewald RA, Sagar HJ (1997) Hallucinosis in idiopathic Parkinson's disease. J Neurol Neurosurg Psychiatry 63: 434–440

Harding AJ, Halliday GM (2001) Cortical Lewy body pathology in the diagnosis of dementia. Acta Neuropathol (Berl) 102: 355–363

Holroyd S, Currie L, Wooten GF (2001) Prospective study of hallucinations and delusions in Parkinson's disease. J Neurol Neurosurg Psychiatry 70: 734–738

Hutchinson M, Fazzini E (1996) Cholinesterase inhibition in Parkinson's disease. J Neurol Neurosurg Psychiatry 61: 324–325

Kaduszkiewicz H, Zimmermann T, Beck-Bornholdt HP, van den Bussche H (2005) Cholinesterase inhibitors for patients with Alzheimer's disease: systematic review of randomised clinical trials. B M J 331: 321–327

Karlsen KH, Larsen JP, Tandberg E, Maland JG (1998) Quality of life measurements in patients with Parkinson's disease: A community-based study. Eur J Neurol 5: 443–450

Kaufer DI, Catt KE, Lopez OL, DeKosky ST (1998) Dementia with Lewy bodies: response of delirium-like features to donepezil. Neurology 51: 1512

Keyser DL, Rodnitzky RL (1991) Neuroleptic malignant syndrome in Parkinson's disease after withdrawal or alteration of dopaminergic therapy. Arch Intern Med 151: 794–796

Klawans HL, Goetz C, Nausieda PA, Weiner WJ (1977) Levodopa-induced dopamine receptor hypersensitivity. Trans Am Neurol Assoc 102: 80–83

Knable MB, Heinz A, Raedler T, Weinberger DR (1997) Extrapyramidal side effects with risperidone and haloperidol at comparable D2 receptor occupancy levels. Psychiatry Res 75: 91–101

Lauterbach EC (1991) Serotonin reuptake inhibitors, paranoia, and the ventral basal ganglia. Clin Neuropharmacol 14: 547–555

McKeith I, Fairbairn A, Perry R, Thompson P, Perry E (1992) Neuroleptic sensitivity in patients with senile dementia of Lewy body type. B M J 305: 673–678

McKeith IG, Ballard CG, Harrison RWS (1995) Neuroleptic sensitivity to risperidone in Lewy body dementia. Lancet 346: 699

McKeith IG, Galasko D, Kosaka K, Perry EK, Dickson DW, Hansen LA, Salmon DP, Lowe J, Mirra SS, Byrne EJ, Lennox G, Quinn NP, Edwardson JA, Ince PG, Bergeron C, Burns A, Miller BL, Lovestone S, Collerton D, Jansen ENH, Ballard C, deVos RAI, Wilcock GK, Jellinger KA, Perry RH (1996) Consensus guidelines for the clinical and pathologic diagnosis of dementia with Lewy bodies (DLB): report of the consortium on DLB international workshop. Neurology 47: 1113–1124

McKeith IG (2000) Spectrum of Parkinson's disease, Parkinson's dementia, and Lewy body dementia. Neurol Clin 18: 865–902

McKeith I, del Ser T, Spano P, Emre M, Wesnes K, Anand R, Cicin-Sain A, Ferrara R, Spiegel R (2000) Efficacy of rivastigmine in dementia with Lewy bodies: a randomised, double-blind, placebo-controlled international study. Lancet 356: 2031–2036

Melamed E, Zoldan J, Friedberg G, Ziv I, Weizmann A (1996) Involvement of serotonin in clinical features of Parkinson's disease and complications of L-DOPA therapy. Adv Neurol 69: 545–550

Meltzer HY, Matsubara S, Lee JC (1989) Classification of typical and atypical antipsychotic drugs on the basis of dopamine D-1, D-2 and serotonin2 pKi values. J Pharmacol Exp Ther 251: 238–246

Meltzer HY, Li Z, Kaneda Y, Ichikawa J (2003) Serotonin receptors : their key role in drugs to treat schizophrenia. Prog Neuropsychopharmacol Biol Psychiatry 27: 1159–1172

Moskovitz C, Moses H III, Klawans HL (1978) Levodopa-induced psychosis: a kindling phenomenon. Am J Psychiatry 135: 669–675

Ondo WG, Levy JK, Vuong KD, Hunter C, Jankovic J (2002) Olanzapine treatment for dopaminergic-induced hallucinations. Mov Disord 17: 1031–1035

Pappert EJ, Goetz CG, Niederman FG, Raman R, Leurgans S (1999) Hallucinations, sleep fragmentation, and altered dream phenomena in Parkinson's disease. Mov Disord 14: 117–121

Paulus W, Jellinger K (1991) The neuropathologic basis of different clinical subgroups of Parkinson's disease. J Neuropathol Exp Neurol 50: 743–755

Perry EK, Curtis M, Dick DJ, Candy JM, Atack JR, Bloxham CA, Blessed G, Fairbairn A, Tomlinson BE, Perry RH (1985) Cholinergic correlates of cognitive impairment in Parkinson's disease: comparisons with Alzheimer's disease. J Neurol Neurosurg Psychiatry 48: 413–421

Perry EK, McKeith I, Thompson P, Marshall E, Kerwin J, Jabeen S, Edwardson JA, Ince P, Blessed G, Irving D, Perry RH (1991) Topography, extent, and clinical relevance of neurochemical deficits in dementia of Lewy body type, Parkinson's disease, and Alzheimer's disease. Ann N Y Acad Sci 640: 197–202

Perry EK, Irving D, Kerwin JM, McKeith I, Thompson P, Collerton D, Fairbairn A, Ince PG, Morris CM, Cheng AV, Perry RH (1993) Cholinergic transmitter and neurotrophic activities in Lewy body dementia: similarity to Parkinson's and distinction from Alzheimer disease. Alzheimer Dis Assoc Disord 7: 69–79

Perry EK, Perry RH (1995) Acetylcholine and hallucinations: disease-related compared to drug-induced alterations in human consciousness. Brain Cogn 28: 240–258

Perry E, Walker M, Grace J, Perry R (1999) Acetylcholine in mind: a neurotransmitter correlate of consciousness? Trends Neurosci 22: 273–280

Poewe W (2003) Psychosis in Parkinson's disease. Mov Disord 18 [Suppl 6]: S80–S87

Poewe W, Wolters E, Emre M, Onofrj M, Hsu C, Tekin S, Lane R (2006) Long term benefits of rivastigmine in dementia associated with Parkinson's disease: an active treatment extension study. Mov Disord: In press

Reading PJ, Luce AK, McKeith IG (2001) Rivastigmine in the treatment of parkinsonian psychosis and cognitive impairment: preliminary findings from an open trial. Mov Disord 16: 1171–1174

Rich SS, Friedman JH, Ott BR (1995) Risperidone versus clozapine in the treatment of psychosis in six patients with Parkinson's disease and other akinetic-rigid syndromes. J Clin Psychiatry 56: 556–559

Rondot P, de Recondo J, Coignet A, Ziegler M (1984) Mental disorders in Parkinson's disease after treatment with L-DOPA. Adv Neurol 40: 259–269

Saint-Cyr JA, Taylor AE, Lang AE (1993) Neuropsychological and psychiatric side effects in the treatment of Parkinson's disease. Neurology 43: S47–S52

Seeman P (2002) Atypical antipsychotics: mechanism of action. Can J Psychiatry 47: 27–38

Shea C, MacKnight C, Rockwood K (1998) Donepezil for treatment of dementia with Lewy bodies: a case series of nine patients. Int Psychogeriatr 10: 229–238

Shimomura T, Mori E, Yamashita H, Imamura T, Hirono N, Hashimoto M, Tanimukai S, Kazui H, Hanihara T (1998) Cognitive loss in dementia with Lewy bodies and Alzheimer disease. Arch Neurol 55: 1547–1552

Stam CJ, Visser SL, Op de Coul AAW, deSonneVille LMJ, Schellens RLLA, Brunia CHM, Desmet JS, Gielen G (1993) Disturbed frontal regulation of attention in Parkinson's disease. Brain 116: 1139–1158

Takeda A, Loveman E, Clegg A, Kirby J, Picot J, Payne E, Green C (2006) A systematic review of the clinical effectiviness of donezepil, rivastigmine and galantamine on cognition, quality of life and adverse events in Alzheimer's disease. Int J Geriatr Psychiatry 21: 17–28

The French Clozapine Parkinson Study Group (1999) Clozapine in drug-induced psychosis in Parkinson's disease. Lancet 353: 2041–2042

The Parkinson Study Group (1999) Low-dose clozapine for the treatment of drug-induced psychosis in Parkinson's disease. N Engl J Med 340: 757–763

Wesnes KA, McKeith I, Edgar C, Emre M, Lane R (2005) benefits of rivastigmine on attention in dementia associated with Parkinson disease. Neurology 65: 1654–1656

Winogrodzka A, Wagenaar RC, Bergmans P, Vellinga A, Booij J, Van Royen EA, Van Emmerik REA, Stoof JC, Wolters ECh (2001) Rigidity decreases resting tremor intensity in Parkinson's disease: a $[^{123}I]$ß-CIT SPECT study in early nonmedicated patients. Mov Disord 16: 1033–1040

Wolters EC, Jansen ENH, Tuynman-Qua HG, Bergmans PLM (1996) Olanzapine in the treatment of dopaminomimetic psychosis in patients with Parkinson's disease. Neurology 47: 1085–1087

Wolters EC, Francot CMJE (1998) Mental dysfunctions in Parkinson's disease. Parkinsonism Relat Disord 4: 107–112

Wolters EC (2001) Psychiatric complications in the treatment of Parkinson's disease. Adv Neurol 86: 385–393

Wolters ECh, Braak (2006) Clinico-pathological correlations in Parkinson's disease. J Neural Transm: In press

Zweig RM, Jankel WR, Hedreen JC, Mayeux R, Price DL (1989) The pedunculopontine nucleus in Parkinson's disease. Ann Neurol 26: 41–46

J Neural Transm (2006) [Suppl] 71: 39–43

Journal of Neural Transmission
Printed in Austria

Antioxidant capacity in postmortem brain tissues of Parkinson's and Alzheimer's diseases

E. Sofic[1], A. Sapcanin[1], I. Tahirovic[1], I. Gavrankapetanovic[2], K. Jellinger[3], G. P. Reynolds[4], T. Tatschner[5], P. Riederer[6]

[1] Department of Chemistry, Faculty of Science, University of Sarajevo, Bosnia & Herzegovina
[2] Clinical Center, University of Sarajevo, Bosnia & Herzegovina
[3] Ludwig Boltzmann Institute for Clinical Neurobiology, Lainz-Hospital, Vienna, Austria
[4] Division of Psychiatry and Neuroscience, Queen's University, Belfast, U.K.
[5] Institute of Forensic Medicine, University of Würzburg, Germany
[6] Clinical Neurochemistry, Clinic and Policlinic for Psychiatry, and NPF Center of Excellence Research Laboratories, University of Wuerzburg, Germany

Summary Oxidative stress has been associated with damage and progressive cell death that occurs in neurodegenerative disorders such as Parkinson's disease (PD) and Alzheimer's disease (AD). The aim of this study was to investigate the antioxidant capacity in postmortem motor cortex (MC), nucleus caudatus (NC), gyrus temporalis (GT) and substantia nigra (SN) from controls (C) and patients with PD and AD. The initial samples consisted of 68 subjects of PD, AD and C. Brains were matched for age, sex and postmortem time. Brain tissue was homogenized in a phosphate buffer pH 7.3 and separated with two-step centrifugation at 15,000 rpm for 30 min and 15,000 rpm for 10 min at 4°C. Antioxidant capacity in the supernatants was measured using the oxygen radical absorbance assay (ORAC). The results showed that in the SN of parkinsonian's brain the balance between production of free radicals and the neutralization by a complex antioxidant system is disturbed. No changes in the antioxidant capacity of postmortem MC and NC of parkinsonian's brain in comparison with C were found. In the SN of parkinsonian's brain, antioxidant capacity seems to be lower in comparison with C ($p < 0.05$). Antioxidant capacity against peroxyl radical showed that MC of AD patients was lower than in the MC of C ($p < 0.005$). In NC of AD patients the antioxidant capacity against hydroxyl radical was increased in comparison with C ($p < 0.04$). No changes in the antioxidant capacity were found in brain tissues of AD in comparison with C, when $CuSO_4$ was used as a free radical generator.

Introduction

Oxidative stress has been associated with damage and progressive cell death that occurs in neurodegenerative disorders such as PD and AD. In PD the SN is most severely affected (Dexter et al., 1987; Sofic et al., 1988, 1991; Riederer et al., 1985, 1990; Mazzio and Soliman, 2004).

Correspondence: Prof. Dr. Emin Sofic, Department of Chemistry, Faculty of Science, University of Sarajevo, Zmaja od Bosne 33-35, 71 000 Sarajevo, Bosnia & Herzegovina
e-mail: esofic@pmf.unsa.ba

The pathogenesis of PD is unknown. Nonetheless, there are some generally accepted hypothesis with respect to the cascade of dopaminergic cell degeneration in SN and particularly in SN zona compacta. Histochemical and biochemical determinations of total iron, iron(II), and iron(III) contents in brain regions from PD and AD diseases have demonstrated a selective increase of total iron content in PD SN zona compacta but not in the zona reticulata (Sofic et al., 1991). Furthermore, there is growing evidence for a cascade of multiple deleterious factors, including oxidative stress and lipid peroxidation (Riederer et al., 1985, 1989; Marcus et al., 1998; Gsell et al., 1995; Goetz et al., 1992), leading to excess free radical (FR) production, mitochondrial dysfunction, as shown by a decrease in respiratory chain complex I activity (Reichmann and Janetzky, 2000) and disturbed calcium homeostasis, which in turn result in cytosceletal damage and cell death in PD and AD.

The abnormality of respiratory chain complex I activity is only found in SN pars compacta but it is currently not known whether this is due to a genetic error of the nuclear or mitochondrial genome or to an exo- or endotoxin. Aging leads to deletions in up to 5% of all mitochondrial genome molecules in the brain. However, to date, no specific changes of the mitochondrial genome has been detected (Reichmann and Janetzky, 2000). FR have been hypothesizes to play a role in the loss of nigrostriatal dopaminergic neurons and dopamine that occur in PD and aging (Halliwell, 1989; Goetz et al., 1994; Serra et al., 2001). Furthermore, brain aging in AD patients is accompanied by the alteration of several neurotransmitter systems with a pronounced deficit in the cholinergic system and abnormal accumulation of amyloid-β peptides and hyperphosphorylated tau (Montine and Morrow, 2005). Nucleus basalis Meynert, hippocampus and cortex are the mostly affected areas in AD brain. In clinical studies where analysis of antioxidant status is important, oxygen radical absorbance capacity assay (ORAC) have been used to evaluate the hydrophilic antioxidants in serum, plasma or other biological samples (Prior et al., 2003; Sofic et al., 2002). The present study has investigated the antioxidant capacity in the postmortem brain MC, NC, GT and SN from control subjects, PD and AD patients using ORAC method. Aim of this work is to proof the ≪oxidative stress≫ hypothesis using the ORAC assay as a screening method in postmortem brain tissues.

Materials and methods

Chemicals

Fluorescein, Standard Fluka for fluoresceine – free acid was obtained from Fluka Chemie GmbH, Steinheim, Germany (FL). 2,2′-azobis (2-amidinopropane) dihydrochloride (AAPH), and 6-hydroxy-2,5,7,8-tetramethylchroman-2-carboxylic acid (Trolox) were purchased from Sigma Aldrich Chemie GmbG Germany. Porphyridium cruentum β-phycoerythrin (β–PE) was obtained from Boehringer Mannheim (Germany). Cupric sulphate penta hydrate and hydrogen peroxide were obtained from Kemika, Zagreb, Croatia. All chemicals were dissolved in phosphate buffer (75 mM) pH = 7.3.

Patients and controls

The initial sample of total 18 subjects consisted of controls (C) and Parkinson's disease (PD). The human brain tissue was collected in the Clinic and Policlinic for Psychiatry and Psychotherapy, School of Medicine, University of Wuerzburg, Germany. Brain motor cortex and corpus nuclei caudati were collected and stored at −80°C until analyzed. Postmortem time of tissue for C was 28.25 ± 22.18 (h) and 20.63 ± 1.95 (h) for PD.

Substantia nigra (SN) from 8 patients with PD [4 males and 4 females; mean age 75.3 years: range 66–86 years, postmortem time, 40.7 ± 26.6 (range 11–78) hours: duration of PD 7.5 ± 3.4 (range: 2–12) years] and from neurologically normal control subjects [4 males and 4 females; mean age 71.3 ± 12.5 years: range 51–91 years, postmortem time, 26.1 ± 23.3 (range 5–79) hours] were obtained at autopsy and dissected according to a standard protocol by a neuroanatomist. The brain areas were quickly frozen at −80°C until analysis.

Diagnosis was confirmed in all cases by pathological and neuropathological examination. In PD drug therapy consisted of combined L-Dopa therapy (L-Dopa plus the peripherally acting decarboxylase inhibitor bensetazide, amantadine sulphate, and anticholinergics). Control had died without any evidence of neurological of psychiatric disease. All brains were examined histologically by routine staining methods and were diagnosed by a neuropathologist. Drug treatment consisted of cardiovascular active drugs and antibiotics. Controls compared to PD examination of DA in the striatum showed a severe depletion of the biogenic amines ranging between 90.4% (NC) and 97% (putamen) indicating a near total denervation. The cause of death (PD group) was bronchopneumonia ($n = 6$), pulmonary embolism after leg vein thrombosis and hypertensive heart disease ($n = 1$), and cardiac arrest after color carcinoma ($n = 1$). In controls the cause of death was bronchopneumonia ($n = 2$), myocardial infarction ($n = 1$), pulmonary thromboembolism and arteriosclerotic cerebro-vascular disease ($n = 1$), coronary arteriosclerosis and old infarction ($n = 1$), coronary thrombosis ($n = 1$), cor pulmonale, chronic bronchitis and emphysema ($n = 1$), and pleural mesothelioma ($n = 1$).

The initial sample of total 50 subjects consisted of C (26) and AD (24). Brain motor cortex, gyrus temporalis (inferior, superior, medialis) and corpus nuclei caudati were collected and stored at −80°C until analyzed. Brains were matched for age (controls 76.6 ± 10.1 years; AD 84.7 ± 7.7) sex and postmortem time (controls 27 ± 18 hours; AD 36.3 ± 24.6).

Control brains did not show any abnormal histopathological changes. The death of control subjects was mainly caused by cardiac and pulmonary arrest and by different tumours. Neuropathological diagnosis was based on histological examination of characteristic Alzheimer's degeneration, the number of senile plaques and neurofibrillary tangles were determined according to the graduation of Khachaturian (1985). Alzheimer's patients died from cardiac and pulmonary deficits. All patients, before death, were underwent psychopharmaceutic therapy and received antibiotics.

Sample preparation

The crude tissue extracts from human brain MC, GT – inferior, superior, medialis and NC were prepared by homogenizing the tissues in a 75 mM phosphate buffer pH = 7.3 (10 ml buffer per gram of tissue). The homogenates were centrifugated and by separating the soluble fractions by two-steps centrifugation (15,000 rpm 30 min, and 15,000 rpm 10 min at 4°C) the supernatant was ready for hydrophilic ORAC analysis after appropriate dilution with buffer solution.

The manual antioxidant radical absorbance capacity (ORAC) assay

Manual ORAC analysis were performed on a Perkin Elmer spectrometer LS 55 with fluorescent filters (Ex: 485 nm; Em: 520 nm). In the final assay mixture (2 ml total volume) fluorescein (FL, 10.5 nM) was used as a target of FR attack, with AAPH (32 mM) as a peroxyl radical generator (ORAC-$_{ROO^\bullet}$ assay), H_2O_2–Cu^{2+} (H_2O_2 0.3%; $CuSO_4 \times 5H_2O$ 0.9 mM) as mainly a hydroxyl radical generator (ORAC-$_{OH^\bullet}$ assay) or Cu^{2+} ($CuSO_4 \times 5H_2O$ 1.8 mM) as a transition metal oxidant. The spectrofluorometer was programmed to record the fluorescence of FL every 10 min after AAPH, H_2O_2–Cu^{2+} or Cu^{2+} were added for as long as 180 min and the samples were thermostated at 37°C (KP 20-D Lauda, Lauda Koenigshofen). All fluorescence measurements were expressed relative to the initial reading. Final results were calculated using the differences of areas under the FL decay curves between the blank and a sample and expressed as a μmol Trolox equivalents per g of human brain tissue.

The automated ORAC assay

The determination of ORAC in SN of PD was done using a modification of the method by Sofic et al. (2002) and the method of Cao et al. (1995).

The automated ORAC assay was carried out on a COBAS FARA II spectrofluorometric analyser (Roche Diagnostic system Inc., Branchburg, NJ, USA) with fluorescent filters (Ex: 540 nm; Em: 565 nm) as previously described (Cao et al., 1995). Briefly, in the final assay mixture (0.4 ml total volume), β-phycoerythrin (β-PE, 16.7 nmol/L) was used as a target of FR attack, with AAPH (4 mmol/L) as a peroxyl radical generator. Trolox, a water soluble vitamin E analog (1 μmol/L) was used as a control standard.

Final results were calculated using the differences of areas under the β-PE decay curves between the blank and a sample. Brain tissue non-protein fraction extracted with perchloric acid (PCA) was used in the ORAC assay. The tissue can also be extracted with pure acetone (for tissue lipid soluble antioxidant). For preparation of the tissue nonprotein fraction, tissue was diluted with 0.5 mol/L PCA (1:1, v/v). The samples were then centrifuged two times (15,000 rpm 30 min and 15,000 rpm 10 min at 4°C) and the supernatant was ready for analysis after appropriate dilution with buffer solution. The final results of ORAC-assay were expressed as μmol Trolox equivalents per g of human brain tissue.

Statistical analysis

For statistical comparisons ANOVA and Student's test was performed.

Results

The ORAC-$_{ROO^\cdot}$ and ORAC-$_{OH^\cdot}$ values from brain NC and MC of C and PD are shown in Table 1. No changes in the antioxidant capacity against peroxyl and hydroxyl radical of postmortem MC and NC of parkinsonian's brain in comparison with C were found.

In the SN of PD antioxidant capacity against peroxyl radical and hydroxyl radical is lower than in C (Table 2), $p < 0.04$ by ANOVA.

The ORAC-$_{ROO^\cdot}$ and ORAC-$_{OH^\cdot}$ values from brain NC, GT and MC of C and AD are shown in Table 3.

In the MC of AD patients antioxidant capacity against peroxyl radical was significantly lower than in the MC of C, $p < 0.005$ by Student's t-test.

In the NC of AD patients antioxidant capacity against hydroxyl radical was increased in comparison with C, $p < 0.04$ by Student's t-test.

Table 1. *The peroxyl and hydroxyl radical absorbance capacity, ORAC-$_{ROO^\cdot}$ and ORAC-$_{OH^\cdot}$ (μmol/g) of C and PD*

Groups	Region	ORAC-$_{ROO^\cdot}$ (μmol/g)	ORAC-$_{OH^\cdot}$ (μmol/g)
C ($n=6$)	Nucleus caudatus	955.35 ± 393.7	386.12 ± 467.17
PD ($n=4$)		732.50 ± 1679.47	486.85 ± 193.78
C ($n=6$)	Motor cortex	1286.03 ± 439.92	411.05 ± 241.01
PD ($n=2$)		544.65 ± 130.32	265.80 ± 87.40

Data are expressed as means ± SD
Numbers in parentheses are number of brain regions

Table 2. *The peroxyl and hydroxyl radical absorbance capacity, ORAC-$_{ROO^\cdot}$ and ORAC-$_{OH^\cdot}$ (μmol/mg protein) of PD and C*

Groups	Region	ORAC-$_{ROO^\cdot}$ (μmol/mg protein)	ORAC-$_{OH^\cdot}$ (μmol/mg protein)
C ($n=8$)	Substantia	607.5 ± 44.0	148.5 ± 22.5
PD ($n=8$)	nigra	511.0 ± 37.0*	112.0 ± 18.0*

Data are expressed as means ± SEM
Numbers in parentheses are number of brain regions
* Significantly different from C using ANOVA, $p < 0.04$

Table 3. *The peroxyl and hydroxyl radical absorbance capacity, ORAC-$_{ROO^\cdot}$ and ORAC-$_{OH^\cdot}$ (μmol/g) of C and AD*

Groups	Region	ORAC-$_{ROO^\cdot}$ (μmol/g)	ORAC-$_{OH^\cdot}$ (μmol/g)
C ($n=11$)	Nucleus caudatus	1043.4 ± 282.7	450.7 ± 253.7
AD ($n=11$)		1017.4 ± 553.3	706.5 ± 391.7*
C ($n=9$)	Gyrus temporalis	1298.2 ± 392.1	871.0 ± 303.2
AD ($n=10$)		972.4 ± 655.7	674.3 ± 480.7
C ($n=7$)	Motor cortex	1248.7 ± 413.5	507.9 ± 169.6
AD ($n=4$)		569.1 ± 111.2**	420.7 ± 119.6

Data are expressed as means ± SD
Numbers in parentheses are number of brain regions
* $p < 0.04$
** $p < 0.005$ by Student's t-test

Table 4. *The transition metal (Cu^{2+}) absorbance capacity, ORAC-$_{Cu^{2+}}$ (μmol/g) for C and AD*

Groups	Region	ORAC-$_{Cu^{2+}}$ (μmol/g)
C ($n=11$)	Nucleus caudatus	608.8 ± 285.0
AD ($n=11$)		454.1 ± 325.1
C ($n=9$)	Gyrus temporalis	328.7 ± 217.2
AD ($n=10$)		506.5 ± 272.1
C ($n=7$)	Motor cortex	492.0 ± 198.4
AD ($n=4$)		417.1 ± 100.0

Data are expressed as means ± SD
Numbers in parentheses are number of brain regions

No changes in the antioxidant capacity were found in brain tissues of AD in comparison with C, when $CuSO_4$ was used as a free radical generator (Table 4).

Discussion

Antioxidant capacity may be defined as the ability of a compound to reduce pro-oxidant activity. Pro-oxidants are oxidants of pathologic importance (Halliwell, 1989).

Several methods have been developed in recent years to evaluate the antioxidant capacity of biological samples (Cao et al., 1993; Glazer, 1990; Ghiselli et al., 1995).

The use of peroxyl and hydroxyl radicals and Cu^{2+} as transition metal oxidants, and fluoresceine and protein β-PE as target of FR attack in the present ORAC method makes it different from other methods for measuring antioxidant capacity in vitro. Using a different FR generator and different biological targets of FR attack can yield different results (Wayner et al., 1985; Whitehead et al., 1992; Cao et al., 1993).

A number of studies have provided evidence that generation of FR contributes to all forms of PD and AD (Halliwell and Gutteridge, 1984; Jenner and Olanow, 1996; Berg et al., 2004; Moreira et al., 2005; Calabrese et al., 2005). The brain is especially susceptible to oxidative stressors than other tissues for several reasons (Cao et al.,

1996). In PD brain the presence of polyunsaturated fatty acids which are easily peroxidizable and highly localized large deposits of iron in SN, NC and globus pallidus are the major reason (Riederer et al.,1989; Sofic et al., 1991; Berg et al., 2004; Zecca et al., 2004). Increased basal lipid peroxidation may result in inhibition of dopamine synthesis and damage to the dopamine synthetic systems. A significant increase of malondialdehyde formation, expressing the rate of lipid peroxidation, has been shown in the SN of PD brain (Dexter et al., 1989). In AD iron accumulation might have a direct impact on plaque formation through its effects on amyloid precursor protein processing (Zecca et al., 2004; Moreira et al., 2005; Valko et al., 2005). Different data from various investigations of human tissue and body fluids have also implicated oxidation products of two fatty acids, arachidonic acid and decosahexaenoic acid as effectors of neurodegeneration and biomarkers of AD (Montine and Morrow, 2005). Sofic et al. (2002) did not show changes of systemic oxidative stress in patients with central nervous system disorders. Although the peripheral and central nervous systems share the same categories of disease (metabolic, vascular, toxic, immune-mediated, heritable, and infectious etiologies), only in the peripheral nervous system disorders alterations of the total serum antioxidant capacity using the ORAC assay were found. However, the findings presented here show that the balance between production of free radicals and the neutralization by a complex antioxidant system is disturbed in the SN of Parkinsonian's brain. The reason that SN is the target of the high degree of oxidative stress in PD may lie in its high energy metabolism and the high content of dopamine in its neuronal cells, although dopaminergic cells are normally endowed with a huge range of protective mechanisms (Berg et al., 2004). The antioxidant capacity, determined using a peroxyl radical generator of the MC in the AD patients was lower than that of the MC in the control subjects. In the NC of AD patients the antioxidant capacity against hydroxyl radical was increased in comparison with C, a probably cause was drug therapy. No changes in the antioxidant capacity were found in brain tissues of AD in comparison with C, when $CuSO_4$ was used as a free radical generator. The present results do not allow any definite conclusion about the total antioxidative capacity of PD and AD brain. Further studies using different methods are necessary to confirm these observations.

Acknowledgements

Research was supported by the DAAD – German Academic Exchange Service, Stability Pact for South East Europe (Referat 324-25.11.2003) and Grant for 2003 of Ministry of Science and Education of Canton Sarajevo, Bosnia and Herzegovina (Grant 11-14-22-814). The author expresses his gratitude to Minister Dr. E. Turkusic for providing laboratory facilities, and to Dr. R. Prior, HNRC Tufts University, in whose laboratory the research was partially conducted.

References

Berg D, Youdim MB, Riederer P (2004) Redox imbalance. Cell Tissue Res 318: 201–213

Calabrese V, Lodi R, Tonon C, D'Agata V, Sapienza M, Scapagnini G, Mangiameli A, Pennisi G, Stella AMG, Buttetfield DA (2005) Oxidative stress, mitochondrial dysfunction and cellular stress response in Friedrich's ataxia. J Neurol Sci 233: 145–162

Cao G, Alessio HM, Cutler RG (1993) Oxygen-radical absorbance capacity assay for antioxidants. Free Rad Biol Med 14: 303–311

Cao G, Verdon C, Wu AHB, Wang H, Prior RL (1995) Automated oxygen radical absorbance capacity assay using the COBAS FARA II. Clin Chem 41: 1738–1744

Cao G, Giovanoni M, Prior R (1996) Antioxidant capacity decreases during growth but not aging in rat serum and brain. Arch Gerontol Geriatr 22: 27–37

Dexter DT, Wells FR, Agid F, Agid Y, Lees AJ, Jenner P, Marsden CD (1987) Increased nigral iron content in postmortem parkinsonian brain. Lancet 341: 1219–1220

Dexter DT Carter CH, Wells FR, Javoy-Agid F, Agid Y, Lees A, Jenner P, Marsden CD (1989) Basal lipid peroxidation in substantia nigra is increased in Parkinson's disease. J Neurochem 52: 381–389

Ghiselli A, Serafini M, Maiani G, Assini E, Ferro-Luzzi A (1995) A fluorescence-based method for measuring total plasma antioxidant capacity. Free Rad Biol Med 18: 29–36

Glazer AN (1990) Phycoerythrin fluorescence-based assay for reactive oxygen species. Methods Enzymol 186: 161–168

Goetz M, Kuenig G, Riederer P, Youdim MBH (1994) Oxidative stress: free radical production in neural degeneration. Pharmac Ther 63: 37–122

Goetz ME, Freyberger A, Hauer E, Burger R, Sofic E, Gsell W, Heckers S, Jellinger K, Hebenstreit G, Froelich L, Beckmann H, Riederer P (1992) Susceptibility of Brains from Patients with Alzheimer's disease to oxygen-stimulated lipid peroxidation and differential scanning calorimetry. Dementia 3: 213–222

Gsell W, Conrad R, Hickethier M, Sofic E, Froelich L, Wichart I, Jellinger K, Moll G, Ransmayr G, Beckmann H, Riederer P (1995) Decreased catalase activity in brains of patients with dementia of Alzheimer type. J Neurochem 64: 1216–1223

Halliwell B (1989) Oxidants and central nervous system: some fundamental questions. Acta Neurol Scand 126: 23–33

Halliwell B, Gutteridge JMC (1984) Oxygen toxicity, transition metals and disease. Biochem J 219: 1–14

Jenner P, Olanow CW (1996) Oxidative stress and the pathogenesis of Parkinsons disease. Neurology 47 [6 Suppl 3]: S161–S170

Khachaturian ZS (1985) Diagnosis of Alzheimer's disease. Arch Neurol 42: 1097–1105

Marcus DL, Thomas C, Rodriguez C, Simberkoff K, Tsai JS, Strafaci JA, Freedman ML (1998) Increased peroxidation and reduced antioxidant enzyme activity in Alzheimer's disease. Exp Neurol 150: 40–44

Mazzio E, Soliman K (2004) Glioma cell antioxidant capacity relative to oxygen species produced by dopamine. J Appl Toxicol 24: 99–106

Montine TJ, Morrow JD (2005) Fatty acid oxidation in the pathogenesis of Alzheimer's disease. Am J Pathol 166: 1283–1289

Moreira PI, Siedlak SL, Aliev G, Zhu X, Cash AD, Smith MA, Perry G (2005) Oxidative stress mechanisms and potential therapeutics in Alzheimer disease. J Neural Transm 112: 921–923

Prior RL, Hoang H, Gu L, Wu X, Bacchiocca M, Howard L, Hampsch-Woodill M, Huang D, Ou B, Jacob R (2003) Assays for hydrophilic and lipophilic antioxidant capacity [oxygen radical absorbance capacity (ORAC-FL)] of plasma and other biological and food samples. J Agric Food Chem 21, 51: 3273–3279

Reichmann H, Janetzky B (2000) Mitochondrial dysfunction – a pathogenetic factor in Parkinson's disease. J Neurol 247 [Suppl 2]: 63–68

Riederer P, Sofic E, Rausch WD, Kruzik P, Youdim MBH (1985) Dopaminforschung heute und morgen – L-DOPA in der zukunft. In: Riederer P, Umek H (eds) L-DOPA-Substitution der Parkinson-Krankheit. Geschichte, Gegenwart-Zukunft. Springer Verlag, Wien, New York, pp 127–144

Riederer P, Sofic E, Moll G, Freyberger A, Wichart I, Gsell W, Jellinger K, Hebenstreit G, Youdim MBH (1990) Senile dementia of Alzheimer's type and Parkinson's disease: neurochemical overlaps and specific differences. In: Dostert P, Riederer P, Strolin M, Roncucci R (eds) Neurochemistry of DAT and PD. New Vistas in Drug Research, vol. 1. Springer-Verlag, Austria, pp 221–232

Riederer P, Sofic E, Rausch WD, Schmidt B, Reynolds GP, Jellinger K, Youdim MBH (1989) Transition metals, ferritin, glutathione, and ascorbic acid in parkinsonian brain. J Neurochem 52: 515–520

Serra JA, Dominquez RO, de Lustig ES, Guareshi EM, Famulari AL, Bartolome EL, Marschoff ER (2001) Parkinson's disease is associated with oxidative stress: comparison of peripheral antioxidant profiles in Living Parkinson's, Alzheimer's and vascular dementia patients. J Neural Transm 108: 1135–1148

Sofic E, Riederer P, Heinsen H, Beckmann H, Reynolds GP, Hebenstreit G, Youdim MBH (1988) Increased iron(III) and total iron content in postmortem substantia nigra of parkinsonian brain. J Neural Transm 74: 199–205

Sofic E, Paulus W, Jellinger K, Riederer P, Youdim MB (1991) Selective increase of iron in substantia nigra zona compacta of parkinsonian brains. J Neurochem 56: 978–982

Sofic E, Rustembegovic A, Kroyer G, Cao G (2002) Serum antioxidant capacity in neurological, psychiatric, renal diseases and cardiomyopathy. J Neural Transm 109: 711–719

Valko M, Morris H, Cronin MTD (2005) Metals, toxicity and oxidative stress. Curr Med Chem 12: 1161–1208

Wayner DDM, Burton GW, Ingold K, Locke S (1985) Quantitative measurement of the total, peroxyl radical-trapping antioxidant capability of human blood plasma by controlled peroxidation. FEBS Lett 187: 33–37

Whitehead TP, Thorpe GHG, Maxwell SRJ (1992) Enhanced chemiluminiscent assay for antioxidant capacity in biological fluids. Anal Chim Acta 266: 265–277

Zecca L, Youdim MB, Riederer P, Conor JR, Crichton RR (2004) Iron, brain ageing and neurodegenerative disorders. Nat Rev Neurosci 5: 863–873

J Neural Transm (2006) [Suppl] 71: 45–51

Journal of
Neural
Transmission
Printed in Austria

Apoptosis inhibition in T cells triggers the expression of proinflammatory cytokines – implications for the CNS

C. Scheller[1], P. Riederer[2], M. Gerlach[3], E. Koutsilieri[1,2]

[1] Institute of Virology and Immunobiology, Würzburg, Germany
[2] Clinical Neurochemistry and NPF Center of Excellence Laboratories, Department of Psychiatry and Psychotherapy, USA
[3] Clinical Neurobiology, Department of Child and Adolescent Psychiatry, Julius-Maximilians-University, Würzburg, Germany

Summary Stimulation of death receptors such as CD95 or TNF-R1 results in rapid onset of apoptosis. Here we show that inhibition of death receptor-induced apoptosis by the broad range caspase inhibitor ZVAD causes a switch from apoptotic to proinflammatory signaling. In previous studies we have reported that caspase inhibitors induce expression of various proinflammatory cytokines in CD95-stimulated primary T cells, such as TNF-α, IFN-γ and GM-CSF. In this study we provide further evidence for the proinflammatory activity of CD95. Stimulation of CD95 by agonistic antibodies (7C11) resulted in expression of IL-2 in primary T cells, which was further enhanced when caspase activity was blocked by ZVAD. Moreover, CD95 triggered expression of IL-4 and IL-8 when caspase activity was inhibited, but not in the absence of ZVAD. Our findings are of significant importance for the CNS as changes in the cytokine pattern in the periphery affects the entry of various immune cells into the brain. Moreover, invading activated T cells can also directly influence the cytokine profile within the brain, triggering signaling cascades that eventually lead to neuronal cell death. The use of caspase inhibitors to prevent apoptotic cell death should be carefully evaluated in the management of systemic and CNS diseases.

Introduction

Apoptosis can be induced by a number of cell surface receptors that are called "death receptors". Some prominent members of this group are CD95 (Fas/Apo-1) and TNF-R1. Once a death receptor has become activated, it catalyzes the formation of a "death inducing signaling complex" (DISC) that forwards the apoptotic signal into the cell by cleavage of caspase-8, which in turn activates downstream effector caspases (for review see Bantel et al., 1998). The death receptors belong to the large group of the tumor necrosis factor receptor superfamily. The members of this family have either proapoptotic or proinflammatory activities, or in some cases, both. For instance, CD95 triggers proapoptotic signaling cascades, whereas TNF-R2 activates only proinflammatory signaling pathways. TNF-R1, in contrast, is known to have both proapoptotic and proinflammatory activity (for review see Baud and Karin, 2001). The proapoptotic signaling cascades are mediated by caspases and can be inhibited by synthetic caspase inhibitors, such as ZVAD (benzyloxycarbonyl-Val-Ala-DL-Asp-fluoromethylketone).

Since active caspases can degrade many enzymes involved in proinflammatory signaling, we hypothesized that other death receptors than TNF-R1 may also have a proinflammatory signaling activity, which, however, remains cryptic. To test this hypothesis, we stimulated CD95 in primary T lymphocytes but blocked apoptosis execution with the broad-range caspase inhibitor ZVAD and analyzed the cells for signs of proinflammatory signaling. In a previous publication we demonstrated a marked expression of the proinflammatory cytokines TNF-α, IFN-γ and GM-CSF in apoptotic primary T cells treated with caspase inhibitors (Scheller et al., 2002b). ZVAD-mediated cytokine expression could also be found in the T cell line A3.01 and was mediated by MEK/ERK and p38 MAP kinases (Scheller et al., 2002b). In addition, we could also show that caspase inhibition in A3.01 T cells was associated with a switch from apoptotic to necrotic cell death (Scheller et al., 2005).

To further investigate the caspase-inhibitor-induced modulation of the cytokine profile expressed by apoptotic T cells, we analyzed expression of additional proinflammartory as well as anti-inflammatory cytokines, such as IL-2, IL-8 and IL-4, respectively.

Correspondence: Dr. C. Scheller, Institute of Virology and Immunobiology, Versbacher Strasse 7, 97078 Würzburg, Germany
e-mail: scheller@vim.uni-wuerzburg.de

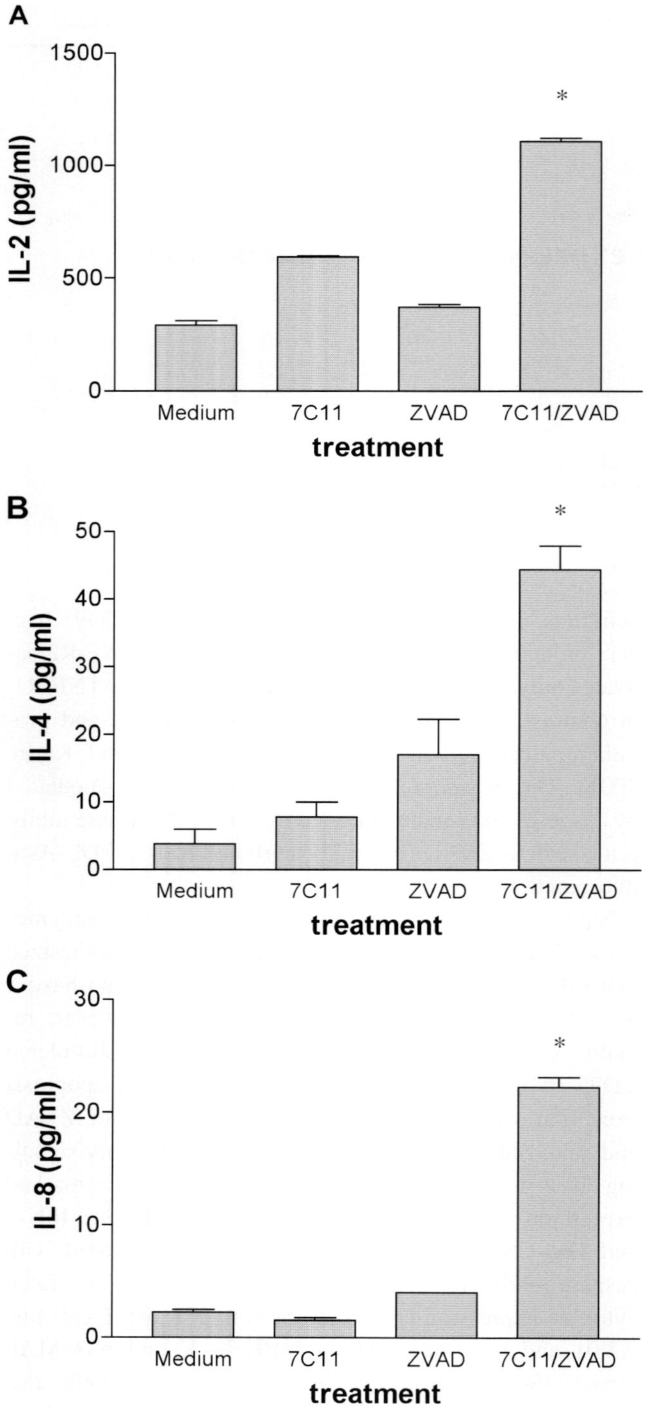

Fig. 1. Stimulation of CD95 in the presence of caspase inhibitors induces expression of various proinflammatory cytokines in mitogen-activated primary T cells. T cells activated with PHA (2 µg/ml) and IL-2 (100 U/ml) for 7 days were cultured for 24 hours in medium alone or in the presence of the agonistic anti-CD95 mAb 7C11 (200 ng/ml), the apoptosis inhibitor ZVADfmk (ZVAD; 100 µM) or both (7C11/ZVAD). Expression of IL-2 (A), IL-4 (B) and IL-8 (C) was monitored by ELISA (A–C). All assays were adjusted to the same solvent (DMSO) concentrations. Values represent means ± S.D. from triplicate analyses. $^{*}p < 0.05$, statistically different from all conditions, Student's *t* test

Materials and methods

Cells, antibodies and reagents

PBMC were prepared by Ficoll-Paque density-gradient centrifugation from heparinized human blood. T cells were enriched to more than 95% using a nylon wool column (NEN, Boston, MA). T cells were stimulated for 7 days with PHA at 2 g/ml and cultured in RPMI, 10% FCS, containing 100 U/ml IL-2 (Proleukin, Eurocetus, Frankfurt, Germany). The anti-CD95 mAb 7C11 was used at 200 ng/ml. The caspase inhibitor ZVAD (Bachem Biochemica, Heidelberg, Germany) was solved in DMSO (100 mM) and used at 100 µM. All experiments were adjusted to identical solvent concentrations.

ELISA

Cells were cultured in a 96-well flat-bottom plate (10^5 cells/well) in a total volume of 200 µl. After culture, 50 µl of the supernatants were used to determine the concentration of IL-2, IL-4 and IL-8 according to the instructions of the manufacturer (OptEia, BD-PharMingen, Heidelberg, Germany).

Results

Stimulation of CD95 with the agonistic apoptosis-inducing antibody 7C11 triggered expression of IL-2 in PHA-activated T lymphoytes isolated from healthy donors (Fig. 1A), indicating that the proinflammatory activity of CD95 is not entirely cryptic in T cells. Consistent with this finding, activation of NF-κB – an important element in proinflammatory signaling cascades – can be observed in CD95-stimulated A3.01 T cells both in the presence and absence of ZVAD (Scheller et al., 2002b). Inhibition of CD95-mediated apoptosis by the broad-range caspase inhibitor ZVAD further enhanced IIL-2 expression, whereas ZVAD had no effects when administered alone (Fig. 1A).

In contrast to IL-2, neither IL-8 nor IL-4 levels were increased in apoptotic cells. However, enhanced cytokine concentrations were observed when apoptosis was inhibited (Fig. 1B, C).

Discussion

Our data demonstrate that other death receptors than TNF-R1, in particular CD95, also mediate signaling activities that lead to cytokine expression. The death-receptor-induced cytokine profile was primarily proinflammatory with IL-4 as the only anti-inflammatory cytokine identified so far. For most of the cytokines tested, this activity remains silent in activated T cells and cytokine expression can only be detected when caspase activity is blocked (Fig. 2). The physiological role for this almost cryptic signaling activity of CD95 is yet unclear. However, under certain circumstances T cells express the caspase inhibitory protein FLIP that may render a cell sensitive for CD95-induced proinflammatory signaling also under natural conditions. Similarly,

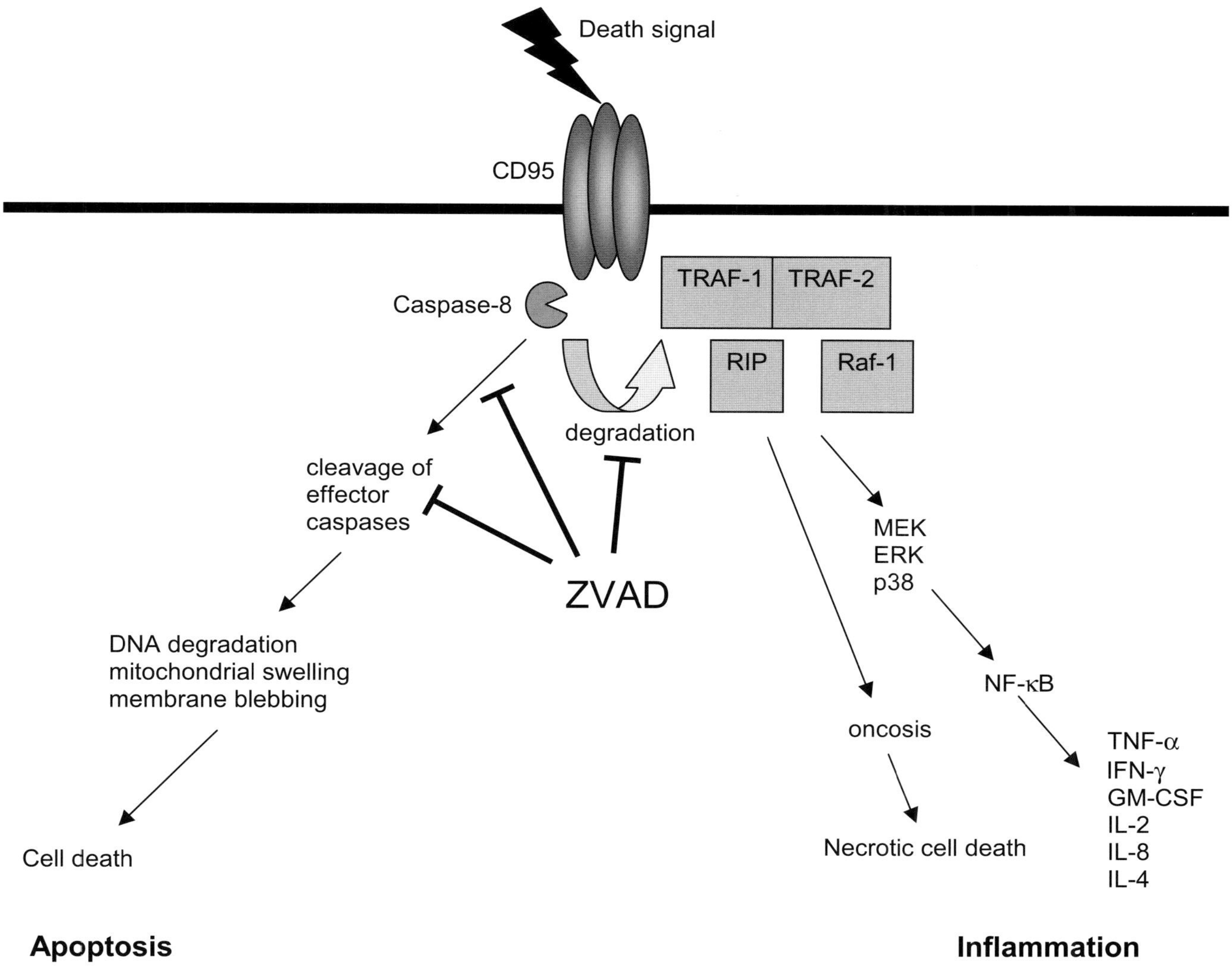

Fig. 2. Caspase inhibition induces a switch from apoptosis to inflammation in CD95-stimulated T cells. Stimulation of CD95 results in activation of caspase-8 that in turn activates downstream effector caspases and induction of apoptotic cell death. Inhibition of caspase-activation by the broad-range caspase inhibitor ZVAD induces expression of proinflammatory cytokines and eventually necrotic cell death. In apoptotic cells, caspases degrade signaling molecules likely involved in CD95-triggered proinflammatory signaling, including TRAF, RIP and Raf. CD95-induced proinflammatory signaling is dependent on activation of MEK/ERK and p38 and triggers the activation of NF-κB

dendritic cells express high levels of FLIP and it has been reported that CD95 stimulation causes cytokine expression in these cells (Rescigno et al., 2000).

In a recent publication we have described that caspase inhibition by ZVAD not only triggers cytokine expression in CD95-stimulated T cells, but similarly activates virus replication of viral genes in T cells latently infected with HIV (Scheller et al., 2002a, 2003). Therefore the observed switch from proapoptotic to proinflammatory signaling induced by caspase inhibitors may be of therapeutic relevance to address the so far unsolved problem to target the latent virus reservoir with current anti-HIV therapy (Chun et al., 1999).

Apoptosis is an important process to maintain cell homeostasis. Dysregulation of apoptosis is associated with multiple disorders, including cancer (Reed, 1999), infections (Reed, 1999; Scheller and Jassoy, 2001) or neurodegenerative disorders (Dragunow et al., 1997), suggesting that caspase inhibitors could be used for the treatment of neurodegenerative diseases such as Parkinson Disease, Alzheimer disease or multiple sclerosis (Pouly et al., 2000; Wellington and Hayden, 2000; Rideout and Stefanis, 2001; Mandel et al., 2003; Fiskum et al., 2003). Traditionally, the CNS has been considered as an "immune-privileged" organ (Wekerle et al., 1986); It is surrounded by bones and it is separated from the blood by a tight endothelial barrier

(Barker and Billingham, 1977). It was this special anatomy together with the lack of dendritic cells within the CNS parenchyma and the rare expression of major histocompatibility complex (MHC) gene products (Vass and Lassmann, 1990) which suggested a reduced activity of the immune system within the brain. However, several lines of evidence indicate that there is a minor but constant influx of immune cells into the healthy CNS (Flugel and Bradl, 2001). Activated T cells regularly enter the CNS, suggesting that there is an ongoing surveillance of the CNS by the immune system. This influx is augmented under pathological conditions like brain infection, autoimmune diseases, neurodegeneration, ischemia or trauma (Neumann and Wekerle, 1998). Several experimental studies have reported on the immune surveillance of the CNS and the properties of T lymphocytes that allow entry into the CNS under normal and inflammatory setup (Bauer et al., 2001). The CNS itself responds to inflammation by regulating local antigen presentation, by its cytokine environment, as well as by terminating inflammation through induction of apoptosis in T cells. Possible mechanisms of apoptosis in the CNS include activation-induced apoptosis, CD95-CD95L interaction, T cell TNFR1 pathway activation, deficiency of IL-2, production of nitric oxide or interaction with regulatory T cells (Pender and Rist, 2001). Both microglia and neurons can induce T cell apoptosis (Ford et al., 1996), e.g. by direct ligation of CD95 on T

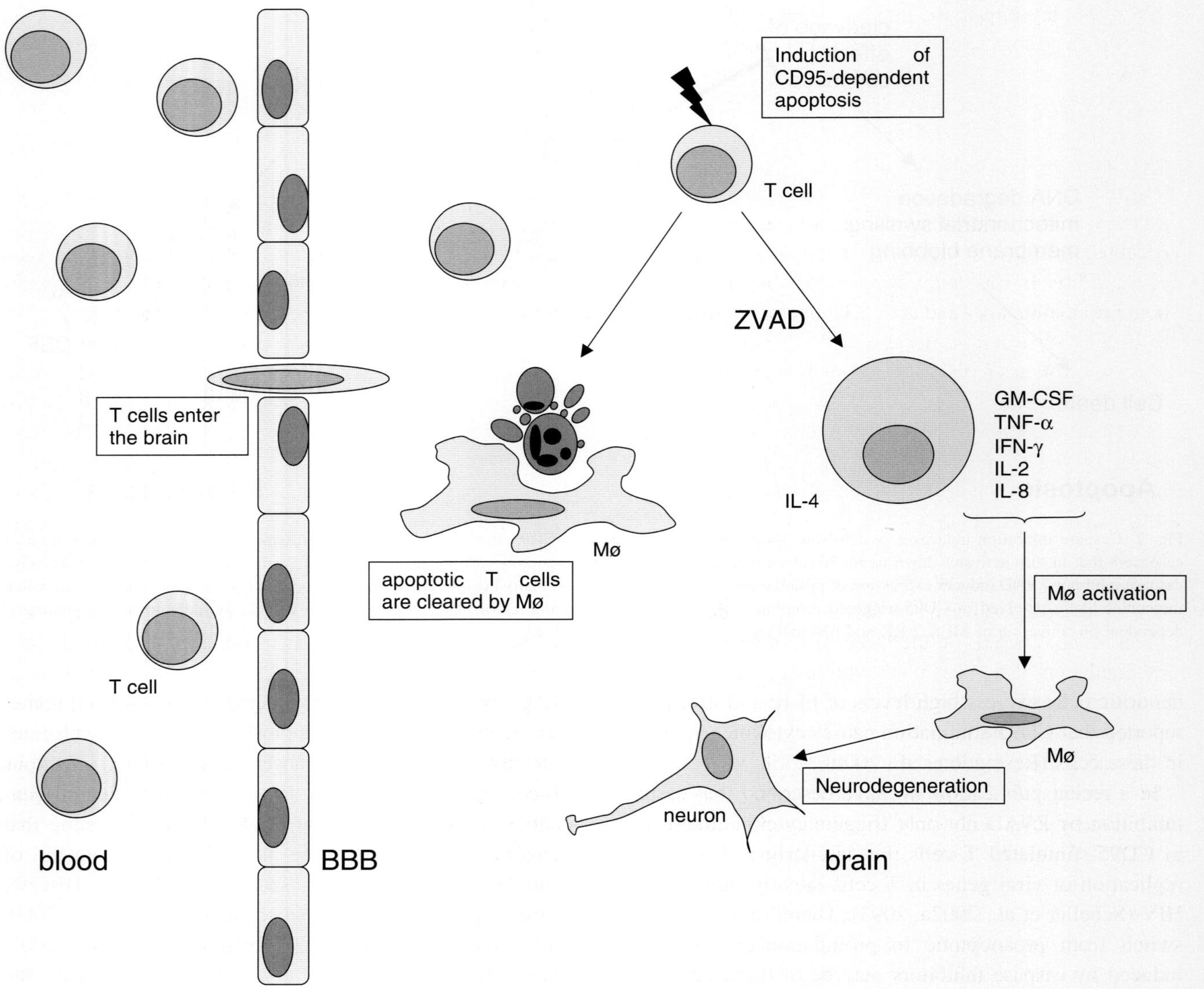

Fig. 3. Implications of CD95-induced proinflammatory T-cell signaling for the CNS. Caspase inhibitors may trigger the release of proinflammatory cytokines in the CNS by inducing a switch from apoptosis to proinflammatory signaling in CD95-stimulated T cells. Proinflammatory cytokines activate macrophages/microglia (Mø) that in turn trigger signaling cascades causing neurodegeneration

cells (Flugel et al., 2000; Frigerio et al., 2000). Apoptotic cells are subsequently cleared so that they cannot induce damage in the surrounding tissue (Magnus et al., 2002; Nguyen and Pender, 1998). The whole immune response cascades from induction of apoptosis to clearance must be precisely regulated, and inappropriate immune and inflammatory responses can lead to disease.

Besides the increase of the anti-apoptotic Bcl-family, both apoptosis inhibition and overexpression of inhibitor of apoptosis protein (IPO), have been shown to protect neurons in neurodegeneration models *in vitro* and *in vivo* (Bilsland et al., 2002; Eberhardt et al., 2000; Mandel et al., 2005). However, our data in this paper and previous publications (Scheller et al., 2002b, 2005), indicate that administration of apoptosis inhibitors may impair the immune balance of the CNS, as they can lead to necrotic processes and change the natural cytokine profile of the system, leading to macrophage/microglia (Mø) activation that in turn may trigger signaling cascades causing neurodegeneration (Fig. 3). Our data are supported by a previous study showing that administration of the apoptosis inhibitor ZVAD impaired recovery and induced earlier relapse in the experimental autoimmune encephalomyelitis, a model for multiple sclerosis (Okuda et al., 2000). In this study, we demonstrated an increase in both proinflammatory and anti-inflammatory cytokines, such as IL-2, IL-8, and IL-4, respectively. The physiological role of these cytokines in the CNS is largely unknown. However, there is accumulating data concerning these cytokines and CNS. IL-2 is a proinflammatory cytokine secreted predominantly by T-cells and has been shown to have proliferative effects as well as enhancing activity on natural killer (NK) cells (Delgado et al., 2003). In normal rodent brain, IL-2 receptors are enriched in the hippocampal formation and IL-2 knockout mice exhibit abnormalities in the cytoarchitecture of the diagonal band of Broca and the dentate gyrus (Beck et al., 2005a). Furthermore, IL-2 deficiency leads to dysregulation of hippocampal cytokine patterns under physiological conditions, causing disturbance of endogenous neurogenesis in the hippocampus (Beck et al., 2005b). IL-2 knockout mice exhibit reduced susceptibility to EAE. On the other hand, IL-2 signaling is necessary for the prevention of autoimmunity and lethal inflammation (Furtado et al., 2002). Whether IL-2 takes part in inflammatory processes during CNS injury responses is uncertain. Increased concentrations of IL-2 have been found in patients with Parkinson's and Alzheimer's disease (Beloosesky et al., 2002; Nagatsu et al., 2000) whereas in ischemic conditions, IL-2 has been reported to remain unchanged.

IL-8, another proinflammatory cytokine, is primarily expressed in astrocytes and microglia. IL-8 receptors have been found in the hippocampus, cerebellum and cortex (Horuk et al., 1997; Meucci et al., 1998). IL-8 has potent trophic actions (Araujo and Cotman, 1993), induces strong survival promoting effects, and is known to be upregulated in neuritic plaques of Alzheimer brains (Horuk et al., 1997; Xia et al., 1997). Short-term intracerebroventricular administration of IL-8 in rats produces anorexia and pyrexia suggesting a role in metabolic control and a feasible relationship to the postinjury syndrome (Plata-Salaman and Borkoski, 1993). IL-8 production is very sensitive to stimulation by IL-1 and TNF (Ehrlich et al., 1998; Hoffmann et al., 2002). Further, evidence has emerged that IL-8 elicit rapid signaling events in neurons, suggesting that IL-8 may be an important factor in intercellular communication between lymphocytes, glia and neurons by altering the excitability of neurons (Puma et al., 2001). Finally, a role of IL-8 in the postinjury syndrom has been postulated, as marked elevations of IL-8 were measured in CSF without parallel increases in serum (Chuang et al., 2005).

IL-4 is regarded as prototypic anti-inflammatory cytokine that regulate tissue inflammation by counteracting the pro-inflammatory responses. IL-4 receptors are found on microglia/macrophages (Hulshof et al., 2002). Moreover, IL-4 induces ramification of microglial cells, the resting phenotype of microglia with reduced phagocytic and antigen-presenting cell functions (Wirjatijasa et al., 2002). IL-4-stimulated astrocytes have been discussed to exert neurotrophic and protective actions in CNS disease (Brodie et al., 1998). In the EAE model, therapeutic upregulation of IL-4 was associated to anti-inflammatory beneficial effects on disease (Khoury et al., 1992). Further, the involvement of IL-4 in brain ischemia or trauma is uncertain (for review see Schroeter and Jander, 2005).

Taken together, therapeutic inhibition of apoptosis is being discussed as a treatment option in various diseases. However, consequences of apoptosis inhibition both in systemic and brain compartments may include a dysregulation in the intercellular communication between immune cells and neurons and induction of inflammation. Therefore, the use of caspase inhibitors to prevent apoptotic cell death should be carefully evaluated in the management of systemic and CNS diseases.

References

Araujo DM, Cotman CW (1993) Trophic effects of interleukin-4, -7 and -8 on hippocampal neuronal cultures: potential involvement of glial-derived factors. Brain Res 600: 49–55

Bantel H, Bruning T, Schulze-Osthoff K (1998) Activation of caspases by death receptors. Eur Cytokine Netw 9: 681–684

Barker CF, Billingham RE (1977) Immunologically privileged sites. Adv Immunol 25: 1–54

Baud V, Karin M (2001) Signal transduction by tumor necrosis factor and its relatives. Trends Cell Biol 11: 372–377

Bauer J, Rauschka H, Lassmann H (2001) Inflammation in the nervous system: the human perspective. Glia 36: 235–243

Beck RD Jr, King MA, Ha GK, Cushman JD, Huang Z, Petitto JM (2005a) IL-2 deficiency results in altered septal and hippocampal cytoarchitecture: relation to development and neurotrophins. J Neuroimmunol 160: 146–153

Beck RD Jr, Wasserfall C, Ha GK, Cushman JD, Huang Z, Atkinson MA, Petitto JM (2005b) Changes in hippocampal IL-15, related cytokines, and neurogenesis in IL-2 deficient mice. Brain Res 1041: 223–230

Beloosesky Y, Salman H, Bergman M, Bessler H, Djaldetti M (2002) Cytokine levels and phagocytic activity in patients with Alzheimer's disease. Gerontology 48: 128–132

Bilsland J, Roy S, Xanthoudakis S, Nicholson DW, Han Y, Grimm E, Hefti F, Harper SJ (2002) Caspase inhibitors attenuate 1-methyl-4-phenylpyridinium toxicity in primary cultures of mesencephalic dopaminergic neurons. J Neurosci 22: 2637–2649

Brodie C, Goldreich N, Haiman T, Kazimirsky G (1998) Functional IL-4 receptors on mouse astrocytes: IL-4 inhibits astrocyte activation and induces NGF secretion. J Neuroimmunol 81: 20–30

Chuang D, Power SE, Dunbar PR, Hill AG (2005) Central nervous system interleukin-8 production following neck of femur fracture. ANZ J Surg 75: 813–816

Chun TW, Fauci AS (1999) Latent reservoirs of HIV: obstacles to the eradication of virus. Proc Natl Acad Sci USA 96: 10958–10961

Delgado AV, McManus AT, Chambers JP (2003) Production of tumor necrosis factor-alpha, interleukin 1-beta, interleukin 2, and interleukin 6 by rat leukocyte subpopulations after exposure to substance P. Neuropeptides 37: 355–361

Dragunow M, MacGibbon GA, Lawlor P, Butterworth N, Connor B, Henderson C, Walton M, Woodgate A, Hughes P, Faull RL (1997) Apoptosis, neurotrophic factors and neurodegeneration. Rev Neurosci 8: 223–265

Eberhardt O, Coelln RV, Kugler S, Lindenau J, Rathke-Hartlieb S, Gerhardt E, Haid S, Isenmann S, Gravel C, Srinivasan A, Bahr M, Weller M, Dichgans J, Schulz JB (2000) Protection by synergistic effects of adenovirus-mediated X-chromosome-linked inhibitor of apoptosis and glial cell line-derived neurotrophic factor gene transfer in the 1-methyl-4-phenyl-1,2,3,6-tetrahydropyridine model of Parkinson's disease. J Neurosci 20: 9126–9134

Ehrlich LC, Hu S, Sheng WS, Sutton RL, Rockswold GL, Peterson PK, Chao CC (1998) Cytokine regulation of human microglial cell IL-8 production. J Immunol 160: 1944–1948

Fiskum G, Starkov A, Polster BM, Chinopoulos C (2003) Mitochondrial mechanisms of neural cell death and neuroprotective interventions in Parkinson's disease. Ann NY Acad Sci 991: 111–119

Flugel A, Bradl M (2001) New tools to trace populations of inflammatory cells in the CNS. Glia 36: 125–136

Flugel A, Schwaiger FW, Neumann H, Medana I, Willem M, Wekerle H, Kreutzberg GW, Graeber MB (2000) Neuronal FasL induces cell death of encephalitogenic T lymphocytes. Brain Pathol 10: 353–364

Ford AL, Foulcher E, Lemckert FA, Sedgwick JD (1996) Microglia induce CD4 T lymphocyte final effector function and death. J Exp Med 184: 1737–1745

Frigerio S, Silei V, Ciusani E, Massa G, Lauro GM, Salmaggi A (2000) Modulation of fas-ligand (Fas-L) on human microglial cells: an in vitro study. J Neuroimmunol 105: 109–114

Furtado GC, Curotto de Lafaille MA, Kutchukhidze N, Lafaille JJ (2002) Interleukin 2 signaling is required for CD4(+) regulatory T cell function. J Exp Med 196: 851–857

Hoffmann E, Dittrich-Breiholz O, Holtmann H, Kracht M (2002) Multiple control of interleukin-8 gene expression. J Leukoc Biol 72: 847–855

Horuk R, Martin AW, Wang Z, Schweitzer L, Gerassimides A, Guo H, Lu Z, Hesselgesser J, Perez HD, Kim J, Parker J, Hadley TJ, Peiper SC (1997) Expression of chemokine receptors by subsets of neurons in the central nervous system. J Immunol 158: 2882–2890

Hulshof S, Montagne L, De Groot CJ, Van Der Valk P (2002) Cellular localization and expression patterns of interleukin-10, interleukin-4, and their receptors in multiple sclerosis lesions. Glia 38: 24–35

Khoury SJ, Hancock WW, Weiner HL (1992) Oral tolerance to myelin basic protein and natural recovery from experimental autoimmune encephalomyelitis are associated with downregulation of inflammatory cytokines and differential upregulation of transforming growth factor beta, interleukin 4, and prostaglandin E expression in the brain. J Exp Med 176: 1355–1364

Magnus T, Chan A, Savill J, Toyka KV, Gold R (2002) Phagocytotic removal of apoptotic, inflammatory lymphocytes in the central nervous system by microglia and its functional implications. J Neuroimmunol 130: 1–9

Mandel S, Grünblatt E, Riederer P, Gerlach M, Levites Y, Youdim MBH (2003) Neuroprotective strategies in Parkinson's disease. An update on progress. CNS Drugs 17: 729–762

Mandel S, Weinreb O, Amit T, Youdim MB (2005) Mechanism of neuroprotective action of the anti-Parkinson drug rasagiline and its derivatives. Brain Res Brain Res Rev 48: 379–387

Meucci O, Fatatis A, Simen AA, Bushell TJ, Gray PW, Miller RJ (1998) Chemokines regulate hippocampal neuronal signaling and gp120 neurotoxicity. Proc Natl Acad Sci USA 95: 14500–14505

Nagatsu T, Mogi M, Ichinose H, Togari A (2000) Changes in cytokines and neurotrophins in Parkinson's disease. J Neural Transm [Suppl]: 277–290

Neumann H, Wekerle H (1998) Neuronal control of the immune response in the central nervous system: linking brain immunity to neurodegeneration. J Neuropathol Exp Neurol 57: 1–9

Nguyen KB, Pender MP (1998) Phagocytosis of apoptotic lymphocytes by oligodendrocytes in experimental autoimmune encephalomyelitis. Acta Neuropathol (Berl) 95: 40–46

Okuda Y, Sakoda S, Fujimura H, Yanagihara T (2000) The effect of apoptosis inhibitors on experimental autoimmune encephalomyelitis: apoptosis as a regulatory factor. Biochem Biophys Res Commun 267: 826–830

Pender MP, Rist MJ (2001) Apoptosis of inflammatory cells in immune control of the nervous system: role of glia. Glia 36: 137–144

Plata-Salaman CR, Borkoski JP (1993) Interleukin-8 modulates feeding by direct action in the central nervous system. Am J Physiol 265: 877–882

Pouly S, Antel JP, Ladiwala U, Nalbantoglu J, Becher B (2000) Mechanisms of tissue injury in multiple sclerosis: opportunities for neuroprotective therapy. J Neural Transm [Suppl]: 193–203

Puma C, Danik M, Quirion R, Ramon F, Williams S (2001) The chemokine interleukin-8 acutely reduces Ca(2+) currents in identified cholinergic septal neurons expressing CXCR1 and CXCR2 receptor mRNAs. J Neurochem 78: 960–971

Reed JC (1999) Dysregulation of apoptosis in cancer. J Clin Oncol 17: 2941–2953

Rescigno M, Piguet V, Valzasina B, Lens S, Zubler R, French L, Kindler V, Tschopp J, Ricciardi-Castagnoli P (2000) Fas engagement induces the maturation of dendritic cells (DCs), the release of interleukin (IL)-1beta, and the production of interferon gamma in the absence of IL-12 during DC-T cell cognate interaction: a new role for Fas ligand in inflammatory responses. J Exp Med 192: 1661–1668

Rideout HJ, Stefanis L (2001) Caspase inhibition: a potential therapeutic strategy in neurological diseases. Histol Histopathol 16: 895–908

Scheller C, Jassoy C (2001) Syncytium formation amplifies apoptotic signals: a new view on apoptosis in HIV infection in vitro. Virology 282: 48–55

Scheller C, Knoferle J, Ullrich A, Prottengeier J, Racek T, Sopper S, Jassoy C, Rethwilm A, Koutsilieri E (2005) Caspase inhibition in apoptotic T cells triggers necrotic cell death depending on the cell type and the proapoptotic stimulus. J Cell Biochem: In press

Scheller C, Sopper S, Chen P, Flory E, Koutsilieri E, Racek T, Ludwig S, ter Meulen V, Jassoy C (2002a) Caspase inhibition activates HIV in latently infected cells. Role of tumor necrosis factor receptor 1 and CD95. J Biol Chem 277: 15459–15464

Scheller C, Sopper S, Ehrhardt C, Flory E, Chen P, Koutsilieri E, Ludwig S, ter Meulen V, Jassoy C (2002b) Caspase inhibitors induce a switch from apoptotic to proinflammatory signaling in CD95-stimulated T lymphocytes. Eur J Immunol 32: 2471–2480

Scheller C, Sopper S, Koutsilieri E, Ludwig S, Ter Meulen V, Jassoy C (2003) Caspase inhibitors as a supplement in immune activation therapies to achieve eradication of HIV in its latent reservoirs. Ann NY Acad Sci 1010: 209–212

Schroeter M, Jander S (2005) T-cell cytokines in injury-induced neural damage and repair. NeuroMolecular Medicine: In press

Vass K, Lassmann H (1990) Intrathecal application of interferon gamma. Progressive appearance of MHC antigens within the rat nervous system. Am J Pathol 137: 789–800

Wellington CL, Hayden MR (2000) Caspases and neurodegeneration: on the cutting edge of new therapeutic approaches. Clin Genet 57: 1–10

Wirjatijasa F, Dehghani F, Blaheta RA, Korf HW, Hailer NP (2002) Interleukin-4, interleukin-10, and interleukin-1-receptor antagonist but not transforming growth factor-beta induce ramification and reduce adhesion molecule expression of rat microglial cells. J Neurosci Res 68: 579–587

Wekerle H, Linington C, Lassmann H, Meyermann R (1986) Cellular immune reactivity within the CNS. Trends Neurosci 9: 271–277

Xia M, Qin S, McNamara M, Mackay C, Hyman BT (1997) Interleukin-8 receptor B immunoreactivity in brain and neuritic plaques of Alzheimer's disease. Am J Pathol 150: 1267–1274

J Neural Transm (2006) [Suppl] 71: 53–65

Journal of Neural Transmission
Printed in Austria

Molecular mechanism of the relation of monoamine oxidase B and its inhibitors to Parkinson's disease: possible implications of glial cells

T. Nagatsu[1,2], M. Sawada[2]

[1] Department of Pharmacology, School of Medicine, Fujita Health University, Toyoake, Aichi, Japan
[2] Research Institute of Environmental Medicine, Nagoya University, Nagoya, Aichi, Japan

Summary Monoamine oxidases A and B (MAO A and MAO B) are the major enzymes that catalyze the oxidative deamination of monoamine neurotaransmitters such as dopamine (DA), noradrenaline, and serotonin in the central and peripheral nervous systems. MAO B is mainly localized in glial cells. MAO B also oxidizes the xenobiotic 1-methyl-4-phenyl-1,2,3,6-tetrahydropyridine (MPTP) to a parkinsonism-producing neurotoxin, 1-methyl-4-phenyl-pyridinium (MPP+). MAO B may be closely related to the pathogenesis of Parkinson's disease (PD), in which neuromelanin-containing DA neurons in the substantia nigra projecting to the striatum in the brain selectively degenerate. MAO B degrades the neurotransmitter DA that is deficient in the nigro-striatal region in PD, and forms H_2O_2 and toxic aldehyde metabolites of DA. H_2O_2 produces highly toxic reactive oxygen species (ROS) by Fenton reaction that is catalyzed by iron and neuromelanin. MAO B inhibitors such as L-(−)-deprenyl (selegiline) and rasagiline are effective for the treatment of PD. Concerning the mechanism of the clinical efficacy of MAO B inhibitors in PD, the inhibition of DA degradation (a symptomatic effect) and also the prevention of the formation of neurotoxic DA metabolites, i.e., ROS and dopamine derived aldehydes have been speculated. As another mechanism of clinical efficacy, MAO B inhibitors such as selegiline are speculated to have neuroprotective effects to prevent progress of PD. The possible mechanism of neuroprotection of MAO B inhibitors may be related not only to MAO B inhibition but also to induction and activation of multiple factors for anti-oxidative stress and anti-apoptosis: i.e., catalase, superoxide dismutase 1 and 2, thioredoxin, Bcl-2, the cellular poly(ADP-ribosyl)ation, and binding to glyceraldehydes-3-phosphate dehydrogenase (GAPDH). Furthermore, it should be noted that selegiline increases production of neurotrophins such as nerve growth factor (NGF), brain-derived neurotrophic factor (BDNF), and glial cell line-derived neurotrphic factor (GDNF), possibly from glial cells, to protect neurons from inflammatory process.

Abbreviations: *BDNF* brain-derived neurotrophic factor, *CSF* cerebrospinal fluid, *DA* dopamine, *GDNF* glial cell line-derived neurotrophic factor, *MAO A* monoamine oxidase A, *MAO B* monoamine oxidase B, *MPDP+* 1-methyl-4-phenyl-2,3-dihydro-pyridinium, *MPP+* 1-methyl-4-phenyl-pyridinium, *MPTP* 1-methyl-4-phenyl-1,2,3,6-tetrahydropyridine, *NGF* nerve growth factor, *PD* Parkinson's disease, *ROS* reactive oxygen species, *TH* tyrosine hydroxylase

Correspondence: T. Nagatsu, Department of Pharmacology, School of Medicine, Fujita Health University, Toyoake, Aichi, Japan
e-mail: tnagatsu@fujita-hu.ac.jp

Parkinson's disease (PD) is an aging-related movement disorder caused by a deficiency of the neurotransmitter dopamine (DA) in the striatum of the brain as a result of selective degeneration of the nigro-striatal DA neurons (A9 neurons). DA deficiency is due to decreased number of DA neurons in the substantia nigra, and the molecular activity (enzyme activity/enzyme protein) of tyrosine 3-monooxygenase (tyrosine hydroxylase, TH) in residual DA neurons increases resulting in compensation for DA deficiency (Mogi et al., 1988). Familial PD for which the causative genes have been identified constitutes a small percentage of PD, and most PD is sporadic (idiopathic) without hereditary history. The molecular mechanism of the DA cell death in sporadic PD is unknown, but monoamine oxidase (MAO), especially type B (MAO B), is speculated to play important roles. In the brain MAO B is mainly localized in glial cells. MAO B activity in the brain increases during aging probably due to increasing numbers of glial cells (Fowler et al., 1980), and aging is a high risk factor of PD. MAO B inhibitors, such as L-(−)-deprenyl (selegiline) and rasagiline, are proved to be clinically effective for the treatment of PD. In the present review, we will examine the molecular mechanism of PD in relation to the mechanism of probable neuroprotection by MAO B inhibitors, and to possible interrelationship between DA neurons and glial cells in the inflammatory process.

Monoamine oxidases A and B (MAO A and MAO B)

Monoamine oxidase (flavin-containing) [amine:oxygen oxidoreductase (deaminating) (flavin-containing); MAO; E.C. 1.4.3.4.] catalyzes the following reaction: $RCH_2NH_2 + H_2O + O_2 = RCHO + NH_3 + H_2O_2$. MAO acts on primary amines, and also on some secondary and tertiary amines. The monoamine substrates for MAO include physiologically and pathologically important neurotransmitters and hormones, such as DA, noradrenaline, adrenaline, and serotonin, which are slow-acting neurotransmitters in the brain and function with rapidly-acting neurotransmitters, i.e., glutamic acid and gamma-aminobutyric acid (GABA), to regulate movement, emotion, reward, cognition, memory, and learning. Thus, MAO is closely related to higher brain functions by regulating the levels of monoamine neurotransmitters and also to the pathogenesis of PD (for reviews, see Nagatsu, 2004; Nicotora et al., 2004; Riederer and Youdim, 1990; Youdim and Riederer, 1997). In the brain, MAO is thought to be important together with catechol O-methyltransferase in regulating the level of DA. The DA level decreases specifically in the nigro-striatal region in PD, which is the characteristic biochemical change (for reviews, see Cookson, 2005; Hornykiewicz, 2001; Nagatsu, 1993).

MAO was first discovered as tyramine oxidase by Hare in 1928, since it catalyzed the oxidative deamination of tyramine. This enzyme was then found to oxidize various monoamines including catecholamines, i.e., DA, noradrenaline, and adrenaline, and serotonine, and was recognized as monoamine oxidase by Blashko, Zeller, Gorkin, and Quastel. The enzyme localizes in the outer membrane of mitochondria (Schneitman et al., 1967). MAO was purified from bovine liver (Gomes et al., 1969; Minamiura and Yasunobu, 1978) and bovine brain (Harada et al., 1971). The cofactor, flavin adenine dinucleotide (FAD), was identified in preparations of purified MAO (Harada and Nagatsu, 1969; Tipton, 1980). Purified MAO was discovered to contain FAD covalently bound as 8-a-cysteinyl-FAD (Walker et al., 1971).

Johnston (1968) pharmacologically discovered that the inhibitor clorgyline was able to distinguish two forms of MAO, i.e., MAO type A (MAO A) and MAO type B (MAO B). The presence of multiple forms of MAO in the human brain was also reported by Collins et al. (1970). The structures and functions of MAO A and MAO B have been elucidated by cDNA cloning, genomic DNA cloning, and genetic engineering (for review, see Shih, 2004; Shih et al., 1999).

Full-length cDNAs encoding human liver MAO A and MAO B and the genomic DNAs were cloned (Bach et al., 1988; Chen et al., 1991; Powell et al., 1991; Weyler et al., 1990). Human placental MAO A (Hsu et al., 1988), and rat liver MAO A and MAO B (Ito et al., 1988; Kwan and Abell, 1992) were also cloned and sequenced, and human and rat MAO A showed 86–88% identity. MAO B from human platelets and frontal cortex were found to have identical amino acid sequences, confirming that human MAO B is a single enzyme in various tissues (Chen et al., 1993).

Human MAO A and MAO B have subunit molecular weights of 59,700 and 58,000, respectively, consisting of 527 and 520 amino acids, respectively, and have a 70% amino acid sequence identity; and both sequences contain the pentapeptide Ser-Gly-Gly-Cys-Tyr, in which the obligatory cofactor FAD is covalently bound through a thio ether linkage to the cysteine (Bach et al., 1988; Chen et al., 1991). MAO is composed of two identical subunits (Minamiura and Yasunobu, 1978), and one FAD couples with each subunit of 60 kDa (Weyler, 1989). FAD is covalently linked to Cys-406 in MAO A and Cys-397 in MAO-B (Abell and Kwan, 2001; Edmondson et al., 2004).

The expression of functional enzymes by transfection of cells with cDNAs provides unequivocal evidence that the different catalytic activities of MAO A and MAO B reside in their primary amino acid sequences. Chimeric enzymes and site-directed mutagenesis studies contributed to elucidating the structure-function relationships of MAO A and MAO B. The enzymatic properties observed for the chimeric MAO enzymes suggest that the internal segment, but not the N- or C-terminal region, confers substrate and inhibitor specificities (Shih et al., 1998; Tsugeno and Ito, 1997; Tsugeno et al., 1995). The catalytic properties and specificity of MAO A were insensitive to substitution of both the NH_2- (up to position 112) and COOH-termini (from residue 395). The replacement of MAO A amino acids 161–375 by the corresponding region of MAO B converted MAO A catalytic properties to ones typical of MAO B; and the converted enzyme did not oxidize serotonin, a preferred substrate of MAO A, and was more sensitive to the MAO B-specific inhibitor, L-(−)-derenyl (selegiline), than to the MAO A-specific inhibitor clorgyline. These results demonstrated that amino acids 152–366 of MAO B contain a domain that confers substrate specificity and inhibitor selectivity on the enzyme (Chen and Shih, 1998; Cesura et al., 1998).

Because MAO A and MAO B are integrated proteins of the outer membrane of mitochondria, their crystallization has been difficult; and so their three-dimensional structure of human MAO B has been only recently elucidated (Binda et al., 2002a, b). Determination of the crystal structure of human MAO B allowed precise modeling of the structure of human MAO A, and preliminary models of human MAO A have been obtained by fold recognition and comparative modeling based on proteins sharing low sequence identity (Leonard et al., 2004). The 50-residue C-terminal tail of human MAO B forms an extended segment that traverses the protein surface and then folds into an alpha-helix, which protrudes from the basal face of the structure to anchor the protein to the mitochondrial outer membrane (Binda et al., 2002a, b).

MAO A and *MAO B* genes are situated on the X chromosome, at Xp 11.23–22.1 (Chen et al., 1992; Kochersperger et al., 1986; Lan et al., 1989; Levy et al., 1989; Pintar et al., 1981). Both genes are closely located and are deleted in patients with Norrie's disease, a rare X-linked recessive neurological disorder characterized by blindness, hearing loss, and mental retardation. Human *MAO A* and *MAO B* genes consist of 15 exons and have an identical exon-intron organization. Exon 12 codes for the covalent FAD-binding site and is the most conserved exon, showing 93.9% amino acid identity between MAO A and MAO B (Chen et al., 1992; Grimsby et al., 1991).

The distribution of MAO in various tissues of various species has been investigated by use of specific inhibitors of MAO A and MAO B enzyme activities, immunohistochemistry, enzyme autoradiography, and in situ hybridization (for review, see Berry et al., 1994; Kitahama et al., 1994; Luque et al., 1998). MAO A and MAO B are distributed in various tissues including the brain of various species. Histochemical localization of MAO A and MAO B was examined in the rat brain (Willonghby et al., 1988). In the rat brain, MAO A was predominantly found in noradrenergic neurons; whereas MAO B was detected in serotonergic and histaminergic neurons and in glial cells (astrocytes) (Arai et al., 1997; Jahung et al., 1997; Levitt et al., 1982; Luque et al., 1995; Saura et al., 1994; Westlund et al., 1988a). However, DA neurons appear not to have MAO A or MAO B, in contrast to the fact that DA is a common substrate of both MAO A and MAO B activity (Arai et al., 1998; Hida et al., 1999). As another puzzling fact on the physiological role of MAO B, serotonin neurons contain only MAO B, but serotonin is a very poor substrate of MAO B (Arai et al., 1997; Levitt et al., 1982).

Most human tissues, including the brain, express both MAO A and MAO B (Konradi et al., 1988; Konradi et al., 1989; Westlund et al., 1988b). However, human placenta contains predominantly MAO A (Egashira and Yamanaka, 1981); and human platelets and lymphocytes express only MAO B (Bond and Cundall, 1997; Donnelly and Murphy, 1977). Thus platelet MAO B can be useful for estimation of brain MAO B (Oreland, 2004). mRNA transcripts of MAO A and MAO B were coexpressed in the same region in the adult human brain; and the relative concentrations of these transcripts were as follows in the decreasing order: frontal cortex, locus coeruleus, temporal cortex, posterior pensylvian cortex-supuramarginal gyri, anterior pensylvian cortex-opercular gyri, hippocampus and thalamus (Grimsby et al., 1990).

Cell-type specific expression of MAO A and MAO B were examined in cultured cells (Donnelly et al., 1976; Hawkins and Breakfield, 1978; Murphy et al., 1976; Nagatsu et al., 1981). The type of MAO activity did not vary through the stage of growth of mouse myoblast G8-1 cells, which contain mostly MAO A (95%) and a small amount of MAO B (5%) (Nagatsu et al., 1981). NG108-15 hybrid cells derived from mouse neuroblastoma $\times$ rat glioma showed both MAO A (65–90%) and MAO B (35–10%), and the total MAO A plus MAO B activity and the ratio of MAO B/MAO A activity increased as a function of time in culture. Prostaglandin E1 and theophylline, the best known combination of agents that increases the intracellular cyclic AMP content of NG-108-15 cells, caused similar increases in MAO and the MAO B/MAO A ratio in NG108-15 cells, suggesting that the activity and expression of MAO B are regulated in a cyclic AMP-dependent manner (Nakano et al., 1985). NCB 20 cells, which are a hybrid of mouse neuroblastoma N18TG-2 and Chinese hamster embryonic brain cells CHB C, had predominantly MAO B activity with a little MAO A activity (Nagatsu et al., 1981). MAO B and MAO A in hybrid NCB 20 cells were determined to be distinct enzyme molecules by peptide mapping (Nakano et al., 1986).

MAO B activity, but not MAO A activity in the brain increases during aging (Fowler et al., 1980). This increase may be due to the increase in the number of glial cells during aging. In the living human brain, MAO B can be detected by positron emission tomography (PET) using deuterium substituted [^{11}C] L-(−)-deprenyl (selegiline) (Fowler et al., 1998). The PET study indicated that MAO levels in the human brain were highest in the basal ganglia and the thalamus, intermediate in the frontal cortex and cingulate gyrus, and lowest in the parietal and temporal cortices and cerebellum. The results of PET confirm post-mortem studies on increases in brain MAO B with age. The whole brain and the cortical regions and the basal ganglia, thalamus, pons, and cerebellum showed an average increase of 7.1 $\pm$ 1.3% per decade. There was also a large variability among subjects in the same age range. Interestingly, inhibition of MAO B was observed by PET study in the brain of smokers (Fowler et al., 1996). Smokers also showed low MAO B in platerets (Olerand, 2004), and are speculated to have a low incidence of PD.

MPTP-induced Parkinsonism and monoamine oxidase B (MAO B)

The discovery of 1-methyl-4-phenyl-1,2,3,6-tetrahydropyridine (MPTP) as the first recognized synthetic neurotoxin that is capable of inducing PD symptoms in humans has greatly contributed to the understanding of the molecular mechanism of sporadic PD. Calne and Langston (1983) reviewed the etiology of PD and pointed out the possibility of involvement of environmental toxic substances as being the important cause of PD, superimposed on a background of slow, sustained neuronal loss due to the process of aging. Humans are highly susceptible to MPTP, and non-human primates are also sensitive to the compound. Various non-primate animals including some strains of the mouse and even the fruit fly Drosophila also show PD-like movement disorder by administration of MPTP. The first human case of PD that appeared after intravenous injection of MPTP as a contaminant of 1-methyl-4-phenyl-piperidine-4-carboxulic acid ethyl ester (meperidine), which is a synthetic heroin, was a 23-year-old chemistry student at Bethesda, MD, USA. He synthesized that meperidine containing MPTP as a by-product and injected it intravenously into himself. L-3,4-Dihydroxyphenylalanine (L-DOPA) to supplement DA in the brain was effective in that patient as in PD patients. Kopin's group at the National Institutes of Health (NIH) identified MPTP in that meperidine preparation and reported the case in 1979 (Davis et al., 1979). Then, in 1983 in California, a group of young drug addicts acutely showed PD-like symptoms after self-administration of street batches of meperidine contaminated by MPTP. Like idiopathic PD, L-DOPA, which supplements DA in the brain as a substrate of aromatic L-amino acid decarboxylase, was an effective cure for the symptoms. These cases were reported by Langston et al. (1983), and since then the molecular mechanism of MPTP-elicited PD and investigation of similar neurotoxins in environment have been extensively studied (for review, see Nagatsu, 1997, 2002b). MPTP is highly lipophilic, and after its systemic injection, it rapidly crosses the blood-brain barrier to enter the brain. Once in the brain, MPTP, which is a pro-neurotoxin, is metabolized to 1-methyl-4-pheny-2,3-dihydro-pyridinium (MPDP+), by MAO B, which is localized in the outer membrane of mitochondria within glial cells. MPDP+ is then probably spontaneously oxidized to 1-methyl-4-phenyl-pyridinium (MPP+), the active PD-producing neurotoxin. MPP+ is then taken up via DA-transporter across the plasma membrane at the nerve terminals of the nigro-striatal DA neurons in the striatum. As acute reactions, MPP+ is taken up into synaptic vesicles from the cytoplasm by vesicular monoamine transporter type 2 (VMAT 2) to release DA from the nerve terminals; it also inhibits and inactivates tyrosine hydroxylase (TH) to decrease DA synthesis. In the chronic phase, MPP+ is transported from the nerve terminals of nigro-striatal DA neurons in the striatum to the cell bodies in the substantia nigra by retrograde axonal flow. MPP+ is also accumulated within the inner mitochondrial membrane, where it inhibits complex I (NADH ubiquinone oxidoreductase), one of the five enzyme complexes of the inner mitochondrial membrane involved in oxidative phosphorylation for ATP fromation, interrupts electron transport, releases reactive oxygen species (ROS) causing oxidative stress, and depletes ATP. Inhibition of mitochondrial complex I opens mitochondrial permeability transition pore, and subsequently triggers apoptotic cell death of the nigro-striatal DA neurons. Thus, MPP+ decreases DA acutely and chronically to produce PD-like symptoms. Oxidation of MPTP to MPP+ by mitochondrial MAO B in glial cells is essential for neurotoxicity, and selegiline as a specific MAO B inhibitor completely prevents the symptom of PD by MPTP. Mitochondrial dysfunction, especially decreased activity of complex I, is confirmed in the nigro-striatal region in the brain in sporadic PD (for review, see Mizuno et al., 1998). However, unlike sporadic PD, Lewy bodies are not observed in the remaining neurons in the substantia nigra in MPTP-induced PD.

Assuming that some MPTP-like neurotoxins in environment may trigger idiopathic PD, endogenous MPTP-like compounds have been investigated in postmortem brains and in the cerebrospinal fluid (CSF) from patients with PD. Two groups of MPTP-like compounds, isoquinolines (IQs) and beta-carbolines, were found in the human brains and CSF from patients with PD.

We found that MPP+ acutely inhibits the TH system in tissue slices of the rat striatum. In screening for various MPTP-like compounds that inhibit the striatal TH system, we found tetrahydroisoquinoline (TIQ) and its derivatives to be active inhibitors (Hirata et al., 1986). Tetrahydroisoquinoline alkaloids were first discovered in the brain as an in vivo metabolite of L-DOPA in humans by Sandler et al. (1973). Various TIQs were found in the brains of patients with PD and in those of non-parkinsonian control patients by gas chromatography/mass spectrometry: TIQ, 1-methyl-TIQ (1-Me-TIQ), N-Me-6,7-$(OH)_2$-TIQ, (N-Me-norsalsolinol), 1,N-$(Me)_2$-6,7-$(OH)_2$-TIQ (N-Me-salsolinol), 1-phenyl-TIQ, N-Me-1-phenyl-TIQ, and 1-benzyl-TIQ (1-Bn-TIQ) (for review, see Nagatsu, 1997, 2002b; Niwa et al., 1993). Exogenously administered TIQ easily crosses the blood-brain barrier and passes into the brain. However, endogenous TIQs in the brain are speculated to be enzymatically synthesized from precursor endogenous monoamines such as phenylethylamine or DA. Only the (R) enantiomer, (R)-N-Me-6,7-$(OH)_2$-TIQ (R-N-Me-salsolinol) is speculated to be enzymatically synthesized in the brain (Naoi et al., 1996). Among these TIQs in the brain, 1,N-$(Me)_2$-6,7-$(OH)_2$-TIQ (N-Me-salsolinol)

(Naoi et al., 1996), N-Me-6,7-$(OH)_2$-TIQ (N-Me-norsalsolinol) (Moser and Koempf, 1992), and 1-Bn-TIQ (Kotake et al., 1995, 1998) have been extensively investigated as probable neurotoxins to cause PD. It was also suggested that some cases of atypical PD in the French West Indies might have a link with the consumption as food of tropical plants that contain Bn-TIQs (Caparros-Lefebvre et al., 1999). Beta-carbolines have structures similar to those of MPTP/MPP+, and may be synthesized in vivo from tryptophan via tryptamine (Collins and Neafsey, 2000; Matsubara, 2000). A neurotoxic 2,9-dimethylated beta-carbonium, 2,9-dimethylated norharman, was found by gas chromatography/mass spectromrtry in CSF in half of the PD patients examined, but was not found in non-PD patients. 1-Trichloromethyl-1,2,3,4-tetrahydro-beta-carboline (TaClo) is another neurotoxic beta-carboline (Bringmann et al., 2000). TaClo can be synthesized in vivo from tryptamine and the synthetic chloral after application of the hypnotic chloral hydrate or after exposure to the widely used industrial solvent trichloroethylene, which is metabolized to chloral (Bringmann et al., 2000). However, since TaClo and the N-methylated derivative had no DA-transporter-mediated neurotoxicity in cultured cells transfected with the human DA-transporter gene, they may not cause neurotoxicity by a mechanism analogous to that of MPTP/MPP+ involving the uptake into DA neurons by DA-transporter.

Like MPTP, the neurotoxicity of 1-Bn-TIQ (Kotake et al., 1998), N-methyl-(R)-salsolinol (Naoi et al., 1996), and beta-carbolines (Collins and Neafsey, 2000; Matsubara, 2000) are suggested to be precursor neurotoxins, and to be protected by MAO B inhibitors. These compounds inhibit complex I to reduce ATP synthesis in agreement with low complex I activity in the brain in PD and may produce ROS.

Rotenone is a naturally occurring, lipophilic compound from the roots of certain plants (Derris species) with the structure not related to amines, and is used as the main component of many insecticides. Rotenone is a specific inhibitor of complex I, and in Lewis rats by the chronic systemic administration causes highly selective degeneration of the nigro-striatal DA neurons with behavioral PD symptoms of hypokinesia and rigidity and with formation of intracytoplasmic inclusions like Lewy bodies, which are mainly composed of alpha-synuclein and a characteristic feature of sporadic PD (Betarbet et al., 2000). The relation of rotenone to MAO B remains to be investigated.

Specific inhibitory activity towards complex I of IQs and beta-carbolines suggests that they might be the possible neurotoxins producing PD. However, the concentrations of IQs and beta-carbolines in postmortem brain and CSF are low (in the order of ng/g tissue), and their in vivo toxicity and clinical significance in human PD remain to be further examined. Also, the question remains; is there any relation between clinical efficacy of MAO B inhibitor L-deprenyl (selegiline) in PD patients, as describes below, and complete prevention of PD symptoms in animal PD-models produced by MPTP- or MPTP-like neurotoxins by the inhibitor?

Clinical efficacy of monoamine oxidase B inhibitors in Parkinson's disease

L-Deprenyl (R-(−)-deprenyl, the generic name selegiline) was the first discovered MAO B specific inhibitor (for review, see Knoll and Magyar, 1972; Knoll, 1980). Selegiline is a suicide inhibitor, i.e., the compound acts as a substrate for the target enzyme MAO B and results in irreversible inhibition (Riederer and Youdim, 1990). Clinical efficacy of the MAO B inhibitor, selegiline, for addition of L-DOPA that supplements deficient DA in PD was first reported by Birkmayer et al. (1985). In a long term (9 years) study of treatment of PD patients with L-DOPA alone or in combination with selegiline, a significant increase of life expectancy in L-DOPA-selegiline group was observed. The results were interpreted as indicating selegiline's ability to prevent or retard the degeneration of striatal DA neurons. This hypothesis was not far fetched since selegiline selectively prevents the degeneration of nigro-striatal DA neurons in animal PD models induced by MPTP, as described above. After the first work on the clinical efficacy of selegiline on Parkinson's disease (Birkmeyer et al., 1985), the Parkinson Study Group in USA (1989) preliminarily reported that the use of selegiline (10 mg per day) delays the onset of disability associated with early, other untreated cases of PD. The Parkinson Study Group (1993) further reported the results of the multicenter controlled clinical trial of Deprenyl and Tocopherol Antioxidative Therapy of Parkinsonism (the "DATATOP" study). Selegiline and tocopherol (vitamin E as an antioxidant) clinical trial from 1987 for 5 years (the US DATATOP study, selegiline momotherapy) suggested that deprenyl (10 mg per day) but not tocopherol (2000 IU per day) dalays the onset of disability associated with early, otherwise untreated PD. However, this remains controversial (Lang and Lees, 2002). Further uncertainty arose in 1995, when a study by the Parkinson's Disease Research Group of the United Kingdom (UK-PDRG) found 57% higher mortality in patients receiving combined selegiline and L-DOPA treatment compared with patients on L-DOPA alone (Lees on behalf of the Parkinson's Disease Research

Group of the United Kingdom, 1995). Other clinical trials have, however, failed to show any increase in mortality and showed neuroprotective effects of selegiline (Counsell, 1998; Olanow and Riederer, 1996; Olanow et al., 1995). Furthermore, another MAO B inhibitor, rasagiline (N-propargyl-R-aminoindan) that is a selsective, irreversible, second-generation MAO B inhibitor, has shown effectiveness in early PD when given as once-daily treatment without dose titration (Parkinson Study Group, 2002). To clarify the role of MAO B inhibitors in the treatment of PD, Ives et al. (2004) did a meta-analysis of data from all published trials, and reported that MAO B inhibitors (selegiline, lazabemide, or rasagiline) with or without L-DOPA, versus placebo, L-DOPA, or both, reduce the need for L-DOPA, and the incidence of motor fluctuations, without substantial side effects or increased mortality. This study supported the efficacy and safety of monotherapy of early PD by MAO B inhibitors such as selegiline.

Molecular mechanism of neuroprotective effects of L-deprenyl (selegiline) against Parkinson's disease

Stimulated by clinical efficacy of selegiline as a MAO B inhibitor for the treatment of early PD as described above, mechanisms of possible neuroprotection by selegiline have been extensively studied. The early hypothesis on the mechanism of clinical efficacy of selegiline in the treatment without or with L-DOPA was the prevention of degradation of DA, which is produced endogenously from tyrosine by TH or from exogenously administered L-DOPA for treatment, by MAO B inhibition (symptomatic effect). However, accumulating results indicate that selegiline may also have neuroprotective effects by several mechanisms that are related or not related to MAO B inhibition.

Neuroprotection due to inhibition of dopamine degradation by MAO B inhibitor selegiline

DA is a common substrate of MAO B and MAO A. However, in PD only MAO B inhibitor is clinically effective. Selegiline may increase the level of DA in the synaptic cleft in the DA nerve endings in the striatum after release from presynaptic terminals by inhibiting MAO B. DA as a substrate of MAO B produces H_2O_2 and 3,4-dihydroxyphenylacetaldehyde as neurotoxic products. However, since presence of MAO activity is not observed in DA neurons (Arai et al., 1998), DA released from DA neurons or produced from exogenously administered L-DOPA in L-DOPA therapy may be oxidized in the outside of DA neurons possibly in glial cells that contain MAO B to produce cytotoxic H_2O_2 and the aldehyde metabolite. Then H_2O_2 may get into the nigro-striatal DA nerons, and may be oxidized to produce cytotoxic oxygen radicals (reactive oxygen species, ROS) by iron presumably catalytically with neuromelanine. Iron accumulates in the DA neurons in the substantia nigra in PD (Dexter et al., 1987; Hirsch et al., 1991; Jellinger et al., 1992; Sofic et al., 1988). ROS may cause lipid membrane peroxidation and finally cell death of DA neurons (Dexter et al., 1993; Youdim et al., 1993). MAO B inhibitors can prevent this neurotoxic process to protect DA neurons.

Another possible mechanism of selegiline related to MAO B inhibition is an amphetamine-like tonic effect due to increased accumulation of phenylethylamine. Phenylethylamine is a good substrate of MAO B and may be produced in glial cells. Phenylethylamine at high concentrations were found in the striatum in the postmortem brain from PD patients treated with selegiline, and may have an endogenous "amphetamine-like activity" to stimulate DA neurons (Gerlach et al., 1992).

Selegiline's neuroprotective mechanism that is not related to MAO B inhibition

It has been known for many years that neuroprotective effects of selegiline can be observed in cell culture experiments at lower concentrations than those for MAO B inhibition, suggesting that selegiline's neuroprotective effects may also be caused by some other mechanisms than MAO B inhibition.

Riederer and Lachenmayer (2003) pointed out the possibility of neuroprotection by selegiline independent from MAO B inhibition by re-examining the clinical studies such as the DATATOP study (1993) based on the half life of selegiline in vivo in humans. In those clinical studies, the efficacy of selegiline was evaluated at the end-point between baseline and the end of the study (14 months including a 2 months wash-out period). Reported data on the half life of seligiline were between about 2–10 days (Gerlach et al., 2003; Youdim and Tipton, 2002) and 40 days (Fowler et al., 1994). Even the slow recovery of MAO B activity as determined by Fowler et al. (1994) would indicate only a 20% recovery of MAO B activity after a 2-week wash-out period and less than 50% recovery after a 4-week period. However, a significant increase in amine neurotransmitter concentrations can only be demonstrated after the MAO activity has been inhibited by at least 80% (Green et al., 1977). Thus a recovery of only 20% of the MAO B activity is already sufficient to prevent an increase in the neurotransmitter concentration. These results would suggest that a safe period of 4 weeks for wash-out of selegiline would be perfectly adequate for avoidance of any residual symptomatic effects by in vivo MAO B inhibition and that the residual efficacy indicates its neuroprotective effectiveness of this class of drugs as a cornerstone of drug development not only for PD but also for neurodegenerative disorders in general (Riederer and Lachenmayer, 2003). In experimental animals selegiline was shown to be protective against the damaging effects of several neurotoxins, including the dopaminergic neurotoxin MPTP and 6-hydroxydopamine (6-OHDA) and the noradrenergic neurotoxin N-(2-chloroethyl)-N-ethyl-2-bromobenzylamine (DSP-4), again suggesting that selegiline may show neuroprotective mechanism of action which is independent of its action on MAO B (Gerlach et al., 1992). Furthermore, selegiline dose-dependently attenuated ethylcholine aziridinium ion-induced memory impairment, and co-administration of selegiline and donepezil, a selective acetylcholinesterase inhibitor, at doses that do not exert efficacy individually, significantly ameliorated scopolamine + p-chlorophenylalanine-induced memory deficits (Takahata et al., 2005a).

There have been several suggestive findings on the molecular mechanism of neuroprotection by MAO B inhibitor selegiline.

First, selegiline and the metabolite desmethylselsegiline stimulated synthesis of neurotrophins, i.e., nerve rrowth factor (NGF), brain- derived neurotrophic factor (BDNF), and glial cell line-derived neurotrophic factor (GDNF), which act for neuroprotection and anti-apoptosis, in cultured mouse astrocytes (Mizuta et al., 2000). Selegiline as well as BDNF showed trophic effects on cultured DA neurons (Kontkanen and Castren, 1999). Besides neuroprotection for DA neurons, in mixed primary cultures of hippocampal neuronal and glial cells, selegiline increased NGF protein content and protected hippocampal neurons from excitotoxic degeneration, suggesting that astrocyte-derived NGF could contribute to the neuroprotective activity (Semkova et al., 1996).

Second, selegiline increased the activity of catalase and Mn-superoxide dismutase (Mn-SOD; SOD 2) in the striatum of 25-week-old rats. In slice cultures, selegiline increased Cu, Zn-superoxide dismutase (Cu, Zn-SOD; SOD 1) and Mn-SOD activities with a maximal effective concentration of 10^{-8} and 10^{-10} M, respectively. Furthermore, selegiline significantly increased glutathione level (Takahata et al., 2005b). Selegiline, at 1 μM or less, induced thioredoxin for protection against oxidative injury caused by MPP + in human SH-SY5Y neroblastoma cells and also in primary neuronal culture of mouse midbrain DA neurons. The redox cycling of thioredoxin may mediate the protective action of selegiline. Thioredoxin at 1 μM increased the expression of mitochondrial proteins Mn-SOD and Bcl-2 supporting cell survival (Andoh et al., 2002). Thus selegiline without modifying MAO B activity may augment the gene induction of thioredoxin leading to elevated expression of anti-oxidative Mn-SOD and anti-apoptotic Bcl-2 protein in the mitochondria for protecting against MPP +-induced neurotoxicity. The induction of thioredoxin was blocked by a protein kinase A (PKA) inhibitor and mediated by a PKA-sensitive phospho-activation of MAP kinase ERK 1/2 and transcription factor c-Myc. Selegiline-induced thioredoxin and associated neuroprotection were concomitantly blocked by the antisense against thioredoxin mRNA (Andoh et al., 2005). These results suggest that selegiline can decrease oxidative stress in the nigro-striatal region by augmenting various anti-oxidant systems.

Third, selegiline was found to alter the cellular poly(ADP-ribosyl)ation response to gamma-irradiation. Because poly(ADP-ribose) formation is catalyzed by the 113-kDa nuclear enzyme poly(ADP-ribose)polymerase 1 (PARP-1), this result suggests that altered cellular PARP-1 activity may contribute to the neuroprotective potential and/or life span extention afforded by selegiline (Brabeck et al., 2003).

Fourth, selegiline and other propargylamines were found to bind to glyceraldehydes-3-phosphate dehydrogenase (GAPDH). The GAPDH binding was associated with decreased synthesis of pro-apoptotic protein, and thus may contribute to neuroprotection (Tatton et al., 2003).

All these results suggest anti-oxidative and anti-apoptotic activity of selegiline, which neuroprotective mechanism may not be related to MAO B inhibition.

Novel MAO B inhibitors as anti-parkinsoian and anti-neurodegenerative drugs

Rasagiline (N-propargyl-1R-aminoindan) is a novel, potent, irreversible MAO B inhibitor designed for use as an anti-perkinsosonian drug. As described above, rasagiline is clinically effective as monotherapy or as an adjunct to L-DOPA for PD (Ives et al., 2004). Youdim et al. (2005) have reported that the neuroprotective activity of rasagiline is associated with the propargylamine moiety, which protects mitochondrial viability and mitochondrial permeability pore by activating Bcl-2 and down-regulating the Bax family of proteins, and that rasagiline processes amyloid precursor protein (APP) into the neuroprotective-neurotrophic soluble APP-alpha by protein kinase C-dependent and mitogen-activated protein kinase-dependent activation of alpha-secretase, and increases expression and proteins of

NGF, GDNF, and BDNF, suggesting its efficacy also in Alzheimer's disease.

Youdim et al. (2004) also reported novel bifunctional drugs targeting MAO inhibition and iron chelation as an approach to neuroprotection in PD and other neurodegenerative diseases. The authors suggest that bi-functional brain penetrable drugs with iron chelating property and MAO inhibitory activity could be the most feasible approach for neuroprotection in neurodegenerative diseases owing to the protection of elevated iron in oxidative stress and also neuroprotective effect by propargylamine moiety.

R-(−)-(Benzofuran-2-yl)-2-propylaminopentane [R-(−)-BPAP], which is a new sensitive enhancer of the impulse propagatin of action potential mediated release of catecholamines and serotonin in the brain (Knoll et al., 1999), was reported to protect apoptosis induced by N-methyl(R)salsolinol, an endogenous DA neurotoxin (Maruyama et al., 2004).

Considering the development of these new neuroprotective drugs, we would be able to expect development of new drugs which are effective against PD, Alzheimer's disease, and various neurodegenerative diseases in preventing or retarding the progress of such diseases.

Neuroprotective effects of MAO B inhibitors and neural growth factors (neurotrophins) and cytokines produced from glial cells in the inflammatory process in Parkinson's disease

Neuroinflammation, especially accompanied by activated microglia in the brain, has been recently noted in PD (for review, see Hirsch et al., 2003; Nagatsu and Sawada, 2005). As the first features of inflammation in PD, McGeer and the collaborators reported an increased number of major histocompatibility complex (MHC) class II antigen [human leukocyte antigen-DR (HLA-DR)]-positive microglial cells in the substantia nigra (McGeer et al., 1988; McGeer and McGeer, 1995). We and other investigators found increased levels of pro-inflammatory cytokines such as tumor necrosis factor (TNF)-alpha (Mogi et al., 1994a), interleukin (IL)-1beta and IL-6 (Mogi et al., 1994b), and decreased levels of neurotrophins such as BDNF and NGF (Mogi et al., 1999a) in the nigro-striatal region of postmortem brains and/or in the ventricular or lumber cerebrospinal fluid (CSF) from patients with sporadic PD, and in animal models, such as MPTP- and 6-hydroxydopamine-induced PD (for review, see Mogi and Nagatsu, 1999b; Nagatsu et al., 1999, 2000a, b; Nagatsu, 2002a). These changes in cytokine and neurotrophin levels may be initiated by activated microglia, which may then proceed to apoptotic cell death and subsequent phagocytosis of DA neurons.

Cytokines such as IL-6, Il-1beta, or TNF-alpha are pleiotropic factors, and promote signals that either exert neuroprotective effects or neurotoxic effects leading to cell death. Neurotrophins such as BDNF and GDNF are strongly neuroprotective for DA neurons. In order to address the question as to whether microglia activation is neurotoxic or neuroprotective in vivo in PD, we examined activated microglia in the autopsy brain from patients with PD by immunohistochemistry using HLA-DR antibody. We (Imamura et al., 2003) found 2 types of activated microglia, one associated with and one without neuronal degeneration: the former was found in the nigro-striatum; and the latter, in the hippocampus and cerebral cortex. We (Imamura et al., 2005) also observed activated microglia in Lewy body disease (LBD), in which neurodegeneration is observed both in the nigro-striatum and hippocampus (Kosaka, 2002), in the nigro-striatum and hippocampus. In normal controls, neuronal loss and activated microglia were not observed in the hippocampus, and neurons were strongly BDNF-positive. In the hippocampus in PD, BDNF-positive neurons were only slightly decreased. In LBD, the number of activated microglia increased more than those in PD, and all neurons were very weakly stained by anti-BDNF. The results suggest activated microglia in the hippocampus to be probably neuroprotective in PD, but in the nigro-striatum to be neurotoxic. As another evidence supporting this hypothesis, two subsets of microglia were isolated from mouse brain by cell sorting: one subset with high production of ROS and the other with no production of ROS. On the other hand, Sawada with coworkers found that a neuroprotective microglia clone in a co-culture experiment converted to a toxic microglia clone by transduction of the HIV-1 Nef protein with increasing NADPH oxidase activity (Vilhardt et al., 2002). Based on these results, we speculate that activated microglia may change in vivo from neuroprotective to neurotoxic subsets as degeneration of DA neurons in the substantia nigra progresses in PD and that the cytokines from activated microglia in the substantia nigra and putamen may be, at least initially, neuroprotective, but then become neurotoxic during the progress of PD (Sawada et al., 2005).

Another interesting question is the possible interrelationship between familial PD and neuroinflammation. Recent discoveries of the causative genes of familial PD (PARK), starting from discoveries of alpha-synuclein in PARK 1 (Polymeropoulos et al., 1997) and parkin in PARK 2 (Kitada et al., 1998) gave a fresh insight to the molecular mechanism of sporadic PD (for review, see Cookson,

2005). Although the function of alpha-synuclein is not yet clear, alpha-synuclein is a main component of cytoplasmic inclusions called Lewy bodies, which are frequently observed in the residual DA neurons in the substantia nigra in PD. The term Lewy body disease (LBD) is proposed by Kosaka (2002) for neurodegenerative diseases with intracellular Lewy bodies. The parkin gene encodes a ubiquitin ligase E3 (Shimura et al., 2000), and the mutated parkin gene results in a faulty ubiquitin-proteasome system. Since misfolded or unfolded proteins in cells are normally degraded by the ubiquitine-proteasome system, dysfunction of the ubiquitine-proteasome system causes accumulation of misfolded proteins, suggesting that PD as well as other neurodegenerative diseases such as LBD and Alzheimer's disease may also be "protein-misfolding diseases". A puzzling question is that Lewy bodies are not observed in PARK 2. Misfolded substrate proteins of parkin accumulated by loss of function, such as Pael receptor (parkin-associated endothelin receptor-like receptor), which is rich in the nigral region, may accumulate in the endoplasmic reticulum (ER) and cause ER stress (Imai et al., 2001). Although the molecular link is not completely clear, ER stress may cause oxidative stress as observed in idiopathic PD, and may ultimately trigger the cascade of apoptotic cell death. A causal link is speculated between oxidative stress and neuroinflammation in sporadic and familial PD (Hald and Lotharius, 2005).

In another experiment using a primary mesencephalic neuron-glia co-culture system, aggregated alpha-synuclein activated microglia, and microglial activation enhanced DA neurodegeneration induced by aggregated alpha-synuclein depending on phagocytosis of alpha-synuclein and activation of NADPH oxidase with production of ROS (Zhang et al., 2005). NADPH activation in activated microglia agrees with the concept of toxic change of activated microglia proposed by Sawada and coworkers (Vilhard et al., 2002).

In addition to microglia, astrocytes are thought to contribute, although to a lesser extent, to the neurodegenerative process in PD (McNaught and Jenner, 1997). Although astrocytes release neurotrophins or small antioxidants with free radical-scavenging properties (reduced glutathione, ascorbic acid, GDNF, BDNF, NGF, basic fibroblast growth factor (bFGF)), in certain disease conditions they may also produce toxic products such as NO, and pro-inflammatory cytokines (Mena et al., 2002).

Astrocytes contain MAO B (Levitt et al., 1982), but the presence of MAO B in microglia has not been examined yet.

The interrelationship between neuroinflamation and the neuroprotective effects of MAO B inhibitors remains to be further elucidated. However, since selegiline, a MAO B inhibitor, increases the production of neurotrophins like BDNF and NGF probably from glial cells, MAO B inhibitors would be expected to prevent the progress of toxic injury by activated toxic microglia or astrocytes and also the progress of the inflammatory process in PD.

Conclusion

MAO, especially MAO B, may play important roles in the pathogenesis of PD. MAO B inhibitors such as selegiline and rasagiline have been shown to prevent the progress of PD either in combination with L-DOPA or alone (monotherapy). Further study on the mechanism of neuroprotection by MAO B inhibitors would contribute both to elucidation of molecular mechanism of PD and to the development of new neuroprotective drugs against PD which could prevent the onset and progress of PD. Such drug development would also be useful not only against PD but also against Alzheimer's disease and other neurodegenerative diseases.

Aknowledgements

We dedicate this paper to Prof. Dr. Moussa Youdim in celebrating his great contribution to basic research on MAO and PD and to development of MAO B inhibitors as new drugs, which are expected to have neuroprotective efficacy to PD, Alzheimer's disease, and other neurodegenerative diseases.

We are grateful to our collaborators in the study of cytokines and microglia in PD: Drs. M. Mogi (Aichi Gakuin University), K. Imamura (Okazaki City Hospital), Y. Hashizume (Aichi Medical University), and Peter Riederer (Wuerzburg University, Wuerzburg), and their collaborators.

References

Abell CW, Kwan SW (2001) Molecular characterization of monoamine oxidase A and B. Prog Nucleic Acid Mol Biol 65: 129–156

Andoh T, Chock PB, Chiueh CC (2002) The roles of thioredoxin in protection against oxidative stress-induced apoptosis in SH-SY5Y cells. J Biol Chem 277: 9655–9660

Ando T, Chock PB, Murphy DL, Chiueh CC (2005) Role of the redox protein thioredoxin in cytoprotective mechanism evoked by (−)-deprenyl. Mol Pharmacol on line publication: 12 August 2005

Arai R, Kimura H, Nagatsu I, Maeda T (1997) Preferential localization of monoamine oxidase type A in neurons of the locus coeruleus and type B activity in neurons of the dorsal raphe nucleus of the rat: a detailed enzyme histochemical study. Brain Res 745: 352–356

Arai R, Horiike K, Hasegawa Y (1998) Dopamine-degrading activity of monoamine oxidase is not detected by histochemistry in neurons of the substantia nigra pars compacta. Brain Res 812: 275–278

Bach AWJ, Lan NC, Johnson DL, Abell CW, Bembenek ME, Kwan SW, Seeburg PH, Shih JC (1988) cDNA cloning of human liver monoamine oxidase A and B: Molecular basis of differences in enzymatic properties. Proc Nat Acad Sci USA 85: 4934–4938

Berry MD, Juorio AV, Peterson IA (1994) The functional role of monoamine oxidase A and B in the mammalian central nervous system. Progr Neurobiol 42: 375–391

Betarbet R, Sherer TB, Mackenzie G, Garcia-Osuna M, Panov AV, Greenamyre JT (2000) Chronic systemic pesticide exposure reproduces features of Parkinson's disease. Nat Neurosci 3: 1301–1306

Binda C, Mattevi A, Edmondson DE (2002a) Structure-function relationship in flavoenzyme-dependent amine oxidase. J Biol Chem 277: 23973–23976

Binda C, Newton-Vinson P, Hubalek F, Edmondson DE, Mattevi A (2002b) Structure of human monoamine oxidase B a drug turget for the treatment of neurological disorders. Nat Struct Biol 9: 22–26

Birkmayer W, Knoll J, Riederer P, Youdim MBH, Hars V, Marton J (1985) Increased life expectancy resulting from addition of L-deprenyl to madopar® treatment in Parkinson's disease: a longterm study. J Neural Transm 64: 113–127

Bond PA, Cundall RL (1977) Properties of monoamine oxidase (MAO) in human blood platelets, plasma, lymphocytes and granulocytes. Clin Chim Acta 80: 317–326

Brabeck C, Pfeiffer R, Leake A, Beneke S, Meyer R, Buerkle A (2003) L-Selegiline potentiates the cellular poly(ADP-ribosyl)ation: Response to ionized radiation. J Pharmacol Exper Ther 306: 973–979

Bringmann G, Brueckner R, Muenchbach M, Feineis D, God R, Wesemann W, Grote C, Herderich M, Diem S, Lesch KP, Moessner R, Storch A (2000) "TaClo", a chloral-derived mammalian alkaloid with neurotoxic properties. In: Storch A, Collins MA (eds) Neurotoxic factors in Parkinson's disease and related disorders. Kluwer Academic Publishing/Plenum, New York, pp 145–149

Calne DB, Langston JW (1983) Aetiology of Parkinson's disease. Lancet 2: 1457–1459

Caparros-Lefebvre D, Elbaz A, The Caribbean Parkinsonism Study Group (1999) Possible relation of atypical parkinsonism in French West Indies with consumption of tropical plants: A case-control study. Lancet 354: 281–285

Cesura AM, Gottowik J, Lang G, Malherbe P, Da Prada MJ (1998) Structure-function relationships of mitochondrial monoamine oxidase A and B: chimaeric enzymes and site-directed mutagenesis studies. J Neural Transm [Suppl 52]: 189–2000

Chen ZY, Hotamisligil GS, Huang JK, Wen L, Ezzeddine D, Aydin-Muderrisoglu N, Powell JF, Huang H, Brealfield XO, Craig I, Hsu YPP (1991) Structure of the human gene for monoamine oxidase type A. Nucleic Acids Res 19: 4537–4541

Chen ZY, Powell JF, Hsu YPP, Breakfield XO, Craig IW (1992) Organization of the human monoamine oxidase genes and long-range physical mapping around them. Genomics 14: 75–82

Chen K, Wu HF, Shih JC (1993) The deduced amino acid sequences of human platelet and frontal cortex monoamine oxidase B are identical. J Neurochem 61: 187–190

Chen K, Shih JC (1998) Monoamine oxidase A and B: structure, function, and behavior. Adv Pharmacol 42: 292–296

Collins GGS, Sandler M, Williams ED, Youdim MBH (1970) Multiple forms of human brain mitochondrial monoamine oxidase. Nature 225: 817–820

Collins MA, Neafsey EJ (2000) Beta-carboline analogues of MPP+ as environmental neurotoxins. In: Storch A, Collins MA (eds) Neurotoxic factors in Parkinson's disease and related disorders. Kluwer Academic Publishing/Plenum, New York, pp 115–130

Cookson MR (2005) The biochemistry of Parkinson's disease. Ann Rev Biochem 74: 29–52

Counsell C (1998) Effect of adding selegiline to levodopa in early, mild Parkinson's disease: formal systematic review of data on patients in all relevant trials is required. Brit Med J 317: 1586

Davis GCB, Williams AC, Markey SP, Ebert MH, Caine ED, Reichert CM, Kopin IJ (1979) Chronic parkinsonism secondary to intravenous injection of meperidine analogues. Psychiatry Res 1: 249–254

Dexter DT, Wells FR, Agid F, Agid Y, Lees AJ, Jenner P, Marsden CD (1987) Increased nigral iron content in postmortem parkinsonian brain. Lancet: 1219–1220

Dexter DT, Sian J, Jenner P, Marsden CD (1993) Implicatios of alterations in trace element levels in brain in Parkinson's disease and other neurological disorders affecting the basal ganglia. In: Narabayashi H, Nagatsu T, Yanagisawa N, Mizuno Y (eds) Parkinson's disease: From basic research to treatmant. Adv Neurol Vol. 60, Raven Press, New York, pp 273–281

Donnelly CH, Richelson E, Murphy DL (1976) Properties of monoamine oxidase in mouse neuroblastoma NIE-115 cells. Biochem Pharmacol 25: 1639–1643

Donnelly CH, Murphy DL (1977) Substrate and inhibitor-related characteristics of human platelet monoamine oxidase. Biochem Pharmacol 26: 853–858

Edmondson DE, Binda C, Mattevi A (2004) The FAD binding sites of human monoamine oxidases A and B. Neuro Toxicology 25: 63–72

Egashira T, Yamanaka Y (1981) Further studies on the synthesis of A-form of MAO. Jap J Pharmacol 31: 763–770

Fowler CJ, Wiberg A, Oreland L, Marcusson J, Winblad B (1980) The effect of age on the activity and molecular properties of human brain monoamine oxidase. J Neural Transm 49: 1–20

Fowler JS, Volkow ND, Logan J, Wang GJ, MacGregor RR, Schlyer Christian D, Wolf AP, Pappaas N, Alexoff D, Shea C, Dorfinger E, Kruchowy L, Yoo K, Fazzini E, Patlak C (1994) Slow recovery of human brain MAO-B after deprenyl (selegiline withdrawal). Synapse 18: 86–93

Fowler JS, Volkow ND, Wang GJ, Pappas N, Logan J, MacGregor RR (1996) Inhibition of MAO B in the brain of smokers. Nature 379: 733–735

Fowler JS, Volkow ND, Wang GJ, Pappas N, Shea C, MacGregor RR (1998) Visualization of monoamine oxidase in human brain. Adv Pharmacol 42: 304–307

Gerlach M, Riederer P, Youdim MBH (1992) The molecular pharmacology of L-deprenyl. Eur J Pharmacol 226: 97–108

Gerlach M, Reichnmann H, Riederer P (2003) Die Parkinson-Krankheit. Grundlagen, Klinik, Therapie, 3rd edn. Springer, Wien New York

Gomes B, Naguwa G, Kloepfer HG, Yasunobu KT (1969) Amine oxidase XV. The sulfhydryl groups of beef liver mitochondrial amine oxidase. Arch Biochem Biophys 132: 28–33

Green AR, Mitchell BD, Tordoff AF, Youdim MBH (1977) Evidence for dopamine deamination by both type A and type B monoamine oxidase in rat brain in vivo and for the degree of inhibition of enzyme necessary for increased functional activity of dopamine and 5-hydroxytryptamine. Br J Pharmacol 60: 343–349

Grimsby J, Lan NC, Neve R, Chen K, Shih JC (1990) Tissue distribution of human monoamine oxidase A and B mRNA. J Neurochem 55: 1166–1169

Grimsby J, Chen K, Wang LJ, Lan NC, Shih JC (1991) Human monoamine oxidase A and B genes exhibit identical exon-intron organization. Proc Nat Acad Sci USA 88: 3637–3641

Hald A, Lotharius J (2005) Oxidative stress and inflammation in Parkinson's disease: Is ther a causal link? Exper Neurol 193: 279–290

Harada M, Nagatsu T (1969) Identification of flavin in the purified beef liver mitochondrial monoamine oxidase. Experientia 25: 538–534

Harada M, Mizutani K, Nagatsu T (1971) Purification and properties of mitochondrial monoamine oxidase in beef brain. J Neurochem 18: 559–569

Hawkins M Jr, Breakfield XO (1978) Monoamine oxidase A and B in cultured cells. J Neurochem 30: 1391–1397

Hida T, Hasegawa Y, Arai R (1999) Histochemical study of dopamine-degrading monoamine oxidase activity in dopaminergic neurons of rat brain. Brain Res 842: 491–495

Hirata Y, Sugimura H, Takei H, Nagatsu T (1986) The effects of pyridinium salts, structurally related compounds of 1-methyl-4-phenylpyridinium ion (MPP+), on tyrosine hydroxylation in rat striatal tissue slices. Brain Res 397: 341–344

Hirsch EC, Brandel JP, Galle P, Javoy-Agid F, Agid Y (1991) Iron and alminum increase in the substantia nigra of patients with Parkinson's disease: an X-ray microanalysis. J Neurochem 56: 446–451

Hirsch EC, Breidert T, Rousselet E, Hunot S, Hartmann A, Michel PP (2003) The role of glial reaction and inflammation in Parkinson's disease. Ann NY Acad Sci 991: 214–228
Hornykiewicz O (2001) Dopamine and Parkinson's disease: A possible personal view of the past, the present, and the future. In: Calne D, Calne SM (eds) Parkinson's disease. Adv Neurol Vol. 86, Lippincott Williams & Wilkins, Philadelphia, pp 1–11
Hsu YP, Weyler W, Chen S, Sims KB, Rinehart WB, Utterback MC, Powell JF (1988) Structural features of human monoamine oxidase A elucidated from cDNA and peptide sequences. J Neurochem 51: 1321–1324
Imai Y, Soda M, Inoue H, Hattori N, Mizuno Y, Takahashi R (2001) An unfolded putative transmembrane polypeptide, which can lead to endoplasmic reticulum stress, is a substrate of parkin. Cell 105: 891–902
Imamura K, Nishikawa N, Sawada M, Nagatsu T, Yoshida M, Hashizume Y (2003) Distribution of major histocompatibility complex class II-positive microglia and cytokine profile of Parkinson's disease brains. Acta Neuropathol 106: 518–526
Imamura K, Hishikawa N, Ono K, Suzuki H, Sawada M, Nagatsu T, Yoshida M, Hashizume Y (2005) Cytokine production of activated microglia and decrease in neurotrophic factors of neurons in the hippocampus of Lewy body disease brains. Acta Neuropatholo 109: 141–150
Ito A, Kuwahara T, Inadome S, Sagara Y (1988) Molecular cloning of a cDNA for rat liver monoamine oxidase B. Biochem Biophys Res Commun 157: 970–976
Ives NJ, Stowe RL, Marro J, Counsell C, Macleod A, Clarke CE, Gray R, Wheatley K (2004) Monoamine oxidase type B inhibitors in early Parkinson's disease: meta-analysis of 17 randomised trials involving 3525 patients. BMJ 329: 593–559
Jahung JW, Houpt TA, Wessel TC, Chen K, Shih JC (1997) Localization of monoamine oxidase A and B mRNA in the rat brain by in situ hybridization. Synapse 25: 30–36
Jellinger K, Kienzl E, Rumpelmair G, Riederer P, Stachelberger H, Ben-Shachar D, Youdim MBH (1992) Iron-melanin complex in substantia nigra of parkinsonian brains: an X-ray microanalysis. J Neurochem 59: 1168–1171
Johnston JP (1968) Some observations upon a new inhibitor of monoamine oxidase in brain tissue. Biochem Pharmacol 17: 1285–1287
Kitada T, Asakawa S, Hattori N, Matsumine H, Yamamura Y, Minoshima S, Yokochi M, Mizuno Y, Shimizu N (1998) Mutations in the parkin gene cause autosomal recessive juvenile parkinsonism. Nature 392: 605–608
Kitahama K, Maeda T, Denney RM, Jouvet M (1994) Monoamine oxidase: distribution in the cat brain studied by enzyme- and immunohistochemistry: recent progress. Progr Neurobiol 42: 53–78
Knoll J (1980) Monoamine oxidase chemistry and pharmacologly. In: Sandler M (ed) Enzyme inhibitors as drugs. Macmillan, London, pp 151–173
Knoll J, Magyar K (1972) Some puzzling pharmacological effect of monoamine oxidase inhibitors. Adv Biochem Psychopharmacol 5: 393–408
Knoll J, Yoneda F, Knoll B, Ohde H, Mikulia I (1999) (−)1-(Benzofuran-2-yl)-2-propylaminopentane, [(−)BPAP], a selective enhancer of the impulse propagation mediated release of catecholamines and serotonin in the brain. Brit J Pharmacol 128: 1723–1732
Kochersperger LM, Parker EL, Siciliano M, Darlington GJ, Denney RM (1986) Assignment of genes for human monoamine oxidase A and B to the X chromosomes. J Neurosci Res 16: 601–616
Konradi C, Svoma E, Jellinger K, Riederer P, Denney R, Thibault J (1988) Tipographic Immunocytochemical mapping of monoamine oxidase-A, monoamine oxidase-B and tyrosine hydroxylase in human post mortem brain stem. Neuroscience 26: 791–802
Konradi C, Kornhuber J, Froelich L, Fritze J, Heisen H, Beckmann H, Schultz E, Riederer P (1989) Demonstration of monoamine oxidase-A and -B in the human brainstem by a histochemical technique. Neuroscience 33: 383–400
Kontkanen O, Castren E (1999) Trophic effects of selegiline on cultured dopaminergic neurons. Brain Res 829: 190–192
Kotake Y, Tasaki Y, Makino Y, Ohta S, Hirobe M (1995) 1-Benzyl-1,2,3,4-tetrahydroisoquinoline as a parkinsonism-inducing agent: A novel endogenous amine in mouse brain and parkinsonian CSF. J Neurochem 65: 2633–2636
Kotake Y, Tasaki Y, Hirobe M, Ohta S (1998) Deprenyl decreases an endogenous parkinsonism-inducing compound, 1-benzyl-1,2,3,4-tetrahydroisoquinoline, in mice: In vivo and in vitro studies. Brain Res 787: 341–343
Kosaka K (2002) Lewy body disease. Neuropathol 20 [Suppl]: 73–78
Kwan SW, Abell CW (1992) cDNA cloning and sequencing of rat monoamine oxidase A: comparison with the human and bovine enzymes. Comp Biochem Physiol 102B: 143–147
Lan NC, Heinzmann C, Gal A, Klisak I, Orth U, Lai E, Grimsby J, Sparkes RS, Mohandas T, Shih JC (1989) Human monoamine oxidase A and B genes map to Xp11.23 and are deleted in a patient with Norrie Disease. Genomics 4: 552–559
Lang AE, Lees AJ (2002) MAO-B inhibitors for the treatment of Parkinson's disease. Mov Disord 17 [Suppl 4]: S38–S44
Langston JW, Ballard P, Tetrud JW, Irwin I (1983) Chronic parkinsonism in humans due to a product of meperidine-analog synthesis. Science 219: 979–980
Lees AJ on behalf of the Parkinson's Disease Research Group of the United Kingdom (1995) Comparison of therapeutic effects and mortality data of levodopa and levodopa combined with selegiline in patients with early mild Parkinson's disease. Brit Med J 311: 1602–1607
Leonard N, Lambert C, Depiereux E, Wouters J (2004) Modeling of human monoamine oxidase A: from low resolution threading models to accurate comparative models based on crystal structures. NeuroToxicology 25: 47–61
Levitt P, Pinter JE, Breakefield XO (1982) Immunocytochemical demonstration of monoamine oxidase B in brain astrocytes and serotonergic neurons. Proc Natl Acad Sci USA 79: 6385–6389
Levy ER, Powell JF, Buckle VJ, Hsu YP, Breakfield XO, Graig IW (1989) Localization of human monoamine oxidase-A gene to Xp11.23-11.4 by in situ hybridization: implication for Norrie disease. Genomics 5: 368–370
Luque JM, Kwan SW, Abell CW, Da Prada M, Richards GJ (1995) Cellular expression of mRNAs encoding monoamine oxidase A and B in the rat central nervous system. J Comp Neurol 363: 665–680
Luque JM, Biou V, Nicholls JG (1998) Three-dimensional visualization of the distribution, growth, and regeneration of monoaminergic neurons in whole mounts of immature mammalian CNS. J Compar Neurol 390: 427–438
Maruyama W, Yi H, Takahashi T, Shimazu S, Ohde H, Yoneda F, Iwase K, Naoi M (2004) Neuroprotective function of R-(−)-1-(benzofuran-2-yl)-2-propylaminopentane, [R-(−)-BPAP], against apoptosis induced by N-methyl(R)salsolinol, an endogenus dopaminergic neurotoxin, in human dopaminergic neuroblastoma SH-SY5Y cells. Life Sci 75: 107–117
Matsubara K (2000) N-Methyl-beta-carbonium neurotoxins in Parkinson's disease. In: Storch A, Collins MA (eds) Neurotoxic factors in Parkinson's disease and related disorders. Kluwer Academic Publishing/Plenum, New York, pp 131–143
McGeer PL, Itagaki S, Boyes BE, McGeer EG (1988) Reactive microglia are positive for HLA-DR in the substantia nigra of Parkinson's disease and Alzheimer's disease brain. Neurology 38: 1285–1291
McGeer PL, McGeer EG (1995) The inflammatory response system of brain: implications for therapy of Alzheimer and other neurodegenerative diseases. Brain Res Rev 21: 195–218
McNaught KS, Jenner P (1997) Altered glia function causes neuronal death and increases neuronal susceptibility to 1-methyl-4-phenylpyridinium-

and 6-hydroxydopamine-induced toxicity in astrocytic/ventral mesencephalic co-cultures. J Neurochem 73: 2469–2476

Mena MA, de Bernardo S, Casarejos MJ, Canals S, Rodriguez-Martin E (2002) The role of astroglia on the survival of dopamine neurons. Mol Neurobiol 25: 245–263

Minamiura N, Yasunobu KT (1978) Bovine liver monoamine oxidase. A modified purification procedure and preliminary evidence for two subunits and one FAD. Arch Biochem Biophys 189: 481–489

Mizuno Y, Hoshino H, Ikebe S, Hattori N, Kobayashi T, Shimoda-Matsubayashi S, Matsumine H, Kondo T (1998) Mitochondrial dysfunction in Parkinson's disease. Ann Neurol 44 [Suppl 1]: S99–S109

Mizuta I, Ohta M, Ohta K, Nishimura M, Mizuta E, Hayashi K, Kuno S (2000) Selegiline and desmethylselegiline stimulate NGF, BDNF, and GDNF synthesis in cultured mouse astrocytes. Biochem Biophys Res Commun 279: 751–755

Mogi M, Harada M, Kiuchi K, Kojima K, Kondo T, Narabayashi H, Rausch D, Riederer P, Jellinger K, Nagatsu T (1988) Homospecific activity (activity per enzyme protein) of tyrosine hydroxylase increases in Parkinsonian brain. J Neural Transm 72: 77–81

Mogi M, Harada M, Riederer P, Narabayashi H, Fujita K, Nagatsu T (1994a) Tumor necrosis factor-alpha (TNF-alpha) increases in the brain and in the cerebrospinal fluid from parkinsonian patients. Neurosci Lett 165: 208–210

Mogi M, Harada M, Kondo T, Riederer P, Inagaki H, Minami M, Nagatsu T (1994b) Interleukin-1beta, interleukin-6, epidermal growth factor and transforming growth factor-alpha are elevated in the brain from parkinsonian patients. Neurosci Lett 180:147–150

Mogi M, Togari A, Kondo T, Mizuno Y, Komure O, Kuno S, Ichinose H, Nagatsu T (1999a) Brain-derived growth factor and nerve growth factor concentrations are decreased in the substantia nigra in Parkinson's disease. Neurosci Lett 270: 45–48

Mogi M, Nagatsu T (1999b) Neurotrophins and cytokines in Parkinson's disease. In: Stern G (ed) Parkinson's disease: Adv Neurol Vol. 80, Lippincott Williams & Wilkins, Philadelpha, pp 135–139

Moser A, Koempf D (1992) Presence of methyl-6,7-dihydroxy-1,2,3,6-tetrarahydroisoquinoline derives of the neurotoxin isoquinoline, in parkinsonian lumbar CSF. Life Sci 50: 1885–1891

Murphy DL, Donnelly CH, Richelson E (1976) Substrate and inhibition-related characteristics of monoamine oxidase in C6 rat glioma cells. J Neurochem 26: 1231–1235

Nagatsu T (1993) Biochemical aspects of Parkinson's disease. In: Narabayashi H, Nagatsu T, Yanagisawa N, Mizuno Y (eds) Parkinson's disease: From basic research to treatment. Adv Neurol Vol. 60, Raven Press, New York, pp 165–174

Nagatsu T (1997) Isoquinoline neurotoxins in the brain and Parkinson's disease. Neurosci Res 29: 99–111

Nagatsu T (2002a) Parkinson's disease: changes in apoptosis-relating factors suggesting possible gene therapy. J Neural Transm 109: 731–745

Nagatsu T (2002b) Amine-related neurotoxins in Parkinson's disesase: Past, present, and future. Neurotoxicology and Teratology 24: 565–569

Nagatsu T (2004) Progress in monoamine oxidase (MAO) research in relation to genetic engineering. Neuro Toxicology 25: 11–20

Nagatsu T, Nakano T, Kato T, Higashida H (1981) Expression of A and B types of monoamine oxidase in neuroblastoma hybrid cells. Neurochem Int 3: 137–142

Nagatsu T, Mogi M, Ichinose H, Togari A, Riedere P (1999) Cytokines in Parkinson's disease. Neuro Sci News 2: 88–90

Nagatsu T, Mogi M, Ichinose H, Togari A (2000a) Cytokines in Parkinson's disease. J Neural Transm [Suppl 58]: 143–151

Nagatsu T, Mogi M, Ichinose H, Togari A (2000b) Changes in cytokines and neurotrophins in Parkinson's disease. J Neural Transm [Suppl 60]: 277–290

Nagatsu T, Sawada M (2005) Inflammatory process in Parkinson's disease: Role for cytokines. Current Pharmaceutical Design 11: 999–1016

Nakano T, Nagatsu T, Higashida H (1985) Expression of A and B types of monoamine oxidase in differentiated neuroblastoma hybrid cells. J Neurochem 44: 755–759

Nakano T, Saito S, Higashida H, Kojima K, Nagatsu T (1986) Assignment of A and B types of monoamine oxidase in NCB 20 hybrid cells to those of the parental hybrid cells. J Neurochem 46: 686–694

Naoi M, Maruyama Y, Dostert P, Hashizume Y, Nakahara D, Takahashi T, Ota M (1996) Dopamine-derived endogenous 1(R), 2(N)-dimethyl-1,2,3,4-tetrahydroisoquinoline, N-methyl-(R)-salsolinol, induced parkinsonism in rats: Biochemical, pathological and behavioral studies. Brain Res 709: 285–295

Nicotra A, Parvez SH, Glover V, Sandler M, Parvez S, Minami M, eds (2004) Monoamine oxidases: molecular, pharmacological and neurotoxicological aspects, Elsevier, Amsterdam, pp 1–335

Niwa T, Takeda N, Yoshizumi H, Tatematsu A, Yoshida M, Dostert P, Naoi M, Nagatsu T (1993) Presence of tetrahydroisoquinoline-related compounds, possible MPTP-like neurotoxins, in Parkinsonian brain. In: Narabayashi H, Nagatsu T, Yanagisawa N, Mizuno Y (eds) Parkinson's disease: From basic research to treatment. Adv Neurol Vol. 60, Raven Press, New York, pp 234–237

Olanow CW, Hauser RA, Gauger L, Malapira T, Koller W, Hubble J, Bushenbark K, Lilienfeld D, Esterlitz J (1995) The effect of deprenyl and levodopa on the progression of Parkinson's dieease. Ann Neurol 38: 771–777

Olanow CW, Riederer P (1996) Selegiline and neuroprotection in Parkinson's disease. Neurology 47 [Suppl 3]: 137–216

Oleland L (2004) Platelet monoamine oxidase, personality and alcoholism: rise, fall and resurrection. Neuro Toxicology 25: 79–89

Parkinson Study Group (2002) A controlled trial of rasagiline in early Parkinson's disease. Arch Neurol 59: 1937–1943

Pintar JE, Barbosa J, Francke U, Castiglione CM Jr, Hawkins M, Breakfield XO (1981) Gene for monoamine oxidase type A assigned to the human X chromosome. J Neurosci 1: 166–175

Polymeropoulos MH, Lavedan C, Leroy E, Ide SE, Dehejia A, Dutra A, Pike B, Root H, Rubenstein J, Boyer R, Stenroos ES, Chandrasekharappa S, Athanassiadoce A, Papapetropoulos T, Johnson WG, Lazzarini AM, Duvoisin RC, DiIoro G, Globe LI, Nussbaum RL (1998) Mutation in the alpha-synuclein gene idetifies in families with Parkinson's disease. Science 276: 2045–2047

Powell JF, Huang RH, Breakefield XO, Craig I, Hsu YPP (1991) Structure of the human gene for monoamine oxidase type A. Nucleic Acids Res 19: 4537–4541

Riederer P, Youdim MBH, eds (1990) Amine oxidases and their impact on neurobiology. J Neural Transm [Suppl 32]: 1–491

Riederer P, Lachenmayer L (2003) Selegiline's neuroprotective capacity revisited. J Neural Transm 110: 1273–1278

Sandler M, Bonham-Carter S, Hunter KR, Stern GM (1973) Tetrahydroisoquinoline alkaloids: in vivo metabolites of L-DOPA in man. Nature 241: 439–443

Saura J, Richards JG, Mahy N (1994) Age-related changes in MAO in Bl/C57 mouse tissues: a quantitative radioautography study. J Neural Transm 41: 89–94

Sawada M, Imamura K, Nagatsu T (2005) Role of cytokines in inflammatory process in Parkinson's disease. J Neural Transm: in press

Schnaitman C, Erwin VG, Greenwalt JW (1967) The submitochondrial localization of monoamine oxidase. An enzymeatic marker for the outer membrane of rat liver mitochondria. J Cell Biol 32: 719–735

Semkova I, Wolz P, Schilling M, Krieglstein J (1996) Selegiline enhances NGF synthesis and protects central nervous system neurons from excitotoxic and ischemic damage. Eur J Pharmacol 315: 19–30

Shih JC, Chen K, Geha RM (1998) Determination of regions important for monoamine oxidase (MAO) A and B substrate and inhibitor selectivities. J Neural Transm [Suppl 52]: 1–8

Shih JC, Chen JC, Ridd MJ (1999) Monoamine oxidase: from gene to behavior. Ann Rev Neurosci 22: 197–217

Shih JC (2004) Cloning, after cloning, knock-out mice, and physiological functions of MAO A and B. Neuro Toxicology 25: 21–30

Shimura H, Hattori N, Kubo S, Mizuno Y, Asakawa A, Minoshima S, Shimizu N, Iwai K, Chiba T, Tanaka K, Suzuki T (2000) Familial Parkinson disease gene product, parkin, is a ubiquitin-protein ligase. Nature Genet 25: 302–305

Sofic E, Riederer P, Heisen H, Beckmann H, Reynolds GP, Hebenstreit G, Youdim MBH (1988) Incresed iron (III) and total iron content in post mortem substantia nigra of parkinsonian brain. J Neural Transm 74: 199–205

Takahata K, Minami A, Kusumoto H, Schimizu S, Yoneda F (2005a) Effects of selegiline alone or with donepezil on memory impairment in rats. Eur J Pharmacol 518: 140–144

Takahata K, Shimizu S, Katsuki H, Yoneda F, Akaike A (2005b) Effects of selegiline on antioxidant systems in the nigrostriatum in rat. J Neural Transm On-line publication, 15 June 2005

Tatton W, Chalmers-Redman R, Tatton N (2003) Neuroprotection by deprenyl and other propargylamines: glyceraldehydes-3-phosphate dehydrogenase rather than monoamone oxidase B. J Neural Transm 110: 509–515

The Parkinson Study Group (1989) Effects of deprenyl on the progression of disability in early Parkinson's disease. New Engl J Med 321: 1364–1371

The Parkinson Study Group (1993) Effects of tocophrol and deprenyl on the progression of disability in early Parkinson's disease. New Engl J Med 328: 176–183

Tipton KF (1980) Monoamine oxidase. In: Jakoby WB (ed) Enzymatic basis of detoxication Vol. 1. Academic Press, New York, pp 355–370

Tsugeno Y, Hirashiki I, Ogata F, Ito A (1995) Regions of the molecule responsible for substrate specificity of monoamine oxidase A and B: a chimeric enzyme analysis. J Biochem 118: 974–980

Tsugeno Y, Ito A (1997) A key amino acid responsible for substrate selectivity of monoamine oxidase A and B. J Biol Chem 272: 14033–14036

Vilhardt F, Plastre O, Sawada M, Suzuki K, Wiznerowicz M, Kiyokawa E, Trono D, Krause K-H (2002) The HIV-1 Nef protein and phagocyte NADPH oxidase activation. J Biol Chem 277: 42136–42143

Walker WH, Kearney EB, Seng RL, Singer TP (1971) Sequence and structure of a cysteinyl flavin peptide from monoamine oxidase. Biochem Biophys Res Commun 44: 287–292

Westlund KN, Denney RM, Rose RM, Abell CW (1988a) Localization of distinct monoamine oxidase A and monoamine oxidase B in rat brain. J Neural Transm 74: 29–42

Westlund KN, Denney RM, Rose RM, Abell CW (1988b) Localization of distinct monoamine oxidase A and monoamine oxidase B cell populations in human brainstem. Neuroscience 25: 439–456

Weyler W (1989) Monoamine oxidase A from human placenta and monoamine oxidase from bovine liver both have one FAD per subunit. An important revision. Biochem J 260: 726–729

Weyler W, Hsu YPP, Breakefield XO (1990) Biochemistry and genetics of monoamine oxidase. Pharmac Ther 47: 391–417

Willonghby J, Glover V, Sandler M (1988) Histochemical localization of monoamine oxidase A and B in rat brain. J Neural Transm 74: 29–42

Youdim BH, Riederer P (1997) Understanding Parkinson's disease. Sci Amer: 82–89

Youdim MBH, Ben-Shachter D, Eshel G, Finberg JPM, Riederer P (1993) The neurotoxicity of iron and nitric oxide: Relevance to etiology of Parkinson's disease. In: Narabayashi H, Nagatsu T, Yanagisawa N, Mizuno Y (eds) Parkinson's disease: From basic research to treatment. Adv Neurol Vol. 60, Raven Press, New York, 259–266

Youdim MBH, Tipton KF (2002) Rat striatal monoamine oxidase-B inhibition by l-deprenyl and rasagiline: its relationship to 2-phenylethylamine-induced stereotypy and Parkinson's disease. Parkinsonism Relat Disord 8: 247–253

Youdim MBH, Fridkin M, Zheng H (2004) Novel bifunctional drugs targeting monoamine oxidase inhibition and iron chelation as an approach to neuroprotection in Parkinson's disease and other neurodegenerative diseases. J Neural Transm 111: 1455–1471

Youdim MBH, Maruyama W, Naoi M (2005) Neuropharmacological, neuroprotective and amyloid precursor processing properties of selective MAO-B inhibitor antiperkinsonian drug, rasagiline. Drugs of Today 41: on line publication

Zhang W, Wang T, Pei Z, Miller DS, Wu X, Block ML, Wilson B, Zhang W, Zhou Y, Hong J-S, Zhang J (2005) Aggregated alpha-synuclein activates microglia: a process leading to disease progression in Parkinson's disease. FASEB J 19: 533–542

J Neural Transm (2006) [Suppl] 71: 67–77

Journal of
Neural
Transmission
Printed in Austria

Involvement of type A monoamine oxidase in neurodegeneration: regulation of mitochondrial signaling leading to cell death or neuroprotection

M. Naoi[1], W. Maruyama[2], Y. Akao[1], H. Yi[1], Y. Yamaoka[1]

[1] Department of Neurosciences, Gifu International Institute of Biotechnology, Kakamigahara, Gifu, and
[2] Department of Geriatric Medicine, National Institute for Geriatrics and Gerontology, Obu, Aichi, Japan

Summary In neurodegenerative diseases, including Parkinson's and Alzheimer's diseases, apoptosis is a common type of cell death, and mitochondria emerge as the major organelle to initiate death cascade. Monoamine oxidase (MAO) in the mitochondrial outer membrane produces hydrogen peroxide by oxidation of monoamine substrates, and induces oxidative stress resulting in neuronal degeneration. On the other hand, a series of inhibitors of type B MAO (MAO-B) protect neurons from cell death. These results suggest that MAO may be involved in the cell death process initiated in mitochondria. However, the direct involvement of MAO in the apoptotic signaling has been scarcely reported. In this paper, we present our recent results on the role of MAO in activating and regulating cell death processing in mitochondria. Type A MAO (MAO-A) was found to bind an endogenous dopaminergic neurotoxin, *N*-methyl(*R*)salsolinol, and induce apoptosis in dopaminergic SH-SY5Y cells containing only MAO-A. To examine the intervention of MAO-B in apoptotic process, human MAO-B cDNA was transfected to SH-SY5Y cells, but the sensitivity to *N*-methyl(*R*)salsolinol was not affected, even though the activity and protein of MAO-B were expressed markedly. MAO-B oxidized dopamine with production of hydrogen peroxide, whereas in control cells expressing only MAO-A, dopamine autoxidation produced superoxide and dopamine-quinone, and induced mitochondrial permeability transition and apoptosis. Rasagiline and other MAO-B inhibitors prevent the activation of apoptotic cascade and induce prosurvival genes, such as bcl-2 and glial cell line-derived neurotrophic factor, in MAO-A-containing cells. These results demonstrate a novel function of MAO-A in the induction and regulation of apoptosis. Future studies will clarify more detailed mechanism behind regulation of mitochondrial death signaling by MAO-A, and bring out new strategies to cure or ameliorate the decline of neurons in neurodegenerative disorders.

Abbreviations: *β-PEA* β-phenylethylamine, *$DiOC_6(3)$* 3,3′-dihexyloxacarbocyanide iodine, *DMEM* Dulbecco's modified Eagle's medium, *$\Delta\Psi m$* mitochondrial membrane potential, *FACS* fluorescence-augmented flow cytometry, *GAPDH* glyceraldehyde-3-phosphate dehydrogenase, *GDNF* glial cell line-derived neurotrophic factor, *HE* hydroethidine, *HPLC-ECD* high-performance liquid chromatography with electrochemical detection, *5-HT* 5-hydroxytryptamine, serotonin, *MAO-A and MAO-B* type A and B monoamine oxidase, *NMRSal and NMSSal* *N*-methyl(*R*)salsolinol and *N*-methyl(*S*)salsolinol, *mPT* mitochondrial permeability transition, *PBS* phosphate-buffered saline, *PD* Parkinson's disease, *PI* propidium iodide, *RNAi* RNA interference, *ROS* reactive oxygen species, *siRNA* small interfering RNA

Correspondence: M. Naoi, Department of Neurosciences, Gifu International Institute of Biotechnology, 1-1 Naka-fudogaoka, Kakamigahara, Gifu 504-0838, Japan
e-mail: mnaoi@giib.or.jp

In neurodegenerative disorders, including Parkinson's disease (PD) and Alzheimer's disease, selective neurons degenerate in specified brain regions in either apoptotic or necrotic process. In PD, the degeneration of dopamine neurons is observed mainly in the substantia nigra. Understanding of the intracellular mechanism of neurodegeneration has been advanced markedly and in the intrinsic pathway to apoptosis mitochondria initiate death signaling. Oxidative and nitrosactive stress, mitochondrial dysfunction, neurotoxins, excitotoxicity, accumulation of misfolded protein and reduced activity of the ubiquitin-proteasome system activate the death cascade (Götz et al., 1990; Andersen, 2004; Bossy-Wetzel et al., 2004; Naoi et al., 2005). The detailed mechanism underlying the cell death in PD has been studied using animal and cellular models, and we found that dopamine-derived *N*-methyl(*R*)-salsolinol [*N*M*R*Sal, 1(*R*),2(*N*)-dimethyl-6,7-dihydroxy-1,2,3,4-tetrahydroisoquinoline] is an endogenous neurotoxin and causes cell death in dopamine neurons (Naoi et al., 2002a, b, 2004). After continuous infusion in the rat striatum, *N*M*R*Sal induces apoptotic cell death in dopamine neurons in the substantia nigra (Naoi et al., 1996). In human dopaminergic neuroblastoma SH-SY5Y cells, *N*M*R*Sal induced apoptosis by sequential activation of death cascade; decline in mitochondrial membrane potential, $\Delta\Psi$m, opening of mitochondrial permeability transition (mPT) pore, release of cytochrome c, activation of caspase 3, nuclear translocation of glyceraldehydes-3-phosphate dehydrogenase [GAPDH, D-glyceraldehyde-3-phosphate: NAD^+ oxidoreductase (phosphorylating), EC 1.2.1.12], and fragmentation of nuclear DNA (Maruyama et al., 1997, 2001a, b; Akao et al., 2002a). Analyses of clinical samples from parkinsonian patients indicate that *NMR*Sal might be involved in the pathogenesis of PD (Maruyama et al., 1996; Naoi et al., 1998).

The mPT is an increase in the permeability of the inner mitochondrial membrane to solutes, by opening of mPT pore, a large proteinaceous pore spanning the outer and inner membrane of mitochondria (Crompton, 1999; Green and Kroemer, 2004). The mPT pore forms a functional micro-compartment with voltage-dependent anion channel in the outer membrane, adenine nucleotide translocator in the inner membrane, and hexokinase at the contact site, but the exact composition has not yet been fully clarified. The (*R*)-enantiomer of *N*-methylsalsolinol (*N*MSal), but not the (*S*)-enantiomer, induces swelling in mitochondrial matrix (Akao et al., 2002a) and $\Delta\Psi$m reduction in SH-SY5Y cells (Maruyama et al., 2001b). The enantio-selective cytotoxicity of *NMR*Sal suggests the occurrence of the specified binding site recognizing *NMR*Sal in mitochondrial membrane. *NMR*Sal was found to inhibit type A, but not type B, monoamine oxidase [MAO-A and MAO-B, monoamine: oxygen oxidoreducatse (deaminating), EC 1.4.3.4]. The inhibition was competitive to the substrate, and the value of the inhibitor constant, K_i, was estimated to be $59.9 \pm 5.4\,\mu$M (mean $\pm$ SD) (Yi et al., 2006b). This suggests that MAO-A may bind *NMR*Sal at or near the substrate-binding site. However, it has never been reported whether MAO is involved directly in apoptotic cascade, or MAO itself is a component of mPT pore.

MAO is localized in the outer membrane of mitochondria and catalyses the oxidative deamination of neuroactive, vasoactive and xenobiotic amines generating hydrogen peroxide and aldehydes. The two MAO isoenzymes, MAO-A and MAO-B, share 70% amino acid sequence identity and are encoded by two closely linked genes in the X chromosome (Bach et al., 1988; Shih et al., 1999). These two isomers have distinct specificities for the substrates and inhibitors (Tipton et al., 2004). MAO-A has substrate preference for 5-hydroxytryptamine (5-HT, serotonin) and norepinephrine, and very high sensitivity to an irreversible inhibitor, clorgyline [*N*-methl-*N*-propargyl-3(2,4-dichlorophenoxy)-propylamine], whereas MAO-B oxidizes β-phenylethylamine (β-PEA) and benzylamine and is inhibited by low concentrations of (−)deprenyl [*N*, α-dimethyl-*N*-2-propynylbenzene-ethanlamine] and rasagiline [*N*-propargl-1(*R*)- aminoindan] (Youdim et al., 2001). In human brain MAO-A is expressed in catecholamine neurons, whereas serotonergic neurons and astrocytes contain MAO-B (Westlund et al., 1988). The studies of MAO-A and MAO-B knockout mice clearly proved that these two MAO isoenzymes have distinct functions in monoamine metabolism and play important roles in neurological and psychiatric disorders, including depression and PD (Cases et al., 1995; Lim et al., 1994; Shih et al., 1999). In human brain MAO-B levels increase 2–3 folds in an age-dependent way, resulting in increased oxidative stress, which may induce vulnerability of the brain in age-dependent neurodegenerative disorders.

A series of MAO-B inhibitors with a propargyl moiety, rasagiline and (−)deprenyl, protect neurons from cell death induced by various insults (Maruyama et al., 2001a; Youdim et al., 2005a, b). Rasagiline is now the most potent in neuro-rescue or -protective function, as shown in animal and cellular models of PD, Alzheimer's disease and brain ischemia, and the neuroprotective effect has been also suggested in clinical trials (Parkinson Study Group, 2004). The anti-apoptotic function is due to the direct stabilization of mPT pore (Maruyama et al., 2001a, 2001b) and induction of prosurvival genes, such as antiapoptotic Bcl-2 and Bcl-xL (Akao et al., 2002a, b) and glial cell line-derived neurotrophic factor (GDNF) (Maruyama et al., 2004). However, the neuroprotective function may not necessarily depend on the inhibition of MAO-B activity, as suggested by the facts that the neuroprotective potency is observed with propargylamines without MAO-inhibition (Maruyama et al., 2001c; Yi et al., 2006a), and at the concentration quite lower than those for MAO inhibition (Akao et al., 2002a; Maruyama et al., 2001a, 2004).

In this paper, the role of MAO in the apoptotic cascade was studied by use of *NMR*Sal in SH-SY5Y cells containing only MAO-A (wild SH), in relation to the *NMR*Sal binding, $\Delta\Psi$M reduction and apoptosis. To confirm the role of MAO-A in apoptotic cascade, the effects of RNA interference (RNAi) targeting MAO was examined by use of small interfering RNA (siRNA) to silence MAO-A in the cells. In addition, the involvement of MAO-B in apoptosis by *NMR*Sal was examined in SH-SY5Y cells transfected with cDNA of human MAO-B (MAO-B-SH). The role of MAO-A and -B in inducing anti-apoptotic genes by rasagiline, a MAO-B inhibitor, was studied by use of these SH cells, and also Caco-2 human colon adenocarcioma cells expressing only MAO-B (Wong et al., 2003). The role of MAO isoenzymes is discussed in relation to the regulation of apoptotic signaling in mitochondria, and their possible involvements in neurodegenerative disorders including PD.

Materials and methods

Materials

*NMR*Sal was synthesized according to Teitel et al. (1972). Kynuramine, 4-quinolinol, dihydroethidine (HE) and dopamine were purchased from Sigma (St. Louis, MO, USA); propidium iodide (PI), MitoTracker Orange and Green, and 3,3′-dihexyloxacarbocyanide iodine [$DiOC_6(3)$] from Molecular Probes (Eugene, OR, USA); 5-hydroxytryptamine (5-HT, serotonin) from Merck (Darmstadt, Germany). Clorgyline, a MAO-A inhibitor, and rasagiline and (−)deprenyl (selegiline), MAO-B inhibitors, were kindly donated by May and Baker (Dagenham, U. K.), TEVA (Netanya, Israel), and Dr. Knoll (Semmellweis University, Budapest, Hungary), respectively. Dulbecco's modified Eagle's medium (DMEM), β-PEA and other drugs were purchased from Nacalai tesque (Kyoto, Japan). SH-SY5Y cells were cultured in Cosmedium-001 tissue culture medium (CosmoBio, Tokyo, Japan) supplemented by 5% fetal calf serum (FCS) in an atmosphere of 95% air-5% CO_2. Mitochondria were prepared according to Desagher et al. (1999). Caco-2 cells were cultured in DMEM supplemented with 10% FCS and 1% nonessential amino acids.

RNAi of MAO-A in SH-SY5Y cells

To reduce MAO-A expression in mitochondria, siRNA targeting MAO-A mRNA (Sc-35874) was purchased from Santa Cruz Biotech (Santa Cruz, CA, USA). The siRNAs were transfected into the cells to be 20–35 nM in the final concentration by use of cationic liposomes TransIT-TKO (Mirus Bio, Madison, WI, USA). The transfection efficiency was evaluated by the transfection of the cells with a duplex siRNA-FITC. Non-specific control duplex (57% GC content; Dharmacon, Lafayette, CO, USA) was used as control for non-specific effects. The effects of RNAi targeting MAO-A on the protein amount and activity of MAO and the binding of *NMR*Sal were determined at 36 h after the transfection. MAO protein was detected by Western blot analyses, using antibody recognizing both MAO-A and -B prepared according to Gargalidis-Moudanos et al. (1997). The polyclonal antisera were isolated from rabbits immunized with the peptide TNGGQ ERKFVGGSGQ, corresponding to amino acids 210–227 in MAO-A and 202–217 in MAO-B, and purified on an affinity column conjugated with the antigen peptide. Bound antibodies were detected using enhanced chemiluminescence detection kit (New England Biolabs, Beverly, MA, USA).

DNA transfection of MAO-B gene in SH-SY5Y cells

To establish transfectants expressing human MAO-B, a pIRES1neo eukaryotic expression vector (Invitrogen, San Diego, CA, USA) was used (Yi et al., 2006b). pIRES1-neo-MAO-B was constructed by including the full-length human MAO-B gene in pECE vector (Lan et al., 1989) and digested with HindIII and inserted into the pIRESneo vector. SH-SY5Y cells were transfected with pIRES1neo or pIRES1neo-MAO-B by using cationic liposomes (Lipofect-AMINE). Selection was started 2 days after the transfection using the culture medium containing geneticin (GIBCO BRL). Individual clones were isolated and characterized by RT-PCR, as described previously (Akao et al., 2002a). Stable clones overexpressing MAO-B protein (MAO-B-SH) were obtained by limiting dilution and confirmed by RT-PCR.

Assay for MAO-A and MAO-B activity

MAO activity in mitochondria was measured fluorometrically by use of kynuramine as a substrate, according to Kraml (1965). Mitochondria prepared from control SH-SY5Y (wild SH) cells were used as a MAO-A sample, and those from MAO-B-SH cells were pre-treated with 1 μM clorgyline at 37°C for 20 min and used as a MAO-B sample. Protein concentration was determined according to Bradford (1976).

Assay for the binding of NMRSal to mitochondria

Mitochondria were suspended in 100 μl of 10 mM Tris-HCl buffer, pH 6.0, and incubated with 10–100 μM *NMR*Sal for 60 min at 4°C. Then, the cells were washed successively with 1.5 ml of phosphate-buffered saline (PBS) containing 1% bovine serum albumin and twice with PBS alone by centrifugation at 6000 *g* for 10 min. The cells were suspended in 200 μl of 10 mM perchloric acid solution containing 0.1 mM EDTA, mixed, centrifuged, filtered through a Millipore HV filter (pore size 0.45 μm), and applied to high-performance liquid chromatography with electrochemical detection (HLC-ECD), as reported previously (Naoi et al., 1996).

Measurement of $\Delta\Psi m$

The effects of *NMR*Sal on $\Delta\Psi$m were quantitatively measured by fluorescence-augmented flow cytometry (FACS) with a FACScaliber 4A and Cell-Quest software (Becton Dickinson, San Jose, CA, USA), and MitoTracker Orange and Green, or 3,3′-dihexylpxacarbocyanide iodine [$DiOC_6(3)$] were used as fluorescent indicators (Yi et al., 2006a, b). The cells were cultured in 6-well poly-L-lysine-coated tissue culture flasks, washed with Cosmedium-001 without FCS, and incubated with 100–500 μM *NMR*Sal or dopamine for 3 h at 37°C. The effects of 5-HT and β-PEA were also examined by addition of 100–500 μM 5-HT and β-PEA. After stained with 100 nM MitoTracker Orange and Green for 30 min at 37°C, or 2.5 nM $DiOC_6(3)$ (Stock solution: 1 μM in ethanol) for 15 min at 37°C. Then, the cells were washed and suspended with PBS and subjected to FACS. The laser emission at 560–640 nm (FL-2) and at shorter than 560 nm (FL-1) with excitation at 488 nm were used for the detection of MitoTracker Orange and Green fluorescence, respectively. $DiO_6(3)$ fluorescence was measured with FL-1.

Assessment of apoptosis induced by NMRSal or dopamine

Apoptosis was quantitatively measured by FACS, as described previously (Yi et al., 2006a). The cells cultured in 6-well poly-L-lysine-coated culture flasks were incubated in DMEM with 100–500 μM *NMR*Sal or 100 μM dopamine at 37°C for 24 h, and treated with trypsin, gathered, and washed with PBS. The cells were stained with 75 μM PI solution in PBS containing 1% Triton X-100 at 24°C for 5 min in the dark, washed and suspended in PBS, then subjected to FACS analysis. Cells with a lower DNA content, as shown by PI staining less than G1, were defined to be apoptotic (subG1 peak) (Eckert et al., 2001).

Rasagiline-induced bcl-2 expression in the cells

Wild SH and MAO-B-SH cells and Caco-2 cells were cultured with 10 μM–10 pM rasagiline overnight and Bcl-2 contents in the cells were quantitatively determined by Western blot analysis as reported (Akao et al., 2002b).

Statistics

Experiments were repeated 3 to 4 times in triplicate, and the results were expressed as the mean and SD. Differences were statistically evaluated by analysis of variance (ANOVA) followed by Sheffe's F-test. A p value less than 0.05 was considered to be statistically significant.

Results

Binding of NMRSal to mitochondrial MAO-A and the effects of siRNA for MAO-A

The binding of *NMR*Sal to mitochondria prepared from control SH-SY5Y (wild SH) cells was kinetically studied

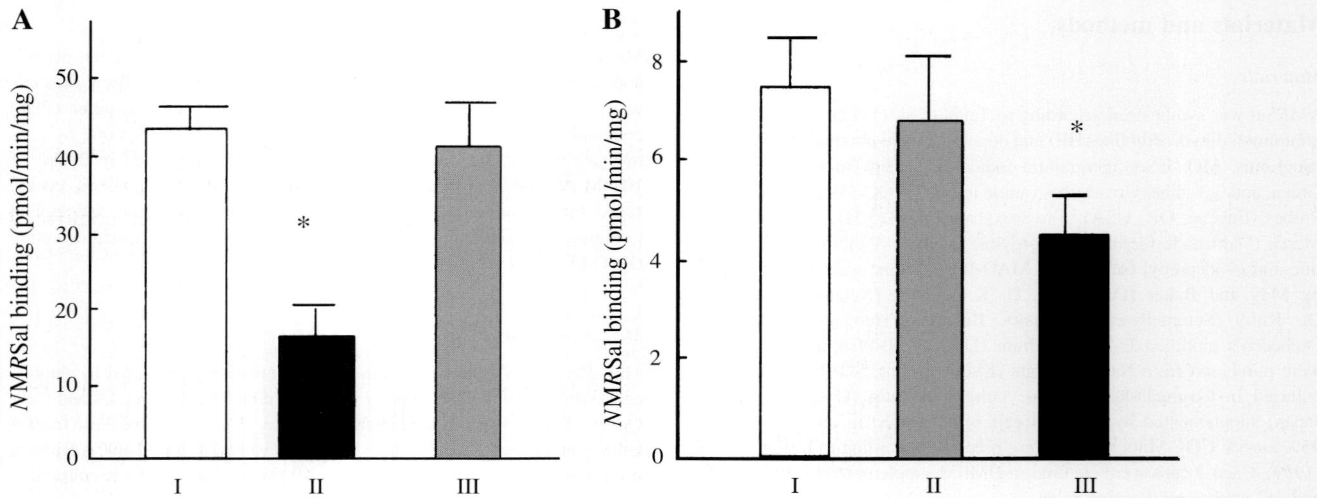

Fig. 1. The effects of MAO-inhibitors and RNAi targeting MAO on *NMR*Sal binding to mitochondria. **A** Effects of clorgyline and (−)deprenyl on the *NMR*Sal binding to mitochondria. Mitochondria were treated with 1 μM MAO inhibitors for 20 min at 37°C, then incubated with 10 μM *NMR*Sal for 1 h at 4°C. The column and bar represent the mean and SD of triplicate measurement of 2 experiments. **B** Effects of MAO-A RNAi. Crude mitochondria were prepared from wild SH (I), negative control (II) and siRNA-treated cells (III), and incubated with *NMR*Sal. *NMR*Sal binding was quantified by HPLC-ECD. The column and bar represent the mean and SD of triplicate measurements. $^{*}p < 0.05$ from control and negative control cells

and the binding kinetics followed the Michaelis-Menten equation. The values of the apparent Michaelis constant, K_m, and the maximal velocity, V_{max}, were obtained to be 80 ± 15 μM and 2.7 ± 0.5 nmol/h/mg protein, respectively. The involvement of MAO in the binding was examined by use of clorgyline and (−)deprenyl, the selective inhibitor of MAO-A and MAO-B, respectively. As shown in Fig. 1A, clorgyline reduced *NMR*Sal binding significantly, but (−)deprenyl did not affect the binding.

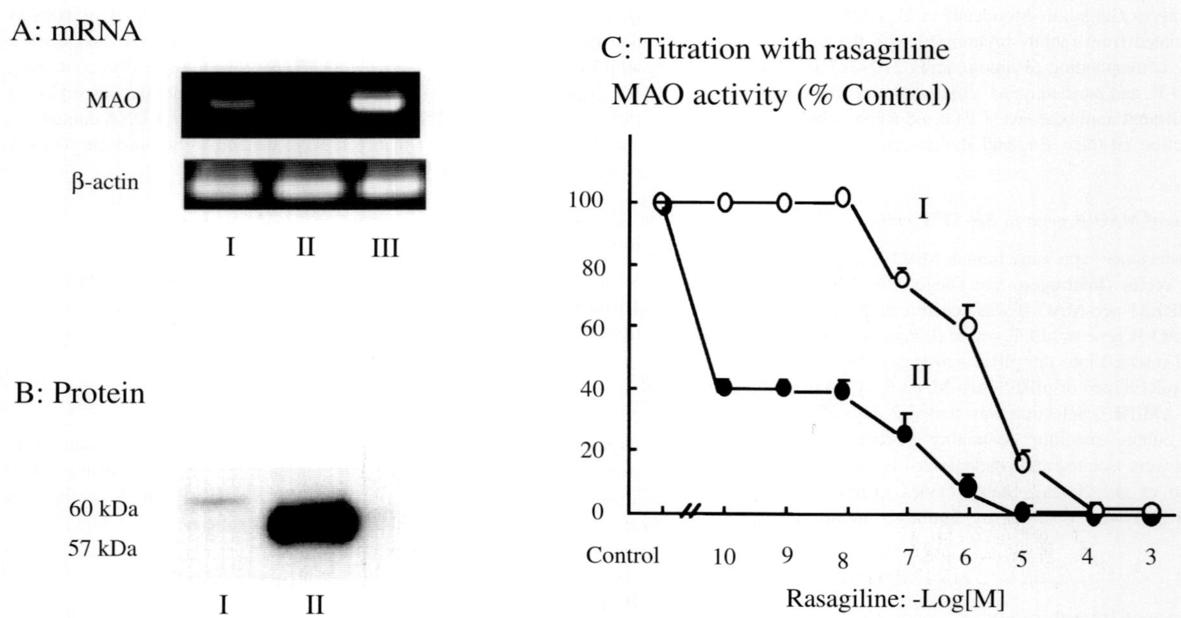

Fig. 2. Establishment of SH-SY5Y cells transfected with human MAO-B. SH-SY5Y cells were transfected with human MAO-B cDNA. **A** mRNA isolated from wild SH cells (I), cells transfected with IRES vector alone (II), and with full length MAO-B cDNA (III). β-Action was used as control. **B** Western blot analyses of MAO protein in mitochondria isolated from wild SH (I) and MAO-B-SH cells (II). MAO protein was detected with the antibody recognizing both MAO-A and -B. **C** Effects of rasagiline, a MAO-B inhibitor, on MAO activity. Mitochondria were prepared from wild SH (I) and MAO-B-SH cells (II), and MAO activities were measured with 100 μM kynuramine as a substrate, after treatment with rasagiline (0.1 nM–1 mM) at 37°C for 20 min. Each point and bar represent the mean and SD of triplicate measurements

In order to confirm whether *NMR*Sal binds to MAO-A in mitochondria, MAO-A expression was inactivated using RNAi. In the siRNA-transfected cells, MAO protein with about 60 kDa was significantly reduced, whereas in non-specific siRNA-transfected cells the protein amount was almost the same as in control. The functional effects of RNAi were confirmed by reduction in MAO activity to 0.22 ± 0.02 nmol/min/mg protein in the siRNA treated-cells from 0.34 ± 0.03 nmol/min/mg protein in control. In non-specific siRNA-transfected cells, the MAO activity was the same as in control, 0.34 ± 0.01 nmol/min/mg protein. Figure 1B shows that RNAi targeting MAO-A markedly reduced *NMR*Sal binding to 4.47 ± 0.88 pmol/mg protein in siRNA-treated cells from 7.46 ± 0.95 and 6.83 ± 1.40 pmol/mg protein in control and non-specific siRNA-treated cells.

Effects of transfected MAO-B on MMRSal binding

To specify the role of MAO-A and -B in the binding of *NMR*Sal and the induction of apoptosis, SH-SY5Y cells transfected with human MAO-B cDNA (MAO-B-SH) were prepared from control cells expressing only MAO-A (wild SH). The expression of mRNA of MAO-B was confirmed in MAO-B-SH cells (Fig. 2A). MAO-A and MAO-B protein in wild SH and MAO-B-SH cells were detected by Western blot analyses and their apparent molecular weights were determined to be approximately 60 and 57 kDa, respectively (Fig. 2B). MAO activity in mitochondria isolated from MAO-B-SH cells increased significantly to be 22.9 ± 0.93 from 2.82 ± 0.18 nmol/min/mg protein in those from wild SH cells. The sensitivity to rasagiline, an irreversible inhibitor of MAO-B, increased by MAO-B transfection, as shown by the inhibitor concentration-ac-

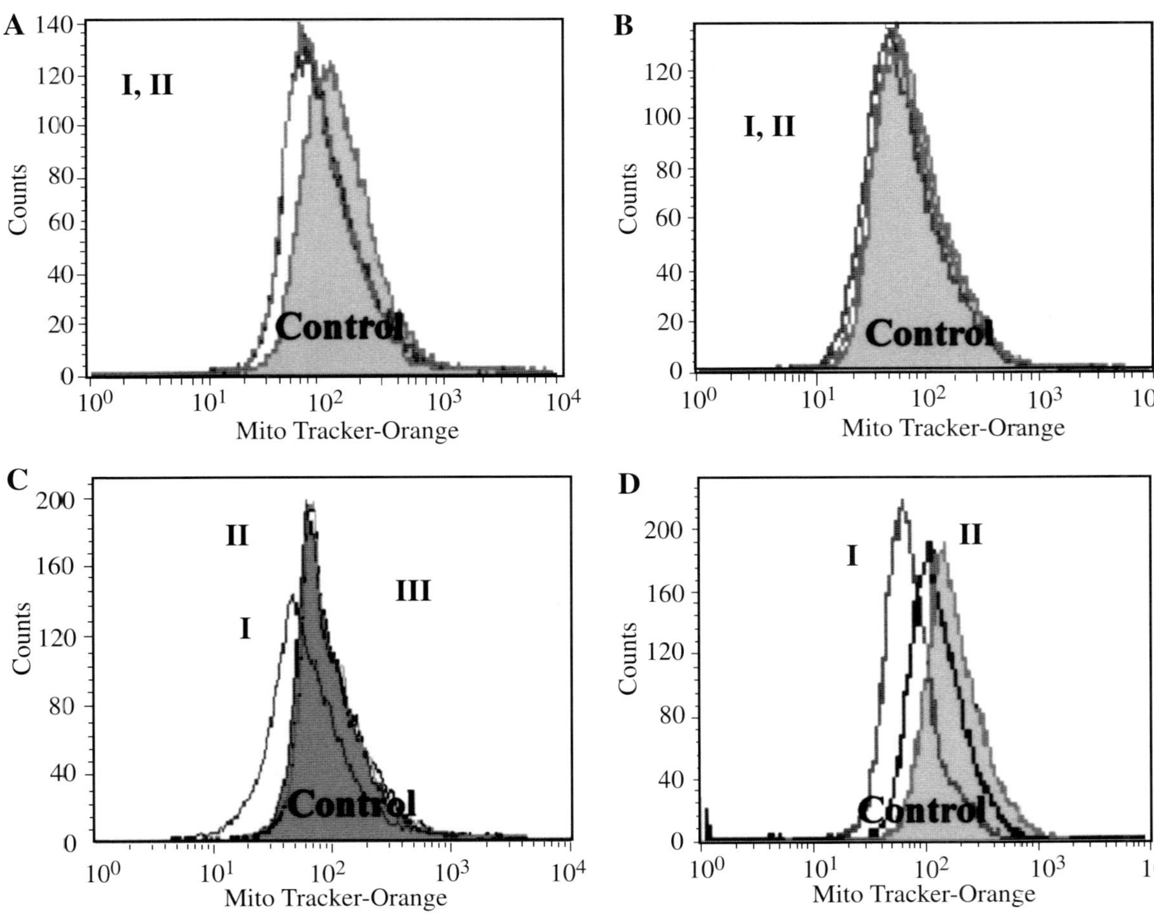

Fig. 3. *NMR*Sal reduced ΔΨm in isolated mitochondria. **A** and **B**: Mitochondria were prepared from wild SH (A) and MAO-B-SH cells (B) and incubated with 500 μM (I) and 250 μM *NMR*Sal (II) at 37°C for 3 h. **C** Mitochondria isolated from wild SH cells were incubated with 100 μM *NMR*Sal in the absence (I) and presence of 100 μM 5-HT (II), or treated with 5-HT alone at 37°C for 3 h. **D** Mitochondria prepared from wild SH were incubated with the anti-MAO antibody diluted by 100-folds (I) or 500-folds (II) at 37°C for 3 h. ΔΨm was measured by FACS after stained with MitoTracker Orange and Green

tivity studies (Fig. 2C), indicating that increased MAO activity was due to transfected MAO-B.

The binding of *NMR*Sal to mitochondria prepared from wild SH and MAO-B-SH cells was examined. The binding velocity of *NMR*Sal to mitochondria isolated from wild SH and MAO-B-SH cells were 163.6 ± 52.6 and 150.1 ± 20.9 pmol/min/mg protein, respectively. The transfection of MAO-B did not increase *NMR*Sal binding, suggesting that *NMR*Sal did not bind to MAO-B, as shown also by the fact *NMR*Sal did not inhibit MAO-B activity.

NMRSal induced $\Delta\Psi m$ decline and apoptosis in MAO-A containing cells

Involvement of MAO-A and -B in apoptosis induced by *NMR*Sal was examined using mitochondria prepared from wild SH and MAO-B-SH cells. Figure 3A and B show that *NMR*Sal reduced $\Delta\Psi$m in mitochondria containing MAO-A, but did not affect $\Delta\Psi$m in those prepared from MAO-B-SH cells. 5-HT, a substrate of MAO-A, prevented $\Delta\Psi$m decline induced by *NMR*Sal (Fig. 3C), whereas β-PEA, a MAO-B substrate, did not. In addition, clorgyline, an irreversible inhibitor of MAO-A reduced $\Delta\Psi$m, which 5-HT prevented. On the other hand, a reversible MAO-A inhibitor moclobemide did not. Figure 3D shows that the antibody against MAO reduced $\Delta\Psi$m in a doe-dependent way.

The role of MAO-A in apoptosis was shown by competition with 5-HT. *NMR*Sal induced apoptosis in wild SH, which 5-HT prevented completely (Fig. 4A). The number of apoptotic cells after *NMR*Sal treatment was 36.9% of the total and reduced to 5.3% by addition of 5-HT, which was almost the same as in control cells or cells treated with 5-HT alone; 5.5 and 4.6%. Clorgyline also induced apoptosis in the cells at the concentration higher than 100 nM (Fig. 4B). Clorgyline (50 μM) increased the number of apoptotic cells to 28.7% of the total from 12.4% and 8.4% in control and 5-HT alone (1 mM)-treated cell, and 5-HT reduced the number of clorgyline-induced apoptotic cells to 14.7%.

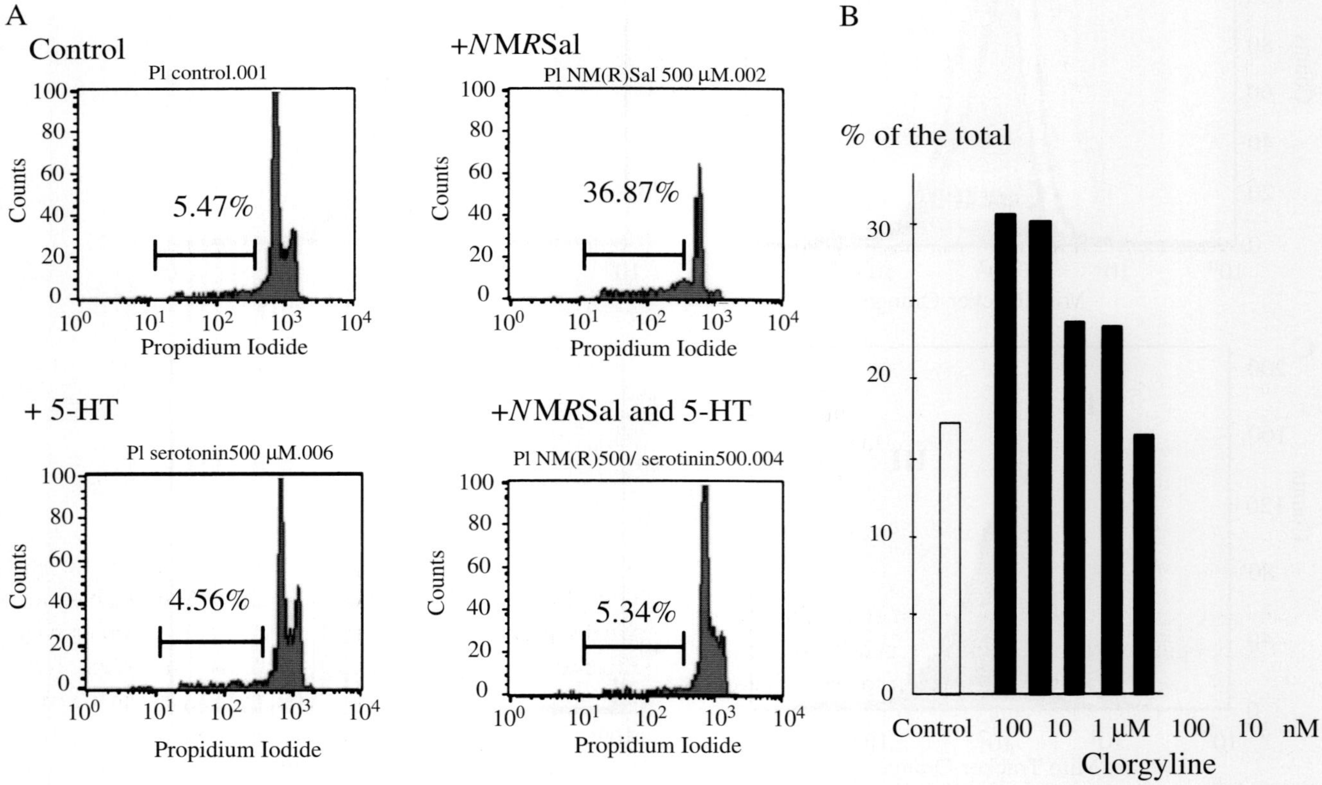

Fig. 4. Effects of 5-HT on *NMR*Sal-induced apoptosis and apoptosis by clorgyline in wild SH cells. **A** Control cells were incubated with *NMR*Sal (+*NMR*Sal) or 500 μM 5-HT (+5-HT) or *NMR*Sal and 5-HT (+*NMR*Sal and 5-HT) at 37°C overnight. Apoptotic cells were quantified by FACS after staining with PI. The cells with lower DNA content showing less PI staining than G1 were defined to be apoptotic. The number in Fig. 4A represents the number of apoptotic cells in the total (%). **B** Wild SH cells were incubated with 10 μM–10 nM clorgyline at 37°C overnight and apoptotic cells were quantified by FACS-PI method. The column represents the number of apoptotic cells as % of the total

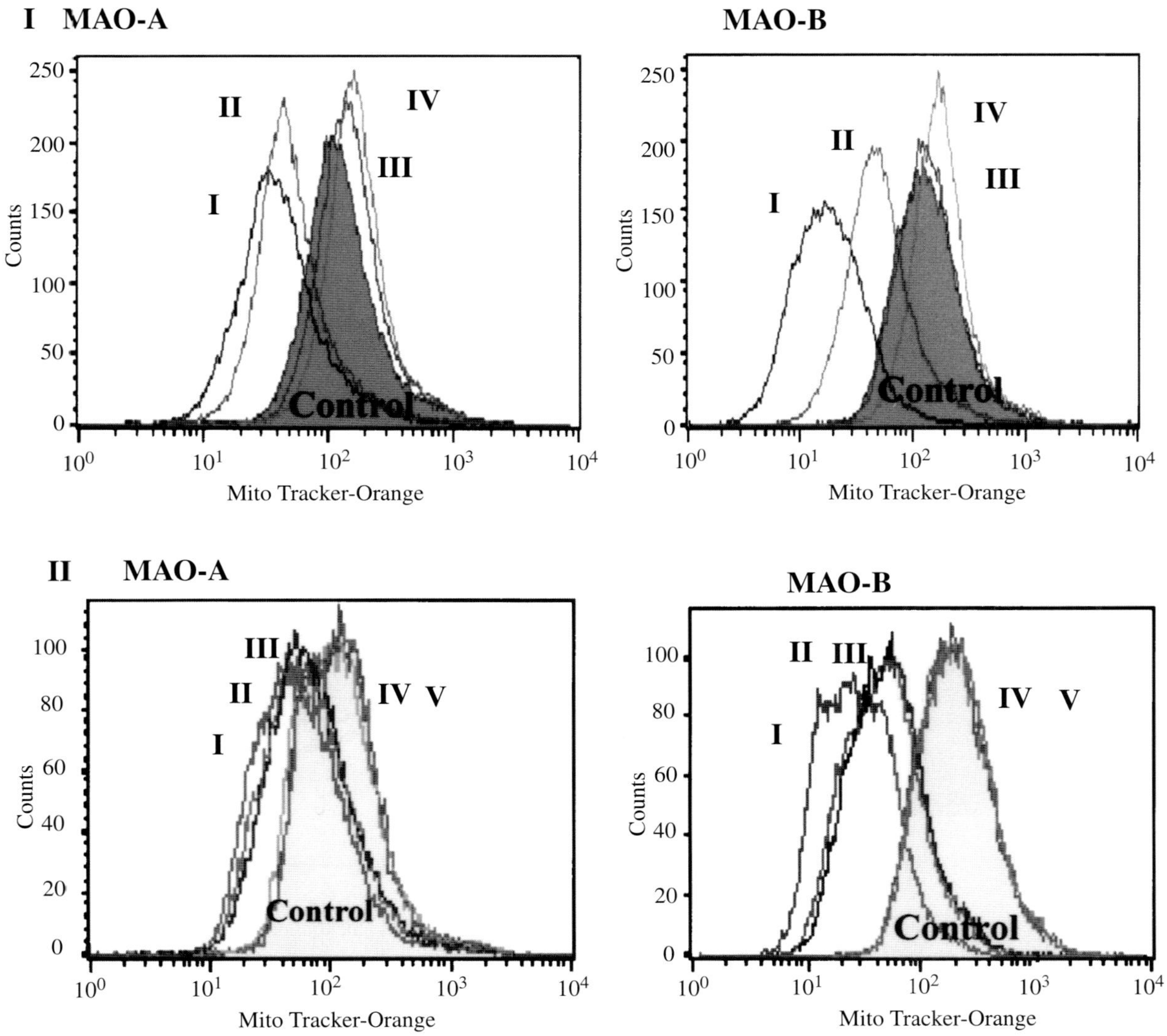

Fig. 5. ΔΨm reduction by dopamine oxidation and effects of MAO inhibitors. Mitochondria were prepared from MAO-A only containing wild SH (**MAO-A**) and MAO-B-SH cells (**MAO-B**). **I** Mitochondria incubated at 37°C for 3 h with 100 μM dopamine (I), 100 μM L-DOPA (II), 1 μM Fe^{2+} (III) and Fe^{3+} (IV). **II** Mitochondria were treated with 100 μM dopamine in the absence (**I**) of 1 μM clorgyline (**II**) or (−)deprenyl (**III**). **IV** and **V**: Mitochondria treated with clorgyline or (−)deprenyl. ΔΨm was measured by FACS with MitoTracker Orange

The role of MAO-A and MAO-B in the cytotoxicity of dopamine oxidation

Dopamine is oxidized either by enzymatic oxidation of MAO to 3,4-dihydrophenylactaldehyde and hydrogen peroxide, or by non-enzymatic autoxidation to dopamine-quinone and superoxide. The role of MAO-A and -B in the dopamine-induced cell death process was studied using mitochondria isolated from wild SH and MAO-B-SH cells. As shown in Fig. 5, I, dopamine and L-DOPA reduced ΔΨm markedly in MAO-A-containing mitochondria, whereas in MAO-B-containing mitochondria dopamine reduced ΔΨm more markedly than by L-DOPA and in MAO-A-containing mitochondria. Clorgyline and (−)deprenyl, inhibitors of MAO-A and MAO-B, did not prevent ΔΨm decline in MAO-A-containing mitochondria, but they partially prevented the ΔΨm decline in MAO-B-containing mitochondria (Fig. 5, II). Using FACS and fluorescent dyes, H_2DCFDA for hydrogen radical, nitric oxide and peroxynitrite (Crow, 1997) and HE for superoxide (Bindokas et al., 1996), ROS produced from dopamine oxidation was confirmed to be superoxide in MAO-A-containing mitochondria, whereas MAO-B produced hydrogen peroxide in addition to superoxide. Reduced glutathione, ascorbic acid and superoxide dismutase prevented ΔΨm decline in

MAO-A and -B-containing-mitochondria, whereas catalase did not. Dopamine oxidation modifies SH residues in mitochondrial complex I with formation of quinoprotein and inhibits the enzymatic activity of mitochondrial oxidative phophorylation (Naoi et al., in preparation).

Involvement of MAO-A in neuroprotection by rasagiline, a MAO-B inhibitor

A series of propargylamine MAO-B inhibitors protect neuronal cells in cellular and animal models of PD and other neurodegenerative disorders. The role of MAO in the neuroprotective function by rasagiline was confirmed in wild SH cells containing only MAO-A. The antiapoptotic, neuroprotective function of rasagiline is ascribed to two mechanisms. One is the stabilization of mitochondrial homeostasis and the prevention of mPT, and the other the induction of anti-apoptotic genes, bcl-2 and GDNF, as shown in Fig. 6. Opening of mPT pore leads to $\Delta\Psi m$ loss and swelling of the matrix, which was completely suppressed by rasagiline. Rasagiline prevents the cytochrome c release from mitochondria caused by rupture of the outer membrane due to the swelling, and suppresses the activation of casspase 3 (Maruyama et al., 2001a; Akao et al., 2002a) and the nuclear translocation of GAPDH (Maruyama et al., 2001b). Rasagiline increases the gene expression and protein amounts of bcl-2 (Aako et al., 2002b) and GDNF (Maruyama et al., 2004) in wild SH cells, and also the activity of catalase and superoxide dismutase in rats (Carrillo et al., 2000). The gene induction has the concen-

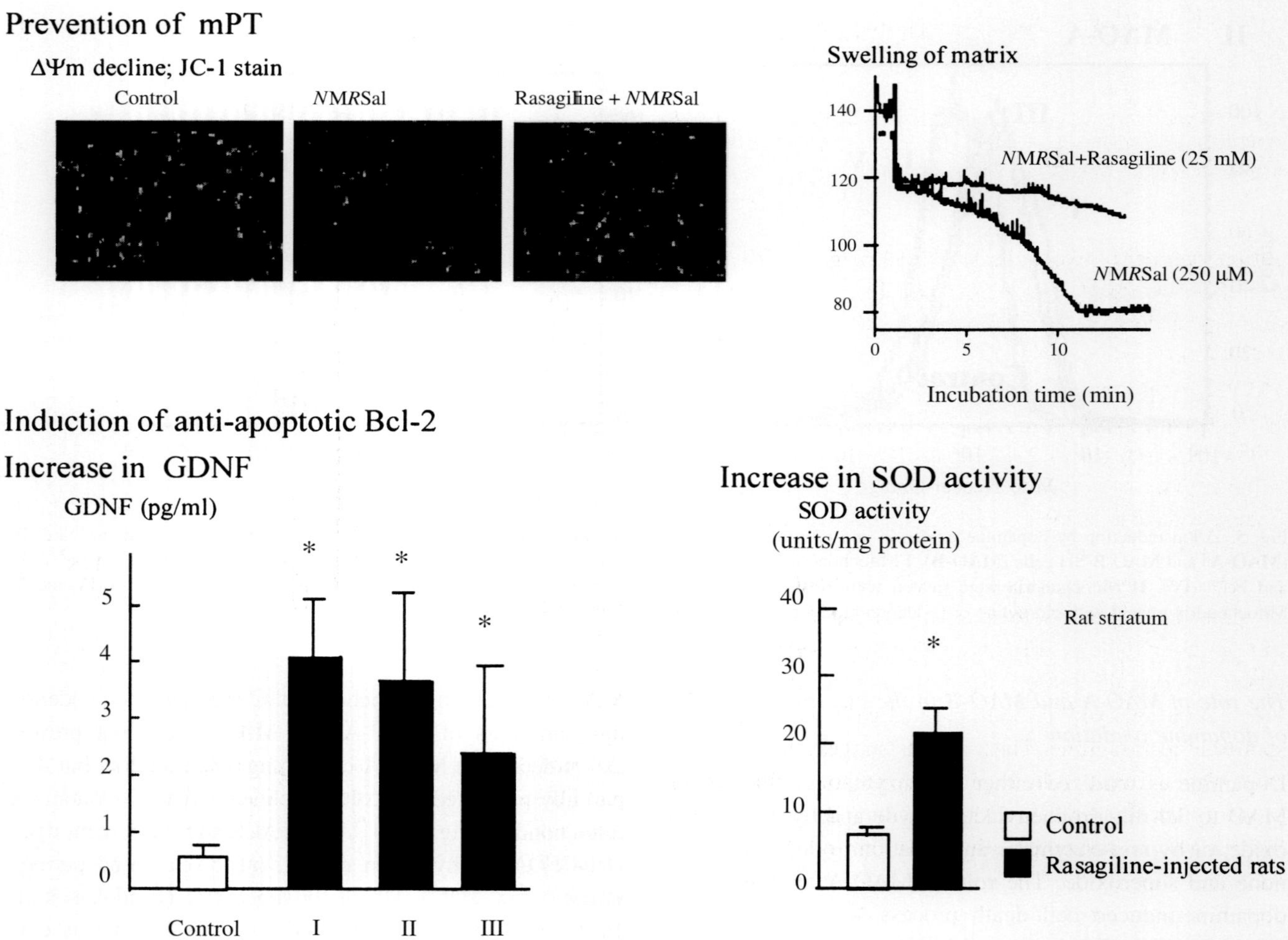

Fig. 6. Intracellular mechanism behind neuroprotective function of rasagiline. Rasagiline stabilizes mPT pore and prevents $\Delta\Psi m$ collapse and swelling of mitochondrial matrix. The activation of following death cascade, release of cytochrome c, activation of caspases and nuclear translocation of GAPDH is completely suppressed. Rasagiline increases GDNF in SH-SY5Y cells in a dose-dependent way. Cells were treated with 1 μM (I), 100 (II) and 10 nM (III) rasagiline at 37°C overnight and GDNF amount was assessed by ELISA. In rat brain regions containing dopamine neurons SOD and catalase activities increases significantly after systematic administration of rasagiline for 3 weeks. $^{*}p < 0.01$

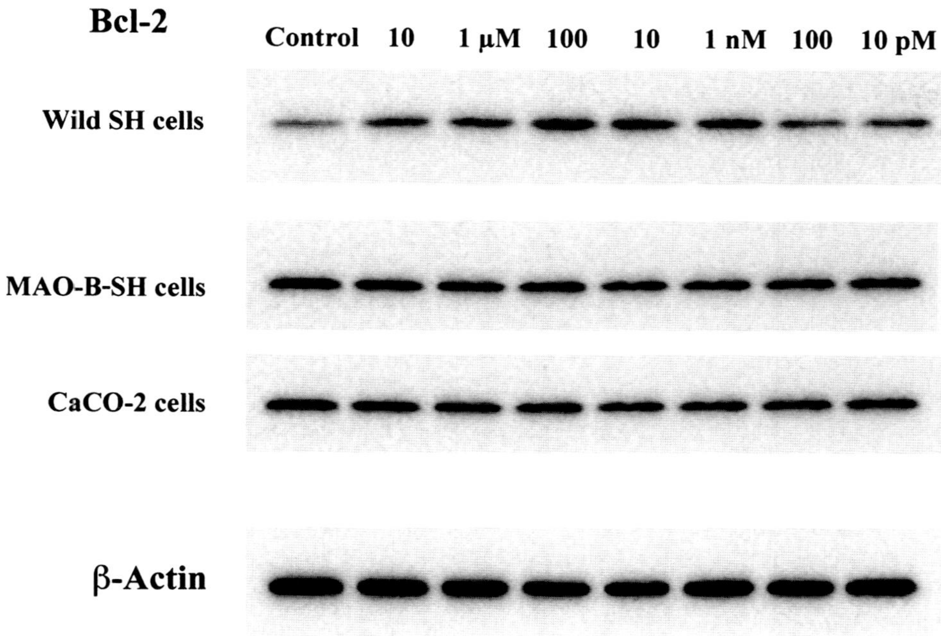

Fig. 7. Induction of Bcl-2 in wild and MAO-B-SH-SY5Y cells, and Caco-2 cells. Only MAO-A containing control and MAO-B transfected cells, and only MAO-B expressing Caco-2 cells were treated with 10 μM-10 pM rasagiline at 37°C overnight and the amount of Bcl-2 was determined by Western blot analysis. β-Action was used as a control

tration optima at two quite different ranges, 100–10 nM and 100–10 pM (Akao et al., 2002b). These concentrations were quite lower than those required for inhibition of MAO-A and -B. The IC_{50} values for inhibition of rat brain MAO activity were reported to be 412 nM and 4.4 nM for MAO-A and -B, respectively (Youdim et al., 2001).

The involvement of MAO-B in the induction of antiapoptotic genes was studied in MAO-B transfected cells and Caco-2 cells expressing only MAO-B. Even though marked expression of MAO-B was confirmed by the increased activity and protein amount, transfected MAO-B did not increase the sensitivity to rasagiline, as shown in Fig. 7. In Caco-2 cells bcl-2 was not induced by rasagiline at the concentrations of 10 μM–10 pM, suggesting that MAO-B may not be involved, or non-neuronal cells may not be responsible to rasagiline. These results suggest that MAO-A may play a major role in the antiapoptotic function of propargylamines, and that MAO-A may have a specified binding site of rasagiline other than that of the substrate and induce antiapoptotic genes. However, these results cannot exclude the possibility that MAO-B itself is involved in regulating apoptotic cascade in other types of cells. In addition, it remains to clarify how the signaling from mitochondria activates the transcription factors, such as NF-κB, which mediates the induction of Bcl-2 and GDNF by rasagiline (Maruyama et al., 2004).

Discussion

This paper reports for the first time the direct involvement of MAO-A in apoptosis. All the hitherto papers discussed the role of MAO in neuronal degeneration mainly in relation to the enzymatic oxidation of monoamines and the induction of oxidative stress (Cohen et al., 1997). In addition, the role of MAO-B in PD was augmented by the fact that MAO-B oxidizes a protoxicant, 1-methyl-4-phenyl-1,2,3,6-tetrahydropyridine (MPTP) into toxic 1-methyl-4-phenylpyridinium ion (MPP^+) (Heikkila et al., 1985). In concern to the role of MAO-A in apoptosis, higher MAO-A levels were expressed in apoptosis induced by depletion of nerve growth factor in PC12 cells, and increased ROS generation was considered to potentiate apoptosis (De Zutter and Davis, 2001). On the other hand, Malorni et al. (1998) reported that clorgyline and pargyline, inhibitors of MAO-A and MAO-A and -B, protected human melanoma M14 cells from apoptosis induced by serum withdrawal. These MAO inhibitors prevented the mPT induced by tyramine, a substrate for MAO-A and -B, in mitochondria isolated from rat liver (Marcocci et al., 2002). The protective function of MAO-A inhibitors was considered to be due to maintaining mitochondrial homeostasis by a direct effect on mPT pore in addition to inhibiting monoamine oxidation, but the detailed mechanisms were not presented in their paper.

Our results point out a novel direct involvement of MAO-A in mitochondrial apoptotic mechanism in addition to the enzymatic generation of ROS. RNAi targeting MAO-A reduced *N*M*R*Sal binding to mitochondria, in almost the same degree as the reduction of MAO protein amount and enzymatic activity. Kinetic studies on the inhibition of MAO-A activity suggest *N*M*R*Sal binding to the substrate binding site in MAO, as shown by competition with 5-HT, a MAO-A substrate, but not β-PEA, a MAO-B substrate. The binding of *N*M*R*Sal to MAO initiates the activation of apoptotic signaling. It is supported further by the fact that overexpression of MAO-B in SH-SY5Y cells did not increase the sensitivity to cytotoxic *N*M*R*Sal, and that *N*M*R*Sal binding to mitochondria inhibited by clorgyline, but not (−)deprenyl. The binding of *N*M*R*Sal to the active site of MAO-A may induce the conformational changes in MAO and the opening of mPT pore. The decline in $\Delta\Psi m$ by anti-MAO antibody suggests the interaction of MAO with mPT pore. However, at present it requires further studies to clarify the mechanism behind the interaction of MAO with other components of mPT pore.

MAO-B is commonly considered to play a major role in the cell death of PD, since in human basal ganglia MAO-B is more abundant than MAO-A and accounts for about 80% of the total MAO activity (O'Carrol et al., 1983). MAO-B in glia cells, but not neurons, may play a major role in the enzymatic oxidation of dopamine and ROS production (Damier et al., 1996). However, in MAO-A only containing cells, superoxide and dopamine quinone produced by dopamine autoxidation induce mPT and apoptosis as well as in MAO-B overexpressed cells. These results suggest again that MAO-A may determine the cell death and survival in neurons. However, we should examine further using *in vivo* and *in vitro* models of neurodegeneration to establish the role of MAO-A and -B in regulation of death cascade and induction of antiapoptotic genes for neuroprotection by rasagiline analogues.

The results in this paper point out the direct involvement of MAO-A in apoptotic mechanism induced by a dopaminergic neurotoxin, *N*M*R*Sal, and similar, but less marked, effects on $\Delta\Psi m$ were observed also with MPP^+. Selective MAO-A inhibitors, *N*M*R*Sal and MPP^+, might activate mitochondrial apoptotic signaling through binding to MAO-A, and induce cell death in MAO-A containing neurons. RNAi effectively reduced MAO in this cell model, suggesting that RNAi can be applied to prepare animal and cellular models by silencing MAO-A gene, and future studies by neurochemical and behavioral analyses may bring new insights on the function of MAO-A in neurodegeneratve and psychiatric disorders, such as bipolar emotional disorders.

Acknowledgements

This work was supported by a Grant-in-Aid on Scientific Research (C) and (A) (W. M.) from Japan Society for the Promotion of Science, Grant for Research on Dementia and Bone Fracture (W. M., M. N.) from the Ministry of Health, Labor and Welfare, Japan.

References

Akao Y, Maruyama W, Shimizu S, Yi H, Nakagawa Y, Shamoto-Nagai M, Youdim MBH, Tsujimoto Y, Naoi M (2002a) Mitochondrial permeability transition mediates apoptosis induced by *N*-methyl(*R*)salsolinol, an endogenous neurotoxin, and is inhibited by Bcl-2 and rasagiline, *N*-propargyl-1(*R*)-aminoindan. J Neurochem 82: 913–923

Akao Y, Maruyama W, Yi H, Shamoto-Nagai M, Youdim MBH, Naoi M (2002b) An anti-Parkinson's disease drug, *N*-propargyl-1(*R*)-aminoindan (rasagiline), enhances expression of anti-apoptotic bcl-2 in human dopaminergic SH-SY5Y cells. Neurosci Lett 326: 10510–10518

Andersen JK (2004) Oxidative stress in neurodegeneration: cause or consequence? Nature Med 10: S18–S25

Bach AWJ, Lan NC, Johnson DL, Abell CW, Bembenek ME, Kwan S-W, Seeburg PH, Shih JC (1988) cDNA cloning of human monoamine oxidase A and B: Molecular basis of differences in enzymatic properties. Proc Natl Acad Sci USA 85: 4934–4938

Bindokas VP, Jordan J, Lee CC, Miller RJ (1996) Superoxide production in rat hippocampal neurons: Selective imaging with hydroethidine. J Neurosci 16: 1324–1336

Bossy-Wetzel E, Schwarzenbacher R, Lipton S (2004) Molecular pathways to neurodegeneration. Nature Med 10: S2–S9

Bradford MM (1976) A rapid and sensitive method for the quantitation of microgram quantities of protein using the principle of protein dye binding. Anal Biochem 72: 248–254

Carrillo MC, Minami C, Kitani K, Maruyama W, Ohashi K, Yamamoto T, Naoi M, Kanai S, Youdim MBH (2000) Enhancing effect of rasagiline on superoxide dismutase and catalase activities in the dopaminergic system in the rat. Life Sci 67: 577–585

Cases O, Seif I, Grimsby J, Gaspa P, Chen K, Pounin S, Müller U, Aguet M, Babinet C, Shih JC, De Maeyer E (1995) Aggressive behavior and altered amounts of brain serotonin and norepinephrine in mice lacking MAOA. Science 268: 1763–1766

Cohen G, Farooqui R, Kesler N (1997) Parkinson disease: a new link between monoamine oxidase and mitochondrial electron flow. Proc Natl Acad Sci USA 94: 4890–4897

Crompton M (1999) The mitochondrial permeability transition pore and its role in the cell death. Biochem J 341: 233–249

Crow JP (1997) Dichlorodihydrofluorescein and dihydrorhodamine 123 are selective indicators of peroxynitrite *in vitro*: Implications for intracellular measurement of reactive nitrogen and oxygen species. Nitric Oxide 1: 145–157

Damier P, Kastner A, Agid Y, Hirsch EC (1996) Does monoamine oxidase type B play a role in dopaminergic nerve cell death in Parkinson's disease? Neurology 46: 1262–1269

Desagher S, Osen-Sand A, Nichols A, Eskes R, Montessuit S, Lauper S, Maundrell K, Amtonsson B, Martinou J-C (1999) Bid-induced conformational change of Bax is responsible for mitochondrial cytochrome c release during apoptosis. J Cell Biol 144: 891–901

DeZutter GS, Davis RJ (2001) Pro-apoptotic gene expression mediated by the p38 mitogen-activated protein kinase signal transduction pathway. Proc Natl Acad Sci USA 98: 6168–6173

Eckert A, Steiner B, Marques C, Leutz S, Roming H, Haass C, Muller WE (2001) Elevated vulnerability to oxidative tress-induced cell death and activation of caspase-3 by the Swedish amyloid precursor protein mutation. J Neurosci Res 64: 183–192

Gargalidis-Moudanos C, Femaury A, Parini A (1997) Predominant expression of monoamine oxidase B isoform in rabbit renal proximal tubule: Regulation by I_2 imidazoline ligands in intact cells. Mol Pharmacol 51: 637–643

Götz MF, Freyberger A, Riederer P (1990) Oxidative stress: a role in the pathogenesis of Parkinson's disease. J Neural Transm [Suppl 29]: 241–249

Green DR, Kroemer G (2004) The pathophysiology of mitochondrial cell death. Science 305: 626–269

Heikkila RE, Manzimo L, Cabbat FS, Duvoisin RC (1985) Studies on the oxidation of the dopaminergic neurotoxin 1-methyl-4-phenyl-1,2,3,5-tetrahydropyridine by monoamine oxidase B. J Neurochem 45: 1049–1054

Kraml M (1965) A rapid microfluorometric determination of monoamine oxidase. Biochem Pharmacol 14: 1684–1686

Lan NC, Chen C, Shih JC (1989) Expression of functional human monoamine oxidase A and B cDNAs in mammalian cells. J Neurochem 52: 1625–1634

Lim LCC, Powell JF, Murray R, Gill M (1994) Monoamine oxidase A gene and bipolar affective disorder. Am J Hum Genet 54: 1122–1124

Malorni W, Giammarioli AM, Matarrese P, Piertrangeli P, Agostinelli E, Ciaccio A, Grassilli E, Mondovi N (1998) Protection against apoptosis by monoamine oxidase A inhibitors. FEBS Lett 426: 155–159

Marcocci L, De Marchi U, Salvi M, Milella ZG, Nocera S, Agostinelli E, Mondovi B, Toninello A (2002) Tyramine and monoamine oxidase inhibitors as modulators of the mitochondrial membrane permeability transition. J Membrane Biol 188: 23–31

Maruyama W, Abe T, Tohgi H, Dostert P, Naoi M (1996) A dopaminergic neurotoxin, (*R*)-*N*-methylsalsolinol, increases in Parkinsonian cerebrospinal fluid. An Neurol 40: 119–122

Maruyama W, Naoi M, Kasamatsu T, Hashizume Y, Takahashi T, Kohda K, Dostert P (1997) An endogenous dopaminergic neurotoxin, *N*-methyl-(*R*)-salsolinol, induces DNA damage in human dopaminergic neuroblastoma SH-SY5Y cells. J Neurochem 69: 322–329

Maruyama W, Akao Y, Youdim MBH, Davis BA, Naoi M (2001a) Transfection-forced Bcl-2 overexpression and anti-Parkinson drug, rasagiline, prevent nuclear translocation of glyceraldehydes-3-phosphate dehydrogenase induced by an endogenous dopaminergic neurotoxin, *N*-methyl(*R*)salsolinol. J Neurochem 78: 727–735

Maruyama W, Boulton AA, Davis BA, Dostert P, Naoi M (2001b) Enantiospecific induction of apoptosis by an endogenous neurotoxin *N*-methyl(*R*)salsolinol, in dopaminergic SH-SY5Y cells: suppression of apoptosis by *N*-(2-heptyl)-*N*-methylpropargylamine. J Neural Transm 108: 11–24

Maruyama W, Youdim MBH, Naoi M (2001c) Antiapoptotic properties of rasagiline, *N*-propargylamine-1(*R*)-aminoindan, and its optical (*S*)-isomer, TV1022. Ann NY Acad Sci 939: 320–329

Maruyama W, Nitta A, Shamoto-Nagai M, Hirata Y, Akao Y, Youdim M, Furukawa S, Nabeshima T, Naoi M (2004) *N*-Propargyl-1(*R*)-aminoindan, rasagiline, increases glial cell line-derived neurotrophic factor (GDNF) in neuroblastoma SH-SY5Y cells through activation of NF-κB transcription factor. Neurochem Int 44: 393–400

Naoi M, Maruyama W, Dostert P, Hashizume Y, Nakahara D, Takahashi T, Ota M (1996) Dopamine-derived endogenous 1(*R*),2(*N*)-dimethyl-6,7-dihydroxy-1,2,3,4-tetrahydroisoquinoline, *N*-methyl-(*R*)-salsolinol, induced parkinsonism in rat: Biochemical, pathological and behavioral studies. Brain Res 709: 285–295

Naoi M, Maruyama W, Nakao N, Ibi T, Sahashi K, Strolin Benedetti M (1998) (*R*)Salsolinol *N*-methyltransferase activity increases in parkinsonian lymphocytes. Ann Neurol 43: 212–216

Naoi M, Maruyama W, Akao Y, Yi H (2002a) Mitochondria determine the survival and death in apoptosis induced by an endogenous neurotoxin, *N*-methyl(*R*)salsolinol, and neuroprotection by propargylamines. J Neural Transm [Suppl 109]: 607–621

Naoi M, Maruyama W, Akao Y, Yi H (2002b) Dopamine-derived endogenous *N*-methyl-(*R*)-salsolinol. Its role in Parkinson's disease. Neurotoxicol Tera 24: 579–591

Naoi M, Maruyama W, Nagy GM (2004) Dopamine-derived salsolinol derivatives as endogenous monoamine oxidase inhibitors: Occurrence. Metabolism and function in human brains. NeuroToxicol 25: 193–204

Naoi M, Maruyama W, Shamoto-Nagai M, Yi H, Akao Y, Tanaka M (2005) Oxidative stress in mitochondria; decision to survival and death of neurons in neurodegenertaion. Mol Neurobiol 31: 81–93

O'Caroll AM, Fowler CJ, Phillips JP, Tobia I, Tipton KF (1988) The deamination of dopamine by human brain monoamine oxidase. Arch Pharmacol 322: 198–223

Parkinson Study Group (2004) A controlled, randomized, delayed-start study of rasagiline in early Parkinson disease. Arch Neurol 61: 561–566

Shih JC, Chen K, Ridd MJ (1999) Monoamine oxidase: from genes to behavior. Annu Rev Neurosci 22: 197–217

Teitel S, O'Brien J, Brossi A (1972) Alkaloids in mammalian tissue II. Synthesis of (+) and (−)substituted 6,7-dihydroxy-1,2,3,4-tetrahydroisoquinolines. J Med Chem 15: 845–846

Tipton KF, Boyce S, O'Sullivan J, Davey GP, Healy J (2004) Monoamine oxidases: Certainties and uncertainties. Curr Med Chem 11: 1965–1982

Westlund KN, Denney RM, Rose RM, Abell CW (1988) Localization of distinct monoamine oxidase A and monoamine oxidase B cell populations in human brainstem. Neuroscience 25: 439–456

Wong WK, Chen K, Shih JC (2003) Decreased methylation and transcription repressor Sp3 up-regulated human monoamine oxidase (MAO) B expression during Caco-2 differentiation. J Biol Chem 278: 36227–36235

Yi H, Maruyama W, Akao Y, Takahashi T, Iwasa K, Youdim MBH, Naoi M (2006) *N*-Propargylamine protects SH-SY5Y cells from apoptosis induced by an endogenous neurotoxin, *N*-methyl(*R*)salsolinol, through stabilization of mitochondrial membrane and induction of anti-apoptotic Bcl-2. J Neural Transm 113: 21–32

Yi H, Akao Y, Maruyama W, Chen K, Shih J, Naoi M (2006) Type A monoamine oxidase is the target of an endogenous dopaminergic neurotoxin, *N*-Methyl(*R*)salsolinol, leading to apoptosis in SH-SY5Y cells. J Neurochem 96: 541–549

Youdim MBH, Gross A, Finberg JPM (2001) Rasagiline [N-propargyl-1R(+)-aminoindan], a selective and potent inhibitor of mitochondrial monoamine oxidase B. Br J Pharmacol 132: 500–506

Youdim MBH, Maruyama W, Naoi M (2005) Neuropharmacological, neuroprotective and amyloid precursor processing properties of selective MAO-B inhibitor antiparkinsonian drug, rasagiline. Drug Today 41: 369–391

Youdim MBH, Bar Am O, Yogev-Falach M, Weinreb O, Maruyama W, Naoi M, Amit T (2005b) Rasagiline: neurodegeneration, neuroprotection, and mitochondrial permeability transition. J Neurochem Res 79: 172–179

J Neural Transm (2006) [Suppl] 71: 79–86

Journal of
Neural
Transmission
Printed in Austria

The relationship of early studies of monoamine oxidase to present concepts

I. J. Kopin

Scientist Emeritus, NINDS, NIH, Bethesda, USA

Summary The development of our understanding of monoamine oxidase (MAO), of its role in the metabolism of amines and of the therapeutic usefulness of MAO inhibitors (MAOIs) have evolved, slowly at times and rapidly at other times, with leaps propelled by new discoveries, new techniques and new insights. Moussa Youdim was one of the major contributors to propulsion of several of these leaps, including the detection of multiple forms of MAO, the descriptions of their properties, active sites and substrates, the use of MAOIs for enhancement of DOPA in treating Parkinson's disease and the evolution of MAO-B inhibitors from mere enzyme inhibitors to lead compounds in the discovery of neuroprotective agents for use in degenerative neurological diseases. Since others will be describing the more recent developments in this field, I thought it would be of interest and instructive to recount the unfolding of our early understanding of MAO, dating from its discovery until the events that first suggested that drugs that inhibit MAO might be neuroprotective. While even the earliest observations about MAO were valid, they were often misinterpreted or confusing, whereas others were predictive of several of our newer concepts of MAO and of side effects encountered in patients treated with MAOIs.

1. Discovery of monoamine oxidase

Nearly 100 years ago, Dale and Dixon (1909) found that 4-hydroxyphenylethylamine (tyramine) was the major in pressor amine found in putrified meat; it seemed to produce adrenaline-like effects. This sparked interest of their colleagues at Cambridge in the metabolic fate of this amine and the following year Ewins and Laidlaw (1910) showed that tyramine was quantitatively converted to p-hydroxyphenylacetic acid by perfused dog liver. Furthermore, orally administered tyramine gave rise to urinary excretion of the acid. They believed that the amine moiety of tyramine was replaced by a hydroxyl and that the resulting alcohol was then metabolized to the corresponding acid:

$$R{-}CH_2{-}NH_2 \rightarrow R{-}CH_2{-}OH \rightarrow R{-}COOH$$

Correspondence: I. J. Kopin, Scientist Emeritus, NINDS, NIH, Bethesda, USA
e-mail: kopini@ninds.nih.gov

Interestingly, tyramine disappeared when perfused through the heart without any evidence of production of the expected acid; they speculated (incorrectly) that the benzene ring of tyramine had been destroyed. The tyramine was probably removed by uptake into the sympathetic nerves, converted to octopamine which remained in the storage veisicles (see below).

Using a Barcroft differential manometer to measure oxygen utilization by liver homogenates, Hare (1928), while a student at Cambridge, was able to show that oxygen uptake corresponded to exactly one atom of oxygen per molecule of tyramine, but only half the expected amount of ammonia was recovered. Furthermore, she demonstrated the production of hydrogen peroxide during the reaction. The thermolability of the reaction indicated that an enzyme, which she named tyramine oxidase, catalyzed the oxidative deamination of tyramine. However, she did not find the expected product, p-hydroxyphenylacetic acid. Several years later, at Duke University, she found that the number of oxygen molecules used in the oxidation of tyramine depended upon factors such as the pH, the age of the preparation and its concentration (Bernheim, see Hare, 1931). With fresh tissue, at physiological pH, two oxygen atoms were required to metabolize tyramine and the product was, as expected, p-hydroxyphenylacetic acid. She explained the discrepancy between the production of ammonia and the disappearance of tyramine in her earlier experiments by suggesting that one molecule of tyramine was converted to p-hydroxyphenylacetaldehyde and that this reacted with a second molecule of tyramine to form a covalent linkage:

$$2R{-}CH_2{-}NH_2 + O_2 \rightarrow 2R{-}CH{=}NH + H_2O_2$$
$$R{-}CH{=}NH + H_2O \rightarrow R{-}CHO + NH_3$$
$$R{-}CH_2{-}NH_2 + R{-}CHO \rightarrow R{-}CH_2{-}N{=}CH{-}R + H_2O$$

Under most conditions, however, the oxidation proceeds further, producing the acid. Ewins and Laidlaw (1910) had shown that both the mono-N-methyl and the dimethyl derivatives of tyramine (hordenine) could be transformed to p-hydroxyphenylacetic acid, albeit at a slower rate. In 1937, several investigators confirmed the production of hydrogen peroxide, ammonia and an aldehyde as a result of oxidative deamination of several primary, secondary and tertiary amines (Kohn, 1937; Richter 1937; Blaschko et al., 1937). The aldehyde was trapped using 2,4-dinitophenylhydrazine. Covalent linkage of the reactive aldehydes formed from catecholamines will show up again, about 60 years later (see below). The competitive interactions among "tyramine oxidase", "adrenaline oxidase" and "aliphatic amine oxidase", suggested that they were all substrates for the same enzyme, subsequently named MAO. The three products formed by the deamination process, hydrogen peroxide, ammonia and an aldehyde, are all potentially toxic.

Bernheim (1931) recognized the potential toxicity of H_2O_2, but assumed that catalase rapidly destroyed this oxidizing agent to generate $H_2O + O_2$. Although Fenton (1894) had described Fe^{++} catalysis of H_2O_2 oxidation reactions, the cycling Haber-Weiss reactions (Haber and Weiss, 1932) and superoxide dismutase (McCord and Fridovich, 1969) had not been discovered. Sixty years after Hare's description of H_2O_2 formation during the oxidative deamination of tyramine, blockade of hydrogen peroxide generation in glia by MAO-B inhibition was suggested as a means to diminish toxicity due to endogenous free radicals. The course of events from that time until the more recent developments in the field have been ably reviewed by Youdim and Riederer (2004).

Blaschko (1952) described at some length covalent bonding of reactive aldehydes formed from deamination of amines. A dozen years later, Holtz et al. (1964) reported that dopamine and the aldehyde derived from its deamination could covalently link to yield tetrahydropapaveroline and later Sandler et al. (1973) found this compound in the urine of parkinsonian patients being treated with DOPA. More recently, covalent bondage of aldehydes formed from the deamination of dopamine, norepinephrine (NE) and epinephrine (EPI) have received increasing attention. Burke et al. (2004) recently reviewed the evidence that reactions of these metabolites with cellular components may be etiological factors in the neurodegenerative processes culminating in death of catecholaminergic neurons in degenerative neurological disorders such as Parkinson's disease.

Ammonia, although a third potential toxin from this source, is formed primarily from transamination of amino acids. It diffuses rapidly and is efficiently converted to urea by the liver. Only under unusual conditions of liver failure has endogenous ammonia formation been considered a hazard.

2. Early indications of in vivo catecholamine deamination

As indicated above, as late as 1950, although the catecholamines had been shown to be substrates for MAO, the role of this enzyme in their metabolism in intact animals had not been convincingly demonstrated. The introduction of radioisotopes and the discovery of an inhibitor of MAO were seminal events that enabled further investigations of the role of MAO in the disposition of catecholamines. Schayer and Smiley (1951) showed that only about one half of the radioactivity in methyl-^{14}C-*dl*-EPI could be recovered in the urine of rats that had received the labeled compound intravenously or subcutaneously, whereas all the administered radioactivity was recovered from β-^{14}C-*dl*-EPI. In a second study, Schayer et al. (1952) showed that this was not due to a difference in the metabolism of the *d*- and *l*-isomers of the catecholamine, indicating that the metabolism of both isomers of EPI involved formation of a breakdown product that lacked the N-methyl group, presumably as a result of deamination. This suggestion was proven correct during the following year (Schayer et al., 1953) when it became possible to inhibit MAO (see below). At that time, Blaschko (1952) described three possible means of inactivation of NE and EPI: oxidative deamination, oxidation to adrenochrome, and conjugation. In that review, he also introduced the concept of "directly" acting sympathomimetic amines, which activated receptors, and "indirectly" acting sympathomimetic amines, which "preserved sympathin in the region of the receptors." He was close to being right, but could not predict the other mechanisms that would be discovered in the next few years, e.g., active neuronal reuptake of the released transmitter as a means of "preserving" the neurotransmitter in the region of the receptor (how cocaine acts) or the release of NE (how tyramine produces its effects) as mechanisms for the adrenergic responses to "indirectly" acting sympathomimetic amines.

3. Discovery of MAO inhibitors

The fortuitous discovery by Chorine (1945) that nicotinamide had a bacteriostatic effect on the tuberculous bacillus led to the investigation of cogeners that might be used for the treatment of tuberculosis. In the course of the next few years, isonicotinylhydrazine (isoniazid) and its isopropyl derivative, 1-isonicotinyl-2-isopropyl hydrazine (marsilid, iproniazid,) emerged as candidates for clinical trials. Since all bases had been reported to inhibit bacterial diamine oxidase, Zeller and Barsky (1952) sought to examine the mode of action of these two hydrazine derivatives by studying their effect on amine oxidases in vitro and found that they inhibited MAO. They found that the more potent of these agents, iproniazid, when administered to animals, inhibited liver and brain MAO. Although MAO inhibition with iproniazid potentiated the actions of administered sympathomimetic amines (such as tyramine), the effects of catecholamines were not altered (Greisemer et al., 1953; Rebnun et al., 1954). These results, combined with the earliest reports of the presence of tyramine in putrified meat (Dale and Dixon, 1910) and the report by Ewins and Laidlaw (1910) that orally administered tyramine is deaminated to p-hydroxyphenylacetic acid might have been predictive of the hypertensive crises evoked by ingestion of foods prepared by bacterial fermentation, e.g., cheese and wine, in patients in whom MAO had been inhibited (see below).

A role for MAO in the metabolism catecholamines was firmly established when Schayer and Smiley (1953) reported that inhibition of MAO with iproniazid prevented the loss of ^{14}C after administration of methyl-^{14}C-*dl*-EPI. These results were confirmed and extended to show that ^{14}C from β-^{14}C-*dl*-NE resulted in the excretion of an acidic metabolite similar to that from β-^{14}C-*dl*-EPI and that the excretion of this compound was markedly diminished when MAO was inhibited (Schayer et al., 1955). Using paper chromatography, they showed that the urine contained five different metabolites of the ^{14}C-labeled catecholamines, but the identity of the products was not determined.

4. The antidepressant effects of MAO inhibitors

In the mid 1950s, the biochemical effects of MAO inhibition were studied independently of clinical studies. By the end of the fifties, however, the discovery of antidepressant activity of MAO inhibitors marked a veritable therapeutic revolution in the world of neuropsychiatry. Iproniazid, the isopropyl derivative of isoniazid, had been introduced into clinical trials seeking a better drug with which to treat tuberculosis (e.g., Bloch et al., 1954; Liechtenstein and Mitzenberg, 1954). It was noted that some of the patients treated with iproniazid felt too good. Their general behavior belied the lack of improvement of their x-rays; they overexerted themselves, generally ignored appropriate medical safeguards, and were inappropriately elated. Some patients became clearly manic. These mental effects, which were reported increasingly by clinicians treating tuberculosis, suggested that iproniazid might be useful in the treatment of depression. In further support of this view, there were reports that the striking sedative effects in animals of reserpine, which had been recently introduced as a treatment for hypertension, were reversed by pretreatment with iproniazid. These observations together with the affective changes in tubercular patients, prompted the initiation of studies of iproniazid in psychiatric patients. The usefulness of iproniazid as a "psychic energizer" in the treatment of depression was first reported by Loomer et al. (1957), The potential market for an effective antidepressant and need for an alternative drug necessitated by the hepatotoxic and other side effects of iproniazid fueled the search for more specific and less toxic MAOIs. During the next few years, over 100 hundred other compounds were reported to inhibit MAO (see, e.g., the papers in a symposium edited by Zeller, 1963) and iproniazid was replaced by other MAOIs.

5. Metabolic products formed from catecholamines

At about the time that iproniazid was introduced as an antidepressant, Armstrong et al. (1957) reported that 3-methoxy-4-hydroxy-D-mandelic acid (vanillylmandelic acid, VMA) was a major urinary metabolite of NE; large amounts of VMA were found in the urine of patients with phaeochomocytoma, a catecholamine-producing tumor, usually of the adrenal medulla. They assumed that VMA was formed from 3,4-dihydroxymandelic acid derived from the deamination of the catecholamine. However, Axelrod and Tomchick (1958) discovered an enzyme that O-methylates EPI and other catechols, catechol-O-methyltransferase (COMT). Axelrod then showed that O-methylation appeared to be the major initial route of metabolic transformation of administered EPI and NE in rats (1958a and 1958b). Quantitative assessment of the relative magnitude of O-methylation of administered EPI in humans showed that about 2/3 of administered EPI was converted to metanephrine before being further metabolized (Kopin, 1960). Although in humans VMA is the major urinary catecholamne metabolite, in rats, administration of ^{3}H-EPI or ^{3}H-NE resulted in the excretion of a compound that was clearly different form the known metabolites of these catecholamines. The new compound was identified as 3-methoxy-4-hydroxy-phenylglycol. (MHPG), excreted as its sulfate conjugate (Axelrod et al., 1959a). Shortly thereafter, we (Kopin and Axelrod, 1960) found that 3,4-dihydroxyphenylglycol. (DHPG) was formed from ^{3}H-EPI administered to rats that had been pretreated with pyrogallol, an inhibitor of COMT (Axelrod and Laroche, 1959). At that time we thought (incorrectly) that the difference between the major urinary metabolites in humans and rats was the result of a species difference in the oxidation versus reduction of the aldehyde formed when NE or EPI was deaminated. Studies carried out over 20 years later showed that VMA was formed mainly from oxidation of plasma MHPG (Blombery et al., 1980; Mardh et al., 1981) and the species difference is in the fate of MHPG; oxidation to VMA vs conjugation with sulfate.

6. MAO vs COMT in terminating the action of catecholamines

Pyrogallol and other catechols had been reported to potentiate the effects of administered EPI and sympathetic nerve stimulation (Bacq, 1936). Although initially Bacq thought to be due to the antioxidant properties of catechols, the demonstration that pyrogallol was a potent inhibitor of COMT (Bacq et al., 1959; Axelrod and Laroche, 1959) strongly suggested that O-methylation was the primary means of inactivation of NE. This view was supported by reports that MAO inhibition with iproniazid prolonged the actions of neither released (Brown and Gillespie, 1957) nor administered catecholamines (Greisemer et al., 1957; Corne and Graham, 1957). The opposite view for the inactivation of NE in brain was based on the effects of MAO inhibition on the effects of reserpine. Shore et al. (1957) thought that MAO was mainly responsible for the physiological inactivation of both serotonin and NE in brain because iproniazid was found to elevate the tissue levels of these amines and to prevent reserpine-induced decline in their levels. Iproniazid also increased cardiac NE levels (Pletscher, 1958). However, Crout (1961) reported that inhibition of both COMT and MAO failed to significantly affect the cardiovascular effects of NE, indicating that alternatives to metabolic inactivation must be sought. The relationships of MAO and COMT to sites of NE metabolism did not become apparent until more information about the storage and release of NE became available.

7. Uptake and storage of NE

After intravenous administration of ^{3}H-EPI or ^{3}H-NE to animals, a major portion of the administered compounds was retained in the tissues and not metabolized (Axelrod et al., 1959b; Whitby et al., 1961). When it was shown that the binding of tritiated catecholamines was markedly diminished after chronic sympathetic denervation, it became evident that presynaptic neuronal reuptake was the major means of terminating the actions of the released neurotransmitter (Hertting et al., 1961). Cocaine potentiation of the actions of EPI, first described by Frölich and Loewi (1910), had been attributed to inhibition of oxidation of the catecholamine (Philpot, 1940). Blaschko (1952) found this explanation unsatisfactory because it "is surprising that the action of tyramine is blocked by cocaine." An alternative to Philpot's explanation was provided when it was shown that cocaine inhibited uptake of ^{3}H-NE (Whitby et al., 1960). Since uptake of tyramine is required for its release of NE, this also explained why cocaine blocked the effects of tyramine. Many other drugs (e.g., imipramine, tyramine, amphetamine, phenoxybenzamine, etc.) were found to inhibit NE uptake and its retention in the tissues (Axelrod et al., 1961, 1962). Determination of the site in the nerve terminals at which the ^{3}H-NE was retained then attracted attention. Because Hillarp (1958) had shown that in the adrenal medulla, catecholamines were stored in granules, a similar site for storage of the catecholamine in sympathetic neurons was suspected. This possibility was examined by combined electron microscopy and autoradiography of sympathetic nerves of the pineal gland of rats that had received ^{3}H-NE (Wolfe et al., 1962). They found a striking localization of photographic grains overlying non-myelinated axons that contained granulated vesicles. The vesicular sequestration of the catecholamine protected it from metabolism by MAO.

The discovery that reserpine, which had recently been introduced as an antihypertensive agent and antipsychotic, depleted tissue levels of serotonin (Pletscher et al., 1955) and NE (Bertler et al., 1956; Holtzbauer and Vogt, 1956) not only spawned hypotheses about the physiological role of these amines, but provided a valuable new pharmacological tool. As indicated earlier, until Blaschko (1952) introduced the concept of "directly" and "indirectly" acting amines, it had been assumed that all sympathomimietic drugs produced their effects by acting on the same receptors as the endogenous catecholamines. When it was shown that pretreatment with reserpine prevented the actions of some sympathomimetic drugs, such as tyramine, it was proposed that such amines acted by releasing NE form the sympathetic nerves (e.g., Burn and Rand, 1958). During reserpine-induced depletion of tissue amines, however, there were no indications that the amines were released at sites at which they normally elicited physiological responses.

The role of MAO in the metabolism of NE became better understood when it was found that the metabolites excreted within 3 hours after intravenously administered ^{3}H-NE and of ^{3}H-NE released by tyramine 10 hours after administration of the labeled catecholamine reflected metabolism primarily by O-methylation, whereas the metabolites of the ^{3}H-NE that had been retained for 10 hours or of stored ^{3}H-NE depleted by the action of reserpine reflected metabolism by MAO (Kopin and Gordon, 1963). NE that is released outside the nerve and escapes reuptake is metabolized by COMT; MAO metabolizes NE released from storage sites into the neuronal cytoplasm. This explains the absence of sympathetic response during reserpine-induced depletion of catecholamines stores. Blocking the vesicular storage of NE exposes the amine to destruction by MAO. Thus, the mechanism for reversal of the effects of reserpine by pretreatment of animals with a MAOI becomes apparent. If vesicular storage is prevented by reserpine and MAO is also blocked, then the catecholamine released into the cytoplasm cannot be deaminated and escapes into the extraneural space to activate receptors. In addition to tyramine causing release of NE into the extracelluar space, but it also competes with reuptake of the released NE (Axelrod et al., 1962), which is then exposed to metabolism by COMT.

Much later it was shown that VMA is formed mainly in the liver from oxidation of plasma MHPG (Blombery et al., 1980; Marde et al., 1981), further studies showed that intraneuronal NE is deaminated and reduced to form 3,4-dihydroxyphenylglycol (DHPG). Eisenhofer et al. (2004) recently reviewed the bases for changes our concepts of the storage and metabolism of NE and some of the misconceptions that have persisted. Vesicular NE stores are not inert but are rather in dynamic equilibrium with the cytoplasmic catecholamine. The avid vesicular amine transporter captures most of the free cytoplasmic catecholamine. Although only a small portion of the cytoplasmic NE is metabolized to DHPG, it is the main source of metabolites of NE. DHPG is readily diffusible, escaping to the plasma or extranneuronal tissues after which it is O-methylated to form MHPG. DHPG and MHPG in plasma are rapidly converted to VMA or MHPG conjugates in the liver. When reserpine blocks the vesicular amine transporter, NE depletion results from deamination to DHPG of the cytoplasmic NE that has been rapidly "leaking" out of the vesicle. Under normal circumstances, more NE is metabolized intraneuronally than is released by exocytosis.

8. Hypotensive effects of MAO inhibition

Orthostatic hypotension was a major side effect of iproniazid treatment. This was unexpected because of the earlier studies that showed that catecholamines were substrates for MAO and that deamination was clearly involved in the metabolism of catecholamines. Furthermore, as indicated above, tissue levels of the amines are generally increased when MAO is inhibited (Shore et al., 1957; Pletscher, 1958). Although the mechanism of the sympatholytic effects was unknown, it was thought that iproniazid might be beneficial for treating hypertension and anginal pain. When Kakimoto and Armstrong (1962) found that octopamine, the β-hydroxylated derivative of tyramine, appeared in the urine of patients and animals treated with iproniazid and was markedly increased in the tissues of animals treated with the MAOI, they suggested that "the beneficial effects of monoamine oxidase inhibitors in the treatment of anginal pain might result from the accumulation of octopamine". Subsequently it was shown that the octopamine that accumulated in the tissue was in sympathetic nerves where it is a "false neurotransmitter" (Kopin et al., 1964). The slow (over several days) accumulation of octopamine is the result of combined failure of MAO in the gastrointestinal tract and the liver to remove the small quantities of tyramine formed by bacterial fermentation in the intestine. This relatively small amount of tyramine reaches the systemic circulation and is taken up into the sympathetic neurons without releasing significant amounts of NE. Because the MAO in the neuron is also inhibited, the tyramine is transported into the synaptic vesicles. The dopamine-β-hydroxylase in the vesicles converts the tyramine to octopamine, which slowly replaces a portion of the NE and is released instead of a portion of the NE. Since octopamine is almost inactive as a transmitter, the effects of nerve stimulation are markedly reduced. Octopamine is among a number of compounds that can serve as false adrenergic neurotransmitters (Kopin, 1968) but is the major amine accumulated in the sympathetic neurons when MAO is inhibited. Although other mechanisms for MOAI-induced orthostatic hypotension have been suggested, e.g., an effect mediated by central nervous system or ganglionic amines, they do not explain the reduced effects of direct stimulation of sympathetic nerves in organ preparations such as the perfused spleen of cats chronically pretreated with a MAO inhibitor.

9. Hypertensive crises from MAO inhibitors

As indicated above, tyramine was identified as the major pressor substance in putrified meat (Dale and Dixon, 1909). Over 60 years later, when hypertensive crises were reported in patients who were being treated with MAO inhibitors (e.g., Blackwell, 1963), the cause of the pressor effect was found to be dietary; as in putrifing meat, tyramine is formed by bacterial decarboxylation of tyrosine during the process of manufacture of cheese, wine, etc., and is present in high concentrations in the ingested products (Horwitz et al., 1964; Blackwell and Mabbitt, 1965). When such foods are ingested, if MAO is inhibited, the concentration of tyramine in the systemic circulation increases rapidly and attains levels that release large quantities of NE. This causes a marked rise in systemic blood pressure, similar to the effects of the tyramine in putrified meat described in 1909 by Dale and Dixon. When MAO in inhibited, but the ingested foods produce only small quantities of tyramine, there are prolonged, relatively low elevations in plasma tyramine concentrations slow displacement of NE stores by octopamine that diminishes sympathetic responsivity, as described above. Avoidance of the hypertensive response to high levels of ingested tyramine became feasible when subtypes of MAO and drugs that selectively inhibit MAO-B were discovered (see Youdim and Finberg, 1987).

10. Multiple forms of MAO

Entirely new perspectives about MAO arose after the demonstration that there are two types of MAO. Although a few previously published evidence suggested that MAO was complex, the first definitive evidence for two different enzymes was present by Johnston (1968), During examination of the kinetics of inhibition of MAO by new potential MAO inhibitors, he noted that one of the compounds being tested, clorgyline (at that time designated as M&B 9302), was strikingly different from most others. Using tyramine as a substrate, graphing of percentage inhibition of MAO activity in a rat brain mitochondrial preparation revealed a pair of sigmoid curves. The midpoints of these curves were separated by over three orders of magnitude. He interpreted this difference as indicating that there were two forms of MAO. The first, MAO-A, was very sensitive to inhibition by clorgyline, whereas the second, MAO-B was relatively resistant to the inhibitor. However, tyramine was an equally good substrate for MAO-A and MAO-B. When tryptamine was used as substrate, only MAO-A activity was apparent, indicating that tryptamine is a poor substrate for MAO-B.

In 1966, Moussa Youdim, working with Ted Sourkes at McGill University in Montreal, sowed the seeds of his remarkably productive career by being the first to solubilize MAO (Youdim and Sourkes, 1966). After joining Merton Sandler in London, Moussa, working with solubilized preparations of MAO subjected to electrophoresis, separated of several isoenzymes of MAO with differing substrate specificities (Youdim et al., 1969) supporting the view that there were several forms of MAO. When a specific inhibitor of MAO-B, deprenyl (selegiline), was discovered (Knoll and Magyar, 1972), it became possible to compare the effects of each of the MAO specific inhibitors on the metabolism and responses elicited by a variety of amines. It had been recognized that the existence of multiple forms of MAO might have important physiological and pharmacological implications (Sandler and Youdim, 1972). After Birkmeyer et al. (1975) reported that deprenyl could potentiate the effects of DOPA in parkinsonian patients, it was found that this MAO inhibitor could be administered without fear of "cheese effect" (Lees et al., 1977; Sandler et al., 1978). Although deprenyl prolonged the effects of administered DOPA, it did not alter the symptoms of depression, when present, in parkinsonian patients (Lees et al., 1977). This was one of the first reports suggesting that inhibition of MAO-A was required for the antidepressant effect, as well as the "cheese effect" of non-specific MAO inhibitors. Thus, the initial use of deprenyl in parkinsonian patients was based on the potentation of DOPA by inhibition of MAO-B. Subsequently molecular genetic approaches definitively established the existence two distinct forms of MAO (Bach et al., 1988). Studies of their tissue distribution, molecular structure, etc. have yielded volumes of new information about the enzymes, but their potentially important role in pathogenic mechanisms was a matter of infrequent speculation.

11. The relationship of MPTP toxicity to MAO

The accidental discovery that a contaminant of an illicit narcotic caused a parkinsonian syndrome in drug addicts and in chemist exposed to the toxin stimulated an entirely new approach to study of the etiology of Parkinson's disease. Soon after 1-methyl-4-phenyl-1,2,5,6-tetrahydropyridine (MPTP) was discovered as the cause of severe chronic Parkinsonism in humans (Davis et al., 1979; Langston et al., 1983) and in primates (Burns et al., 1973), the mechanism of its toxicity was found to require its conversion to 1-methyl-4-phenylpyridinium (MPP^+) by the action of MAO (Chiba et al., 1984). This unleashed a flood of research seeking environmental or endogenous agents (see review by Tanner, 1989) that might mimic MPTP. Others focused on determination of how MPP^+ caused cell death and how these mechanisms might explain the degeneration of stiatal dopaminergic neurons in Parkinson's disease.

12. MAO and neurotoxicity

As described above, H_2O_2 formation as a product of deamination was discovered over about 80 years ago, but it was assumed that the ubiquitous catalase would rapidly destroy this potentially toxic agent. This view has been questioned. The cycles of oxidative stress, free radicals and the catalysis by iron in generating them, mitochondrial damage that has been demonstrated in Parkinson's disease, the cascade of events that terminate in cell death, the relationship of genetic abnormalities in the a-synuclein or parkin (defects that are the bases of heritable forms of Parkinson's disease) and the aldehydes formed from catecholamine deamination are all pieces of a puzzle that continues to challenge investigators. The mechanism(s) of neuronal degeneration remain poorly defined, but there are numerous active approaches to development of agents that target MAO (particularly the B form) and other potential participants in the events terminating in cell death (see e.g., Youdim and Riederer, 2004). The rationale for targeting multiple sites with a single drug that would prevent or retard the progression of neurodegenerative diseases has been championed by Moussa Youdim and his collaborators (see e.g., Youdim and Buccafusco, 2005).

13. Moussa Youdim and the future

Since his first paper describing solubilization of MAO, Moussa Youdim has contributed hundreds of papers dealing with many of these MAO-associated issues. He has been an imaginative scientist, inspired leader and highly valued collaborator in the pharmacological approaches to the alleviation, retardation the progress or prevention of the development of Parkinson's and Alzheimer's diseases. We wish him well in all his future endeavors, knowing that he will not shirk from trying to meet the new challenges.

References

Armstrong MD, McMillan A, Shaw KN (1957) 3-Methoxy-4-hydroxy-D-mandelic acid, a urinary metabolite of norepinephrine. Biochim Biophys Acta 25: 422–423

Axelrod J, Hertting G, Potter L (1962) Effect of drugs on the uptake and release of 3H-norepinephrine in the rat heart. Nature 194: 297

Axelrod J, Inscoe JK, Senoh S, Witkop B (1958a) O-methylation, the principal pathway for the metabolism of epinephrine and norepinephrine in the rat. Biochim Biophys Acta 27: 210–201

Axelrod J, Kopin IJ, Mann JD (1959) 3-Methoxy-4-hydroxyphenylglycol sulfate, a new metabolite of epinephrine and norepinephrine. Biochim Biophys Acta 36: 576–577

Axelrod J, Laroche MJ (1959) Inhibitor of O-methylation of epinephrine and norepinephrine in vitro and in vivo. Science 130: 800

Axelrod J, Senoh S, Witkop B (1958b) O-Methylation of catechol amines in vivo. J Biol Chem 233: 697–701

Axelrod J, Tomchick R (1958) Enzymatic O-methylation of epinephrine and other catechols. J Biol Chem 233: 702–705

Axelrod J, Weil-Malherbe H Tomchick R (1959) The physiological disposition of H3-epinephrine and its metabolite metanephrine. J Pharmacol Exp Ther 127: 251–256

Axelrod J, Whitby LG, Hertting G (1961) Effect of psychotropic drugs on the uptake of H3-norepinephrine by tissues. Science 133: 383–384

Bach AW, Lan NC, Johnson DL, Abell CW, Bembenek ME, Kwan SW, Seeburg PH, Shih JC (1988) cDNA cloning of human liver monoamine oxidase A and B: molecular basis of differences in enzymatic properties. Proc Natl Acad Sci USA 85: 4934–4938

Bacq ZM (1936) Sensibilisation ae l'adrenaline et ae l'excitatiou des nerfs adrenergiques par les antioxygenes. Arch intern Physiol 42: 340, 44: 15

Bacq, ZM, Gosselin L, Dresse A, Renson J (1959) Inhibition of *O*-methyltransferase by catechol and sensitization to epinephrine. Science 130: 453–454

Bernheim MLC (1931) Tyramine oxidase II Course of the oxidation. J Biol Chem 93: 299–314

Bertler A, Carlsson A, Rosengren E (1956) Release by reserpine of catecholamines from rabbit's hearts. Naturwissenschaften 22: 521–522

Birkmayer W, Riederer P, Youdim MB, Linauer W (1975) The potentiation of the anti akinetic effect after L-dopa treatment by an inhibitor of MAO-B, Deprenil. J Neural Transm 36: 303–326

Blackwell B (1963) Hypertensive Crisis Due to Monoamine Oxidase Inhibitors. Lancet 1: 849–850

Blackwell B, Mabbitt LA (1965) Tyramine in Cheese Related to Hypertensive Crises after Monoamine Oxidase Inhibitions. Lancet 1: 938–940

Blaschko H (1952) Amine oxidase and amine metabolism. Pharm Rev 4: 415–458

Blaschko H, Richter D, Schlossman H (1937) The oxidation of adrenaline and other amines. Biochem J 31: 2187–2196

Bloch RG, Dooneieff AS, Buchberg AS, Spellman S (1954) The clinical effect of isoniazid and iproniazid in the treatment of pulmonary tuberculosis. Ann Intern Med 40: 881–900

Blombery PA, Kopin IJ, Gordon EK, Markey SP, Ebert MH (1980) Conversion of MHPG to vanillylmandelic acid. Implications for the importance of urinary MHPG. Arch Gen Psychiatry 37: 1095–1098

Brown GL, Gillespie JS (1957) The output of sympathetic transmitter from the spleen of the cat. J Physiol 138: 81–102

Burke WJ, Li SW, Chung HD, Ruggiero DA, Kristal BS, Johnson EM, Lampe P, Kumar VB, Franko M, Williams EA, Zahm DS (2004) Neurotoxicity of MAO metabolites of catecholamine neurotransmitters: role in neurodegenerative diseases. Neurotoxicology 25: 101–115

Burn JH, Rand MJ (1958) The action of sympathomimetic amines in animals treated with reserpine. J Physiol 144: 314–336

Burns RS, Chiueh CC, Markey SP, Ebert MH, Jacobowitz DM, Kopin IJ (1983) A primate model of parkinsonism: selective destruction of dopaminergic neurons in the pars compacta of the substantia nigra by N-methyl-4-phenyl-1,2,3,6-tetrahydropyridine. Proc Natl Acad Sci USA 80: 4546–4550

Chiba K, Trevor A, Castagnoli N Jr (1984) Metabolism of the neurotoxic tertiary amine, MPTP, by brain monoamine oxidase. Biochem Biophys Res Commun 20: 574–578

Chorine V (1945) Action de l'amide nicotinique sur les bacilles du genre Mycobacterium. Comptes Rendus de l'Academie des Sciences (Paris) 220: 150–151

Corne SJ, Graham JD (1957) The effect of inhibition of amine oxidase in vivo on administered adrenaline, noradrenaline, tyramine and serotonin. J Physiol 135: 339–349

Crout JR (1961) Effect of inhibiting both catechol-O-methyl transferase and monoamine oxidase on cardiovascular responses to norepinephrine. Proc Soc Exp Biol Med 108: 482–484

Dale HH Dixon WE (1909) The action of Pressor Amines Produced by Putrifaction J Physiol 25: 78–87

Davis GC, Williams AC, Markey SP, Ebert MH, Caine ED, Reichert CM, Kopin IJ (1979) Chronic Parkinsonism secondary to intravenous injection of meperidine analogues. Psychiatry Res 1: 249–254

Eisenhofer G, Kopin IJ, Goldstein DS (2004) Catecholamine metabolism: a contemporary view with implications for physiology and medicine. Pharmacol Rev 56: 331–349

Ewins AJ, Laidlaw PP (1910) The fate of parahydroxyphenylethylamine in the organism. J Physiol 41: 78–87

Fenton HJH (1894) The oxidation of tartaric acid in the presence of iron. J Chem Soc 65: 899–910
Frölich A, Loewi O (1910) Über eine Steigerung der Adrenalinempfindlichkeit durch Cocaine. Arch f exper Path u Pharmakol 62: 159–169
Griesemer EC, Barsky J, dragstedt CA, Wells JA, Zeller EA (1953) Potentiating effect of iproniazid on the pharmacological action of sympathomimetic amines. Proc Soc Exp Biol Med 84: 699–701
Haber F, Weiss J (1932) Über die Katalyse des Hydroperoxydes. Naturwiss 51: 948–950
Hare MLC (1928) Tyramine Oxidase. I. A new enzyme system in the liver. Biochem J 22: 968–979
Hertting G, Axelrod J, Kopin IJ, Whitby LG (1961) Lack of uptake of catecholamines after chronic denervation of sympathetic nerves. Nature 189: 66–67
Hillarp NA (1958) Isolation and some biochemical properties of the catecholamine granules in the cow adrenal medulla. Acta Physiol Scand 43: 82–96
Holtz P, Stock K, Westermann E (1964) Pharmacology of Tetrahydropapaveroline and its Formation from Dopamine. NaunynSchmiedebergs Arch Exp Pathol Pharmakol 248: 387–405
Holtzbauer M, Vogt (1956) Depression by reserpine of the noradrenaline concentration in the hypothalamus of the cat. J Neurochem 1: 8–11
Horwitz D, Lovenberg W, Engelman K, Sjoerdsma A (1964) Monoamine Oxidase Inhibitors, Tyramine, and Cheese. JAMA 188: 1108–1010
Johnston JP (1968) Some observations upon a new inhibitor of monoamine oxidase in brain tissue. Biochem Pharmacol 17: 1285–1297
Kakimoto Y, Armstrong MD (1962) On the identification of octopamine in mammals. J Biol Chem 237: 208–214
Knoll J, Magyar K (1972) Some puzzling pharmacological effects of monoamine oxidase inhibitors. Adv Biochem Psychopharmacol 5: 393–408
Kohn HI (1937) Tyramine oxidase. Biochem J 31: 1693–1704
Kopin IJ (1960) Technique for the study of alternate metabolic pathways: Epinephrine metabolism in man. Science 131: 1372–1374
Kopin IJ (1964) Storage and Metabolism of Catecholamines: the Role of Monoamine Oxidase. Pharmacol Rev 16: 179–191
Kopin IJ (1968) False adrenergic transmitters. Annu Rev Pharmacol 8: 377–394
Kopin IJ, Axelrod J (1960) 3,4-Dihydroxyphenylglycol, a metabolite of epinephrine. Arch Biochem Biophys 89: 148
Kopin IJ, Fischer JE, Musacchio J, Horst WD (1964) Evidence for a false neurochemical transmitter as a mechanism for the hypotensive effect of monoamine oxidase inhibitors. Proc Natl Acad Sci USA 52: 716–721
Kopin IJ, Gordon EK (1963) Metabolism of administered and drug-released norepinephrine-7-H3 in the rat. J Pharmacol Exp Ther 140: 207–216
Langston JW, Ballard P, Tetrud JW, Irwin I (1983) Chronic Parkinsonism in humans due to a product of meperidine-analog synthesis. Science 219: 979–980
Lees AJ, Shaw KM, Kohout LJ, Stern GM, Elsworth JD, Sandler M, Youdim MB (1977) Deprenyl in Parkinson's disease. Lancet 2: 791–795
Liechtenstein MR, Mizenberg E (1954) A controlled study of isoniazid and iproniazid. Dis Chest 25: 573–579
Loomer HP, Saunders JC, Kline NS (1957) A clinical and pharmacodynamic evaluation of iproniazid as a psychic energizer. Psychiatr Res Rep Am Psychiatr Assoc 135: 129–141
Mardh G, Sjoquist B, Anggard E (1981) Norepinephrine metabolism in man using deuterium labelling: the conversion of 4-hydroxy-3-methoxyphenylglycol to 4-hydroxy-3-methoxymandelic acid. J Neurochem 36: 1181–1185
Marley E, Blackwell B (1970) Interactions of monoamine oxidase inhibitors, amines, and foodstuffs. Adv Pharmacol Chemother 8: 185–349
McCord JM, Fridovich I (1969) Superoxide dismutase. An enzymic function for erythrocuprein (hemocuprein). J Biol Chem 244: 6049–6055
Philpot FT (1940) The Inhibition of Oxidation of Adrenaline Oxidation by Local Anaesthetics. J Physiol 97: 301–318
Pletscher A (1958) Einfluss von Isopropyl-isonocotinsaurehydrazid auf den Catecholamingehalt des myocards. Experientia 14: 73
Pletscher A, Shore PA, Brodie BB (1955) Serotonin release as a possible mechanism of reserpine action. Science 122: 374–375
Rebhun J, Feinberg SM, Zeller EA (1954) Potentiating effect of iproniazid on action of some sympathicomimetic amines. Proc Soc Exp Biol Med 87: 218–220
Richter D (1937) Adrenaline and amine oxidase. Biochem J 31: 2022–2028
Sandler M, Carter SB, Hunter KR, Stern GM (1973) Tetrahydroisoquinoline alkaloids: in vivo metabolites of L-dopa in man. Nature 241: 439–443
Sandler M, Glover V, Ashford A, Stern GM (1978) Absence of "cheese effect" during deprenyl therapy: some recent studies. J Neural Transm 43: 209–215
Sandler M, Youdim MB (1972) Multiple forms of monoamine oxidase: functional significance. Pharmacol Rev 24: 331–348
Schayer RW (1951) Studies on the metabolism of β-C^{14}-dl-adrenaline. J Biol Chem 189: 301–306
Schayer RW, Smiley RL (1951) The metabolism of adrenalin containing isotopic carbon. J Biol Chem 192: 875–881
Schayer RW, Smiley RL (1953) III Metabolism of epinephrine containing isotopic carbon. III. J Biol Chem 202: 425–430
Schayer RW, Smiley RL, Davis KJ, Kobayashi Y (1955) Role of monoamine oxidase in nor-adrenaline metabolism. Am J Physiol 82: 285–286
Schayer RW, Smiley RL, Kaplan EH (1952) The metabolism of epinephrine containing isotopic carbon. II. J Biol Chem 198: 545–551
Shore PA Mead JAR, Kuntzman, RG, Spector, S, Brodie, BB (1957) On the physiological significance of monoamine oxidase in brain. Science 126: 1063–1064
Tanner CM (1989) The role of environmental toxins in the etiology of Parkinson's disease. Trends Neurosci 12: 49–54
Whitby LG, Axelrod J, Weil-Malherbe H (1961) The fate of H3-norepinephrine in animals. J Pharmacol Exp Ther 132: 193–201
Whitby LG, Hertting G, Axelrod J (1960) Effect of cocaine on the disposition of noradrenaline labelled with tritium. Nature 187: 604
Wolfe DE, Potter LT, Richardson KC, Axelrod J (1962) Localizing tritiated norepinephrine in sympathetic axons by electron microscopic autoradiography. Science 138: 440–442
Youdim MB, Buccafusco JJ (2005) Multi-functional drugs for various CNS targets in the treatment of neurodegenerative disorders. Trends Pharmacol Sci 26: 27–35
Youdim MB, Collins GG, Sandler M (1969) Multiple forms of rat brain monoamine oxidase. Nature 223: 626–628
Youdim MB, Finberg JP (1987) Monoamine oxidase B inhibition and the "cheese effect". J Neural Transm 25 [Suppl]: 27–33
Youdim MB, Riederer PF (2004) A review of the mechanisms and role of monoamine oxidase inhibitors in Parkinson's disease. Neurology 63 [Suppl 2]: S32–S35
Youdim MB, Sourkes TL (1966) Properties of purified, soluble monoamine oxidase. Can J Biochem 44: 1397–1400
Zeller EA (1963) New reflections on monoamine oxidase inhibition. Ann NY Acad Sci 107: 809–1158
Zeller EA, Barsky J (1952) In vivo inhibition of liver and brain monoamine oxidase by 1-Isonicotinyl-2-isopropyl hydrazine. Proc Soc Exp Biol Med 81: 459–461

J Neural Transm (2006) [Suppl] 71: 87–95

Journal of Neural Transmission
Printed in Austria

Isatin, an endogenous MAO inhibitor, and a rat model of Parkinson's disease induced by the Japanese encephalitis virus

M. Minami[1], N. Hamaue[1], M. Hirafuji[1], H. Saito[1], T. Hiroshige[1], A. Ogata[2], K. Tashiro[2], S. H. Parvez[3]

[1] The Research Institute of Personalized Health Science, Health Science University of Hokkaido, Ishikari-Tobetsu, Japan
[2] Department of Neurology, Hokkaido University Graduate School of Medicine, Sapporo, Japan
[3] Alfred Fressard Institute of Neuroscience, CNRS UPR, Gif Sur Yvette, France

Summary A single dose of isatin (indole-2,3-dione)(i.p.), an endogenous MAO inhibitor, significantly increased norepinephrine and 5-hydroxytryptamine concentrations in the rat brain and also significantly increased acetylcholine and dopamine (DA) levels in the rat striatum. Urinary isatin concentrations in patients with Parkinson's disease tend to increase according to the severity of disease. We have developed a rat model of Parkinson's disease induced by the Japanese encephalitis virus (JEV). The distribution of the pathological lesions of JEV-rats resemble those found in Parkinson's disease. Significant behavioral improvement was observed in JEV-rats after isatin, L-DOPA and selegiline administration using a pole test. Both isatin and selegiline prevented the decrease in striatum DA levels of JEV-rats. The increased turnover of DA (DOPAC/DA) induced by JEV was significantly inhibited by isatin, but not selegiline. These findings suggest that JEV-infected rats may serve as a model of Parkinson's disease and that exogenously administered isatin and selegiline can improve JEV-induced parkinsonism by increasing DA concentrations in the striatum.

Endogenous monoamine oxidase (MAO) inhibitory component was first discovered in normal human urine by Glover et al. (1980) and the compound responsible for the MAO activity was subsequently given the name "tribulin" (Sandler, 1982). In 1988, isatin was identified as a major constituent of tribulin (Glover et al., 1988). We also identified isatin as one of the extracts in the urine of stroke-prone spontaneously hypertensive rats (SHRSP) (Hamaue et al., 1992) and in SHRSP brains (Hamaue et al., 1994) using gaschromatography-mass spectrometry (GC-MS). Tribulin may be responsible for the metabolites of isatin-related compounds (McIntyre and Norman, 1990). MAO inhibitory drugs such as selegiline have been widely used in clinical practice, originally for depressive illness, anxiety and for Parkinson's disease. There is, however, virtually no information regarding the detailed central nervous system (CNS) function of isatin. Some experiments suggested that isatin can serve as a marker of stress and anxiety (Glover et al., 1991; Tozawa et al., 1998). We previously reported that exogenously administered isatin increased dopamine (DA) levels in the rat striatum (Hamaue et al., 1999a) and recently demonstrated that a significant increase in urinary isatin excretion was present in patients with Parkinson's disease (Yahr's classifications III, IV, V) (Hamaue et al., 2000). These results suggest that isatin may be associated with the pathogenic process in Parkinson's disease. In this study, we analyzed neurochemical and pathological changes in our rat model of Parkinson's disease induced by the Japanese encephalitis virus (JEV). By analyzing the DA levels together with movement problems, we evaluated the potential treatment of JEV-induced parkinsonism by endogenous MAO inhibitor isatin and synthesized MAO-B inhibitor selegiline. Furthermore, we analyzed and evaluated the MAO-inhibitor effects on neurochemical and pathological changes in our rat model of Parkinson's disease induced by JEV.

Chemistry and MAO activity of isatin, an endogenous MAO inhibitor

Several previous reports have shown that stress can induce a decrease in MAO inhibitory activity (Clow et al., 1988). Isatin was identified as a major constituent of tribulin, a low-molecular-mass inhibitor of MAO type B (Glover et al., 1988). Tribulin output in human urine increases during various conditions of stress and anxiety (Clow et al., 1988). Cold immobilization stress has been shown to be associated

Correspondence: M. Minami, MD, PhD, (Professor of Emeritus, Health Science University of Hokkaido), Chief Director, Unit of Geriatrics: Ohzora, Touei Hospital, Higashi-ku, Okadama 167-10, Sapporo 007-0880, Japan
e-mail: minami-m@touei.or.jp

with the serotonergic system (Oxenkrug and McIntyre, 1985). Cold-restraint stress increases the tribulin content in the rat heart and kidney (Armando et al., 1988).

Tribulin, which acts on central benzodiazepine receptors, has been proposed as an anxiety-promoting agent (Sandler, 1982). The MAO inhibitory and benzodiazepine receptor binding inhibitory components of tribulin are roughly equipotent (Clow et al., 1983). Tribulin differs from most other benzodiazepine receptor ligands in that it is not a peptide, because tribulin is extracted with ethyl acetate (Elsworth et al., 1986). Glover et al. (1988) reported that endogenous isatin has properties similar to tribulin. Isatin emerged as one of the major MAO inhibitory compounds to be isolated from human urine. Substantial concentrations of isatin are present in urine and tissues of both the rat and human.

Isatin is well known as a pharmacological agent and its effects have been studied in a variety of systems. It is a selective MAO-B inhibitor. At much higher concentrations it inhibits a variety of other enzymes, such as alkaline phosphatase (Bansal et al., 1988). There are also several reports of its *in vivo* effects. In rodents, isatin is anxiogenic and urinary excretion is increased after cold exposure (Tozawa et al., 1998). It remains unclear, however, whether all of the MAO inhibitory and benzodiazepine displacing activity attributed to tribulin is due to isatin (Glover et al., 1988). Jarman et al. (1990) have measured urinary tribulin and isatin in parallel and found a highly significant but not complete correlation between the two ($r = 0.68$, $n = 18$, $p < 0.001$ in migraine patients). Tribulin may be responsible for metabolites of isatin or related endogenous compounds (McIntyre and Norman, 1990). The physiological and pathological roles of isatin are not yet clear. Its molecular formula and weight are $C_8H_5NO_2$ and 147.14. It dissolves easily in water as well as in organic solvents such as ethyl acetate, although not in acetone (Glover et al., 1991).

In our *in vitro* study, isatin was found to be a potent MAO inhibitor that was more active against MAO-B than MAO-A. The IC_{50} of the MAO total, the MAO-A and the MAO-B, was 1.5×10^{-5}, 5.8×10^{-5} and 1.4×10^{-5} M, respectively (Hamaue et al., 1992). Line Weaver-Burk plot and Dixon analysis indicated that isatin competitively inhibited the MAO activity of the rat liver homogenate in a concentration-dependent manner (Hamaue et al., 1992).

Tribulin has endogenous MAO and benzodiazepine binding inhibitory activity. It is extractable from biological tissues and body fluids into ethyl acetate. Research (Glover et al., 1988) on tribulin (low molecular weight endogenous inhibitory activity of MAO) has confirmed that its level is increased in both human urine and rat tissues by stress or anxiety, and by anxiogenic drugs. Isatin is thought to be a portion of tribulin that is a selective inhibitor of MAO-B. Other portions of tribulin, the ethyl and methyl esters of indoleacetic and 4-hydroxyphenylacetic acids, selectively inhibit MAO-A (Medvedev et al., 1996). Pathways for the synthesis and metabolism of isatin have not been established. One possible source would be via the action of the gut flora. It has been suggested that dietary tryptophan may be converted into indole by the gut flora and then transported to the liver where it is oxidized. Urinary isatin excretion is significantly reduced in germ free rat urine (0.22 μg/ml) compared with the urine of control rats (0.66 μg/ml) (Glover et al., 1991). This suggests that isatin is derived, at least in part, from the gut flora, which act perhaps on tryptophan containing food.

The stroke-prone spontaneously hypertensive rat (SHRSP)-stroke model in which stroke was clearly detected by pathological examination had significantly higher plasma norepinephrine (NE) levels than the controls. Plasma NE levels of the Wistar Kyoto rats (WKY), SHRSP-control and SHRSP-stroke groups were 248.8 ± 23.2, 346.9 ± 35.2 and 466.0 ± 85.7 pg/ml, respectively, while the mitochondrial MAO activity of the three groups was 146.4 ± 13.3, 87.1 ± 11.2 and 72.1 ± 8.64 (mean $\pm$ SE, $n = 12$) nmol/hr/mg protein, respectively. An inverse relationship was demonstrated between plasma NE levels and kidney MAO activity in SHRSP and WKY. Parvez and Parvez (1973) reported that catechol-o-methyltransferase (COMT) activity was related to the amount of substrate present in normotensive rats. It was assumed that the relative increase in red cell COMT activity was due to an increased level of circulating catecholamines. A compensatory increase in COMT and MAO activity may be an important factor in the control of plasma catecholamines in normotensive rats.

In brain and kidney extracts (Hamaue et al., 1992), tribulin-like activity was found to be significantly higher in SHRSP than in WKY. Tribulin activity was also significantly greater in the extract of SHRSP urine than in that of WKY (Hamaue et al., 1992). It has been suggested that impairment of the central adrenergic neurons is associated with blood pressure control and MAO activity in SHRSP (Minami et al., 1988). Thus, it is important in the regulation of monoamine concentrations (Blaschko, 1973). Although mechanisms other than enzyme concentration have been postulated for the regulation of MAO activity *in vivo*, evidence of short term regulation of the enzyme is scarce. Normal human urine inhibits MAO (Glover et al., 1988). This inhibitory activity is also present in SHRSP urine (Hamaue et al., 1992). Although the mechanism of decreased MAO activity induced by tribulin (or isatin) has not yet been elucidated, it was postulated that increased blood pressure may be associated with increased monoamine concentrations induced by tribulin (or isatin) in SHRSP.

In line with the above, we isolated and identified isatin as one of the extracts in SHRSP urine (Hamaue et al., 1992) and in SHRSP brains (Hamaue et al., 1994) using GC-MS.

Characteristics of the biological properties of isatin

Isatin has a wide spectrum of biological properties against stress and certain infections (Glover et al., 1991). Isatin has been shown to inhibit a number of enzymes such as acid phosphatase (Singh et al., 1977), alkaline phosphatase (Bansal et al., 1988), hyaluronidase (Kumar et al., 1977), xanthine oxidase (Susheela et al., 1969), as well as MAO.

Isatin has been found to act as an antiseizure agent in a variety of tests (Chocholova and Kolinova, 1979). It potentiates the antiseizure action of propranolol (Muller and Schramek, 1989). It also appears to increase vigilance and reduce slow wave sleep (Chocholova and Kolinova, 1981), yet Yumiler (1990) found some indirect evidence to support that isatin acts as a benzodiazepine receptor blocker *in vivo*. The most potent action of isatin *in vitro* determined to date is the inhibition of the atrial natriuretic peptide (ANP) binding to its receptor (IC_{50}: 0.4 μM) (Glover et al., 1995). Isatin also attenuates ANP-stimulated guanylate cyclase activity in the rat brain, heart and kidney (Glover et al., 1995). Recent studies also suggest that the anxiogenic effect of isatin may be explained by its antagonism to ANP (Battacharya et al., 1996). Thus isatin may provide a link between the function of the monoamines involved in stress and the control of the natriuretic system by ANP (Medvedev et al., 1996). Isatin-induced anxiogenic action can be blocked by 5-HT_3 receptor antagonists (Glover et al., 1993). *In vivo* studies suggest that isatin may function as an agonist at the 5-HT_3 receptors, although this was not evident in recent *in vitro* binding studies (Hota and Acharya, 1994).

In human urine, tribulin increases as a result of exercise (Armando et al., 1984) and old age (Ueki et al., 1989). Urinary tribulin excretion was found to be significantly higher in females than in males (Clow et al., 1988). Tribulin output is transiently raised following alcohol withdrawal (Battacharya et al., 1982), benzodiazepine withdrawal (Peturson et al., 1982), lactate-induced panic attacks (Clow et al., 1988) and migraine attacks (Jarman et al., 1990). Tribulin output thus appears to be raised in a variety of different conditions related to stress, agitation or anxiety.

Acute food deprivation and acute cold exposure induced a marked increase in rat urinary isatin excretion during the 24 hrs following the initiation of stress (Tozawa et al., 1998). Dexamethasone administration prevented this increase in urinary isatin excretion induced by acute food deprivation and cold exposure. Furthermore, administration of either diazepam or the tyrosine hydroxylase inhibitor α-methyl-p-tyrosine prevented the increase in urinary isatin excretion induced by acute food deprivation, whereas the dopamine-beta-hydroxylase (DBH) inhibitor diethyldithiocarbamate proved ineffective. These observations suggest that during stress, activated catecholamine synthesizing cells and corticotropin-releasing factor cells, both of which play central roles in stress responses, may be involved in isatin production (Tozawa et al., 1998). Thus, isatin may serve as an endogenously generated maker for some types of stress.

Acute effect of exogenously administered isatin on tissue monoamine concentrations in the rat

A single dose of isatin (50 or 200 mg/kg, i.p.) increased 5-HT concentrations measured 2 hours later in various brain regions of WKY and SHRSP (Hamaue et al., 1994). The magnitude of changes caused by isatin in SHRSP was lower than that observed in WKY. The ratio of 5-hydroxyindoleacetic acid (5-HIAA)/5-HT was significantly decreased by isatin in both WKY and SHRSP. *In vitro*, 5-HT is primarily metabolised by MAO-A (Yang and Neff, 1974). These data indicate that isatin significantly affects 5-HT activity which may, in turn, have an important physiological effect on CNS function. Several studies have shown that acute peripheral administration of isatin causes an increase of monoamines such as NE and 5-HT in the brain (Battacharya and Acharya, 1993; Hamaue et al., 1994; McIntyre and Norman, 1990; Yumier, 1990). Isatin passes into the brain from the periphery, but a peripheral dose of 50 or 100 mg/kg results in a brain concentration of about 9 mg/kg (Battacharya et al., 1993). The dose of isatin for these experiments was selected on the basis of previous reports that doses of higher than 40 mg/kg produced physiological changes (Chocholova et al., 1981; McIntyre and Norman, 1990). A single injection of isatin (50 or 200 mg/kg, i.p.) did not induce any significant cardiovascular or behavioral effects in either WKY or SHRSP.

Effects of isatin on acetylcholine and dopamine concentrations in the rat brain

Kumar et al. (1993) first reported that isatin inhibits acetylcholine esterase (AChE) activity in the rat brain and erythrocytes. We determined the levels of ACh, choline

Table 1. *Acetylcholine (ACh), choline (Ch), and dopamine (DA) concentration in the striatum of Wistar Kyoto rats after isatin administration*

Treatment	ACh	Ch	DA
Control	42.7 ± 2.8	14.7 ± 1.7	25.7 ± 4.1
50 mg/kg	38.5 ± 0.7	12.4 ± 0.3	$39.8 \pm 4.0^{*}$
200 mg/kg	$53.1 \pm 3.2^{*}$	$20.5 \pm 1.5^{*}$	$53.6 \pm 4.6^{**}$

Mean ± SEM, $n = 5$–7; *ACh, Ch, DA* pmol/mg wet tissue; $^{*}p<0.05$; $^{**}p<0.01$ vs control

(Ch) and DA in the rat brain 2 hrs after isatin administration (Hamaue et al., 1999a) using HPLC-ECD according to the method of Matsumoto et al. (1990). As shown in Table 1, ACh and Ch levels in the striatum of the group receiving isatin (50 or 200 mg/kg, i.p.) significantly increased. Striatal DA levels also increased after isatin treatment (Hamaue et al., 1999a). In other words, isatin simultaneously increased ACh and DA levels in the WKY striatum. In our *in vitro* study, 10^{-4} M of isatin induced an approximate 93% inhibition of MAO and a 5% inhibition of AChE in the rat brain. It is clear that isatin has a higher affinity to MAO than to AChE. Isatin administration also increased Ch, an AChE metabolite of ACh, in various brain regions. These results suggested that isatin increased ACh levels not by inhibiting AChE activity, but rather through another pathway.

In the microdialysis study, rats were placed in a stereotaxic apparatus and their right striatum were implanted with a guide cannula (0.8 mm outer diameter) under pentobarbital anesthesia (60 mg/kg, i.v.) according to the method of Paxinos and Watson (1980). Isatin administration (10^{-4} M) caused a significant rise in the extracellular levels of ACh and DA (Hamaue et al., 1999a). During microdialysis with isatin, the DA release from the WKY striatum was greater than the ACh release. Many reports have demonstrated that D_2 dopaminergic receptors increase ACh release (Gorell and Czarnecki, 1986; Imperato et al., 1993; Scatton, 1992; Wedzong et al., 1988). Ohue et al. (1992) reported that perfusion with DA increased the release of ACh from the hippocampus. Apomorphine also increases ACh release (Nilsson et al., 1992), indicating that ACh release from the striatal cholinergic interneuron is induced by D_2 receptor stimulation. The output of striatal ACh is inhibited by D_2 receptors (Lehmann and Langer, 1983; Stoof et al., 1992). The pronounced stimulatory effects of DA antagonists on the release of striatal ACh and their opposite effect on tissue concentration have been reported (Sethy and van Woert, 1974; Stadler et al., 1973). ACh release, therefore, may be increased by DA rise after isatin administration.

Urinary isatin excretion in patients with Parkinson's disease

We have reported that exogenously administered isatin significantly increased ACh and DA levels in the rat striatum (Hamaue et al., 1999b). In order to elucidate the relation between isatin and Parkinson's disease, we measured the urinary isatin excretion of patients with Parkinson's disease (Hamaue et al., 2000). We have developed a convenient, alternative method for the determination of isatin by high-performance liquid chromatography (HPLC) (Hamaue et al., 1998) to replace the GC-MS determination (Hamaue et al., 1994).

Urinary isatin concentration in Parkinson's disease tended to increase in accordance to the degree of Hoehn and Yahr criteria (1967). A significant increase in urinary isatin excretion was observed in patients with Stage III (102.71 ± 28.29, $p<0.05$, $n=13$), VI (129.29 ± 65.92, $p<0.05$, $n=6$) and V (267.05 ± 154.48, $p<0.01$, $n=8$) Parkinson's disease as compared with that of healthy control subjects (52.00 ± 24.29, $n=11$). At these stages, Parkinson's patients demonstrate severe clinical symptoms such as tremor, spastic gait, freezing and masked face. One of the reasons for increased urinary isatin in Parkinson's disease might be due to the stress of this disease or to the compensatory increase response to a lower level of cerebral dopamine content. Patients taking drugs for the treatment of Parkinson's disease were included in this study. Urinary isatin concentrations in drug-treated patients with Parkinson's disease at Stages I (38.11 ± 25.22, $n=6$) and II (62.97 ± 27.64, $n=15$) tended to decrease compared with those of patients without medication. These results suggest that urinary isatin is an endogenous marker for the clinical severity of Parkinson's disease.

A rat model of Parkinson's disease induced by the Japanese encephalitis virus

Animals and virus

The virus strain used was the JaGAr-01 strain of JEV. The supernate from 10% homogenates of infected mouse brains (10^9 PFU/ml) were diluted with 20% Hemaccel (Hoechst) in Eagle's minimum essential medium and stored at −70°C until use. The virus (0.03 ml containing 3×10^6 PFU) was inoculated intracerebrally with a specially designed two-step thin 27 gauge needle (Hoshimori Iryoki KK, Tokyo, Japan) with a stopper 3 mm from the tip. The site of inoculation was located at the midpoint of the line connecting the left eye to the midpoint between the right and left ears of Albino rats of the Fischer strain. We used animals older than 17 days because the mortality rate of animals infected when they were older than 12 days decreased with age, with 13-day-old rats having a 50% mortality rate and 14-day-old rats having 8.3%. Animals inoculated when they were older the 17 days showed 0% mortality.

Neuropathologic study

The topographical distribution of JEV antigen in the developing rat brain was determined 3 days after JEV inoculation (Ogata et al., 1991). The neuropathologic changes in rats infected with JEV on days 12, 13 and 14 after birth were examined. Animals were sacrified 3 days, 10 days, 12 weeks or one year after inoculation under ether anesthesia by perfusion fixation via the aorta with 4% freshly prepared paraformaldehyde in 0.1 M phosphate buffer. Coronal brain sections were taken from the frontal tip to the medulla, embedded in paraffin and stained with hematoxylin-eosin, Luxol fast blue-cresyl violet (Klüver-Barrera method), anti-JEV antibody and anti-tyrosine hydroxylase (TH) monoclonal antibody (Chemicon). The avidin-biotin-peroxidase complex (ABC) method was used in this immunohistochemical study (Hsu et al., 1981). After deparaffinization, the specimens were treated with 0.3% H_2O_2-methanol to suppress endogenous peroxidase activity, incubated with 10% normal goat serum, and allowed to react with anti-JEV rabbit serum or anti-TH monoclonal antibody, diluted in 1% bovine serum albumin (BSA) at 4°C overnight. Incubation with 1% BSA was used as a negative control. The sections were reacted with anti-JEV antibody. Anti-TH monoclonal antibody were then reacted with biotinylated goat anti-rabbit IgG and biotinylated goat anti-mouse IgG (Vecstain), respectively. ABC reaction products were visualized with 3,3′-diaminobenzidine tetrahydrochloride (Sigma) and counterstained with hematoxylin.

Assessment of motor function

A pole test (Ogawa et al., 1985) was performed to evaluate bradykinesia in the rats. The time it took the rats to descend from the top of a rough-surfaced pole (2.5 cm in diameter and 100 cm in height) to the floor was recorded in JEV-infected adult rats and control adult rats. We measured the motor activity of the adult rats (12 weeks after infection) infected with JEV at the age of 13 days and age-matched control rats. The difference between the JEV-infected rats and the control rats was significant ($p < 0.001$). The pole test showed a marked bradykinesia in the JEV-infected rats. Masked faces or tremor could not be assessed in the rats.

Characteristics of the model for Parkinson's disease induced by the Japanese encephalitis virus

The pathogenesis of Parkinson's disease currently is thought to depend upon hereditary, aging and environmental factors (Burns et al., 1983; Calne and Langston, 1983; Ballard et al., 1985; Cohen, 1986; Nagatsu and Yoshida, 1988; Dexter et al., 1989; Riederer et al., 1989; Adams and Odunze, 1991). Among the toxic factors, exogenous toxins such as MPTP and endogenous toxins such as free radicals or tetrahydroisoquinoline (Yoshida et al., 1990) have been implicated. Viruses can also selectively attack the substantia nigra and induce parkinsonism (Duvoisin and Yahr, 1965; Kristensson, 1992). Post-encephalitic parkinsonism is well documented (von Economo, 1917; Yahr, 1978). Walters (1960) described a 54-year-old woman who manifested symptoms of parkinsonism while convalescing from meningoencephalitis due to Coxsackie B virus. Influenza A virus (Hudson and Rice, 1990), poliovirus (Bojinov, 1971) and measles virus (Alves et al., 1992) have also been suspected from case reports as possible viral causes. Fishman et al. (1980) reported an experimental model with a selective attack on the substantia nigra and subthalamic nucleus induced by a strain of mouse hepatitis virus which is a coronavirus that causes persistent CNS infection. Recently similar features have been described in rats infected with influenza virus (Takahashi et al., 1995).

JEV is a positive-strand enveloped RNA virus that belongs to the family of the flaviviruses and is the most common cause of arthropod-borne human encephalitis worldwide. Goto (1962) detected parkinsonian sequelae in 11.6% of 143 unselected patients five years after they had Japanese encephalitis. The parkinsonian syndrome after Japanese encephalitis differs from that which follows encephalitis lethargica in several respects. In general, parkinsonism following Japanese encephalitis is mild, develops in the acute phase and occasionally improves slightly over a long period. Recently, it was reported that MRI abnormalities were seen mainly in the substantia nigra and putamen in a case of typical parkinsonism following Japanese encephalitis (Shoji et al., 1993). Patients without a clear history of encephalitis who follow the clinical course and have pathologic findings consistent with postencephalitic parkinsonism have been reported (Gibb and Lees, 1987; Geddes et al., 1993). Although there were no Lewy bodies found in the substantia nigra in the JEV-treated rats, the pathologic findings otherwise resembled those of idiopathic Parkinson's disease. Furthermore, the immunohistochemical data using anti-TH antibody suggested that the function of the dopaminergic system might have deteriorated with age in the absence of ongoing or persistent JEV infection. McGeer et al. (1988) showed that the rate of neuronal cell degeneration was considerably higher in parkinsonian patients than could be accounted for on the basis of normal age-related neuronal degeneration alone. It seems likely that neuronal cell degeneration progressed more rapidly in the JEV-treated rats than in the controls. This observation raises the possibility that post-encephalitic parkinsonism as well as Parkinson's disease is a continuing degenerative process rather than an acute illness on which the effects of aging or decompensation are superimposed. Such late deterioration might be due to a resurgence of viral-mediated damage (Appel et al., 1992), although our model does not support this view.

The complete nucleotide sequence of JEV genome RNA has been determined (Sumiyoshi et al., 1987). Our RT-PCR study for NS3 region amplification (Morita et al., 1991) of the JEV genome showed that the JEV genome was undetectable in rats sacrificed 12 weeks after JEV infection at the age of 13 days. Moreover, JEV antigen as well as the JEV genome disappeared from the brain. These findings indicate that there is no persistent infection in the brain and suggest that following the acute phase, JEV-infected rats are a safe model for researchers.

Thus far, no virus has been isolated from patients with Parkinson's disease, and there are no data that directly link known viruses to idiopathic Parkinson's disease. However, our findings support the possibility that as yet unidentified specific pathogens could cause similar pathologic lesions in man, resulting in Parkinson's disease. Why neurons of the subtantia nigra remain susceptible to JEV infection longer than in other parts of the brain is unclear. One possibility is that virus receptors on the substantia nigra neurons persist longer. Certainly, the capacity of viruses to attack specific tissues selectively depends on an interaction between viral genes or proteins and host factors. An immune mechanism following an infection or other factors could be associated with the destruction of the substantia nigra. A more detailed understanding of JEV tropism for the substantia nigra in this experimental model might reveal mechanisms that aid in unraveling the degeneration of nigral dopaminergic neurons that is central to Parkinson's disease.

The JEV-induced parkinsonism in rats is characterized by selective destruction of neurons in the bilateral substantia nigra, especially in the zona compacta of the substantia nigra, similar to the lesions found in Parkinson's disease.

The effects of isatin and selegiline on bradykinesia and dopamine levels in a rat model of Parkinson's disease induced by the Japanese encephalitis virus

JEV is the most common cause of arthropod-borne human encephalitis in Asia (Johnson et al., 1985) and may also be a cause of post-encephalitis parkinsonism (Dickerson et al., 1952). Ogata et al. (1997, 1998) have reported pathological results that in adult Fisher rats sacrificed 12 weeks after infection with JEV at 13 days, the number of tyrosine hydroxylase (TH)-positive cells was decreased in the substantia nigra, suggesting post-encephalitis parkinsonism. Many of the existing therapies of Parkinson's disease counteract the detection of DA levels in the stratum as a result of the disease. The JEV-infected rat model showed marked bradykinesia, with significant behavioral improvement being observed following administration of L-DOPA (Ogata et al., 1997). Next, we compared the effects of isatin, an endogenous MAO-inhibitor, on the motor function and DA levels of JEV-induced Parkinson's model rats with those of selegiline, a selective MAO-B inhibitor (Hamaue et al., 2004).

It is an important observation that exogenously administered isatin or selegiline ameliorated the bradykinesia observed in JEV-induced parkinsonism rats. Also, isatin or selegiline significantly increased striatum DA levels in the JEV-infected rats. Selegiline was found to be a potent inhibitor that is more active against MAO-B than MAO-A. Selegiline competitively inhibited the MAO-B activity of the rat brain in a dose-dependent manner (Tipton et al., 1976). This drug is frequently used as an adjunct therapy in the treatment of Parkinson's disease (Berry et al., 1994; Gerlach et al., 1996). As a MAO-B inhibitor and a derivative of amphetamine, selegiline can alter catecholaminergic neurotransmission resulting in a neuroprotective effect (Bursey and Eichenbaum, 1996). The dose of selegiline used in the treatment of parkinsonism (5–10 mg daily in tablet) is considered to be low enough to block MAO-B selectively while leaving MAO-A activity unaffected (Knoll, 1978). We medicated the JEV rat with 0.2 mg/kg selegiline. Selegiline recovered movement function. The striatum DA concentrations in JEV-infected rats were increased by selegiline medication. These results suggest a high efficacy and a therapeutic role in Parkinson's disease. In conclusion, both MAO-B inhibitor isatin and selegiline prevented the decrease in striatum DA levels in JEV-rats. The increased turnover of DA (DOPAC/DA) induced by JEV was significantly inhibited by isatin, but not by selegiline. The effect of isatin on DA turnover may be one of its main roles as an endogenous MAO-B inhibitor. Hence, isatin could be a new treatment for Parkinson's disease as an endogenous MAO-B inhibitor, despite the fact that isatin is unlikely to be directly related to the etiology of Parkinson's disease (Ogata et al., 2002) by increasing DA levels in the striatum.

Acknowledgement

This work was supported in part by the Academic Science Frontier Project of the Ministry of Education, Culture, Sports, Sciences, and Technology of Japan.

References

Adams JD, Odunze IN (1991) Oxygen free radicals and Parkinson's disease. Free Radical Biol Med 10: 161–169

Alves RSC, Barbosa ER, Scaff M (1992) Postvaccinial parkinsonism. Movement Disorders 7: 178–180

Appel SH, Le WD, Tajti J, Haverkamp LJ, Engelhardt JI (1992) Nigral damage and dopaminergic hypofunction in mesencephalon-immunized guinea pigs. Ann Neurol 32: 494–501

Armando I, Barontini M, Levin G, Simsolo R, Glover V, Sandler M (1984) Exercise increases endogenous urinary monoamine oxidase benzodiazepine receptor ligand inhibitory activity in normal children. J Auton Nerv Syst 11: 95–100

Armando I, Levin G, Barontini M (1988) Stress increases endogenous benzodiazepine receptor ligand-monoamine oxidase inhibitory activity (tribulin) in rat tissues. J Neural Transm 71: 29–37

Battacharya SK, Glover V, Sandler M, Clow A, Topham A, Bernadt M, Murray R (1982) Raised endogenous monoamine oxidase inhibitor output in postwithdrawal alcoholics: effects of L-dopa and ethanol. Biol Psychiat 17: 829–836

Battacharya SK, Acharya SB (1993) Further investigations on the anxiogenic effects of isatin. Biog Amines 9: 453–463

Battacharya SK, Chakrabarti A, Sandler M, Glover V (1996) Anxyolytic activity of intraventricularly administered atrial natriuretic peptide in the rat. Neuropsycho-pharmacol 15: 199–206

Ballard PA, Tetrud JW, Langston JW (1985) Permanent human parkinsonism due to 1-methyl-4-phenyl-1,2,3,6-tetrahydropyridine (MPTP): seven cases. Neurology 35: 949–956

Bansal RC, Kaur P, Kiran R (1988) Mode of interaction of isatin with rat liver alkaline phosphatase. Res Bull (Science) PU Chandigarh 39: 71–76

Berry MD, Juorio AV, Paterson IA (1994) Possible mechanisms of action of (−)deprenyl and other MAO-B inhibitors in some neurologic and psychiatric disorders. Prog Neurobiol 44: 141–161

Blaschko H (1973) Amine oxidase. In: Boyer PD, Lardy H, Myrback K (eds) The Enzymes. 3rd ed, vol 8, Academic Press, New York, pp 337–351

Bojincv S (1971) Encephalitis with acute parkinsonian syndrome and bilateral inflammatory necrosis of the substantia nigra. J Neurol Sci 12: 383–415

Burns RS, Chiueh CC, Markey SP, Ebert MH, Jacobowitz DM, Kopin IJ (1983) A primate model of parkinsonism: Selective destruction of dopaminergic neurons in the pars compacta of the substantia nigra by N-methyl-4-phenyl-1,2,3,6-tetrahydropyridine. Proc Natl Acad Sci USA 80: 4546–4550

Bursey M, Eichenbaum H (1996) Conservation of hippocampal memory function in rats and humans. Nature 379: 255–257

Calne DB, Langston JW (1983) Aetiology of Parkinson's disease. Lancet 2: 1457–1459

Chocholova L, Kolinova M (1979) Effect of isatin on audiogenic seizures in rats and its relationship to electrographic and behavioral phenomena. Physiol Bohemoslov 28: 495–502

Chocholova L, Kolinova M (1981) Effect of isatin (2, 3 dioxyindoline) on physiological and pathological electrographic manifestations of vigilance. Physiol Bohemoslov 30: 129–137

Clow A, Glover V, Armando I, Sandler M (1983) New endogenous benzodiazepine receptor ligand in human urine: identity with endogenous MAO inhibitor? Life Sci 33: 735–741

Clow A, Glover V, Weg MW, Walker PL, Sheehan DV, Carr DB, Sandler M (1988a) Urinary catecholamine metabolite and tribulin output during lactate infusion. Br J Psychiatry 152: 122–126

Clow A, Glover V, Sandler M, Tiller J (1988b) Increased urinary tribulin output in generalized anxiety disorder. Psychopharmacol 95: 378–380

Cohen G (1986) Monoamine oxidase, hydrogen peroxidase and Parkinson's disease. Adv Neurol 45: 119–125

Dexter DT, Wells FR, Lees AJ, Agid F, Agid Y, Jenner P, Marsden CD (1989) Increased nigral iron content and alterations in other metal ions occurring in brain in Parkinson's disease. J Neurochem 52: 1830–1836

Dickerson RB, Newton JR, Hansen JE (1952) Diagnosis and immediate prognosis of Japanese B encephalitis. Am J Med 12: 277–288

Duvoisin RC, Yahr MD (1965) Encephalitis and parkinsonism. Arch Neurol 12: 227–239

Elsworth JD, Dewar D, Glover V, Goodwin BL, Clow A, Sandler M (1986) Purification and characterization of tribulin, an endogenous inhibitor of monoamine oxidase and benzodiazepine receptor binding. J Neural Transm 67: 45–56

Fishman PS, Gass JS, Swoveland PT, Lavi E, Highkin MK, Weiss SR (1985) Infection of the basal ganglia by a murine coronavirus. Science 229: 877–879

Geddes JF, Hughes AJ, Lees AJ, Daniel SE (1993) Pathological overlap in cases of parkinsonism associated with neurofibrillary tangles. A study of recent cases of postencephalitic parkinsonism and comparison with progressive supranuclear palsy and Guamanian parkinsonism-dementia complex. Brain 116: 281–302

Gerlach M, Youdim MB, Riederer P (1996) Pharmacology of selegiline. Neurology 47 [Suppl 3]: S137–S145

Gibb WRG, Lees AJ (1987) The progression of idiopathic Parkinson's disease is not explained by age-related changes. Clinical and pathological comparisons with post-encephalitic parkinsonian syndrome. Acta Neuropathol (Berl) 73: 195–201

Glover V, Reveley MA, Sandler M (1980) A monoamine oxidase inhibitor in human urine. Biochem Pharmacol 29: 467–470

Glover V, Halket JM, Watkins PJ, Clow A, Goodwin BL, Sandler M (1988) Isatin: identity with the purified endogenous monoamine oxidase inhibitor tribulin. J Neurochem 51: 656–659

Glover V, Bhattacharya SK, Sandler M (1991) Isatin-a new biological factor. Indian J Exp Biol 29: 1–5

Glover V, Clow A, Sandler M (1993) Effects of dopaminergic drugs on superoxide dismutase: implications for senescence. J Neurol Transm 40 [Suppl]: 37–45

Glover V, Medvedev A, Sandler M (1995) Isatin is a potent endogenous antagonist of guanylate cyclase-coupled atrial natriuretic peptide receptors. Life Sci 57: 2073–2079

Gorell JM, Czarnecki B (1986) Pharmacological evidence for direct dopaminergic regulation of striatal acetylcholine release. Life Sci 38: 2239–2246

Goto A (1962) Follow-up study of Japanese B encephalitis. Psychiat Neurol Jpn (Tokyo) 64: 236–266

Hamaue N, Minami M, Kanamaru Y, Togashi M, Monma Y, Ishikura M, Mahara R, Yamazaki N, Togashi H, Saito H, Parvez SH (1992) Endogenous monoamine oxidase (MAO) inhibitor (tribulin-like activity) in the brain and urine of stroke-prone SHR. Biog Amines 8: 401–412

Hamaue N, Minami M, Kanamaru Y, Ishikura M, Yamazaki N, Saito H, Parvez SH (1994) Identification of isatin, an endogenous MAO inhibitor, in the brain of stroke-prone SHR. Biog Amines 10: 99–110

Hamaue N, Yamazaki N, Minami M, Endo T, Hirafuji M, Monma Y, Togashi H (1998) Determination of isatin, an endogenous monoamine oxidase inhibitor, in urine and tissues of rats by HPLC. Gen Pharmacol 30: 387–391

Hamaue N, Yamazaki N, Minami M, Endo T, Hirafuji M, Monma Y, Togashi H, Saito H, Parvez SH (1999a) Effects of isatin, an endogenous MAO inhibitor, on acetylcholine and dopamine levels in the rat striatum. Biog Amines 15: 367–377

Hamaue N, Minami M, Hirafuji M, Terado M, Machida M, Yamazaki N, Yoshioka M, Ogata A, Tashiro K (1999b) Isatin, an endogenous MAO inhibitor, as a new biological modulator. CNS Drug Rev 5: 331–346

Hamaue N, Yamazaki N, Terado M, Minami M, Ohno K, Ide H, Ogata A, Honma S, Tashiro K (2000) Urinary isatin concentrations in patients with Parkinson's disease determined by a newly developed HPLC-UV method. Res Commun Mol Pathol Pharmacol 108: 63–73

Hamaue N, Minami M, Terado M, Hirafuji M, Endo T, Machida M, Hiroshige T, Ogata A, Tashiro K, Saito H, Parvez SH (2004) Comparative study of the effects of isatin, an endogenous MAO-inhibitor, and selegiline on bradykinesia and dopamine levels in a rat model of Parkinson's disease induced by the Japanese encephalitis virus. NeuroToxicology 25: 205–213

Hoehn MM, Yarh MD (1967) Parkinsonism: onset, progression and mortality. Neurolol 17: 427–442

Hota D, Acharya SB (1994) Studies on peripheral actions of isatin. Ind J Exp Biol 32: 710–717

Hsu SM, Raine L, Fanger H (1981) Use of avidin-biotin-peroxidase complex (ABC) in immunoperoxidase techniques: a comparison between ABC and unlabeled antibody (PAP) procedures. J Histochem Cytochem 29: 577–580

Hudson AJ, Rice GPA (1990) Similarities of Guamanian ALS/PD to post-encephalitic parkinsonism/ALS: possible viral cause. Can J Neurol Sci 17: 427–433

Imperato A, Obinu MC, Casu A, Mascia S, Dazzi L, Gessa GL (1993) Evidence that neuroleptics increase striatal acetylcholine release though stimulation of dopamine D_1 receptors. J Pharmacol Exp Ther 266: 557–562

Jarman J, Przylorowska A, Glover V, Halket J, Davies PT, Rose FC, Sandler M (1991) Urinary output of endogenous monoamine oxidase inhibitor and isatin during acute migraine attack. J Neural Transm Gen Sect 84: 129–134

Johnson RT, Burke DS, Elwell M, Leake CJ, Nisalak A, Hoke CH, Lorsomrudee W (1985) Japanese encephalitis: immunocytochemical studies of viral antigen and inflammatory cells in fatal cases. Ann Neurol 18: 567–573

Knoll J (1978) The possible mechanisms of action of (−)deprenyl in Parkinson's disease. J Neural Transm 43: 177–198

Kristensson K (1992) Potential role of viruses in neuro-degeneration. Mol Chem Neuropathol 16: 45–58

Kumar P, Dani HM, Trehan S (1977) Effect of isatin testicular hyaluronidase. Ind J Exp Biol 15: 655–656

Kumar P, Bansal RC, Mahmood A (1993) Isatin, an inhibitor of acetylcholinesterase activity in rat brain. Biog Amines 9: 281–289

Lehmann J, Langer SZ (1983) The striatal cholinergic interneuron: Synaptic target of dopaminergic terminals? Neurosci 10: 1105–1120

Matsumoto M, Togashi H, Yoshioka M, Hirokami M, Morii K, Saito H (1990) Simultaneous high-performance liquid chromatographic determination of norepinephrine, serotonin, acetylcholine and their metabolites in the cerebrospinal fluid of anaesthetized normotensive rats. J Chromatogr 526: 1–10

McIntyre IM, Norman TR (1990) Serotonergic effects of isatin: an endogenous MAO inhibitor related to tribulin. J Neural Transm 79: 35–40

McGeer PL, Itagaki S, Akiyama H, McGeer EG (1988) Rate of cell death in parkinsonism indicates active neuropathological process. Ann Neurol 24: 574–576

Medvedev AE, Clow A, Sandler M, Glover V (1996) Isatin: A link between natriuretic peptides and monoamines? Biochem Pharmacol 52: 385–391

Minami M, Senjo M, Togashi H, Yoshioka M, Saito H, Kawaguchi H, Takebayashi K, Parvez H (1988) Kidney glutathione S-transferase activity and kidney monoamine oxidase activity in stroke cases of SHRSP. Biog Amines 5: 517–526

Morita K, Tanaka M, Igarashi A (1991) Rapid identification of dengue virus serotypes by using polymerase chain reaction. J Clin Microbiol 29: 2107–2110

Muller M, Schramek J (1989) Combined application of propranolol and local anesthetics: enhanced anticonvulsant action. Biomed Biochim Acta 4: 333–336

Nagatsu T, Yoshida M (1988) An endogenous substance of the brain, tetrahydroisoquinoline, produces parkinsonism in primate with decreased dopamine, tyrosine hydroxylase and biopterin in the nigrostriatal regions. Neurosci Lett 87: 178–182

Nilsson OG, Leanza G, Bjkölund A (1992) Acetylcholine release in the hippocampus: regulation by monoaminergic afferents as assessed by in vivo microdialysis. Brain Res 584: 132–140

Ogata A, Nagashima K, Hall WW, Ichikawa M, Kimura-Kuroda J, Yasui K (1991) Japanese encephalitis virus neurotropism is dependent on the degree of neuronal maturity. J Virol 65: 880–886.

Ogata A, Tashiro K, Nukuzuma S, Nagashima K, Hall WW (1997) A rat model of Parkinson's disease induced by Japanese encephalitis virus. J Neurol Virol 3: 141–147

Ogata A, Nagashima K, Yasui K, Matsuura T, Tashiro K (1998) Sustained release dosage of thyrotropin-releasing hormone improves experimental Japanese encephalitis virus-induced parkinsonism in rats. J Neurol Sci 159: 135–139

Ogata A, Hamaue N, Terado M, Minami M, Nagashima K, Tashiro K (2003) Isatin, an endogenous MAO inhibitor, improves bradykinesia and dopamine levels in a rat model of Parkinson's disease induced by Japanese encephalitis virus. J Neurol Sci 206: 79–83

Ogata A, Hamaue N, Minami M, Yabe I, Kikuchi S, Sasaki H, Tashiro K (2004) Post-encephalitis parkinsonism: clinical features and experimental model. Biog Amines 18: 339–347

Ogawa N, Hirose Y, Ohara S, Ono T, Watanabe Y (1985) A simple quantitative bradykinesia test in MPTP-treated mice. Res Commun Chem Pathol Pharmaco 50: 435–441

Ohue T, Koshimura K, Akiyama Y, Ito A, Kido T, Takagi Y, Miwa S (1992) Regulation of acetylcholine release in vivo from rat hippocampus by monoamines as revealed by novel column-switching HPLC with electrochemical detection. Brain Res 572: 340–344

Oxenkrug G, McIntyre I (1985) Stress-induced synthesis of melatonin; possible involvement of the endogenous monoamine oxidase inhibitor (tribulin). Life Sci 37: 1743–1746

Parvez H, Parvez S (1973) The effects of metopirone and adrenectomy on the regulation of the enzymes monoamine oxidase and catechol-O-methyl transferase in different brain regions. J Neurochem 20: 1011–1020

Paxinos G, Wason C (1980) The rat brain in stereotaxic coordinates. 2nd ed, New York, Academic Press Inc

Peturson H, Bhattacharya SK, Glover V, Sandler M, Lader MH (1982) Urinary monoamine oxidase inhibitor and benzodiazepine withdrawal. Br J Psychiat 140: 7–10

Riederer P, Sotic E, Rausch WD, Schmidt B, Reynolds GP, Jellinger K, Youdim MB (1989) Transition metals ferritin, glutathione and ascorbic acid in Parkinsonian brain. J Neurochem 52: 515–520

Sandler M (1982) The emergence of tribulin. Trends Pharmacol Sci 3: 471–472

Scatton B (1992) Further evidence for the involvement of D_2, but not D_1 dopamine receptors in dopaminergic control of striatal cholinergic transmission. Life Sci 31: 2883–2890

Sethy VH, van Woert MH (1974) Regulation of striatal acetylcholine concentration by dopamine receptors. Nature 251: 529–530

Shoji H, Watanabe M, Itoh S, Kuwahara H, Hattori F (1993) Japanese encephalitis and parkinsonism. J Neurol 240: 59–60
Singh B, Sharma R, Sareen K, Sareen KN, Sohal MS (1977) Isatin enzyme interaction V. Activation of rat liver acid phosphatase. Enzyme 22: 256–261
Stadler H, Lloyd KG, Gadea-Ciria M, Bartholini G (1973) Enhanced striatal acetylcholine release by chlorpromazine and its reversal by apomorphine. Brain Res 55: 476–480
Stoof JC, Drukarch B, DeBoer P, Westerink BHC, Groenewegen HJ (1992) Regulation of the activity of striatal cholinergic neurons by L-DOPA. Neurosci 47: 755–770
Sumiyoshi H, Mori C, Fuke I, Morita K, Kuhara S, Kondou J, Kikuchi Y, Nagamatu H, Igarashi A (1987) Complete nucleotide sequence of the Japanese encephalitis virus genome RNA. Virology 161: 497–510
Susheela I, Singh B, Dani HM, Amma MKP, Sareen K (1969) Enzyme inhibition by isatin I. Inhibition of rat liver xanthine oxidase. Enzymol 37: 325–334
Takahashi M, Yamada T, Nakajima S, Nakajima K, Yamamoto T, Okada H (1995) The substantia nigra is a major target for neurovirulent influenza A virus. J Exp Med 181: 2161–2169
Tipton KF, Housy MD, Mantle TJ (1976) The nature and locations of the multiple forms of monoamine oxidase. In: Mary LC (ed) Monoamine oxidase: its inhibition. Elsevier, New York, pp 5–31
Tozawa Y, Ueki A, Manabe S, Matsushima K (1998) Stress-induced increase in urinary isatin excretion in rats: reversal by both dexamethasone and α-methyl-p-tyrosine. Biochem Pharmacol 56: 1041–1046
Ueki A, Willoughby J, Glover V, Sandler M, Stibbe K, Stern GM (1989) Endogenous urinary monoamine oxidase inhibitor excretion in Parkinson's disease and other neurological disorders. J Neural Transm 1: 263–268
Von Economo C (1917) Encephalitis lethargica. Wien klin Wschr 30: 581–585
Walters JH (1960) Post-encephalitic parkinson syndrome after meningoencephalitis due to coxsackie virus group B, type 2. New Eng J Med 263: 744–747
Wedzong K, Limberger N, Spath L, Wichman T, Stare K (1988) Acethylcholine release in rat nucleus accumbens is regulated though dopamine D_2-receptor. Naunym-Schmied Arch Pharmacol 338: 250–255
Yahr MD (1978) Encephalitis lethargica (Von Economo's disease, epidemic encephalitis). In: Vinken PJ, Bruyn GW (eds) Handbook of clinical neurology vol 34 Elsevier, Amsterdam, pp 451–457
Yang HYT, Neff NH (1974) The monoamine oxidases of brain: selective inhibition with drugs and the consequences for the metabolism of the biogenic amines. J Pharmacol Exp Ther 189: 733–740
Yoshida M, Miwa T, Nagatsu T (1990) Parkinsonism in monkeys produced by chronic administration of an endogenous substance of the brain, tetrahy droisoquinoline: the behavioral and biochemical changes. Neurosci Lett 119: 109–113
Yumiler A (1990) The effect of isatin (tribulin) on metabolism of indoles in the rat brain and pineal: *in vitro* and pineal: *in vitro* and *in vivo* studies. Neurochem Res 15: 95–100

J Neural Transm (2006) [Suppl] 71: 97–103

Journal of Neural Transmission
Printed in Austria

Isatin interaction with glyceraldehyde-3-phosphate dehydrogenase, a putative target of neuroprotective drugs: partial agonism with deprenyl

A. Medvedev[1], O. Buneeva[1], O. Gnedenko[1], V. Fedchenko[1], M. Medvedeva[2], Y. Ivanov[1], V. Glover[3], M. Sandler[3]

[1] Institute of Biomedical Chemistry, Russian Academy of Medical Sciences, Moscow, Russia
[2] School of Biology, Moscow State University, Moscow, Russia
[3] Hammersmith Campus, Institute of Reproductive and Developmental Biology, Imperial College London, London, UK

Summary There is evidence that the binding of deprenyl, a monoamine oxidase (MAO) B inhibitor, and other propargylamines to glyceraldehyde-3-phosphate dehydrogenase (GAPDH) is primarily responsible for their neuroprotective and antiapoptotic effects. Thus, GAPDH may be a target for other neuroprotective drugs. Using two independent approaches, radioligand analysis and an optical biosensor technique, we demonstrate here that GAPDH also interacts with the endogenous, reversible MAO B inhibitor, isatin. Deprenyl inhibited both [^{3}H]isatin binding to GAPDH, and the binding of this enzyme to an isatin analogue, 5-aminoisatin, immobilized on to an optical biosensor cell. Another MAO inhibitor, tranylcypromine, was ineffective. Both deprenyl and isatin inhibited GAPDH-mediated cleavage of *E. coli* tRNA, and their effects were not additive. We suggest that isatin may be an endogenous partial functional agonist of deprenyl in its effect on GAPDH and GAPDH-mediated RNA cleavage. Changes in level of endogenous isatin may influence the neuroprotective effect of deprenyl in vivo.

Introduction

(−)-Deprenyl was the first selective mechanism-based inhibitor of monoamine oxidase B (MAO-B) to be synthesized (Knoll and Magyar, 1972). It exhibits neuroprotective and antiapoptotic properties in several experimental models (e.g. Carlile et al., 1998; Kragten et al., 1998; Suuronen et al., 2000; Qin et al., 2003). However, the neuroprotective effect of deprenyl, observed in the picomolar concentration range in vitro (Tatton et al., 2003; Szende, 2004), cannot be attributed to selective inhibition of MAO-B, which requires nanomolar-submicromolar concentrations (Singer, 1979). Moreover, recent data suggest that neuroprotection by deprenyl and other propargylamines involves glyceraldehyde-3-phosphate dehydrogenase (GAPDH) rather than MAO B (Tatton et al., 2003).

GAPDH (EC 1.2.1.12) has long been known as a classical glycolytic cytosolic enzyme. However, good evidence now exists that it is a multifunctional protein, exhibiting diverse cytoplasmic, membrane and nuclear activities, influencing cell survival and death (Sirover, 1996; Tatton et al., 2003; Berry, 2004). GAPDH specifically interacts with different RNAs in vivo and it vitro (Nagy and Rigby, 1995; De et al., 1996; Lin et al., 2000; Yi et al., 2000; Evguenieva-Hackenberg et al., 2002) and may cleave some of them (Evguenieva-Hackenberg et al., 2002). Several groups have also demonstrated that the overexpression of GAPDH and its subsequent nuclear translocation are implicated in the initiation of one or more apoptotic cascades and also in the aetiology of some neurological diseases (Tatton et al., 2003; Berry, 2004).

The translocation of GAPDH into the nucleus can be an important event leading to apoptosis (Tatton et al., 2003; Berry, 2004) especially in neuronal cells. Deprenyl and its structurally related analogue, the compound CGP 3466, lacking MAO B inhibitory activity, were able to bind to GAPDH and reduce apoptosis induced by nerve growth factor and serum withdrawal (Carlile et al., 1998; Kragten et al., 1998). Another anti-Parkinson drug, rasagiline, similarly brought about decreased GAPDH translocation into the nucleus and reduce apoptosis initiated in cell cultures by the endogenous dopaminergic neurotoxin, N-methyl(R)salsolinol (Maruyama et al., 2001). Thus the interaction of certain antiapoptotic drugs with GAPDH is likely to be an early event important for the manifestation of the antiapoptotic

Correspondence: Prof. A. Medvedev, Institute of Biomedical Chemistry, Russian Academy of Medical Sciences, 10 Pogodinskaya str., Moscow 119121, Russia
e-mail: Alexei.Medvedev@ibmc.msk.ru

effect. Some authors reasonably consider GAPDH to be a putative molecular target for the development of antiapoptotic therapeutic agents for the treatment of certain neurodegenerative disorders (Ishitani et al., 2003).

The interaction of exogenous pharmacological agents with their molecular targets may be modified by the presence of endogenous compounds, which can potentially interact with the same targets. One putative endogenous ligand which may influence deprenyl activity is isatin (2,3-indole-dione). Isatin is an endogenously generated indole, widely distributed in tissues and body fluids at concentrations from 0.1–10 μM (Glover et al., 1988; Watkins et al., 1990; Medvedev et al., 1996; Medvedev and Glover 2004). It is an effective competitive inhibitor of MAO B in vitro (Glover et al., 1988; Medvedev et al., 1996; Medvedev and Glover, 2004). Recently, it has been demonstrated that non-physiologically high isatin concentrations (50–100 μM) may be proapoptotic in some cell lines (Cane et al., 2000; Igosheva et al., 2005).

Thus, there is evidence that isatin and deprenyl may share some common molecular targets, particularly MAO B, but may have opposite effects on programmed cell death in some cell cultures. We therefore suggest that GAPDH represents a potential target not only for the exogenous antiapoptotic agent deprenyl, but also for the endogenous (pro?)apoptotic compound isatin. Thus, in the present study we have investigated the binding of isatin to GAPDH, the possible consequence of this binding as far as GAPDH-mediated RNA cleavage is concerned and the effect of deprenyl on these processes.

Materials and methods

Materials

5-Aminoisatin was synthesized by Dr. Brian L. Goodwin (Queen Charlotte's and Chelsea Hospital, London) using standard methods (Medvedev et al., 1999). (−)Deprenyl was kindly provided by Professor J. Knoll (Semmelweis University, Budapest). Carboxymethyl-dextran sample cells were obtained from Affinity sensors (Division of Labsystems, Cambridge, UK). [^{3}H]Isatin (26 Ci/mmol) was prepared by Amersham (Buckinghamshire, UK; custom-made order). Rabbit muscle GAPDH was purified by the method of Scopes and Stoter (1982). The resulting enzyme preparation (specific activity 52 ± 5 μmole/min per 1 mg of protein) showed one band during electrophoresis in the Laemmli system. Before use, the purified enzyme was kept as ammonium sulphate solution at +4°C. Other chemicals were from Sigma-Aldrich (Russia).

Binding of rabbit muscle GAPDH to immobilized 5-amino isatin monitored

On the IAsys optical biosensor chip. 5-Aminoisatin (see Fig. 1) was covalently linked to the surface of a carboxymethylated dextran cell by the following procedure (Ivanov et al., 2002). The sensor chip was initially

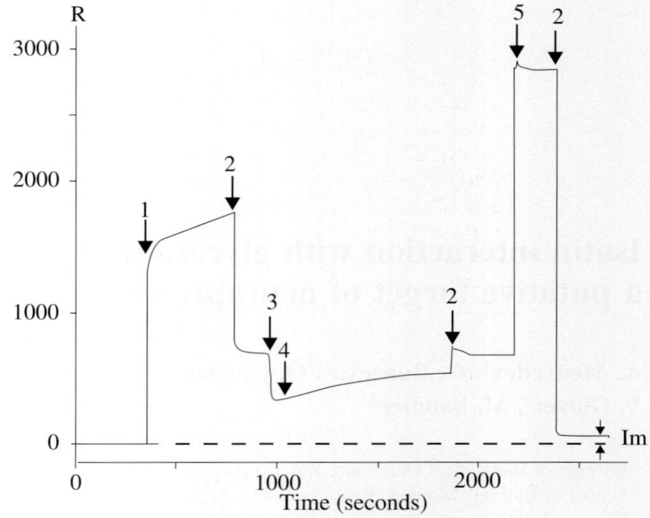

Fig. 1. Immobilization of 5-aminoisatin on the optical biosensor chip. Arrows indicate: *1* NHS + EDC, *2* PBS/t, *3* 10 mM formiate buffer, pH 3.0, *4* 0.4 mM, 5-aminoisatin, *5* 1 M ethanolamine-HCl, pH 8.5, *Im* quantity of immobilized 5-aminoisatin. Other explanations are in the text

activated by 0.4 M 1-ethyl-3(3-dimethylaminopropyl)carbodiimide (EDC) and 0.1 M N-hydroxysuccinimide (NHS) for 7 min and washed with 10 mM sodium phosphate buffer, pH 7.4, containing 138 mM NaCl, 2.7 mM KCl and 0.05% Tween-20 (PBS/t). A solution of 0.4 mM 5-aminoisatin was then added and immobilization was carried out for 20 min in 10 mM formiate buffer, pH 3.0. Unreacted activated sites on the chip were subsequently blocked by adding 1 M ethanolamine-HCl, pH 8.5, for 2 min. Figure 1 shows a typical profile of 5-aminoisatin immobilization on the IAsys optical biosensor chip.

The sensor chip surface, with immobilized 5-aminoisatin, was washed with 50 mM potassium phosphate buffer containing 1 M NaCl and 2% sodium cholate and then with 50 mM potassium phosphate buffer, pH 7.4, containing 1% Triton X-100. In all cases the volume added to the cell was 200 μl. After adding 180 μl of working buffer the baseline was stabilized for 3 min and 20 μl of GAPD preparation (+ various additives) was included; the biosensor response was then registered for 10 min. Then the sensor chip surface was sequentially washed with 50 mM potassium phosphate buffer, pH 7.4, containing 1 M NaCl and with 50 mM potassium phosphate buffer, pH 7.4, containing 1 M NaCl and 2% sodium cholate.

Prior to injection on to the IAsys chip, salts were removed from the enzyme preparations by gel centrifugation chromatography (Andersen and Vaughan, 1982) using Sephadex G-50 (fine) equilibrated with 50 mM glycine buffer, pH 8.9.

Nonspecific binding was evaluated using the sensor chips run throughout the whole operation described above but without 5-aminoisatin. All procedures were carried out at 25°C using a thermostated cell.

Binding of [^{3}H]isatin to rabbit muscle GAPDH

Binding of [^{3}H]isatin to 1.875 μM GAPDH was investigated in the following medium: 0.2 M sucrose, 10 mM Hepes-KOH buffer, pH 7.2, using 20 and 200 nM [^{3}H]isatin (final volume 200 μl). For Scatchard analysis, a range of [^{3}H]isatin concentrations from 10 nM to 200 nM was used. The incubation was carried out at 0°C for 60 min. Non-specific binding was determined in the presence of 0.2 mM unlabelled isatin. The reaction was terminated by rapid filtration on to Whatman glass fibre filters presoaked with a solution of polyethyleneimine. Radioactivity, trapped onto the filters, was measured with a scintillation cocktail (Medvedev et al., 2005).

Determination of GAPDH-mediated cleavage of RNA

RNA hydrolyzing activity was assayed under conditions described by Evguenieva-Hackenberg et al. (2002) by analyzing the amount of *E. coli* tRNA remaining after incubation with GAPDH for 10 min at 56°C. The reaction mixture contained 30 mM Tris–HCl buffer, pH 7.5, 130 mM KCl, 5 mM $MgCl_2$, 5% glycerol, 0.01 mg/ml *E. coli* tRNA and 2 mg/ml GAPDH. The RNA content of the reaction mixture supernatant was evaluated by electrophoresis on 10% polyacrylamide gel stained with ethidium bromide and scanned on a Typhoon 9400 Fluorescent Densitometer (Amersham Bioscience, UK). Each track was scanned twice at different positions and the average areas of the peaks were calculated. A pilot experiment revealed that RNA-cleaving activity of GAPDH was insensitive to the ribonuclease inhibitor, RNasin, suggesting that the RNase activity represents an intrinsic property of GAPDH.

Determination of glycolytic activity of GAPDH

Glycolytic activity was assayed spectrophotometrically by recording NAD^+ reduction at 340 nm in the reaction glyceraldehyde-3-phosphate + $NAD^+ + P_i =$ 1,3-diphosphoglycerate + NADH (Carlile et al., 2000). The enzyme assay was carried out at 25°C in 50 mM glycine buffer, pH 8.9, in the presence of 50 mM sodium phosphate, 0.6 mM glyceraldehyde-3-phosphate, 5 mM EDTA, and various concentrations of NAD^+ (2.5 μM–1 mM). Reaction was initiated by adding 1–2 μg/ml GAPDH.

The values of k_{ass} and k_{diss} were calculated using the standard method of non-linear regression. Statistical significance of differences was evaluated by paired Student's *t*-test.

Results

Injection of a solution of rabbit muscle GAPDH in binding buffer into a CarboxymethylDextran chip containing covalently bound 5-aminoisatin resulted in the appearance of a characteristic response (Fig. 2). Its magnitude depended on the amount of enzyme protein added. Some non-specific binding of GAPDH was also observed in the control chip (without immobilised isatin analogue). This non-specific binding also depended on the amount of protein added. Therefore, in subsequent experiments we usually selected a protein concentration providing at least 70% specific binding. Calculated values of association (k_{on}) and dissociation (k_{off}) rate constants were $(0.79 \pm 0.03) \times 10^3\,M^{-1} \cdot sec^{-1}$ and $(9.3 \pm 1.8) \times 10^{-3} \cdot sec^{-1}$, respectively. The K_d value calculated by the ratio k_{off}/k_{on} was 12 μM.

The existence of specific isatin binding sites on the GAPDH molecule was confirmed in independent experiments using [^{3}H]isatin. A Scatchard analysis of GAPDH interaction with [^{3}H]isatin revealed a single type of isatin binding (Fig. 3) with K_d value of 3.1 μM.

Another cytosolic NAD-dependent oligomeric dehydrogenase, lactate dehydrogenase, failed to bind to the immobilized isatin analogue (Fig. 4) providing some evidence for the specificity of the interaction of GAPDH with isatin.

The binding of GAPDH to the immobilised 5-aminoisatin was strongly inhibited by NAD (Fig. 5). Similar results were obtained using [^{3}H]isatin (Fig. 6). This finding points to the possible involvement of an NAD-binding site in the interaction with isatin. To explore this possibility further, we investigated the effect of isatin on the catalytic activity of GAPD. The presence of 10 μM isatin increased the apparent K_m for NAD from 30.5 ± 2.3 to 77.5 ± 11.2 μM ($n = 4$), without any influence on V_{max}. This observation also supports the possible involvement of an NAD-binding site in the GAPDH interaction with isatin. Higher concentrations of isatin (0.1 and 1 mM) did not influence the K_m

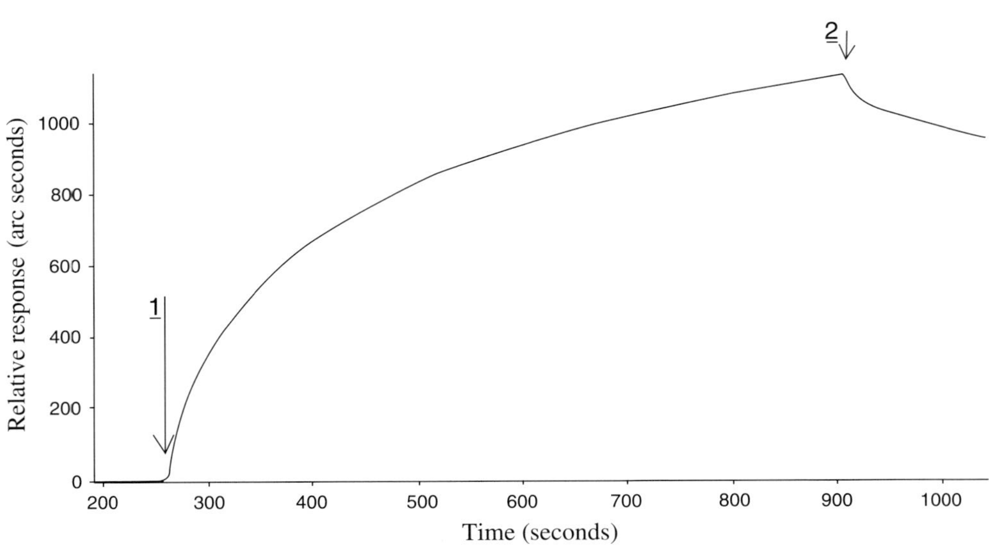

Fig. 2. Sensogram of specific binding of GAPDH to the CarboxymethylDextran chip with immobilized isatin analogue (Total-nonspecific). Asterisk 1 indicates addition of enzyme, asterisk 2 indicates addition of buffer

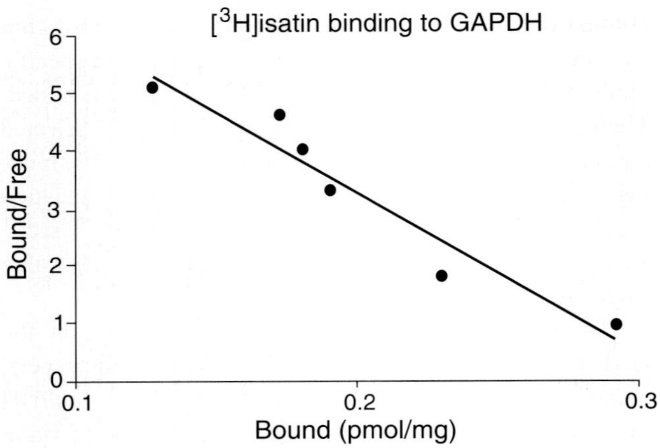

Fig. 3. Scatchard analysis of [^{3}H]isatin binding to GAPDH

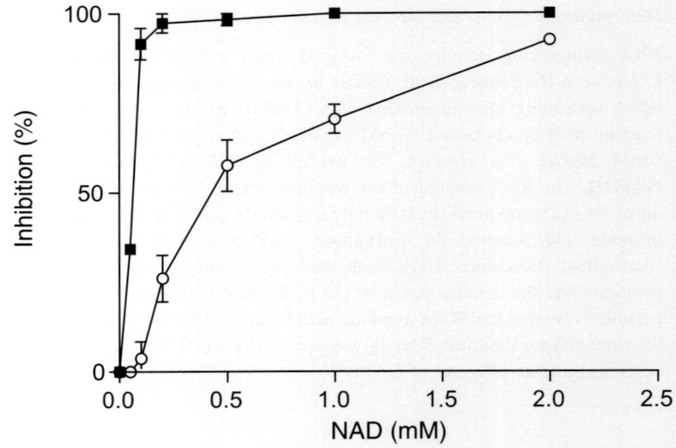

Fig. 6. Inhibition of 10 (closed symbol) and 100 (open symbol) nM [^{3}H]isatin binding to GAPDH by NAD. Data represent mean $\pm$ SEM of 5 experiments

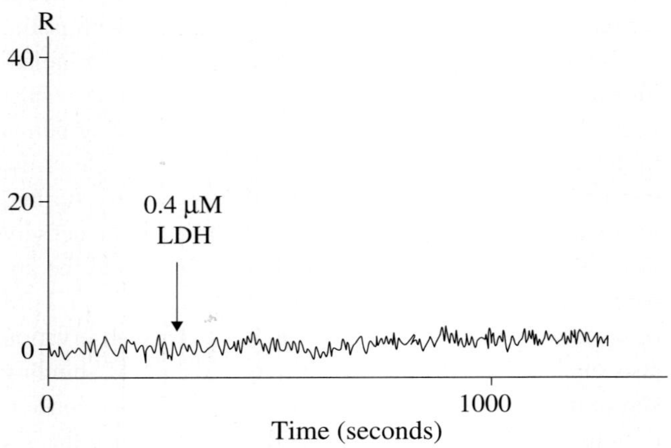

Fig. 4. Lack of binding of lactate dehydrogenase to the immobilized isatin analogue

value for NAD but decreased the V_{max} in a concentration dependent manner by 44 ± 5 and $58 \pm 5\%$, in the presence of 0.1 and 1.0 mM isatin, respectively.

(−)Deprenyl effectively brought about a decrease in GAPDH binding to the immobilized isatin analogue in dose dependent fashion (Fig. 6). This effect appeared to be specific, in that another MAO inhibitor, tranylcypromine did not influence GAPDH binding to the immobilized isatin analogue. Inhibition of isatin binding to GAPDH was also demonstrated using two concentrations of [^{3}H]isatin (Fig. 7). The higher concentration of [^{3}H]isatin required correspondingly higher concentration of deprenyl for inhibition of GAPD binding. The IC_{50} values for deprenyl inhibition of GAPDH binding obtained at 10 and 100 nM [^{3}H]isatin were 13 and 140 nM, suggesting competitive interaction for

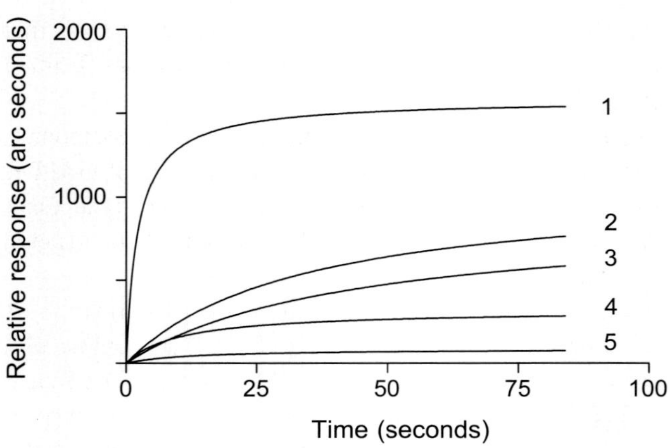

Fig. 5. The effect of NAD^+on the GAPDH interaction with isatin: *1* without NAD^+, *2* 1 μM NAD^+, *3* 5 μM NAD^+, *4* 50 μM NAD^+, *5* 100 μM NAD^+

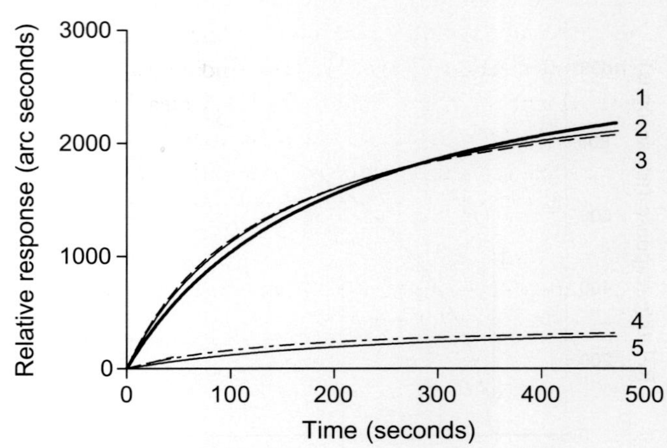

Fig. 7. The effect of deprenyl and tranylcypromine on GAPDH interaction with the immobilized isatin analogue: *1* without deprenyl, *2* 10 μM tranylcypromine, *3* 1000 μM tranylcypromine, *4* 10 μM deprenyl, *5* 1000 μM deprenyl

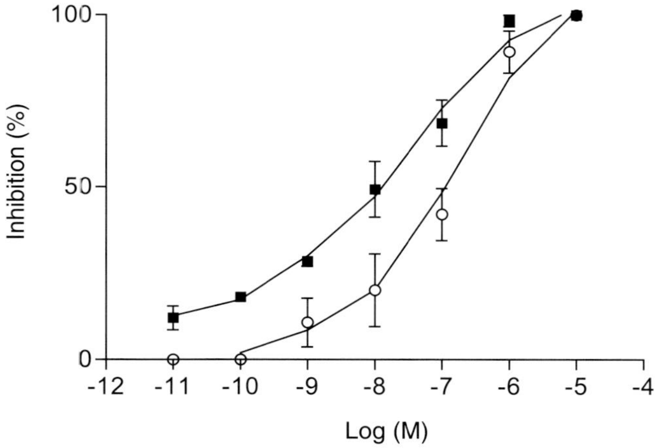

Fig. 8. The effect of deprenyl on binding of 10 (closed symbol) and 100 (open symbol) nM [^{3}H]isatin to GAPDH. Data represent mean ± SEM of 6–9 experiments

GAPDH binding. Kinetic data for GAPDH inhibition by deprenyl revealed that a micromolar concentration of deprenyl (10 μM) did not influence K_m for NAD, but decreased V_{max} by 35 ± 13%. Higher concentrations of deprenyl (0.1 and 1 mM) did not cause a further decrease of V_{max}, and 1 mM deprenyl brought about a 2-fold increase of K_m for NAD^+. Taken together, these results indicate that binding of isatin and deprenyl to GAPDH involves the NAD-binding site.

Binding experiments cannot determine whether isatin and deprenyl act as agonists or antagonists. We therefore investigated their effect on GAPDH-mediated cleavage of RNA. In accordance with the literature (Evguenieva-Hackenberg et al., 2002) rabbit muscle GAPDH cleaved *E.coli* tRNA, measured as a decrease of RNA in the incubation mixture (Fig. 8). Addition of optimal amounts of deprenyl and isatin, 1 μM and 0.1 mM, respectively, caused an increase of RNA contentration (Table 1). This finding suggests that deprenyl and isatin both inhibit the RNA cleaving activity of GAPDH. Although the optimal concentration of deprenyl resulted in a more pronounced inhibition of RNA cleavage than did isatin their effects were not additive.

Table 1. *Residual amount of E. coli tRNA after treatment (0.01 mg/ml) with GAPDH (2 mg/ml) for 10 min at 56°C*

GAPDH	GAPDH + Isatin 0.1 mM	GAPDH + Deprenyl 1 μM	GAPDH + Isatin 0.1 mM + Deprenyl 1 μM
17.6 ± 3.2	31.6 ± 4.9*	58.8 ± 11.1**	35.8 ± 8.1*

Data represent mean ± SEM of four independent experiments employing different GAPDH samples. Asterisks show statistical significance of differences compared with control: *$P < 0.05$; **$P < 0.02$

Discussion

Glyceraldehyde-3-phosphate dehydrogenase is a classical glycolytic enzyme, which exhibits diverse nonglycolytic functions depending on its subcellular localization (Sirover, 1996; Tatton et al., 2003; Berry, 2004). Release of cytoplasmic GAPDH followed by its subsequent translocation into the nucleus is thought to be an early event of the GAPDH-mediated programmed cell death cascade (Tatton et al., 2003; Berry, 2004).

There is increasing evidence that GAPDH may serve as a target for small-molecule anti-apoptotic compounds slowing/preventing progression of neurodegenerative disorders (Berry, 2004). GAPDH is thus a promising target for various neuroprotective drugs and good evidence now exists that the binding of deprenyl and other propargylamines to GAPDH is primarily responsible for the neuroprotective and antiapoptotic effects of these substances (Carlile et al., 1998; Kragten et al., 1998; Maruyama et al., 2001; Tatton et al., 2003; Berry, 2004).

We have demonstrated here that isatin, an endogenous indole may also bind to GAPDH. Two independent approaches, an optical biosensor technique and a Scatchard analysis of [^{3}H]isatin binding to GAPDH, gave similar K_d values (12 and 3.1 μM, respectively) which are within the upper physiological limit of isatin concentrations. The effect of isatin on this enzyme was relatively specific because another oligomeric cytosolic NAD-dependent enzyme, lactate dehydrogenase, did not bind to the immobilized isatin analogue. Deprenyl inhibited isatin binding in a concentration dependent manner and this effect was not reproduced by the other MAO inhibitor, tranylcypromine. Interestingly, deprenyl but not tranylcypromine and some other MAO inhibitors lacking MAO-independent neuroprotective properties inhibited monocytic THP-1 cell neurotoxicity (Klegeris and McGeer, 2000). This seems to support hypothesis that GAPDH is a target for some neuroprotective drugs (Ishitani et al., 2003).

Data in the present study indicate that both compounds apparently interact with the NAD-binding site of GAPDH which is responsible for most of the nonglycolytic functions of this protein (Sioud and Jespersen, 1996; Kragten et al., 1998).

Binding experiments cannot provide any information on the functional effects of ligands bound to a macromolecular receptor target. We have compared the effects of isatin and deprenyl on the nonglycolytic RNA-cleaving activity of GAPDH. It is known that dehydrogenases and other metabolic enzymes can bind RNA. In numerous studies on RNA binding GAPDH was identified as a major RNA-binding

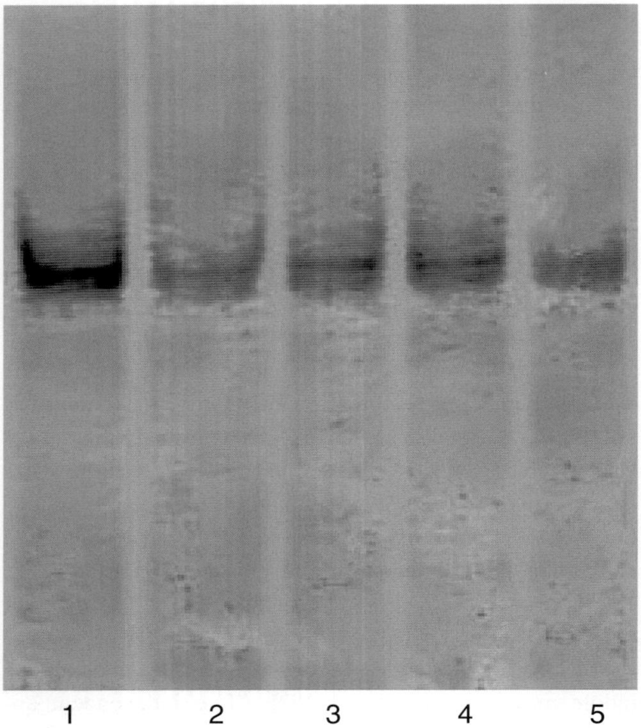

Fig. 9. The effect of isatin and deprenyl on RNA cleavage by GAPDH: Tracks: *1* tRNA, *2* tRNA + GAPDH, *3* tRNA + GAPDH + 0.1 mM isatin, *4* tRNA + GAPDH + 1 μM deprenyl, *5* tRNA + GAPDH + 0.1 mM isatin + 1 μM deprenyl

protein and the selectivity of GAPDH binding to RNA has been demonstrated in vitro and in vivo (Singh and Green, 1993; De et al., 1996; Yi et al., 2000). GAPDH selectively binds tRNA and the cofactor, NAD, disrupted the complex formation between tRNA and GAPDH (Singh and Green, 1993). Evguenieva-Hackenberg et al. (2002) demonstrated that rabbit muscle GAPDH cleaved different RNA transcripts derived from 23°S rRNA of α-proteobacteria. Under our experimental conditions rabbit muscle GAPDH also cleaved *E. coli* tRNA (Fig. 9, Table 1) and this resulted in a decrease in band intensity of tRNA on the electrophoretogram. Optimal concentrations of the compounds studied, 0.1 mM isatin and 1 μM deprenyl, inhibited RNase activity of GAPDH. This inhibition was detected by an increase of the residual amount of tRNA remaining after incubation with GAPDH. Deprenyl was a more effective inhibitor of GAPDH-dependent RNA cleavage than isatin and their effects were not additive (Table 1).

Since both compounds inhibited the GAPDH-mediated cleavage of *E. coli* tRNA, it is possible that they exerted the same type of regulatory effect on GAPDH. The IC_{50} values deprenyl inhibition of [3H]isatin binding to GAPDH were close to the radioligand concentrations. However, it should be noted that isatin was less effective in inhibiting GAPDH-dependent *E. coli* tRNA cleavage than deprenyl. It is therefore possible that being less effective than deprenyl, isatin may actually attenuate some (neuroprotective) effects of deprenyl. Thus, the present study suggests that isatin may be a partial functional agonist of deprenyl in its effect on GAPDH and GAPDH-mediated RNA cleavage. A partial agonist is usually defined (e.g. Ross, 2003) as a compound, which possesses affinity for a receptor, but unlike a full agonist, elicits only a small degree of the pharmacological response.

The evidence concerning the effects of isatin in intact cells, organs and whole organisms is clearly more complex. In some cell cultures prolonged incubation (48–72 h) with high concentrations of isatin (≥50 μM) caused antiproliferative and proapoptotic effects in N1E-115, BALB/c3T3, BBC (Cane et al., 2000) and neuroblastoma SH-SY5Y cells (Igosheva et al., 2005). However, rats or mice treated with a low dose (20 mg/kg) or high dose (200–300 mg/kg) of isatin for 3–4 weeks (Val'dman et al., 2004; Kumar et al., 1994; Hamaue et al., 1996) did not develop any impairment of neurochemical parameters. Moreover, isatin (100 mg/kg) improved parkinsonism induced by Japanese encephalitis virus in a similar manner to deprenyl (0.2 mg/kg) (Hamaue et al., 2004).

In conclusion, the results of the current study suggest that while isatin inself may be anti-apoptotic under some circumstances, it may also interfere with such effects of deprenyl. These suppositions clearly need experimental validation in vivo.

Acknowledgements

The authors are grateful to Professor Alexander Archakov for constructive criticism and valuable discussion of this paper.

Authors thank Dr. Natalia Panova for her excellent work during pilot studies of GAPDH interaction with the immobilized isatin analogue. This work was supported by grants from INTAS (grant No. 97-1818), Russian Foundation for Basic Research (grant 03-04-48244), Royal Society and The Wellcome Trust (grant No. 072381/Z/03).

References

Andersen KB, Vaughan MH (1982) Gel centrifugation chromatography for macromolecular separation. J Chromatogr 240: 1–8

Berry MD (2004) Glyceraldehyde-3-phosphate dehydrogenase as a target for small-molecule disease-modifying therapies in human neurodegenerative disorders. J Psychiatry Neurosci 29: 337–345

Cane A, Tournaire MC, Barritault D, Crumeyrolle-Arias M (2000) The endogenous oxindoles 5-hydroxyoxindole and isatin are antiproliferative and proapoptotic. Biochem Biophys Res Commun 276: 379–384

Carlile GW, Tatton WG, Borden KL (1998) Demonstration of a RNA-dependent nuclear interaction between the promyelocytic leukaemia protein and glyceraldehyde-3-phosphate dehydrogenase. J Biochem 335: 691–696

Carlile GW, Chalmers-Redman RME, Tatton NA, Pong A, Borden KLB, Tatton WG (2000) Reduced apoptosis after nerve growth factor and serum withdrawal: conversion of tetrameric glyceraldehyde-3-phosphate dehydrogenase to a dimer. Mol Pharmacol 57: 2–12

De BP, Gupta S, Zhao H, Drazba JA, Banerjee AK (1996) Specific interaction *in vitro* and *in vivo* of glyceraldehyde-3-phosphate dehydrogenase and LA protein with Cis-acting RNAs of human parainfluenza Virus Type 3. J Biol Chem 271: 24728–24735

Evguenieva-Hackenberg E, Schiltz E, Klug G (2002) Dehydrogenases from all three domains of life cleave RNA. J Biol Chem 277: 46145–46150

Glover V, Halket JM, Watkins PJ, Clow A, Goodwin BL, Sandler M (1988) Isatin: identity with the purified monoamine oxidase inhibitor, tribulin. J Neurochem 51: 656–659

Hamaue N, Minami M, Hirafuji M, Monma Y, Yamazaki N, Togashi H, Saito H, Parvez SH (1996) Significance of isatin, an endogenous MAO inhibitor, on blood pressure control and monoamine levels in rats. Biogenic Amines 12: 305–405

Hamaue N, Minami M, Terado M, Hirafuji M, Endo T, Machida M, Hiroshige T, Ogata A, Tashiro K, Saito H, Parvez SH (2004) Comparative study of the effects of isatin, an endogenous MAO-inhibitor, and selegiline on bradykinesia and dopamine levels in a rat model of Parkinson's disease induced by the Japanese encephalitis virus. Neurotoxicology 25: 205–213

Igosheva N, Lorz C, O'Conner E, Glover V, Mehmet H (2005) Isatin, an endogenous monoamine oxidase inhibitor, triggers a dose- and time-dependent switch from apoptosis to necrosis in human neuroblastoma cells. Neurosci Int 47: 216–224

Ishitani R, Tajima H, Takata H, Tsuchiya K, Kuwae T, Yamada M, Takahashi H, Tatton NA, Katsube N (2003) Proapoptotic protein glyceraldehyde-3-phosphate dehydrogenase: a possible site of action of antiapoptotic drugs. Prog. Neuropsychopharmacol. Biol Psychiatry 27: 291–301

Ivanov ID, Panova NG, Gnedenko OV, Buneeva OA, Medvedev AE, Archakov AI (2002) Study of the tissue and subcellular distribution of isatin-binding proteins with optical biosensor Vopr. Med Khim 48: 73–83

Klegeris A, McGeer PL (2000) R-(−)-Deprenyl inhibits monocytic THP-1 cell neurotoxicity independently of monoamine oxidase inhibition. Exp Neurol 66: 458–464

Knoll J, Magyar K (1972) Some puzzling pharmacological effects of monoamine oxidase inhibitors. Adv Biochem Pharmacol 5: 393–408

Kragten E, Lalande I, Zimmermann K, Roggo S, Schindler P, Muller D, van Oostrum J, Waldmeier P, Furst P (1998) Glyceraldehyde-3-phosphate dehydrogenase, the putative target of the antiapoptotic compounds CGP 3466 and R-(−)-deprenyl. J Biol Chem 273: 5821–5828

Lin SS, Chang SC, Wang YH, Sun CY, Chang MF (2000) Specific interaction between the hepatitis delta virus RNA and glyceraldehyde 3-phosphate dehydrogenase: an enhancement on ribozyme catalysis. Virology 271: 46–57

Kumar R, Bansal RC, Mahmood A (1994) In vivo effects of isatin on certain enzymes, lipids & serotonergic system of rat brain. Indian J Med Res 100: 246–250

Maruyama W, Akao Y, Youdim MB, Davis BA, Naoi M (2001) Transfection-enforced Bcl-2 overexpression and an anti-Parkinson drug, rasagiline, prevent nuclear accumulation of glyceraldehyde-3-phosphate dehydrogenase induced by an endogenous dopaminergic neurotoxin, N-methyl(R)salsolinol. J Neurochem 78: 727–735

Medvedev AE, Glover V (2004) Tribulin and endogenous MAO-inhibitory regulation in vivo. Neurotoxicology 25: 185–192

Medvedev AE, Clow A, Sandler M, Glover V (1996) Isatin – a link between natriuretic peptides and monoamines? Biochem Pharmacol 52: 385–391

Medvedev AE, Goodwin DL, Sandler M, Glover V (1999) Efficacy of isatin analogues as antagonists of rat brain and heart atrial natriuretic peptide receptors coupled to particulate guanylate cyclase. Biochem Pharmacol 57: 913–915

Medvedev A, Crumeyrolle-Arias M, Cardona A, Sandler M, Glover V (2005) Natriuretic peptide interaction with [^{3}H]isatin binding sites in rat brain. Brain Res 1042: 119–124

Nagy E, Rigby WF (1995) Glyceraldehyde-3-phosphate dehydrogenase selectively binds AU-rich RNA in the NAD(+)-binding region (Rossmann fold). J Biol Chem 270: 2755–2763

Qin F, Shite J, Mao W, Liang CS (2003) Selegiline attenuates cardiac oxidative stress and apoptosis in heart failure: association with improvement of cardiac function. Eur. J Pharmacol 461: 149–158

Ross RA (2003) Anandamide and vanilloid TRPV1 receptors. Br J Pharmacol 140: 790–801

Scopes RK, Stoter A (1982) Purification of all glycolytic enzymes from one muscle extract. Methods Enzymol 90: 479–490

Singer TP (1979) Active site directed, irreversible inhibitors of monoamine oxidase. In: Singer TP, von Korff RW, Murphy DL (eds) Monoamine oxidase: structure, function and altered functions. R Academic Press, New York, London, pp 7–24

Singh R, Green MR (1993) Sequence-specific binding of transfer RNA by glyceraldehyde-3-phosphate dehydrogenase. Science 259: 365–368

Sioud M, Jespersen L (1996) Enhancement of hammerhead ribozyme catalysis by glyceraldehyde-3-phosphate dehydrogenase. J Mol Biol 257: 775–789

Sirover MA (1996) Emerging new functions of the glycolytic protein, glyceraldehyde-3-phosphate dehydrogenase, in mammalian cells. Life Sci 58: 2271–2277

Suuronen T, Kolehmainen P, Salminen A (2000) Protective effect of L-deprenyl against apoptosis induced by okadaic acid in cultured neuronal cells. Biochem Pharmacol 59: 1589–1595

Szende B (2004) Cell proliferation and cell death in relation to dose of various chemical substances. In: Torok TL, Klebovich L (eds) Monoamine oxidase inhibitors and their role in neurotransmission (drug development). Medicina Publishing House Co., Budapest, pp 133–140

Tatton W, Chalmers-Redman R, Tatton N (2003) Neuroprotection by deprenyl and other propargylamines: glyceraldehyde-3-phosphate dehydrogenase rather than monoamine oxidase B. J Neural Transm 110: 509–515

Val'dman EA, Kapitsa IG, Nerobkova LN, Axenova LN, Buneeva OA, Medvedev AE (2004) The effect of long-term administration of isatin and himantan to mice on sensitivity of brain monoamine oxidase B to inhibition by deprenyl *in vivo* and *in vitro*. Biomed Khim 50: 509–513

Watkins P, Clow A, Glover V, Halket J, Przyborowska A, Sandler M (1990) Isatin, regional distribution in rat brain and tissues. Neurochem Int 17: 321–323

Yi M-K, Schultz DE, Lemon SM (2000) Functional significance of the interaction of hepatitis A virus RNA with glyceraldehyde 3-phosphate dehydrogenase (GAPDH): Opposing effects of GAPDH and polypyrimidine tract binding protein on internal ribosome entry site function. J Virol 74: 6459–6468

J Neural Transm (2006) [Suppl] 71: 105–112

Journal of Neural Transmission
Printed in Austria

Inhibition of amine oxidases by the histamine-1 receptor antagonist hydroxyzine

J. O'Sullivan[1,2], **M. I. O'Sullivan**[2], **K. F. Tipton**[1], **G. Davey**[1]

[1] Department of Biochemistry, and
[2] Dublin Dental School and Hospital, Trinity College, Dublin, Ireland

Summary The effects of the drug hydroxyzine on the activities of the rat liver monoamine oxidases (EC 1.4.3.6; MAO) and the membrane-bound and soluble forms of bovine semicarbazide-sensitive amine oxidase (EC 1.4.3.6; SSAO) were studied. Hydroxyzine was found to be a competitive inhibitor of MAO-B ($K_i \sim 38\,\mu M$), whereas it had a low potency towards MAO-A ($IC_{50} > 630\,\mu M$). Although it was a relatively potent competitive inhibitor of bovine plasma SSAO ($K_i \sim 1.5\,\mu M$), it was a weak inhibitor of the membrane-bound form of the enzyme from bovine lung ($IC_{50} \sim 1$ mM). These findings extend our knowledge of the drug binding capabilities of the amine oxidases and suggest that these interactions may contribute to the complex actions of this drug.

Abbreviations: *MAO* monoamine oxidase, *SSAO* semicarbazide-sensitive amine oxidase.

Introduction

The semicarbazide sensitive amine oxidases (SSAO) belong to the copper-containing group of amine oxidases (EC 1.4.3.6; amine: oxygen oxidoreductase (deaminating) (copper containing)). They catalyse the oxidative deamination of primary amines according to the overall reaction:

$$RCH_2NH_2 + O_2 + H_2O \longrightarrow RCHO + NH_3 + H_2O_2.$$

Their sensitivity to inhibition by semicarbazide and other carbonyl reagents results from the presence of a 3,4,6,trihydroxyphenylalanine (TOPA) residue that serves as a cofactor in the reaction.

They have been known by several different names, including benzylamine oxidase, owing to their preference for benzylamine as a substrate, and clorgyline-resistant amine oxidases, as they are not inhibited by the monoamine oxidase (MAO; EC 1.4.3.6) inhibitor clorgyline. They are a ubiquitous group of enzymes found in plants, animals and microbes (Lewinsohn, 1984; Callingham et al., 1995; Lyles, 1996; Houen, 1999). Most mammalian species contain a soluble form of SSAO in the blood plasma plus a membrane bound form of the enzyme that has a relatively high activity in cardiovascular tissue, lung and adipocytes (Boomsma et al., 2000; Lyles, 1995, 1996).

Although the physiological functions of SSAO are by no means fully understood, a primary role of SSAO is believed to be the scavenging of primary amines, either endogenous or xenobiotic (Tipton and Strolin Benedetti, 2001). The active site of the membrane bound form of the enzyme appears to be externally facing, thus allowing the metabolism of extracellular amines. Methylamine and aminoacetone are specific substrates for SSAO, in that MAO does not oxidise them (Lyles and Chalmers, 1992; Lizcano et al., 1994). SSAO and MAO, which is an intracellular enzyme, have been shown to work in concert to facilitate the removal of tyramine in the isolated perfused mesenteric arterial bed of the rat (Elliott et al., 1989). The metabolism of dopamine may also involve both SSAO and MAO, as shown in rat vas deferens (Lizcano et al., 1991).

Several other functions of SSAO have been identified (O'Sullivan et al., 2004; Tipton et al., 2003, for reviews). At least in some tissues, it functions as a vascular-adhesion protein (vascular-adhesion protein-1; VAP-1) (Jalkanen and Salmi, 2001). It may also modulate cellular glucose transport by stimulating membrane glucose transporter recruitment (Enrique-Tarancon et al., 1998, 2000). Roles for SSAO/VAP-1 have also been identified in adipocyte

Correspondence: Dr. J. O'Sullivan, Department of Biochemistry, Trinity College, Dublin 2, Ireland
e-mail: josulli@tcd.ie

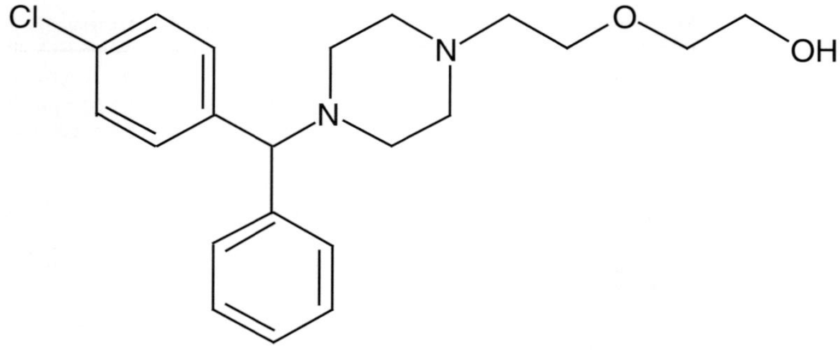

Fig. 1. Chemical structure of hydroxyzine (2-[2-[4-[(4-chlorophenyl)phenylmethyl]-1-piperazinyl]ethoxy]ethanol)

development (Mercier et al., 2001) and in extracellular matrix formation (Langford et al., 2002; Gokturk et al., 2003). It appears that SSAO, may also function as a drug-binding protein. Imidazolines, such as amiloride, and guanidine compounds, which are used clinically, as diuretic and hypertensive agents have been shown to bind to MAO, SSAO and other amine oxidases (Mu et al., 1994; Remaury et al., 2000; Holt et al., 2004). However the physiological significance of these drug-binding sites remains obscure (e.g., Eglen et al., 1988).

The heterocyclic piperazine derivative hydroxyzine 2-[2-[4-[(4-chlorophenyl)phenyl-methyl]-1-piperazinyl]ethoxy]ethanol) (Fig. 1) is a histamine-1 receptor antagonist, with anticholinergic properties, which has a wide variety of therapeutic applications, including the treatment of allergic skin disorders and the control the nausea and vomiting caused by various conditions, including motion sickness. It is also used as a tranquilliser for the symptomatic management of conditions, such as generalised anxiety disorder (GAD) and the tension associated with psychoneuroses (Lader et al., 1998; Ferreri and Hantouche, 1988), as well as in the treatment of the symptoms of alcohol withdrawal. It is also used in the management of pruritis associated with allergic conditions, such as chronic urticaria and histamine-mediated pruritus. Hydroxyzine has been shown to inhibit neurogenic mast-cell activation by a mechanism that is unrelated to its H-1 receptor antagonistic properties (Minogiannis et al., 1998). It has also been shown to inhibit experimental allergic encephalomyelitis and the associated brain mast cell activation and may also be effective in the prevention of relapsing/remitting multiple sclerosis (Dimitriadou et al., 2000).

Cetirizine, the carboxylic acid metabolite of hydroxyzine, may also suppress inflammatory responses, as it possesses an ability to inhibit both macrophage inhibitory factor (MIF) and IL-8 production (Shimizu et al., 2004; Giustizieri et al., 2004). It has been also been suggested to be effective against autoimmune diseases (Namazi, 2004). The carboxyl group results in this derivative having high selectivity as an antagonist of the histamine H-1 receptor resulting in a reduction in sedation and brain penetration (Gillard et al., 2001).

Since, histamine is a substrate for semicarbazide-sensitive amine oxidase whereas MAO-B oxidizes its metabolite N^T-methylhistamine, we have investigated the possibility that hydroxyzine, might interact with these amine oxidases.

Materials and methods

[7-^{14}C] Benzylamine hydrochloride (Specific activity 59 mCi/mmol), 5-Hydoxy [side-chain 2-^{14}C]tryptamine creatine sulphate (Specific activity 57 mCi/mmol) and 2-Phenylethylamine[ethyl-1-^{14}C]hydrochloride (Specific activity 57 mCi/mmol) were from Amersham. *l*-Deprenyl HCl was from Fluka and unlabelled substrates and other chemicals were from Sigma. Rat liver mitochondria, prepared as previously described (Fowler and Tipton, 1981) were used as the source of MAO. Bovine lung microsomes were prepared as a source of membrane-bound SSAO (Lizcano et al., 1998) and bovine plasma SSAO was from Sigma.

More highly purified bovine plasma SSAO was prepared by a modification of the procedure of Wang et al. (1994). 10 L of bovine blood were mixed with 1 L of 2.5% sodium citrate solution and centrifuged at 3000 *g* for 20 min. Ammonium sulphate was added, with continuous stirring, to 4 L of the supernatant to give 35% saturation. Stirring was continued for 2 h before centrifugation at 10,000 *g* for 20 min. The supernatant was retained and ammonium sulphate was added, with continuous stirring, to give 55% saturation. Stirring was continued for 30 min before centrifugation at 10,000 *g* for 20 min. The precipitate taken up in 200 ml of 100 mM potassium phosphate buffer, pH 7.2 and applied, at a flow rate of 150 ml/h, to a Q-Sepharose column (30 × 2.5 cm), which had been equilibrated with 10 mM potassium phosphate buffer, pH 7.5. After washing with 500 ml of the 10 mM phosphate buffer, SSAO was eluted, at a flow rate of 150 ml/h, with a linear concentration gradient from 0.05 to 0.35 M NaCl in the same buffer. Fractions with a specific activity equal to or higher than 0.4 μmol/min/mg protein were pooled, mixed with an equal volume of 100 mM potassium phosphate buffer, pH 7.2, and applied to a Con A-Sepharose column (30 × 2.0 cm) that had been equilibrated with the same buffer. The column was washed with 500 ml of 100 mM phosphate buffer and then with 300 ml of 20 mM methyl-α-D-glucopyranoside in that buffer before the SSAO was eluted with 200 ml of 0.5 M methyl-α-D-mannopyranoside in the same potassium buffer. Fractions (6 ml) with specific activities equal or higher than 0.95 μmol/min/mg were pooled and applied to a Q-Sepharose (30 × 2.5 cm) column, previously equilibrated with 20 mM potassium phosphate buffer (pH 6.8). The column was then washed with 300 ml of the buffer and eluted with a continuous gradient from 0.05 to 0.35 M NaCl in that. The fractions with SSAO specific activity higher than equal or higher than 15 μmol/min/mg protein were then pooled, dialysed against 20 mM potassium phosphate buffer, pH 6.8, for 6 h and stored in aliquots of 300 µl in 20% glycerol at −20°C.

Assay of SSAO and MAO activities

All enzyme assays were performed at 37°C and at pH 7.2, unless otherwise stated. For the determination of the SSAO activity in the microsomal preparation it was preincubated at 37°C for 30 min with clorgyline plus deprenyl (1 µM each), to inhibit MAO. It was found that MAO-B contributed approximately 22% of the total activity of the microsomal preparation in the absence of these inhibitors. Mitochondrial samples were incubated with 1 mM semicarbazide, to inhibit SSAO, before assay of MAO activity.

The oxidation of 5-hydroxytrypamine, 2-phenethylamine (substrates for MAO A and MAO B, respectfully) was determined according to the method of Tipton et al. (2000). SSAO activity was assayed with benzylamine as the substrate by the radiochemical method of Tipton et al. (2000) or by a modification of the method of Tabor et al. (1954). The standard reaction mixture contained 50 mM potassium phosphate buffer, pH 7.2, and 0.024 mg/ml SSAO in a final volume of 1 ml. The reaction was initiated by the addition of the substrate benzylamine and the rate of change of absorbance at 250 nm was monitored using a Cary 300-Biospectrophotometer.

The oxidation of methylamine by SSAO was determined by coupling the formation of formaldehyde to the reduction of NAD^+ in the presence of formaldehyde dehydrogenase (Lizcano et al., 2000). The ability of hydroxyzine to act as a substrate for the amine oxidase was assessed by the determination of hydrogen peroxide formation. Both the fluorimetric method of Tipton (1969) and by the spectrophotometric procedure of Holt et al. (1997) were used.

In all cases, assay conditions used were those determined from preliminary studies to correspond to the linear, initial velocity, period of product formation and a linear dependence of this velocity on the concentration of

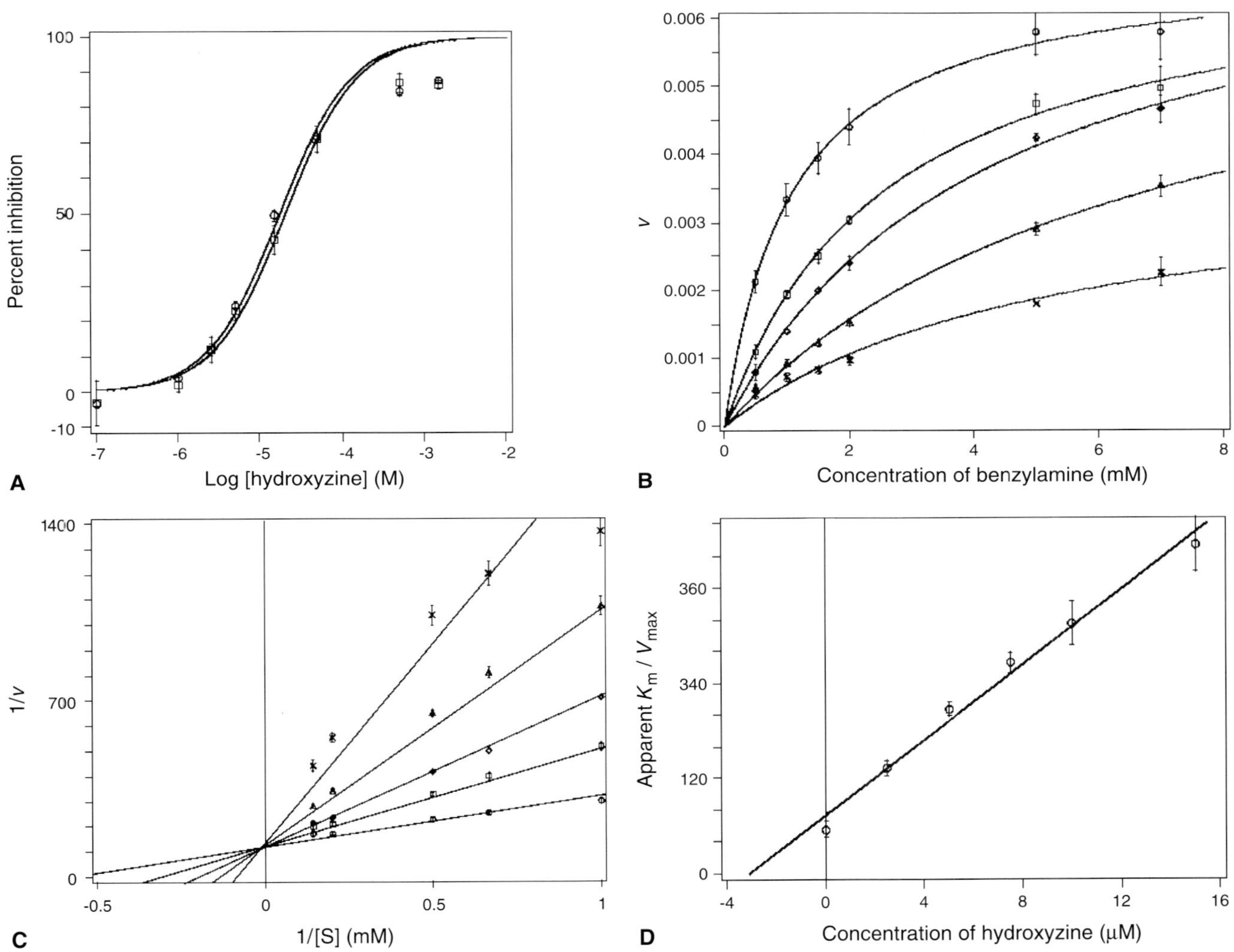

Fig. 2. The kinetics of the inhibition of bovine plasma SSAO by hydroxyzine. All data were obtained using the enzyme from Sigma. Data points are mean values±s.e.m. from triplicate determinations. A The enzyme was preincubated with hydroxyzine for 0 (O) and 60 (□) min at 37°C before the reaction was started by the addition of benzylamine. The curves are those obtained by fitting to the inhibition equation described in the text by non-linear regression. B Michaelis-Menten curves for the oxidation of benzylamine in the presence of following fixed concentrations of hydroxyzine 0 (O), 2.5 (△), 7.5 (◊), 10 (ρ) and 15 (×) µM. The curves are those obtained by non-linear regression. C Double-reciprocal plots of the data in B, presented to illustrate the type of inhibition. D. Plot of the apparent values of K_m/V_{max} values, determined from B, as a function of the hydroxyzine concentration

the tissue sample. Samples were assayed in triplicate. Protein concentrations were determined according to the method of Markwell et al. (1978). For kinetic studies, initial rates were determined by varying the substrate concentration at a constant specific radioactivity and kinetic parameters were determined by non-linear regression, using the programme MacCurveFit, Version 1.5 (Kevin Raner Software, Australia). IC_{50} values (the inhibitor concentration that gives 50% inhibition of the reaction) were also determined by using the same software to fit data to the equation.

$$F(x) = \frac{100(10^{(x+a)})}{10^{(x+a)} + 1}$$

Reversibility of inhibition was assessed by dilution experiments. The enzyme (bovine plasma amine oxidase) from Sigma or partially purified enzyme, at a concentration of 1.2 mg protein ml^{-1}, was incubated with inhibitor until inhibition was essentially complete, using previous time-course experiments as a guide. 20 µl samples were then removed and diluted into the standard benzylamine assay mixture, to give a final protein concentration of 0.024 mg · ml^{-1}, for activity determinations. SSAO activity was then assayed as described above. A control sample was also taken through the same procedure where inhibitor was added to the desired final concentration after dilution.

Reversibility of MAO inhibition was assessed by centrifugation and resuspension. 1 ml of a 10 mg/ml suspension of rat liver mitochondria was incubated for 1 hour with sufficient inhibitor to give essentially complete inhibition. The inhibitor was then depleted by centrifugation at 14000 rpm for 10 min. The supernatant was discarded and the mitochondrial pellet was resuspended in a fresh phosphate buffer (100 mM, pH 7.5) to give a concentration of approximately 10 mg/ml. The MAO activity was then assayed as described previously.

Results

The inhibition of bovine plasma SSAO (from Sigma) by hydroxyzine was found to be time-independent, with no significant change in the extent of inhibition occurring over a 60 min period of enzyme-inhibitor preincubation (Fig. 2A and Table 1). The K_i value for the inhibition of benzylamine oxidation by bovine plasma SSAO was determined, by nonlinear regression of the curves shown in Fig. 2B, to be 3.8 ± 0.39 µM. As illustrated by the double-reciprocal and secondary plots in Fig. 2C and D, the inhibition was simple competitive in nature.

Table 1. *The inhibition of amine oxidases by hydroxyzine*

Enzyme preparation	IC_{50} (µM) 0 min	IC_{50} (µM) 60 min	Inhibition	K_i (µM)
Bovine plasma SSAO (Sigma)	17 ± 0.83	20 ± 0.85	Competitive	1.8 ± 0.39
Bovine plasma SSAO (Purified)	23 ± 0.5	20 ± 0.42	Competitive	1.47 ± 0.79
Bovine lung microsomal SSAO	1050 ± 43	870 ± 28	n.d.	n.d.
Rat liver MAO-A	631 ± 13	676 ± 16	n.d.	n.d.
Rat liver MAO-B	40 ± 1.5	38 ± 0.9	Competitive	19 ± 1.3

The microsomal membrane-bound SSAO was found to be considerably less sensitive to inhibition by hydroxyzine. There was no time-dependence, with IC_{50} values determined as 1.0 ± 0.04 and 0.870 ± 0.03 mM after enzyme-inhibitor preincubation for 0 min and 60 min respectively (Fig. 3). The high IC_{50} value made determination of the K_i impractical.

Since the SSAO preparation obtained from Sigma was found, by polyacrylamide-gel electrophoresis in the presence of sodium dodecyl sulphate (SDS-PAGE), to contain multiple impurities (data not shown), the possibility was

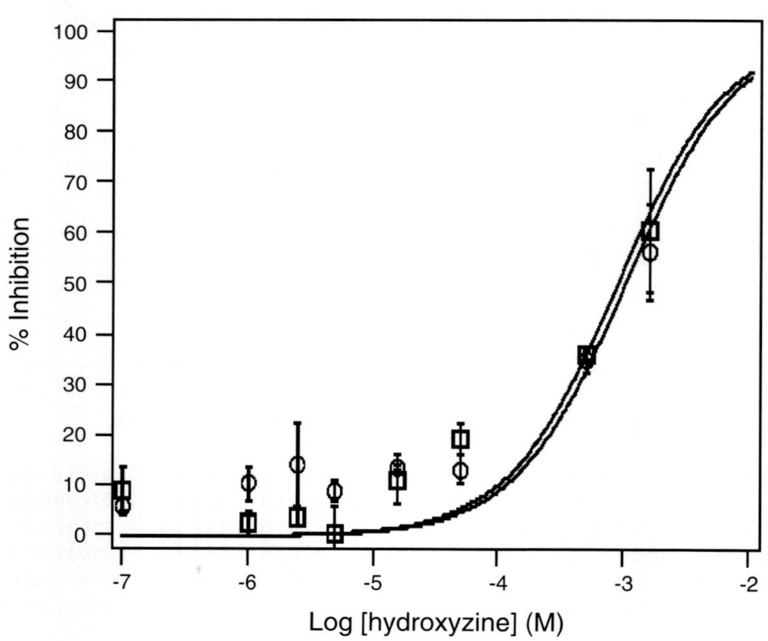

Fig. 3. The inhibition of bovine lung membrane-bound SSAO by hydroxyzine. The enzyme was preincubated with hydroxyzine for ○ = 0 min and □ = 60 min at 37°C before the reaction was started by the addition of benzylamine. The curves are those obtained by fitting to the inhibition equation described in the text by non-linear regression. Data points are mean values ± s.e.m. from triplicate determinations

considered that degradation during the purification procedure used might have contributed to the higher sensitivity of the plasma enzyme. The bovine plasma SSAO, purified as described above, which showed only minor impurities on SDS-PAGE, was studied for comparison. The purified and Sigma SSAO preparations showed similar K_m values towards benzylamine, $1088 \pm 73\,\mu M$ and $997 \pm 59\,\mu M$, respectively, and methylamine, $317 \pm 64\,\mu M$ and $305 \pm 32\,\mu M$, respectively. For comparison, the K_m for the microsomal membrane bound SSAO towards benzylamine was determined as $76 \pm 29\,\mu M$. The two preparations of the plasma enzyme also behaved similarly in their sensitivities to inhibition by hydroxyzine, as shown in Table 1. Incubation of the microsomal fraction in the presence of endoglycosidase-H (1 unit) for 20 h at 37°C before assay decreased the sensitivity to inhibition by hydroxyzine; an IC_{50} value of 2.9 ± 0.79 mM being obtained. Incubation of the purified plasma SSAO with endoglycosidase-H under similar conditions did not significantly affect the activity towards benzylamine or the sensitivity towards inhibition by 20 μM hydroxyzine, as compared to a control incubated under the same conditions in the absence of the endoglycosidase (Fig. 4).

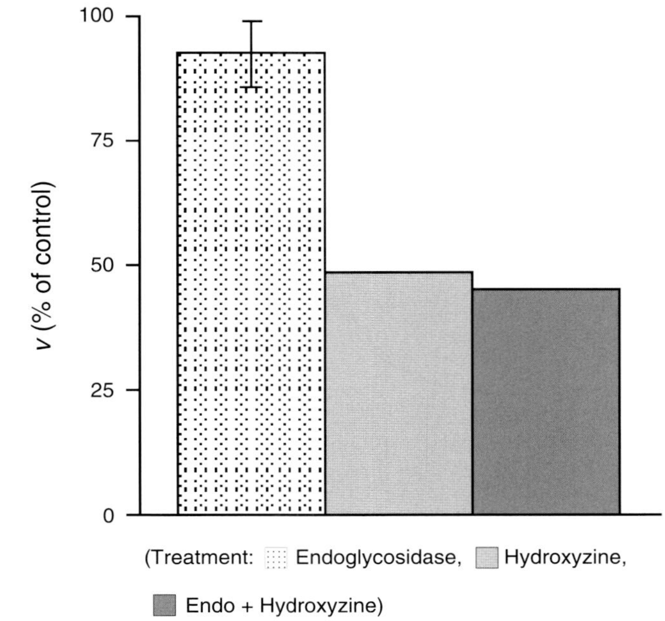

Fig. 4. The effects of pretreatment with endoglycosidase-H (Endo) on the inhibition of purified beef plasma SSAO by hydroxyzine. Experimental details are described in the text. Values are means ± s.e.m. from triplicate determinations

Rat liver MAO-A, determined towards 5-HT, was relatively insensitive to inhibition by hydroxyzine, which was not time dependent (Fig. 5). The high IC_{50} value, shown in Table 1, made determination of the K_i impractical. In contrast, hydroxyzine was a much more potent inhibitor of MAO-B (Fig. 6) The inhibition, which showed no time dependence, was found to be competitive, with respect to 2-phenylethylamine, as shown, for illustrative purposes, in Fig. 6B and C. The K_i value indicated it to be about 10 times less potent an inhibitor of MAO-B, as compared to the plasma SSAO (Table 1).

The inhibition of the amine oxidase preparations, used in this study, by hydroxyzine was found to be freely reversible with essentially complete recoveries of activity after removal of the inhibitor, by dilution in the case of SSAO and by sedimentation for MAO. Hydroxyzine was found not to be a substrate for any of the enzymes studied, as determined by H_2O_2 release.

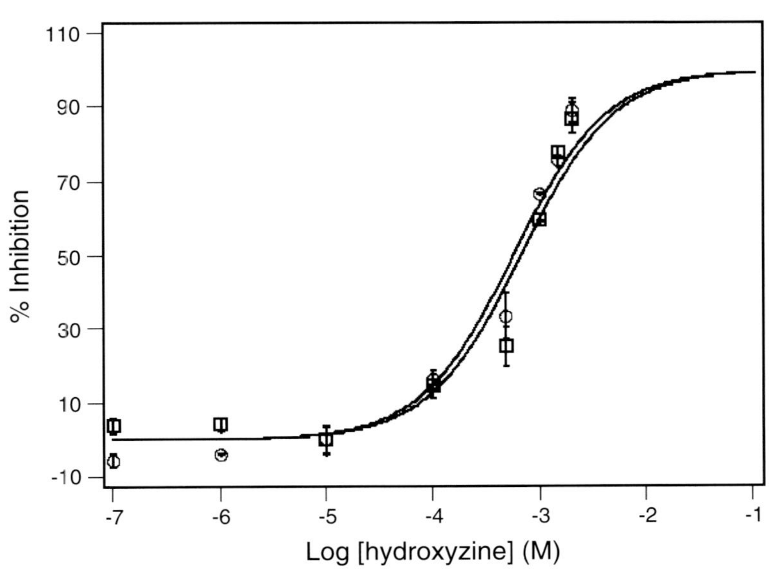

Fig. 5. The inhibition of rat liver mitochondrial MAO-A by hydroxyzine. The enzyme was preincubated with hydroxyzine for O = 0 min and □ = 60 min at 37°C before the reaction was started by the addition of 5-hydroxytryptamine. The curves are those obtained by fitting to the inhibition equation described in the text by non-linear regression. Data points are mean values ± s.e.m. from triplicate determinations

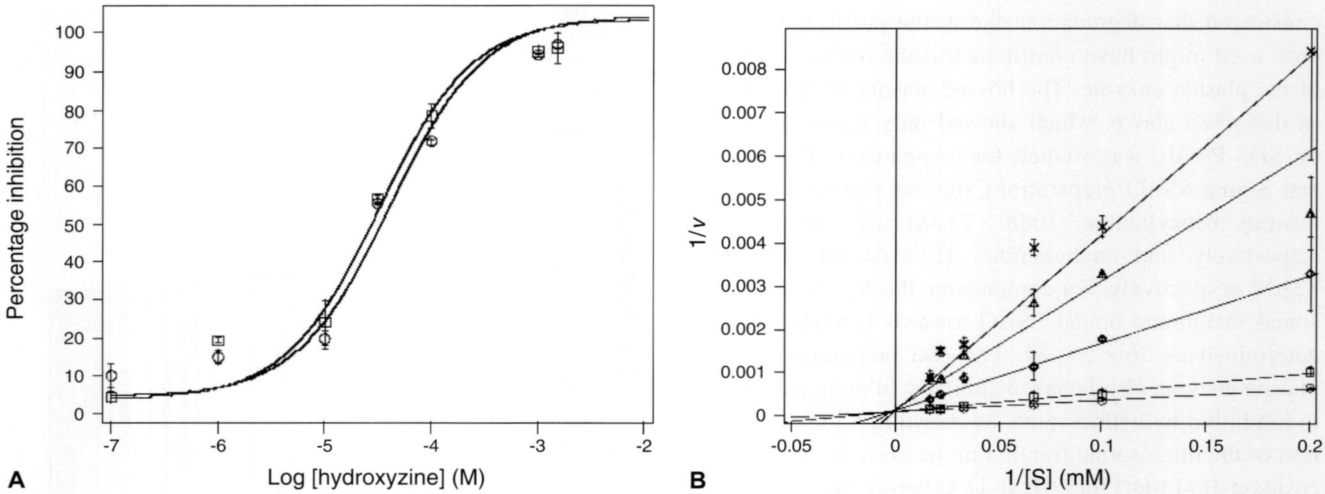

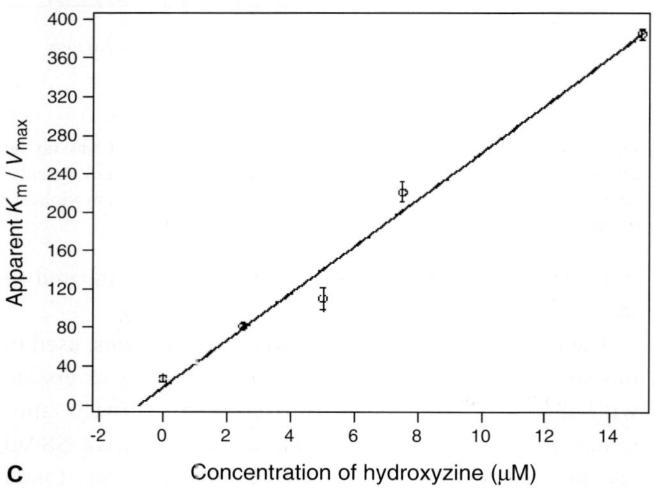

Fig. 6. The inhibition of rat liver mitochondrial MAO-B by hydroxyzine. A. The enzyme was preincubated with hydroxyzine for O = 0 min and □ = 60 min at 37°C before the reaction was started by the addition of 2-phenylethylamine. The curves are those obtained by fitting to the inhibition equation described in the text by non-linear regression. Data points are mean values ± s.e.m. from triplicate determinations. B. Double-reciprocal plots of the data of the initial rates of 2-phenylethylamine oxidation at the following fixed concentrations of hydroxyzine 0 (O), 10 (△), 100 (◊), 175 (ρ) and 250 (×) μM, presented to illustrate the type of inhibition. Plot of the apparent values of K_m/V_{max} values, determined from non-linear regression fitting of the initial-rate data, as a function of the hydroxyzine concentration

Discussion

The reversible inhibition of bovine plasma SSAO and MAO-B by hydroxyzine adds a further potential complexity to the mechanism of action of this drug. In contrast, the low inhibitory potency towards MAO-A and the membrane-bound SSAO suggests that the interactions with these enzymes are unlikely to be important. The difference between the behaviour of the plasma and membrane-bound SSAO is likely to be a result of some processing event, since it appears that they are both encoded by the same gene (Zhang and McIntire, 1996). It does not appear that artefactual degradation during purification of the plasma enzyme may have resulted in a greater sensitivity, since two different preparations gave similar results. Since SSAO is a heavily glycosylated protein, differences in glycosylation between membrane-bound SSAO and the plasma form, which are believed to be associated with cleavage of the membrane form (Kurkijärvi et al., 1998), might be involved. However, treatment of the microsomal preparation with endoglycosidase-H resulted in a decreased sensitivity to inhibition by hydroxyzine. Thus, although the glycosylation of SSAO may affect the accessibility of hydroxyzine it would appear to enhance, rather than impede, access.

The membrane location may play a role in this difference. Lizcano et al. (1998) have reported inhibitor-sensitivity differences between bovine membrane-bound and plasma SSAO. For example, amiloride to be ineffective as an inhibitor of membrane bound SSAO ($IC_{50} > 50$ mM), mM), although the inhibitor sensitivity increased somewhat after extraction and purification ($K_i = 750 \pm 100$ μM). Purification also resulted in a 50-fold increase in the sensitivity of the bovine lung enzyme to inhibition by phenylhydrazine (Lizcano et al., 1998).

The competitive nature of the inhibition of plasma SSAO and mitochondrial MAO-A might suggest that hydroxyzine binds to the active sites of these amine oxidases, although it showed no detectable activity as a substrate. These results extend our knowledge of the drug-binding capabilities of these enzymes, which are already known to include the imidazolines. β-Carbolines and harmala alkaloids bind to MAO (Miralles et al., 2005; Herraiz and Chaparro, 2006) and a number of transport-inhibiting antidepressants, such as imipramine, maprotiline, nomifensine and zimeldine, bind as inhibitors both to MAO (Egashira et al., 1999) and SSAO (Obata and Yamanaka, 2000), although the nature of these interactions appears to show considerable species differences. In none of these cases is it known whether or not this binding significantly affects the bioavailability of these drugs or might give rise to undesirable drug-drug interactions.

Histamine, which may play important role in cell adhesion (Andriopoulou et al., 1999; Winter et al., 1999), is a relatively poor substrate for semicarbazide-sensitive amine oxidase (Raimondi et al., 1997; Lizcano et al., 1998) and is not oxidized by MAO, although its metabolite, N^T-methylhistamine, is a substrate for MAO-B (Waldmeier et al., 1997) and SSAO (Gitomer and Tipton, 1983). Inhibition of SSAO might affect its other diverse functions and a major consequence of MAO-B inhibition is the elevation of 2-phenylethylamine. Further work would be necessary to show whether the amine oxidase inhibition contributes significantly to the diverse actions of hydroxyzine.

Acknowledgement

Financial assistance from the Health Research Board (Ireland) is gratefully acknowledged.

References

Andriopoulou P, Navarro P, Zanetti A, Lampugnani MG, Dejana E (1999) Histamine induces tyrosine phosphorylation of endothelial cell-to-cell adherens junctions. Arterioscler Thromb Vasc Biol 19: 2286–2297

Boomsma F, van Dijk J, Bhaggoe UM, Bouhuizen AM, van den Meiracker AH (2000) Variation in semicarbazide-sensitive amine oxidase activity in plasma and tissues of mammals. Comp Biochem Physiol C 126: 69–78

Callingham BA, Crosbie AE, Rous BA (1995) Some aspects of the pathophysiology of semicarbazide-sensitive amine oxidase enzymes. Prog Brain Res 106: 305–321

Dimitriadou V, Pang X, Theohardies TC (2000) Hydroxyzine inhibits experimental allergic encephalomyelitis (EAE) and associated brain mast cell function. Int J Immunopharmacol 22: 673–684

Egashira T, Takayama F, Yamanaka Y (1999) The inhibition of monoamine oxidase activity by various antidepressants: differences found in various mammalian species. Jpn J Pharmacol 81: 115–121

Eglen RM, Hudson AL, Kendall DA, Nutt DJ, Morgan NG, Wilson VG, Dillon MP (1988) 'Seeing through a glass darkly': casting light on imidazoline 'I' sites. Trends Pharmacol Sci 19: 381–390

Elliott J, Callingham BA, Sharman DF (1989) Semicarbazide-sensitive amine oxidase (SSAO) of the rat aorta. Interactions with some naturally occurring amines and their structural analogues. Biochem Pharmacol 38: 1507–1515

Enrique-Tarancon G, Marti L, Morin N, Lizcano JM, Unzeta M, Sevilla L, Camps M, Palacin M, Testar X, Carpene C, Zorzano A (1998) Role of semicarbazide-sensitive amine oxidase on glucose transport and GLUT4 recruitment to the cell surface in adipose cells. J Biol Chem 273: 8025–8032

Enrique-Tarancon G, Castan I, Morin N, Marti L, Abella A, Camps M, Casamitjana R, Palacin M, Testar X, Degerman E, Carpene C, Zorzano A (2000) Substrates of semicarbazide-sensitive amine oxidase co-operate with vanadate to stimulate tyrosine phosphorylation of insulin-receptor-substrate proteins, phosphoinositide 3-kinase activity and GLUT4 translocation in adipose cells. Biochem J 350: 171–180

Ferreri M, Hantouche EG (1988) Recent clinical trials of hydroxyzine in generalized anxiety disorder. Acta Psychiatr Scand [Suppl 393]: 102–108

Fowler CJ, Tipton KF (1981) Concentration dependence of the oxidation of tyramine by the two forms of rat liver mitochondrial monoamine oxidase. Biochem Pharmacol 30: 3329–3332

Gillard M, van der Perren C, Moguilevsky N, Massingham R, Chatelain P (2002) Binding characteristics of cetirizine and levocetirizine to human H1 histamine receptors: contribution of Lys191 and Thr194. Mol Pharmacol 61: 392–399

Gitomer WL, Tipton KF (1983) Determination of K_m and V of an enzyme for an unstable substrate and its application to the oxidation of N^T-methylimidazol-3-ylacetaldehyde by aldehyde dehydrogenase. J Biochem 211: 277–280

Giustizieri ML, Albanesi C, Fluhr J, Gisondi P, Norgauer J, Girolomoni G (2004) H1 histamine receptor mediates inflammatory responses in human keratinocytes. J Allergy Clin Immunol 114: 1176–1182

Gokturk C, Nilsson J, Nordquist J, Kristensson M, Svensson K, Soderberg C, Israelson M, Garpenstrand H, Sjoquist M, Oreland L, Forsberg-Nilsson K (2003) Overexpression of semicarbazide-sensitive amine oxidase in smooth muscle cells leads to an abnormal structure of the aortic elastic laminas. Am J Pathol 163: 1921–1928

Herraiz T, Chaparro C (2006) Human monoamine oxidase enzyme inhibition by coffee and beta-carbolines norharman and harman isolated from coffee. Life Sci 178: 795–802

Holt A, Wieland B, Baker GB (2004) Allosteric modulation of semicarbazide-sensitive amine oxidase activities in vitro by imidazoline receptor ligands. Br J Pharmacol 143: 495–507

Holt A, Sharman DF, Baker GB, Palcic MM (1997) A continuous spectrophotometric assay for monoamine oxidase and related enzymes in tissue homogenates. Anal Biochem 244: 384–392

Houen G (1999) Mammalian Cu-containing amine oxidases (CAOs): new methods of analysis, structural relationships, and possible functions. APMIS [Suppl 96]: 1–46

Jalkanen S, Salmi M (2001) Cell surface monoamine oxidases: enzymes in search of a function. EMBO J 20: 3893–3901

Kurkijärvi R, Adams DH, Leino R, Mottonen T, Jalkanen S, Salmi M (1998) Circulating form of human vascular adhesion protein-1 (VAP-1): increased serum levels in inflammatory liver diseases. J Immunol 161: 1549–1557

Langford SD, Trent MB, Boor PJ (2002) Semicarbazide-sensitive amine oxidase and extracellular matrix deposition by smooth-muscle cells. Cardiovasc Toxicol 2: 141–150

Lader M, Scotto JC (1998) A multicentre double-blind comparison of hydroxyzine, buspirone and placebo in patients with generalised anxiety disorder. Psychopharamcol 139: 402–406

Lewinsohn R (1984) Mammalian monoamine-oxidizing enzymes, with special reference to benzylamine oxidase in human tissues. Brazil J Med Biol Res 17: 223–256

Lizcano JM, Fernandez de Arriba A, Lyles GA, Unzeta M (1994) Several aspects on the amine oxidation by semicarbazide-sensitive amine

oxidase (SSAO) from bovine lung. J Neural Transm [Suppl 41]: 415–420
Lizcano JM, Tipton KF, Unzeta M (1998) Purification and characterization of membrane-bound semicarbazide-sensitive amine oxidase (SSAO) from bovine lung. J Biochem 331: 69–78
Lizcano JM, Unzeta M, Tipton KF (2000) A spectrophotometric method for determining the oxidative deamination of methylamine by the amine oxidases. Anal Biochem 286: 75–79
Lizcano JM, Balsa D, Tipton KF, Unzeta M (1991) The oxidation of dopamine by the semicarbazide-sensitive amine oxidase (SSAO) from rat vas deferens. Biochem Pharmacol 41: 1107–1110
Lyles GA (1995) Substrate-specificity of mammalian tissue-bound semicarbazide-sensitive amine oxidase. Prog Brain Res 106: 293–303
Lyles GA (1996) Mammalian plasma and tissue-bound semicarbazide-sensitive amine oxidases: biochemical, pharmacological and toxicological aspects. Int J Biochem Cell Biol 28: 259–274
Lyles GA, Chalmers J (1995) Aminoacetone metabolism by semicarbazide-sensitive amine oxidase in rat aorta. Biochem Pharmacol 49: 416–419
Markwell MA, Haas SM, Bieber LL, Tolbert NE (1978) A modification of the Lowry procedure to simplify protein determination in membrane and lipoprotein samples. Anal Biochem 87: 206–210
Mercier N, Moldes M, El Hadri K, Feve B (2001) Semicarbazide-sensitive amine oxidase activation promotes adipose conversion of 3T3-L1 cells. J Biochem 358: 335–342
Minogiannis P, El-mansoury M, Betances JA, Sant GR, Theoharides TC (1998) hydroxyzine inhibits neurogenic bladder mast cell activation. Int J Immunopharmacol 20: 553–563
Miralles A, Esteban S, Sastre-Coll A, Moranta D, Asensio VJ, Garcia-Sevilla JA (2005) High-affinity binding of beta-carbolines to imidazoline I2B receptors and MAO-A in rat tissues: norharman blocks the effect of morphine withdrawal on DOPA/noradrenaline synthesis in the brain. Eur J Pharmacol 518: 234–242
Mu D, Medzihradszky KF, Adams GW, Mayer P, Hines WM, Burlingame AL, Smith AJ, Cai D, Klinman JP (1994) Primary structures for a mammalian cellular and serum copper amine oxidase. J Biol Chem 269: 9926–9932
Namazi MR (2004) Cetirizine and allopurinol as novel weapons against cellular autoimmune disorders. Int Immunopharmacol 4: 349–353
Raimondi L, Banchelli G, Ignesti G, Pirisino R, Conforti L (1997) The histaminase activity of rat white adipocytes. Inflamm Res 46: 125–131
Remaury A, Raddatz R, Ordener C, Savic S, Shih JC, Chen K, Seif I, De Maeyer E, Lanier SM, Parini A (2000) Analysis of the pharmacological and molecular heterogeneity of I(2)-imidazoline-binding proteins using monoamine oxidase-deficient mouse models. Mol Pharmacol 58: 1085–1090
Obata T, Yamanaka Y (2000) Inhibition of monkey brain semicarbazide-sensitive amine oxidase by various antidepressants. Neurosci Lett 286: 131–133
O'Sullivan J, Unzeta M, Healy J, O'Sullivan MI, Davey G, Tipton KF (2004) Semicarbazide-sensitive amine oxidases: enzymes with quite a lot to do. Neurotoxicology 25: 303–315
Tabor CW, Tabor H, Rosenthal SM (1954) Purification of amine oxidase from beef plasma. J Biol Chem 208: 645–661
Tipton KF (1969) A sensitive fluorometric assay for monoamine oxidase. Anal Biochem 28: 318–325
Tipton KF, Strolin Benedetti M (2001) Amine Oxidases and the metabolism of xenobiotics. In: Ioannides C (ed) Enzyme Systems that Metabolise Drugs and Other Xenobiotics. John Wiley & Sons, Chichester, pp 95–146
Tipton KF, Davey G, Motherway M (2000) Monoamine oxidase assays. In: Enna SJ, Willias M, Ferkany JW, Kenakin T, Porsolt RE, Sullivan JP (eds) Current protocols in pharmacology. John Wiley & Sons, New York, pp 3.61–3.6.42
Tipton KF, Boyce S, O'Sullivan J, Davey GP, Healy J (2004) Monoamine oxidases: certainties and uncertainties. Curr Med Chem 11: 1965–1982
Tipton KF, O'Sullivan MI, Davey GP, O'Sullivan J (2003) It can be a complicated life being an enzyme. Biochem Soc Trans 31: 711–715
Wang XT, Dumoulin MJ, Befani O, Mondovi B, Mateescu MA (1994) Joint chromatographic purification of bovine serum ceruloplasmin and amineoxidase. Prep Biochem 24: 237–250
Winter MC, Kamath AM, Ries DR, Shasby SS, Chen YT, Shasby DM (1999) Histamine alters cadherin-mediated sites of endothelial adhesion. Am J Physiol 277: L988–L995
Waldmeier PC, Feldtrauer JJ, Maitre L (1977) Methylhistamine: evidence for selective deamination by MAO B in the rat brain *in vivo*. J Neurochem 29: 785–790
Zhang X, McIntire WS (1996) Cloning and sequencing of a copper-containing, TOPA quinone-containing monoamine oxidase from human placenta. Gene 179: 279–286

J Neural Transm (2006) [Suppl] 71: 113–122

Journal of
Neural
Transmission
Printed in Austria

Neuroprotection for Parkinson's disease

P. A. LeWitt

Departments of Neurology, Psychiatry and Behavioral Neuroscience, Wayne State University School of Medicine, The William Beaumont Hospital Research Institute, Royal Oak Michigan, and The Clinical Neuroscience Program, Southfield, Michigan, USA

Summary Although still a disorder of unknown etiology, Parkinson's disease (PD) has provided a number of clues that have led to clinical trials of neuroprotection. For example, defects in mitochondrial metabolism and evidence for oxidative stress in PD have fostered therapeutic interventions aimed at slowing disease progression. More than a dozen compounds already have been tested in PD for disease modification, and others are in planning stages for clinical trials. The challenge is to find a highly effective therapy halting disease progression (beyond the relatively modest clinical effect exemplified by recent findings with coenzyme Q-10 treatment administered at 1200 mg/day). Clinical exam-based ratings and disability assessments still serve at providing the primary evidence of efficacy. However, with surrogate biomarkers such as radiotracer neuroimaging of the dopaminergic system, the pace of clinical investigation can be increased. Recent years have seen the utilization of more sensitive study methods in PD neuroprotection research, such as staggered wash-in, 2 × 2 factorial, and "futility" trial designs. The results of several ongoing PD neuroprotection trials are planned for release in the near future.

Introduction

For most patients with Parkinson's disease (PD) over the past four decades, highly effective symptomatic treatment with levodopa has been a routine experience. At their best, such medications have permitted most patients to achieve near-normalization of most Parkinsonian signs and symptoms. Only for some advanced cases of PD does significant disability evolve, and this typically occurs with at least some degree of continuing benefit from levodopa and other drugs that can mask most of PD's motor features. Therapeutics for Parkinsonism has capitalized on an increasingly thorough understanding of the key pathophysiology behind PD's motor deficits: a marked decrease of dopaminergic neurotransmission normally provided by neurons projecting to the striatum from the substantia nigra pars compacta (SNpc). For some fortunate patients, the relief of motor disabilities by medications can continue indefinitely. However, over time, the consistency of such benefits tends to diminish and problems such as involuntary movements can develop. Since mild PD tends to be so responsive to medication, treatment strategies to maintain this disorder in its mild stage are desirable. Such therapies, if applied to PD at its preclinical stage, might even prevent the loss of SNpc neurons and so would serve as the equivalent of a cure. Protective therapy against the progression of PD might also help to avert problems of advanced disease that are currently untreatable, such as impairments of posture, balance, and cognition.

Correspondence: P. A. LeWitt, MD, Clinical Neuroscience Center, 26400 West Twelve Mile Road, Suite 180, Southfield, Michigan 48034, USA
e-mail: palewitt@ameritech.net

The search for a neuroprotective therapy of PD has captured the interest of thousands of clinicians and basic neuroscience researchers. A leader in this quest has been Professor Moussa Youdim, who has contributed a wealth of ideas and discoveries to finding the cause(s) and treatments of PD. Readers of this Festschrift should be well aware of Professor Youdim's influential role at investigating the most promising directions of PD pathogenesis, including oxidative stress, apoptosis, and toxicities of iron and neuromelanin. Through his own laboratory's efforts and from numerous collaborations established throughout the world, Professor Youdim has also maintained a longstanding interest in the discovery of potential neuroprotective agents for PD. Each of his lectures on the topic (and Moussa has never been shy about placing himself in the thick of debate!) has aimed at bring together the multiple strands of the etiological puzzle into a unifying theme. The challenge is to find rational therapeutic interventions for PD in the current absence of evidence that unequivocally points to a particular cause (or causes) of PD. Contemporary efforts to slow or halt the disease are guided primarily by analogies to animal models and a few insights into the disorder's pathophysiology. Nonetheless, a growing list of hypothetical targets for definitive treatment of PD has been developed. Reflecting this diversity of options, a recent initiative by the National Institutes of Health considered 59 possible therapies against the progression of PD (Ravina et al., 2003) (a list that does not include the option of mercury treatment as originally proposed by James Parkinson (Parkinson, 1817)). The diversity of possible anti-Parkinsonian therapies has expanded greatly from an earlier focus limited to anti-oxidant strategies (Spencer et al., 1996). In this article, the results of several clinical trials and ongoing studies of neuroprotection in PD will be reviewed.

Although cognitive and autonomic disturbances can develop as later features in many cases of PD, the increasing severity of motor impairments generally provides the most obvious evidence for disease progression over time. These motor features can be linked to loss of the majority of dopaminergic neurons in the SNpc (Fearnley and Lees, 1991). Parkinsonian features correlate to the extent of SNpc neuronal dropout after reaching a theshold of greater than 60% of the original cellular complement. Although no biological marker unequivocally gauges these changes in the living patient, neuroimaging techniques utilizing radiotracers have shown a linear rate of decline in the striatal dopaminergic system as PD worsens (Ravina et al., 2005). These neuroimaging techniques have been utilized in clinical trials as potential surrogate markers, although their possible role in replacing or even supplementing clinical indicators is still in question.

The elusive goal of disease modification

Initially, the specific goal of an effective PD neuroprotective treatment would seem to be obvious, especially if the therapeutic perspective is guided from studies of neurotoxins such as MPTP and 6-hydroxydopamine (Heikkila et al., 1990). Like the pathological outcome in PD, these neurotoxins produce a relatively selective loss of dopaminergic neurons in the SNpc. The analogy these neurotoxins have provided to the development of neuroprotective therapies has been pervasive. Sparing the further loss of dopaminergic SNpc neurons would seem to be the means to accomplish slowing of disease progression and leads to conceptualizing the appropriate treatment of PD as inhibiting a toxic mechanism. This is exemplified in some of thinking behind proposals for studying selegiline as a neuroprotective strategy, based on outcome of selegiline pre-treatment in the animal model of MPTP toxicity (Heikkila et al., 1990). However, whether there actually is a similar neurotoxicity mechanism to target in PD is not known. Another challenge ahead is the interpretation of results from a successful clinical trial. For example, a therapy associated with less worsening on clinical criteria might reflect either the halting of further neuronal dropout or else the initiation of recovery processes (such as neuronal sprouting or increased output of dopamine from remaining SNpc neurons). These alternative therapeutic mechanisms are obviously quite different though the clinical result is the same. Other challenges await the interpretation of successful disease-modifying therapies. For example, an effective treatment preventing clinical deterioration might be quite distinct from the mechanisms initiating the disorder. Intervening at a common final pathway of neurodegeneration, such as at steps in inflammatory processes observed in PD (Miklossy et al., 2006) or apoptotic mechanisms (Tatton et al., 2003) might be successful without having targeted the specific causative mechanism. For these reasons, inferring a disease process from the outcomes of clinical studies will continue to be problems, even now that more than a dozen neuroprotection trials have been undertaken (LeWitt, 2004).

Monoamine oxidase inhibitors in Parkinson's disease

As clinicians and researchers in the 1980s set their sights on more than symptomatic relief of PD, the predominant viewpoint was that this disorder was the result of unprotected oxidant stress causing progressive damage to SNpc neurons. The selective vulnerability of these neurons was thought to be partly a consequence of their dopamine metabolism. Dopamine produced by SNpc neurons can convert to quinones, semiquinones, and other byproducts of autooxidation. The action of monoamine oxidase (MAO) generates hydrogen peroxide, which can then further react to produce various reactive oxyradicals (Spencer et al., 1996; Jenner, 2003). Consequences of these processes include oxidant reactions against vital cell constituents such as lipid membranes, nucleic acids, and proteins. The unique relationship between dopamine metabolism and SNpc neurons led to speculation that blocking MAO might offer one means for slowing a plausible mechanism for progressive damage to dopaminergic neurons. With this thought in mind, a clinical trial was designed by clinicians who formed the Parkinson Study Group in North America in the mid 1980s (Parkinson Study Group, 1989a). Their study, the first large neuroprotective clinical trial in PD, incorporated a trial of a selective MAO inhibitor, selegiline (deprenyl), as one of two antioxidant strategies to be tested. Blockade of the type B species of MAO (MAO-B) was chosen to be the appropriate target since, at that time, this enzyme was thought to be the predominant source of dopamine catabolism. Selective MAO-B can be accomplished with selegiline at 10 mg per day, the dose chosen for this study. A 2-year randomized clinical trial of 800 subjects tested whether selegiline might protect against progression of PD. This study, titled "deprenyl and tocopherol antioxidative therapy of Parkinsonism" (DATATOP), was also conducted with a biologically active form of vitamin E, alpha-tocopherol. The study was a 2×2 factorial randomization between for treatment arms, including placebo and a combination of alpha-tocopherol and selegiline (Parkinson Study Group, 1989a, b; 1993). Otherwise untreated PD subjects were followed to a primary endpoint defined as the need for symptomatic treatment of worsening parkinsonism. Other secondary endpoints included the unified Parkinson disease rating scale (UPDRS), other clinical and neuropsychological assessments, and measurement of CSF homovanillic acid and other neurochemicals as biomarkers of change over time in dopamine metabolism (Parkinson Study Group, 1995; LeWitt et al., 1992).

The DATATOP trial was halted prior to its planned two-year duration because of initial findings suggesting a neuroprotective effect from selegiline. A major treatment effect, observed at a mean of 12 $\pm$ five months after start of selegiline, was that 170 of 401 subjects receiving placebo but only 97 of 399 receiving selegiline reached the study endpoint. The two treatment arms had a highly significant difference ($p < 10^{-8}$) and led to initial conclusions of a disease modifying effect that could evolve rapidly following the start of selegiline treatment (Parkinson Study Group, 1989b). A Kaplan-Meier analysis of subjects reaching the need-for-levodopa endpoint demonstrated reduction in the risk by approximately half in the selegiline-treated group. No benefit occurred for the alpha-tocopherol-treated group, however (Parkinson Study Group, 1993). Although exciting in its implications for the hypothesis of oxidant stress as a mechanism for PD, subsequent analysis of the DATATOP study revealed that the rate of reaching endpoint did not differ from placebo if the assessment was evaluated just a few months later. Furthermore, there was an alternative explanation for the apparent reduction in rate of progression. Unsuspected at the design of the study was a small symptomatic effect exerted by selegiline. Although these symptomatic actions against mild Parkinsonism didn't necessarily account for all of the clinical improvements found in the selegiline-treated group, as compared to placebo, any further analysis of the study data was compromised by this confound. The DATATOP study has continued to be a challenge for interpretation of its findings (Ward, 1994; Maki-Ikola and Heinonen, Goetz et al., 2002) and emphasizes the complexities implicit in clinical research for neuroprotection against PD (Clarke, 2004). It has offered researchers considerable information on the natural history of untreated PD and yielded the unexpected finding that selegiline treatment was associated with decreased risk for eventually developing "freezing" of gait (Giladi et al., 2001).

The DATATOP trial provided useful insights into the development of study designs for neuroprotection in PD. Although the "need for levodopa" endpoint may appear unduly subjective and imprecise for studying the progression of PD (LeWitt et al., 1997), this endpoint, along with DATATOP findings from UPDRS scores have found their way to guide subsequent neuroprotection clinical trials. The expectation that CSF homovanillic acid (derived from CNS dopamine metabolism) would provide a useful biomarker of disease progression was not supported by comparisons of homovanillic acid concentrations measured before and after the study was completed. Furthermore, the CSF findings also demonstrated that selegiline treatment did not completely block the oxidative deamination of dopamine as was initially hypothesized (LeWitt et al., 1992). As one of the largest clinical studies ever carried out with PD patients, the DATATOP trial provided the groundwork for future studies of MAO-B inhibitors (Parkinson Study Group, 1996, 2002) and other potential neuroprotective therapies.

Selegiline has been studied in several smaller investigations using study formats similar to the DATATOP trial. In 2 of them, also using selegiline as a monotherapy (10 mg/day) in 54 PD subjects, progression and delay to the need for levodopa was demonstrated (Tetrud and Langston, 1989; Myllylä et al., 1991). Other studies attempted to assess for symptomatic effects of selegiline by prolonging drug washout for eight weeks, and concluded that this drug may have conferred a neuroprotective effect (Palhagen et al., 1998). One study found that the ability of selegiline-treated subjects remained milder than placebo for up to 12 months, although as in the DATATOP study, the apparent protective action was lost by 12 months after the start of treatment (Myllylä et al., 1991). In another study, conducted over five-years with a randomized and placebo-controlled format involving selegiline together with levodopa therapy, an attempt was made to discern neuroprotective form the symptomatic actions of the MAO-B inhibitor (Larsen et al., 1999). The statistically significant slower rate of PD progression found in the selegiline-treated group provided evidence for a possible protective effect. In the background of studies suggesting that selegiline might be disease-modifying were laboratory findings indicating that, beyond inhibition of MAO, the drug's metabolite desmethylselegiline might offer neuroprotective actions including anti-apoptotic effects (Tatton et al., 2003).

The initial reports of possible neuroprotective benefits from selegiline prompted consideration of other MAO inhibitors. The next compound to be investigated was lazabemide, a reversible inhibitor of MAO-B with greater selectivity and no amphetamine metabolites. The possibility of fully washing out the drug in a short period of time offered a better opportunity to sort out symptomatic from neuroprotective actions. Lazabemide provided a similar degree of mild anti-Parkinsonian action to the effects of selegiline (LeWitt et al., 1994). In a randomized placebo-controlled study of 321 subjects lasting up to one year, the results were strikingly similar to those of the DATATOP trial. In addition to small symptomatic effects, a Kaplan-Meier analysis revealed that the several might reduce the risk for reaching the "need for levodopa" endpoint by 51% ($p = 0.008$) (Parkinson Study Group, 1996). With lazabemide, a disease-modifying effect linked to inhibition of MAO-B was starting to appear all the more likely. However, further opportunities for the study of this drug were halted despite the promising results.

Selective inhibition of MAO-B was the target of rasagiline, another compound that was developed for a trial of neuroprotection for PD. Rasagiline is, like selegiline, a propylpargyline structure that is an irreversible inhibitor of MAO-B (Akao et al., 2001). In laboratory research conducted by Professor Youdim and his colleagues, it has demonstrated a number of properties beyond MAO-B inhibition that show promise for achieving neuroprotection (Maruyama et al., 2002; Mandel et al., 2003; Youdim et al., 2003). Rasagiline at 1 and 2 mg/day was studied in a randomized, placebo-controlled clinical trial of 404 otherwise untreated PD subjects. In addition to a secondary endpoint of "need for levodopa", the primary measure of efficacy was a magnitude of change in total UPDRS from baseline to 26 weeks. A "staggered start" study design was utilized in an effort to minimize the potentially confounding effect of an insufficient drug washout. Results of the trial (termed the TEMPO study) revealed that both doses of rasagiline produced small but potentially meaningful improvements, as compared to placebo ($p < 0.001$) (Parkinson Study Group, 2002). The magnitude of this effect (approximately 4 points improvement in total UPDRS scores as compared to placebo) was comparable to the results of selegiline in the DATATOP study (Parkinson Study Group, 1989). Statistically significant improvement in UPDRS activities of daily living scores and in a quality-of-life measure indicated improvements were more than derived from motor improvements. However, Kaplan-Meier survival analysis showed no statistically significant changes between placebo and rasagiline in delayed need for the start of symptomatic treatment (Parkinson Study Group, 2002).

Dopaminergic agonists and levodopa

Medications that have symptomatic effects against PD have also been studied as to their possible role as neuroprotective agents. For many years there have been hypotheses that an exogenous source of dopaminergic stimulation may lessen the progression of PD. Although this line of reasoning has rested upon more intuitive than experimental evidence, laboratory research has in fact supported a potential neuroprotective role for several dopaminergic agonists. For example, dopaminergic agonists such as apomorphine and pramipexole have been shown to exert free radical scavenging properties that might be beneficial if an oxidant stress mechanism is demonstrated to be involved in the progression of PD (Grunblatt et al., 2001; Le and Jankovic, 2001). Other evidence has also connected dopaminergic agonists currently in use for PD with experimental properties in support of neuroprotection. The ergoline compound pergolide, when administered chronically to Fischer 344 rats, leads to diminished age-related attrition of dopaminergic nigrostriatal neurons (Felten et al., 1992). Another dopaminergic compounds, pramipexole, has been studied in a number of models in which neuronal damage has been produced, including methamphetamine, 6-hydroxydopamine, 3-acetylpyridine, and MPTP (Hall et al., 1996; Vu et al., 2000; Sethi et al., 1997; Cassarino et al., 1998; Kitamura et al., 1998; Zou et al., 2000; Le et al., 2000; Carvey et al., 1997; Ling et al., 1999; Anderson et al., 2001). The protective actions noted with pramipexole, as suggested by studies of cultured dopaminergic mesencephalic neurons, may be related to inactivation of specific dopaminergic receptors (Ling et al., 2002) or by anti-apoptotic actions (Abramova et al., 2001, 2002). Protection against 6-hydroxydopamine-induced damage of dopaminergic nigrostriatal projections in mice has also been demonstrated with ropinirole, another dopaminergic agonist (Takata et al., 2000, 2001). These and other results from studies with dopaminergic compounds have supported the notion that various agonists in clinical use might also add to their value by neuroprotective actions.

Clinical trials have provided intriguing findings suggesting possible protective actions of dopaminergic therapy. Two clinical trials have been carried out in which radiotracer neuroimaging techniques have helped to gauge the progression of PD over time as a surrogate of degeneration in the dopaminergic nigrostriatal system. Imaging the presynaptic dopamine nerve terminal with a positron emission tomography [PET] ligand, [^{18}F]-dihydroxyphenylalanine (fluorodopa), has permitted the comparison of long-term outcomes from ropinirole to levodopa therapy in PD patients (Brooks et al., 2003; Marek et al., 2002). Survival of dopaminergic nerve terminals is a correlate of remaining neurons based in the SNpc. In the clinical trial termed REAL-PET (Whone et al., 2003), 86 mildly affected PD patients were randomized to monotherapy with either ropinirole or carbidopa/levodopa. The PET data indicated less loss of dopaminergic nerve terminals at two years from ropinirole treatment as compared to levodopa. Overall uptake of fluorodopa in the putamen showed a 13% loss in the ropinirole group, as compared to a 20% reduction in the group randomized to levodopa ($p = 0.034$). In addition, statistical parametric mapping detected slower progression of dopaminergic loss in the putamen and the substantia nigra (which showed a +3% change in the ropinirole treated PD patients as compared to a −8% loss in the levodopa treated group ($p = 0.035$).

Another randomized clinical trial comparing outcomes of pramipexole and levodopa has also concluded that the dopaminergic agonist conferred an apparent neuroprotective action, as judged by less change in a biomarker of striatal dopaminergic terminals (Parkinson Study Group, 2000a and b, 2002). This study used single proton emission computed tomography (SPECT) with the ligand imaging the dopamine transporter, [^{123}I]-2β-carboxymethoxy-3β(4-iodophenyl)tropane (β-CIT). The 82 PD patients in this study (a subset of the CALM-PD trial) were followed up to 46 months after baseline assessments with two β-CIT SPECT studies. The data in this investigation, which showed linear decline in imaging of the dopamine transporter for both treatment arms, showed significantly less loss of transporter sites in the pramipexole-treated group compared to patients randomized for levodopa. Changes from baseline scan showed $16.0 \pm 13.3\%$ decline versus $25.5 \pm 14.1\%$ decline in the pramipexole group compared to levodopa ($p < 0.01$). The similar direction of results with both pramipexole and ropinirole point to a "class" effect of dopaminergic agonists in conferring protection against the advance of PD. Since these clinical studies did not involve washout of the dopaminergic drugs to permit assessment of a drug-free state, the clinical relevance of the neuroimaging changes has not been determined.

Although levodopa has been thought of as nothing more than the amino acid precursor of dopamine, the possibility that chronic treatment might promote disease progression remains at the background of interpreting the dopaminergic agonist studies. There is little evidence in support of the latter assertion and some evidence supports the possibility that levodopa might confer an anti-oxidative neuroprotectant effect (Camp et al., 2000). A formal investigation of this matter was recently conducted to study disease progression and possible relation to levodopa dose. This was explored in a 40-week clinical trial of levodopa treatment in which baseline UPDRS status was compared to Parkinsonian state following a 2-week drug washout (Fahn et al., 2004). For the 361 mildly-affected PD subjects, randomized assignment to levodopa regimens of 150, 300, and 600 mg/day was compared to placebo treatment. This study (the ELLDOPA trial) was complemented with a SPECT study of β-CIT comparing baseline and post-washout status at 42 weeks in a subset of 142 subjects. The clinical results showed that all levodopa regimens yielded improvement even after washout, with the greatest effect at levodopa intake of 600 mg/day. In contrast, the placebo group showed some deterioration. While the UPDRS findings were compatible with a protective effect (and not indicative of increasing the rate of disease progression as compared to placebo), the outcome of striatal β-CIT uptake showed significantly more decline in the levodopa-treated groups. β-CIT measures the integrity of the dopamine transporter located in the nigrostriatal nerve terminals in the striatum and has been proposed to be a correlate of progressive loss in dopaminergic SNpc neurons. Since long-term PD treatment effects might confound the analysis of dopaminergic nigrostriatal projections, the validity of using β-CIT (and other radiotracer imaging in this and other studies) still remains questionable (Ravina et al., 2005).

Neuroprotection by enhancement of mitochondrial metabolism

The only identified systemic biochemical marker of PD is and alteration in the mitochondrial chain of electron transport (Shults et al., 1999). The finding of diminished complex I activity in PD brain prompted clinical investigation of coenzyme Q-10, which serves as an antioxidant as well as electron acceptor. Impaired mitochondrial function is a biologically plausible mechanism of slow neuronal damage as well as oxidative stress. On this basis, a clinical trial was carried out to test supplementation with coenzyme Q10 in order to enhance complex I activity. This placebo-controlled study involved doses of 300, 600, and 1200 mg per day for 16 months in 80 otherwise untreated PD subjects (Shults et al., 2002). Total adjusted mean UPDRS scores for the highest dose indicated an improvement of 6.69 points ($p = 0.0416$). Improvements were not seen for the lower doses. Most of the benefit on total UPDRS was attributable to less decline in the activities of daily living component of this scale, rather than change in motor features of Parkinsonism. This study has prompted a second clinical trial investigating the use of coenzyme Q-10 at 2400 mg per day. Although the latter study will be conducted as a "futility" trial (see below) (Elm et al., 2005), it should provide some indication whether the initial trial's positive findings represented a dose threshold affect. The beneficial outcome of the first trial, however small, is intriguing but does not necessarily point to enhancement of mitochondrial metabolism as the only explanation.

Enhancing impaired mitochondrial metabolism is the theme behind another clinical trial targeting the defect in mitochondrial complex I in PD. Creatine is a precursor for the formation of phosphocreatine, an energy intermediate that serves to transfer phosphoryl groups in the synthesis of mitochondrial ATP. The mechanism by which increase dietary intake of creatine might be beneficial through enhancing phosphocreatine production includes an overall reduction in mitochondrial oxidative stress (through stabilizing creatine kinase). Creatine kinase acts to inhibit opening of the mitochondrial transition pore, a step in the initiation of apoptosis, which, in turn, has been hypothesized to be a possible contributing factor to neurodegeneration in PD (Tarnopolsky and Beal, 2001). Laboratory studies have suggested the potential for dietary supplementation with creatine to spare MPTP-induced SNpc degeneration in mice (Matthews et al., 1999). To test the hypothesis that the progression of otherwise untreated PD might be slowed by daily supplementation with 10 grams of creatine, a clinical trial in a "futility" study format (see below) has been carried out. The results of the study, conducted by a North American research consortium under the direction of the National Institutes of Health (Ravina et al., 2003), are planned to be released shortly.

Neuroprotection from glutamate antagonism

For a number of neurodegenerative disorders, excitotoxicity via activation of glutamate receptors has been hypothesized (Wu et al., 2002). In PD, the possibility that activation of NMDA receptors might be a pathway for neurodegeneration has led to a search for compounds potentially blocking endogenous glutamate stimulation (Matthews et al., 1999). Many of the pharmacological agents achieving glutamatergic blockade confer their own neurotoxicity. However, riluzole has been well tolerated in its clinical application for slowing progression of amyotrophic lateral sclerosis. Riluzole was studied in conventional doses as a possible means for slowing the progression of otherwise untreated PD in a multicenter clinical trial. Because of lack of efficacy determined in an interim analysis, this trial was halted before its planned duration (Rascol et al., 2002).

Neuroprotection by inhibition of microglial activation

In the PD brain, activation of microglial is a prominent feature suggesting an inflammatory component to the pathogenesis of neurodegeneration in this disorder (Vila et al., 2001). Similar findings can be produced from experimental lesioning of dopaminergic SNpc neurons. Attempts to block microglial activation have been explored using the tetracycline compound minocycline. In rodent models of Parkinsonism induced by the neurotoxins MPTP and 6-hydroxydopamine, increased survival of dopaminergic SNpc neurons has been achieved by administration of minocycline (Du et al., 2001; Wu et al., 2002; He et al., 2001). The beneficial effects of minocycline may also be due to its properties of blocking caspases 1 and 3 as well as other factors that mediate apoptosis (Du et al., 2001). On the basis of these effects as well as its action against microglial activation, a clinical trial of minocycline at 200 mg per day has been carried out as a futility study (in the same 2×2 factorial study also investigating creatine, discussed above). The results of the study are planned for reporting shortly.

Neuroprotection by neurotrophin-like compounds

In the past 15 years there have been several studies investigating compounds with neurotrophin-like properties. One of these, GM1-ganglioside, has shown promise against MPTP-induced Parkinsonism in nonhuman primates (Schneider, 1992; Schneider et al., 1998) and has undergone limited human testing. Another clinical trial involved oral administration of AMG-474, a compound designated as a *neuroimmunophyllin* and an analogue of the immunosupressant FK-506 (which selectively enhances regeneration in damaged nerves). Although lacking the immunosuppressive actions of FK-506, AMG-474 attached to the same binding proteins and showed effectiveness at promoting recovery from animal models of neurotoxin-induced Parkinsonism. AMG-474 (also designated as NIL-A) penetrates the blood-brain barrier and was investigated in a 24-week clinical trial at 800 or 4000 mg per day. This placebo-controlled study enrolled 300 PD patients.

Although the results of this investigation were not been formally reported, it was discontinued after the sponsor (Amgen) reported that the study results were negative. AMG-474 returned to neuroprotection study in PD under the sponsorship of Guilford Pharmaceuticals and designated as GPI-1485. This compound is undergoing investigation as part of the NET-PD futility study (as one of the treatments in a multicenter, placebo-controlled 2×2 factorial study together with Coenzyme Q-10).

Another compound recently studied for its neuroprotective potential is CEP-1347 (a synthetic compound also designated as KT7515). This small molecule acts to inhibit mixed lineage kinase-3, which is a major component of the transcription factor c-Jun-mediated terminal kinase signaling pathway involved in apoptotic cell death (Harris et al., 2002; Saporito et al., 2002). With the hypothesis that SNpc neuronal loss in PD might be spared by use of CEP-1347, a randomized placebo-controlled clinical study has been carried out to determine feasibility for a larger scale investigation (Schwid et al., 2002). With the finding of good tolerability and safety at 100 mg per day, more extensive testing has been underway in a randomized clinical trial termed the PRECEPT study by the Parkinson Study Group.

Clinical trials have been carried out with TCH346 (also designated in laboratory research reports as CGP3466 and as CGP 3466B), a small molecule with structural similarities to selegiline but without MAO inhibitory properties. TCH346 was developed to target a key step in programmed cell death involving the glycolytic enzyme glyceraldehyde-3-phosphate dehydrogenase (GAPDH). Inhibition of GAPDH is also a property of rasagiline (see above) and other interventions by other neurotrophic-like compounds. Studies in cultured PC12 cells and in MPTP-treated monkeys have supported the neuroprotective potential for TCH346 (Ishitani et al., 1996; Kragten et al., 1998; Andringa et al., 2000). A large-scale randomized clinical trial in early PD was carried out and its results will be reported shortly.

Discussion

There has been an expanding range of therapeutic options for halting the progression of PD since the first neuroprotection study, the DATATOP trial, was conducted almost 2 decades ago. This study, which focused upon anti-oxidative treatment strategies, was instrumental in developing techniques and learning the pitfalls involved in clinical trials. Its influence continues to current investigations and has also generated concern as to whether clinical trials can provide proof of neuroprotection in PD (Clarke, 2004). To answer the simple question of whether a drug is neuroprotective or not requires dozens (if not hundreds) of PD patients and careful attention to placebo effects, the choice of clinical endpoints, and clinically meaningful outcomes. Clinical trials that investigated outcomes from inhibitors of MAO-B have not a final answer as to whether this is an appropriate target for neuroprotection. Since both selegiline and rasagiline treatments have anti-apoptotic effects and additional pharmacological actions, the question remains unanswered as to whether these properties beyond MAO-B inhibition provide the basis for the observed clinical results.

One recent development that has impacted upon accelerating the pace of neuroprotection investigation in PD is the incorporation of *futility trial* study designs. This methodology, utilized in the ongoing NET-PD studies (Ravina et al., 2003), serves as a screening tool for promising therapies. If a study does not demonstrate a futility outcome, then it would be appropriate to plan and conduct a study designed for clinical benefit. In contrast, futility trials are powered only to indicate whether a treatment would be futile to extend into a larger scale study and, as a result, involve fewer patients and often require shorter study duration (Elm et al., 2005). The guidance from a futility analysis can help to prioritize utilization of the limited resources of funding, time, and available PD patients, especially when there is a long list of possible protective therapies in need of testing.

Other issues needing resolution by further research include the possible intermingling of symptomatic and neuroprotective actions, the value and limitations of surrogate biomarkers, and ways to differentiate compensatory responses from genuine reversal of the disease process. In particular, there is a need for SPECT and PET radiotracer neuroimaging to be validated, if possible, as to how well these techniques correlate to progression of PD. The ultimate target of neuroprotection is, of course, the relief of disability and improvement in quality of life, whose ideal rating methodology has been elusive. Fortunately, with the tremendous productivity of recent research, the PD patient is entitled to take an optimistic stance towards a future in which curing the disease may become a reality.

References

Abramova NA, Cassarino DS, Khan SM, Painter TW, Bennett JP Jr (2002) Inhibition by R(+) or S(−) pramipexole of caspase activation and cell death induced by methylpyridinium ion or beta amyloid peptide in SH-SY5Y neuroblastoma. J Neurosci Res 67: 494–500

Akao Y, Youdim MB, Davis BA, Naoi M, Rabey JM (2001) Rasagiline mesylate, a new MAO-B inhibitor for the treatment of Parkinson's disease: a double-blind study as adjunctive therapy to levodopa. J Neurochem 78: 727–735

Anderson DW, Neavin T, Smith JA, Schneider JS (2001) Neuroprotective effects of pramipexole in young and aged MPTP-treated mice. Brain Res 905: 44–53

Andringa G, Cools AR (2000) The neuroprotective effects of CGP 3466B in the best *in vivo* model of Parkinson's disease, the bilaterally MPTP-treated rhesus monkey. J Neural Transm [Suppl 60]: 215–225

Bara-Jimenez W, Sherzai A, Dimitrova T, Favit A, Bibbiani F, Gillespie M, Morris MJ, Mouradian MM, Chase TN (2003) Adenosine A_{2A} receptor antagonist treatment of Parkinson's disease. Neurology 61: 293–296

Besirli CG, Johnson EM Jr (2003) JNK-independent activation of c-Jun during neuronal apoptosis induced by multiple DNA-damaging agents. J Biol Chem 278: 22357–22366

Bilsland JG, Harper SJ (2003) CEP-1347 promotes survival of NGF responsive neurones in primary DRG explants. Neuroreport 14: 995–999

Bjorklund A, Lindvall O (2000) Cell replacement therapies for central nervous system disorders. Nat Neurosci 6: 537–544

Brooks DJ, Frey KA, Marek KL (2003) Assessment of neuroimaging techniques as biomarkers of the progression of Parkinson's disease. Exp Neurol 184 [Suppl 1]: S68–S79

Camp DM, Loeffler DA, LeWitt PA (2000) Levodopa does not enhance hydroxyl radical formation in the nigrostriatal dopamine system of rats with a unilateral 6-hydroxydopamine lesion. J Neurochem 74: 1229–1240

Carlile GW, Chalmers-Redman RME, Tatton NA, et al. (2000) Reduced apoptosis after nerve growth factor and serum withdrawal: conversion of tetrameric gluteraldehyde-3-phosphate dehydrogenase to a dimer. Mol Pharmacol 57: 2–12

Carvey P, Pieri S, Ling Z (1997) Attenuation of levodopa-induced toxicity in mesencephalic cultures by pramipexole. J Neural Transm 104: 209–228

Cassarino DS, Fall CP, Smith TS, Bennett JP Jr (1998) Pramipexole reduces reactive oxygen species production in vivo and in vitro and inhibits the mitochondrial permeability transition produced by the Parkinsonian neurotoxin methylpyridinium ion. J Neurochem 71: 295–301

Chase TN, Oh JD (2000) Striatal mechanisms and pathogenesis of parkinsonian signs and motor complications. Ann Neurol 47 [Suppl 4]: S122–S129

Chen JF, Xu K, Petzer JP, Staal R, Xu YH, Beilstein M, Sonsalla PK, Castagnoli K, Castagnoli N Jr, Schwarzschild MA (2001) Neuroprotection by caffeine and A_{2A} adenosine receptor inactivation in a model of Parkinson's disease. J Neurosci 21: RC143

Clarke CE (2004) A "cure" for Parkinson's disease: can neuroprotection be proven with current trial designs? Mov Disord 19: 491–498

Djaldetti R, Ziv I, Melamed E (2002) The effect of deprenyl washout in patients with longstanding Parkinson's disease. J Neural Transm 109: 797–803

Elm JJ, Goetz CG, Ravina B, et al. (2005) A responsive outcome for Parkinson's disease neuroprotection futility studies. Ann Neurol 57: 197–203

Fahn S, Oakes D, Shoulson I, et al. (2004) Levodopa and the progression of Parkinson's disease. N Engl J Med 351: 2498–2508

Fearnley J, Lees AJ (1991) Aging and Parkinson's disease: substantia nigra regional selectivity. Brain 114: 2283–2301

Felten DL, Felten SY, Fuller RW, et al. (1992) Chronic dietary pergolide preserves nigrostriatal neuronal integrity in aged Fischer 344 rats. Neurobiol Aging 13: 339–351

Ferger B, Teismann P, Mierau J (2000) The dopamine agonist pramipexole scavenges hydroxyl free radicals induced by striatal application of 6-hydroxydopamine in rats: an in vivo microdialysis study. Brain Res 883: 216–223

Giladi N, McDermott MP, Fahn S, et al. (2001) Freezing of gait in PD: prospective assessment in the DATATOP cohort. Neurology 56: 1712–1721

Gill SS, Patel NK, Hotton GR, O'Sullivan K, McCarter R, Bunnage M, Brooks DJ, Svendsen CN, Heywood P (2003) Direct brain infusion of glial derived neurotrophic factor (GDNF) in Parkinson's disease. Nature Med 9: 589–595

Goetz CG, Leurgans S, Raman R, Parkinson Study Group (2002) Placebo-associated improvements in motor function: comparison of subjective and objective sections of the UPDRS in early Parkinson's disease. Mov Disord 17: 283–288

Grunblatt E, Mandel S, Maor G, Youdim MB (2001) Effects of R- and S-apomorphine on MPTP-induced nigro-striatal dopamine neuronal loss. J Neurochem 77: 146–156

Hall ED, Andrus PK, Oostveen JA, et al. (1996) Neuroprotective effects of ramipexole against post-ischemic or methamphetamine-induced degeneration of nigrostriatal neurons. Mov Disord 11 [Suppl 1]: 191

Harris CA, Deshmukh M, Tsui-Pierchala B, et al. (2002) Inhibition of the c-Jun N-terminal kinase signaling pathway by the mixed lineage kinase inhibitor CEP-1347 (KT7515) preserves metabolism and growth of trophic factor-deprived neurons. J Neurosci 22: 103–113

He Y, Appel S, Le W (2001) Minocycline inhibits microglial activation and protects nigral cells after 6-hydroxydopamine injection in mouse striatum. Brain Res 909: 187–193

Heikkila RE, Terleckyj I, Sieber BA (1990) Monoamine oxidase and the bioactivation of MPTP and related neurotoxins: relevance to DATATOP. J Neural Transm [Suppl 32]: 217–227

Hettinger BD, Lee A, Linden J, Rosin DL (2001) Ultatrstructural localization of adenosine A_{2A} receptors suggests multiple cellular sites for modulation of GABAergic neurons in rat striatum. J Comp Neurol 431: 331–346

Hilker R, Schweitzer K, Coburger S, et al. (2005) Nonlinear progression of Parkinson disease as determined by serial positron emission tomographic imaging of striatal fluorodopa ^{18}F-activity. Arch Neurol 62: 378–382

Hirsch EC, Breidert T, Rousselet E, et al. (2003) The role of glial reaction and inflammation in Parkinson's disease. Ann N Y Acad Sci 991: 214–228

Hocherman S, Levin G, Giladi N, Youdim MB (1998) Deprenyl monotherapy improves visuo-motor control in early parkinsonism. J Neural Transm [Suppl 52]: 63–69

Ikeda K, Kurokawa M, Aoyama S, Kuwana Y (2002) Neuroprotection by adenosine A2A receptor blockade in experimental models of Parkinson's disease. J Neurochem 80: 262–270

Ishitani R, Kimura M, Sunaga K, Katsube N, Tanaka M, Chuang DM (1996a) An antisense oligonucleotide to glyceraldehyde-3-phosphate-dehydrogenase blocks age-induced apoptosis of mature cerebrocortical neurons in culture. J Pharmacol Exptl Therap 278: 447–454

Ishitani R, Sunaga K, Hirano A, Saunders P, Katsube N, Chuang DM (1996b) Evidence that glyceraldehyde-3-phosphatedehydrogenase is involved in age-induced apoptosis in mature cerebellar neurons in culture. J Neurochem 66: 928–935

Jellinger KA (2000) Cell death mechanism in Parkinson's disease. J Neural Transm 107: 1–27

Jenner P (2003) Oxidative stress in Parkinson's disease. Ann Neurol 53 [Suppl 3]: S26–S38

Kitamura Y, Kosaka T, Kakimura JI, Matsuoka Y, Kohno Y, Nomura Y, Taniguchi T (1998) Protective effects of the antiparkinsonian drugs talipexole and pramipexole against 1-methyl-4-phenylpyridinium-induced apoptotic death in human neuroblastoma SH-SY5Y cells. Mol Pharmacol 54: 1046–1054

Kragten E, Lalande I, Zimmerman K, et al. (1998) Glyceraldehyde-3-phosphate dehydrogenase, the putative target of the antiapoptotic compounds CGP 3466 and R-(−)-deprenyl. J Biol Chem 273: 5821–5828

Larsen JP, Boas J, Erdal JE (1999) Does selegiline modify the progression of early Parkinson's disease? Results from a five-year study. The Norwegian-Danish Study Group. Eur J Neurol 6: 539–547

Le WD, Jankovic J, Xie W, Appel SH (2000) Antioxidant property of pramipexole independent of dopamine receptor activation in neuroprotection. J Neural Transm 107: 1165–1173
Le W-D, Jankovic J (2001) Are dopamine receptor agonists neuroprotective in Parkinson's disease? Drugs and Aging 18: 389–396
LeWitt PA, Galloway M, Matson W, Milbury P, McDermott M, Srivastava DK, Oakes D, Parkinson Study Group (1992) Markers of dopamine metabolism in Parkinson's disease. Neurology 42: 2111–2117
LeWitt PA (2004) Clinical trials of neuroprotection for Parkinson's disease. Neurology 63 [7 Suppl 2]: S23–S31
LeWitt PA, Segel SA, Mistura KL, Schork MA (1993) Symptomatic anti-Parkinsonian effects of monoamine oxidase-B inhibition: comparison of selegiline and lazabemide. Clin Neuropharmacol 16: 332–337
LeWitt PA, Oakes D, Cui L, Parkinson Study Group (1997) The need for levodopa as an endpoint of Parkinson's disease progression in a clinical trial of selegiline and alphatocopherol. Mov Disord 12: 183–189
Ling ZD, Robie HC, Tong CW, Carvey PM (1999) Both the antioxidant and D3 agonist actions of pramipexole mediate its neuroprotective actions in mesencephalic cultures. J Pharmacol Exp Ther 289: 202–210
Lipton SA, Rosenberg PA (1994) Excitatory amino acids as a final common pathway for neurologic disorders. N Engl J Med 330: 613–622
Maki-Ikola O, Heinonen E (1986) Study design problems of DATATOP study analysis. Ann Neurol 40: 946–948
Mandel S, Grunblatt E, Riederer P, Gerlach M, Levites Y, Youdim MB (2003) Neuroprotective strategies in Parkinson's disease: an update on progress. CNS Drugs 17: 729–762
Marek K, Jennings D, Seibyl J (2002) Do dopamine agonists or levodopa modify Parkinson's disease progression? Eur J Neurol 9 [Suppl 3]: 15–22
Maroney AC, Glicksman MC, Basma AN, et al. (1998) Motoneuron apoptosis is blocked by CEP-1347 (KT 7515), a novel inhibitor of the JNK signaling pathway. J Neurosci 18: 104–111
Maroney AC, Finn JP, Bozyczko-Coyne D, et al. (1999) CEP-1347 (KT 7515), an inhibitor of JNK activation, rescues sympathetic neurons and neuronally differentiated PC12 cells from death evoked by three distinct insults. J Neurochem 73: 1–12
Maruyama W, Akao Y, Youdim MB, et al. (2001) Transfection-enforced Bcl-2 overexpression and an anti-Parkinson drug, rasagiline, prevent nuclear accumulation of glyceraldehyde-3-phosphate dehydrogenase induced by an endogenous dopaminergic neurotoxin, N-methyl(R)-salsolinol. J Neurochem 78: 727–735
Maruyama W, Akao Y, Carrillo MC, et al. (2002) Neuroprotection by propylargylamines in Parkinson's disease. Suppression of apoptosis and induction of prosurvival genes. Neurotoxicol Teratol 24: 675–682
Miklossy J, Doudet DD, Schwab C, et al. (2006) Role of ICAM-1 in persisting inflammation in Parkinson disease and MPTP monkeys. Exp Neurol 197: 275–283
Muriel MP, Orieux G, Hirsch EC (2002) Levodopa but not ropinirole induces an internalization of Dl dopamine receptors in parkinsonian rats. Mov Disord 17: 1174–1179
Myllylä VV, Sotaniemi KA, Vuorinen JA, Heinonen EH (1991) Selegiline as a primary treatment of Parkinson's disease. Acta Neurol Stand [Suppl 136]: 70–72
NINDS NET-PD Investigators (2006) A randomized, double-blind, futility clinical trial of creatine and minocycline in early Parkinson disease. Neurology 66: 664–671
Nutt JG, Burchiel KJ, Comella CL, et al. (2003) Randomized double-blind trial of glial cell line-derived neurotrophic factor (GDNF) in PD. Neurology 60: 69–73
Palhagen S, Heinonen EH, Hagglund J, et al. (1998) Selegiline delays the onset of disability in *de novo* parkinsonian patients. Swedish Parkinson Study Group. Neurology 51: 520–525
Parkinson J (1817) An essay on the shaking palsy. Sherwood, Neely, and Jones, London
Parkinson Study Group (1989a) DATATOP: a multicenter controlled clinical trial in early Parkinson's disease. Arch Neurol 46: 1052–1060
Parkinson Study Group (1989b) Effect of deprenyl on the progression of disability in early Parkinson's disease. N Engl J Med 321: 1364–1371
Parkinson Study Group (1993) Effects of tocopherol and deprenyl on the progression of disability in early Parkinson's disease. N Engl J Med 328: 176–183
Parkinson Study Group (1994) A controlled trial of lazabemide (Ro 19-6327) in levodopa-treated Parkinson's disease. Arch Neurol 51: 342–347
Parkinson Study Group (1995) CSF homovanillic acid in the DATATOP study on Parkinson's disease. Arch Neurol 52: 237–245
Parkinson Study Group (1996) Effect of lazabemide on the progression of disability in early Parkinson's disease. Ann Neurol 40: 99–107
Parkinson Study Group (2000a) Design of a clinical trial comparing pramipexole to levodopa in early PD (CALM-PD). Clin Neuropharmacol 23: 34–44
Parkinson Study Group (2000b) Pramipexole vs. levodopa as initial treatment for Parkinson disease. JAMA 284: 1931–1938
Parkinson Study Group (2002) Dopamine transporter brain imaging to assess the effects of pramipexole vs. levodopa on Parkinson disease progression. JAMA 287: 1653–1661
Pope-Coleman A, Schneider JS (1998) Effects of chronic GM1 ganglioside treatment on cognitieve and motor deficits in a slowly progressing model of Parkinsonism in non-human primates. Restor Neurol Neurosci 12: 255–266
Przedborski S (2005) Pathogenesis of nigral cell death in Parkinson's disease. Parkinsonism Relat Disord 11 [Suppl 1]: S3–S7
Rascal O, Brooks D, Korczyn A, et al. (2000) A five-year study of the incidence of dyskinesia in patients with early Parkinson's disease who were treated with ropinirole or levodopa. N Engl J Med 342: 1484–1491
Rascal O, Olanow CW, Brooks D, et al. (2002) A 2-year multicenter placebo-controlled, double-blind parallel group study of the effect of riluzole in Parkinson's disease. Mov Disord 17: 39
Ravina BM, Fagan SC, Hart RG, et al. (2003) Neuroprotective agents for clinical trials in Parkinson's disease: A systematic assessment. Neurology 60: 1234–1240
Ravina B, Eidelberg D, Ahlskog JE, et al. (2005) The role of radiotracer imaging in Parkinson disease. Neurology 64: 208–215
Saporito MS, Brown EM, Miller MS, Carswell S (1999) CEP-1347/KT-7515, an inhibitor of c-Jun N-terminal kinase activation, attenuates the l-methyl-4-phenyl tetrahydropyridine-mediated loss of nigrostriatal dopaminergic neurons in vivo. J Pharmacol Exp Ther 288: 421–427
Saporito MS, Thomas BA, Scott RW (2000) MPTP activates c-Jun NH(2)-terminal kinase (JNK) and its upstream regulatory kinase MKK4 in nigrostriatal neurons in vivo. J Neurochem 75: 1200–1208
Saporito MS, Hudkins RL, Maroney AC (2002) Discovery of CEP-1347/KT-7515, an inhibitor of the JNK/SAPK pathway for the treatment of neurodegenerative diseases. Prog Med Chem 40: 23–62
Schneider JS (1992) Effects of age on GM1 ganglioside-induced recovery of concentrations of dopamine in the striatum in 1-methyl-4-phenyl-1,2,3,6-tetrahydropyridine-treated mice. Neuropharmacology 31: 185–202
Schwid SR, Parkinson Study Group (2002) CEP-1347 in Parkinson's disease: a pilot study. Presented at the 7th International Congress of Parkinson's disease and Movement Disorders (Miami, Florida), November 10–14, 2002
Sethy VH, Wu H, Oostveen JA (1997) Neuroprotective effects of the dopamine agonists. pramipexole and bromocriptine in 3-acetylpyridine-terted rats. Brain Res 754: 181–186
Shults CW, Oakes D, Kieburtz K, et al. (2002) Effects of coenzyme Q10 in early Parkinson's disease: evidence for slowing of the functional decline. Arch Neural 59: 1541–1550
Spencer JP, Jenner A, Butler J, et al. (1996) Evaluation of the pro-oxidant and antioxidant actions of L-DOPA and dopamine in vitro: implications for Parkinson's disease. Free Radic Res 24: 95–105

Studer L, Tabar V, McKay RDG (1998) Transplantation of expanded mesencephalic precursor lead to recovery in parkinsonian rats. Nature Neurosci 1: 290–295

Takata K, Kitamura Y, Kakimura J, et al. (2000) Increase of bcl-2 protein in neuronal dendritic processes of cerebral cortex and hippocampus by the antiparkinsonian drugs, talipexole and pramipexole. Brain Res 872: 236–241

Tanaka K, Miyazaki I, Fujita N, et al. (2001) Molecular mechanism in activation of glutathione system by ropinirole, a selective dopamine D2 agonist. Neurochem Res 26: 31–36

Tatton W, Chalmers-Redman R, Tatton N (2003) Neuroprotection by deprenyl and other propargylamines: glyceraldehyde-3-phosphate dehydrogenase rather than monoamine oxidase B. J Neural Transm 110: 509–515

Tetrud JW, Langston JW (1989) The effect of deprenyl (selegiline) on the natural history of Parkinson's disease. Science 245: 519–522

Thomas M, Le WD (2004) Minocycline: neuroprotective mechanisms in Parkinson's disease. Curr Pharm Des 10: 679–686

Tilley BC, Palesch YY, Kieburtz K, et al. (2006) Optimizing the ongoing search for new treatments for Parkinson disease: using futility designs. Neurololgy 66: 628–633

Vila M, Jackson-Lewis V, Guegan C, et al. (2001) The role of glial cells in Parkinson's disease. Curr Opin Neurol 14: 483–489

Vu TQ, Ling ZD, Ma SY, et al. (2000) Pramipexole attenuates the dopaminergic cell loss induced by intraventricular 6-hydroxydopamine. J Neural Transm 107: 159–176

Ward CD (1994) Does selegiline delay progression of Parkinson's disease? A critical re-evaluation of the DATATOP study. J Neurol Neurosurg Psychiatry 57: 217–220

Whone AL, Watts RL, Stoessl AJ, et al. (2003) Slower progression of Parkinson's disease with ropinirole versus levodopa: The REAL-PET study. Ann Neurol 54: 93–101

Wu DC, Jackson-Lewis V, Vila M, et al. (2002) Blockade of microglial activation is neuroprotective in the 1-methyl-4-phenyl-1,2,3,6-tetrahydropyridine mouse model of Parkinson disease. J Neurosci 22: 1763–1771

Youdim MB, Amit T, Bar-Am O, et al. (2003) Amyloid processing and signal transduction properties of antiparkinson-antialzheimer neuroprotective drugs rasagiline and TV3326. Ann NY Acad Sci 993: 378–386

Zemke D, Majid A (2004) The potential of minocycline for neuroprotection in human neurologic disease. Clin Neuropharmacol 27: 293–298

Zou L, Xu J, Jankovic J, He Y, et al. (2000) Pramipexole inhibits lipid peroxidation and reduces injury in the substantia nigra induced by the dopaminergic neurotoxin 1-methyl-4-phenyl-1,2,3,6-tetrahydropyridine in C57BL/G mice. Neurosci Lett 281: 167–170

J Neural Transm (2006) [Suppl] 71: 123–132

Journal of Neural Transmission
Printed in Austria

Marker for a preclinical diagnosis of Parkinson's disease as a basis for neuroprotection

Daniela Berg

Hertie Institute of Clinical Brain Research, University of Tübingen, Tübingen, Germany

Summary Neuroprotective therapy is a pivotal aim in the treatment of the relentlessly progressive disorder Parkinson's disease. However, more than 60% of the dopaminergic neurons of the substantia nigra have already degenerated, when the diagnosis may be established. At this "advanced stage" neuroprotective strategies will – if at all – only have limited effect. It is, therefore, essential to establish markers to identify subjects at risk before motor manifestation. A number of such "premotor" signs have been discovered and investigated lately. Such signs include a genetic vulnerability and hyperechogenicity of the substantia nigra as well as premotor symptoms like olfactory and autonomic dysfunction, depression, REM sleep behaviour disorder, visual and neuropsychological impairment. Moreover, first signs of affection of the substantia nigra like PET and SPECT abnormalities and slight motor signs can be included, as they may be detected before a definite diagnosis can be made.

Although most of these signs and symptoms are unspecific if singularly evaluated a combination of these features may indeed be valuable to detect a subgroup of the population at risk for PD. However, future studies are necessary to establish the predictive value of these "markers" singularly and in combination.

Introduction

Parkinson's disease is the second most common movement disorder. Growing incidence with increasing age leads to an increment of prevalence in the aging population of many countries. There is still no cure for the relentlessy progressive disorder. Nor has any therapeutic strategy applied in affected individuals so far shown any relevant neuroprotection or postponing of cell death, although a number of therapeutic agents proved to be highly effective in *in vitro* and animal experiments (Ben-Shachar et al., 1991; Blum-Degen et al., 1998; Beal, 2001; Gal et al., 2005; Zheng et al., 2005). One reason for the lack of neuroprotective effect may be the fact that in PD patients the neurodegenerative process has proceeded substantially when first motor symptoms allow the clinical diagnosis of PD. At this time point a 60–70% degeneration of SN dopaminergic neurons and a reduction of dopamine content of about 80% has been documented (Bernheimer et al., 1973; Riederer and Wuketich, 1976), indicating that neurodegeneration has advanced too far for effective neuroprotection. For the application of potentially neuroprotective therapies identification of subjects at an earlier stage of neurodegeneration is therefore essential. At this time point, no motor symptoms are at hand to allow the diagnosis. Therefore other, preclinical markers need to be established.

For the establishment of a preclinical marker either a risk group or at least the duration of the preclinical period would be helpful to be known. Thanks to genetic research of the past decade a number of monogentic forms of PD have been identified. In these and other forms of documented familial PD subjects at risk may be considered. However, for the general population there is no obvious genetic predisposition. Therefore, knowledge of the preclinical period would be helpful. Estimations concerning the duartion of this period are derived from post mortem as well as functional neuroimaging studies. Unfortunately, these estimations vary by large, suggesting a preclinical period between 3 to 7 (Fearnley and Lees, 1991; Morrish et al., 1996; Nurmi et al., 2001) and 40 to 50 years (Gibb and Lees, 1988; Scherman et al., 1989; Vingerhoets et al., 1994; Schwarz et al., 1997; Hardie, 1999). All of these estimations are based on the assumption of a linear progressive neuronal cell loss. However, one could also assume a nonlinear progression of cell loss as assumed by Hilker et al. (2005). Moreover, if besides linear or nonlinear neuronal cell loss a genetic predisposition to a reduced number of dopaminergic neurons is also taken into consideration, it seems impossible to define a preclinical period for an individual

Correspondence: D. Berg, M.D., Hertie Institute of Clincial Brain Research, Hoppe-Seyler-Strasse 3, 72076 Tübingen, Germany
e-mail: daniela.berg@uni-tuebingen.de

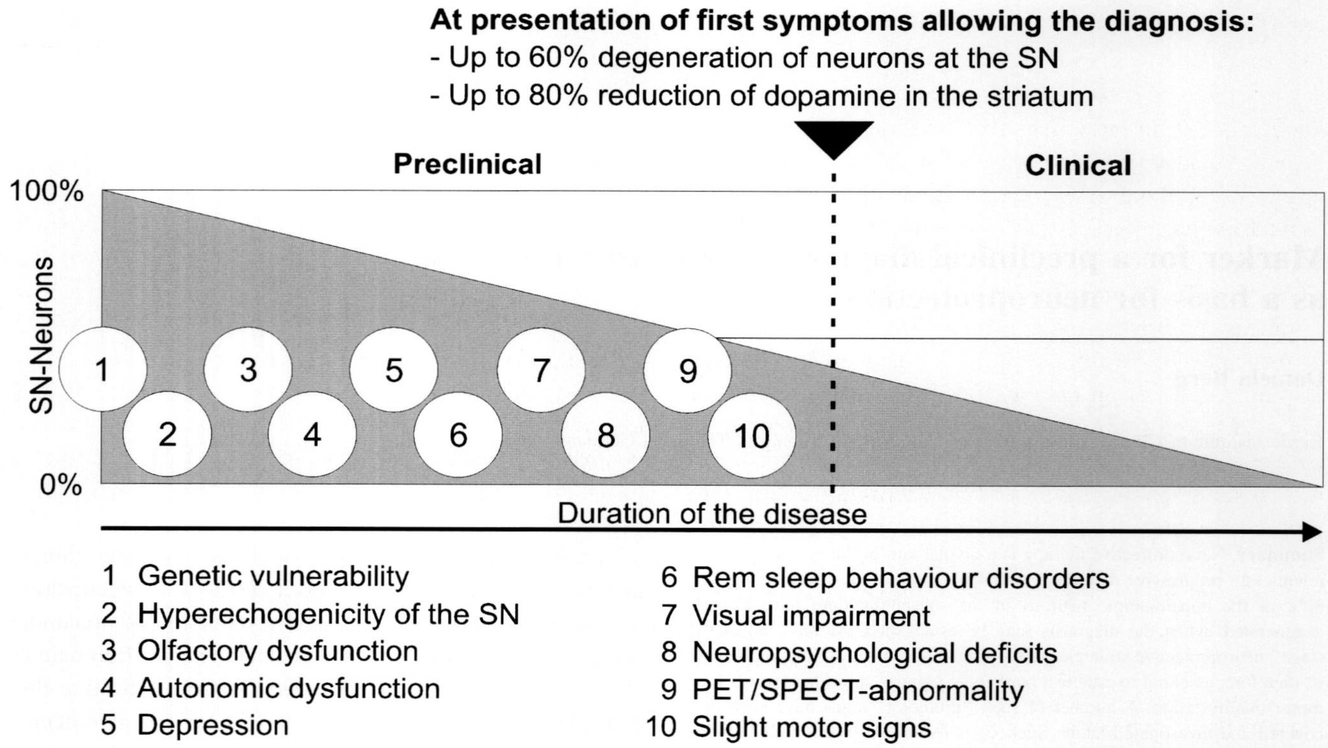

Fig. 1. Course of neurodegeneration and possible preclinical signs and symptoms. Typical motor symptoms indicating Parkinson's disease (PD) occur, when about 60% of the initially 100% of dopaminergic neurons of the substantia nigra (SN) have degenerated. In the preclinical period, however, a number of signs may become evident that may serve as markers for persons at risk for nigrostriatal vulnerability. From birth on a genetic predisposition may be such a vulnerability marker. Also very early in life, hyperechogenicity of the SN may be detected, which may also constitute a marker for predisposition. Other symptoms like olfactory and autonomic dysfunction, depression, Rem sleep behaviour disorder as well as visual and neuropsychological deficits are already signs of the beginning neurodegenerative process which has not reached the SN yet. The order in which these symptoms occur may vary and not all individuals who will finally develop PD will recognize all of these sympotms beforehand. Slight motor signs and PET and SPECT abnormalities indicate an affection of the SN, which has not proceeded to a stage, which allows the diagnosis of PD. A combination of several of these markers may be helpful to identify persons at risk for the development of PD

person. Therefore, risk markers should be applicable independent of age.

In recent years a number of markers have been identified, that have been shown to be associated with an impairment of the nigrostriatal system and may precede the development of PD by decades (Fig. 1). Current knowledge about the value of the most widely discussed markers for a predisposition to nigrostriatal impairment is summarized in this paper.

1. Family history and genetic markers

Parkinson's disease has long been regarded as a sporadic disease, triggered and finally brought to manifestation by different endo- or exotoxins. However, over the last few years several genes for monogenetically inherited forms of PD have been mapped and cloned. To date, 10 gene loci have been found to be causative for monogenetical PD and 6 genes have been identified, which in the case of point mutations, deletions, insertions or multiplications lead to the clinical picture of familial PD.

The gene most commonly responsible for the recessively inherited form of PD is the PARKIN gene. Almost 50% of affected sibling show mutations in this gene (Lücking et al., 2000). In seemingly sporadic PD with onset between 20 and 30 years of age, prevalence is about 25%, while in older patients a prevalence under 5% can be expected (Lücking et al., 2000). All other recessively inherited forms of PD are far more seldom. The question whether heterozygous mutations conribute to the development of PD is still under investigation.

In autosomal dominantly inherited forms of PD only mutations in the LRRK2 gene account for a representative number of affected families. In our own cohort of 99 apparently autosomal dominant families, we identified variations in the LRRK2 gene in 13% (Berg et al., 2005).

Although more genes are expected to be identified in families with PD inherited in a Mendelian trait, only the minority of PD cases will be found to be caused monogenetically. The vast majority of PD cases seems to be sporadic.

Still, there also seems to be a genetic contribution to idiopathic PD. In more than 10% of patients with PD one or more relatives are also affected by this disorder (Elbaz et al., 1999; Kang et al., 2005). Epidemiological studies provide evidence for a three to four times higher prevalence of clinical PD in first degree relatives of PD patients (Payami et al., 1994; Marder et al., 1996; Uitti et al., 1997). A genetic contribution to idiopathic PD is strongly supported by neuroimaging studies using 18-F-Dopa PET, SPECT or transcranial sonography in both first degree relatives or twins of patients with idiopathic PD (see also below). To date, it is believed that idiopathic PD is a genetically complex disorder involving several susceptibility genes with presumably only a slight risk. However, interaction of several of these with other genetic factors or with endo- or exotoxins may be responsible for the development of PD (Gasser, 2005). Large series of total genome screens as well as the investigation of candidate genes have been performed to identify some of these genes. However, inspite of many initially positive results findings could not be confirmed beyond any doubt in any of the genes investigated (Gasser, 2005; Riess et al., 2005). This might be due to the fact, that the clinical presentation of PD comprises a large variety of factors contributing to its etiology to differing extent.

Still, knowledge about the genetic contribution to both familiar and sporadic PD implies that family history should be regarded as one, in the case of sporadic PD only small, risk marker for PD.

2. Non-motor symptoms

a. Olfactory dyfunction

Olfactory dysfunction was first documented in PD in 1975 (Ansari and Johnson, 1975). Since then, a number of studies have been performed confirming that olfactory dysfunction is present in 80–100% of PD patients (Ward et al., 1983; Quinn et al., 1987; Hawkes et al., 1997; Müller et al., 2002). The olfactory impairment in PD comprises a significantly increased olfactory threshold as well as deficits in odour identification and discrimination (Tissingh et al., 2001; Zucco et al., 1991). Already in the very early disease stages olfactory deficits have been described (Doty et al., 1988, 1992; Tissingh et al., 2001) leading to the investigation of relatives of at risk individuals with familial autosomal dominant parkinsonism. The finding that 41% of these at risk individuals presented with olfactory deficits implies that olfactory dysfunction may precede the onset of motor symptoms (Markopoulou et al., 1997). Also, first degree relatives of patients with sporadic PD were found to have olfactory deficits (Montgomery et al., 1999). The hypothesis, that smelling deficits in these subjects may indicate subclinical nigrostriatal dysfunction has been confirmed by functional neuroimaging data (see below) and is underlined by the neuropathological staging of Braak and coworkers (2003). Braak proposes 6 neuropathological stages of PD. In stage 1 and 2 there is no affection of the substantia nigra (SN). Therefore, no motor signs can be expected. However, stage 1 affects the anterior olfactory nucleus and/or the olfactory bulb, while in stage 2 additional involvement of the lower brain stem confined to the medulla oblongata and pontine tegmentum can be found. Therefore, the clinical symptom of olfactory deficits may well be a premotor sign for Parkinson's disease in individuals at risk.

However, one must be careful, since numerous health conditions including rhinitis, Alzheimers's disease and others as well as certain lifestyles, e.g. smoking, may lead to olfactory dysfunction.

b. REM sleep behaviour disorder

REM sleep behaviour disorder (RBD) is common in PD. It has been described in 15% (Comella et al., 1998) to 33% (Gagnon et al., 2002) of PD patients. Subclinical RBD is found as frequently as 58% (Gagnon et al., 2002). In a longitudinal study Schenk et al. could show, that 38% of older patients with the initial diagnosis of idiopathic RBD developed a Parksinonian syndrome on average 12.7 years after onset of RBD (Schenck et al., 1996). Further follow up 7 years later, disclosed that 65.4% developed Parkinsonism (Schenck et al., 2003). In accordance with this follow up studies, a decreased dopamine transporter binding was found in patients diagnosed as idiopathic RBD (Eisensehr et al., 2000, 2003). The neuropathological hallmarks of PD affect in stage 2 according to Braak et al., the pontine and medullary area (Braak et al., 2003). These areas are mainly responsible for sleep control and eye movements (Hendricks et al., 1982; Schenkel and Siegel, 1989; Sanford et al., 1994). The fact that exactly in these areas Lewy bodies have been found in patients diagnosed as idiopathic PD (Uchiyama et al., 1995; Turner et al., 2000) underlines the hypothesis, that RBD may be a premotor sign of PD in a subgroup of patients.

c. Depression

The prevalence of depression in PD is estimated to be 40% (range 4–70% in different studies) (Cummings et al., 1992; Becker et al., 2001). Already in the early stages of the disease, abnormal results have been found in the Beck Depression Inventory in 40% of PD patients (Montgomery et al., 2000a, b). Moreover, about 20% of patients with PD report mood disturbances years before onset of the disease (Mindham, 1970; Robins et al., 1976; Santamaria et al., 1986). Of course it has to be considered that some symptoms overlap between early PD and depression (Hoogendijk et al., 1998). Also, it may be argued that depressive symptoms are reactive to the beginning motor symptoms. However, it has been shown that depressive symptoms do not correlate with the severity of motor features and are far more frequent in PD than in disorders with similar motor disability (Mayeux et al., 1981; Santamaria et al., 1986).

Moreover, brainstem alterations including lesions in the ventral tegmental area, the raphe nuclei (especially the serotonergic raphe nuclei), and the locus ceruleus have been shown to be associated with depression (Chan-Palay and Asan, 1989; D'Amato et al., 1987; Torack and Morris, 1986; Berg et al., 1999b; Becker et al., 1997, 2001) – and correspond to areas with neurodegeneration claimed to represent stage 2 of PD. Therefore, depression may also be considered as a possible premotor sign in persons at risk for PD.

d. Neuropsychological impairment

Neuropsychological impairment is frequent in early non-demented PD patients. As neuropsychological dysfunction in PD mainly comprises tasks requiring the internal regulation of behavioural repsonses (Lees and Smith, 1983; Brown and Marsden, 1988, 1990; Cooper et al., 1991; Owen et al., 1993; Dubois and Pillon, 1997) these deficits may not become obvious in daily life, in which external signals and information may guide behaviour. However, neuropsychological testing excluding any external cues or guidelines may disclose impairment in working memory or establishment of internally generated strategies to solve a problem. There is no correlation of kind or extent of neuropsychological impairment and motor disability in early PD (Cooper et al., 1991), indicating that cognitive dysfunction is largely independent of frontostriatal dopamine deficiency underlying motor disability. In a slowly progressing model of Parkinsonism in monkeys it has been shown, that cognitive deficits may even precede motor disability (Schneider and Pope-Coleman, 1995). Also, unaffected co-twins of patients with PD showed modification in cognitive performance (Holthoff et al., 1994). Based on these findings Dujardin et al. (1999) investigated first degree relatives of patients with well documented familial PD. Of 41 first degree relatives, 15 showed deviations of executive functions. Among them, 9 presented with a global executive impairment, while the six others showed only signs of limited executive dysfunction. Although the relevance of these findings in the affected subjects still needs to be determined, the similarity in kind of cognitive dysfunction in comparison to the cognitive impairment found in early PD is striking. Therefore, further investigations are needed to evaluate whether impaired executive functions may serve as a possible premotor sign in persons at risk for PD.

e. Autonomic symptoms

Although frequency and severity of autonomic dysfunction is more pronounced in atypical Parkinsonian syndromes like multiple system atrophy, a variety of autonomic symptoms also occur in the course of PD (Goetz et al., 1986). Changes in the integrity of the autonomic systems can not only be assessed clinically. Radio labeled metaiodobenzylguanidine (MIBG) may be used to visualize the function of sympathetic cardiac neurons by scintigraphy. Already very early in the disease course a gross reduction of MIBG uptake by sympathetic cardiac neurons can be seen in PD patients (Braune, 2001). At present it remains to be determined whether these alterations may even be detected prior to the onset of motor symptoms. However, there are anamnestic hints for a premotor affection of the autonomic system. Some patients report to have suffered of constipation, bladder dysfunction and seborrheic dermatitis long before first motor symptoms occurred (Koller, 1992; Becker et al., 2002).

This is not astonishing, as important supraspinal and spinal autonomic centers show neurodegeneration and the pathologic hallmarks Lewy bodies and Lewy neurites already very early in the neurodegerenrative process of PD (Braak et al., 2003). Supraspinally, affected autonomic centers include the dorsal motor nucleus of the vagal nerve and the medullary tegmentum. According to Braak et al., these centers are always affected before the SN is reached by the ascending pathologic process (Braak et al., 2003). Therefore, autonomic dysfunction may well occur before the onset of motor symptoms. Moreover, as Lewy bodies have been reported in autonomic ganglia in subjects without Parkinsonism during life time (Braak et al., 2002), it can be speculated that autonomic ganglia may be affected prior to the manifestation of motor symptoms.

f. Visual impairment

Visual impairment is common in PD (Bodis-Wollner et al., 1987; Bodis-Wollner and Onofri, 1987). Deficits in achromatic visual contrast sensitivity, color discrimination, color perception as well as pathological findings in visual evoked potentials and electroretinography have been reported (Bodis-Wollner et al., 1987; Bodis-Wollner and Onofri, 1987; Buttner et al., 1994, 1995; Price et al., 1992; Bandini et al., 2001; Antal et al., 2002). In general, a relation of visual dysfunction and severity of motor symptoms has been described (Bodis-Wollner and Onofri, 1987; Buttner et al., 1995). However, it has been shown, that color discrimination is disturbed in the majority of PD patients at the very early clinical stages (Buttner et al., 1995a, b). It has been proposed that both, a retinal dopaminergic deficiency as well as an additional pathology beyond the retina may be responsible for the visual changes in PD (Bodis-Wollner, 1987). As data on the diagnostic value of visual dysfunction in PD is still limited, further studies are warranted to proof the value of color vision impairment as an early or even preclinical diagnostic marker.

3. Motor symptoms

The combination of brady- or akinesia and one of the other cardinal symptoms of PD (resting tremor, rigidity or impairment of postural reflexes) is usually suggestive for PD. However, frequently slight motor symptoms may precede these definite criteria. Subtle signs of slowness, stiffness, trouble with handwriting, and slightly flexed posture are often reported by patients or their relatives long before a diagnosis is made with certainty. These symptoms are usually intermittend, sometimes they only occur during periods of stress. Monosymptomatic resting tremor is another feature, that may present as a single symptom years before other motor symptoms of PD occur (Deuschl, 1999; Ghaemi et al., 2002). One impressive example of preceding subtle motor signs is the analysis of disease manifestation in the British football star Ray Kennedy. He was 35 years old, when PD was diagnosed. Videos taken during football games 10 years and more beforehand, however, already showed a reduced swinging of the right arm as well as mild facial immobility of the star (Lees, 1992). Still he made some of the most sensational goals for Liverpool.

It is known, that 60–70% of neurons of the SN have degenerated with a reduction of striatal dopamine of 80% when the clinical diagnosis of PD can be made (Bernheimer et al., 1973; Riederer and Wuketich, 1976). However, less severe neurodegeneration may manifest in only subtle symptoms or may become clinically evident only in periods of stress requring more dopaminergic transmission.

Also, it has been shown that PD patients suffer from a failure of the visuomotor co-ordination of hand movements (Benecke et al., 1987; Morris et al., 1988). These high level motor-control systems control among others movement direction and velocity. It has been suggested that visuomotor impairment may become relevant, even before executive motor functions become affected, as patients with hemiparkinsonism showed significant deficits in control of movement direction and movement velocity in both the affected and unaffected hand (Hocherman and Giladi, 1998).

Therefore, even if it may not be possible to use special visuomotor testing procedures in all persons at risk for PD anamnesis and assessment of subtle motor signs should definitely be included in a list of markers predicting a vulnerability to PD.

4. Neuroimaging markers

a. Visualizing the dopaminergic system by PET and SPECT examinations

The application of radiotracers to visualize the function of the dopaminergic system has been a brakethrough in the understanding of the pathogenesis of the disorder.

Positron emission tomography (PET) studies have mainly been performed with the radioligand [^{18}F]6-fluoro-Dopa (F-Dopa). Its accumulation measures L-Dopa uptake through the blood brain barrier and into the dopaminergic neurons as well as its conversion to dopamine, providing thereby a measurement for nigral cell count (Snow et al., 1993). For single photon emission computed tomography (SPECT) the radioligands [^{123}I]β-CIT and (123)I-FP-CIT have mainly been applied to visualize the density of dopamine transporters. Several lines of evidence indicate that these techniques are capable to detect a preclinical impairment of the nigrostriatal system. In patients with hemiparkinsonism a reduced radiotracer uptake was not only found contralateral to the clinically affected side but also ipsilateral, anticipating the clinical involvement of the other side (Morrish et al., 1995; Nagasawa et al., 1996; Schwarz et al., 2000; Filippi et al., 2005). Moreover, clinically unaffected twins of PD patients showed markedly reduced radiotrancer binding, indicating a sub- or preclinical alteration (Burn et al., 1992; Brooks, 1998; Laihinen et al., 2000; Piccini et al., 1999). Follow-up examination of some of these subjects revealed that some of them developed typical PD (Piccini et al., 1999). Also SPECT and PET studies in well documented familial and monogentic forms of PD showed that a genetically determined vulnerability may be visualized by these functional neuroimaging techniques years before the disease manifests in clinically unaffected mutation carriers (Piccini et al., 1997; Maraganore et al., 1999; Hilker et al., 2002). However, it needs to be considered that especially in the early stages of the disease compensatory processes may influence neuroimaging data. Moreover, it is not clear, yet, at what stage neuronal cell loss becomes evident in PET and SPECT neuroimaging, as at onset of symptoms a 30% loss of putaminal F-Dopa uptake has been documented, while histological examinations provide evidence for a 60–70% degeneration of SN dopaminergic neurons and a reduction of dopamine content of about 80% (Bernheimer et al., 1973; Riederer and Wuketich, 1976).

Still, these nuclear medicine methods seem to provide valuable instruments for the dection of a subclinical nigrostriatal impairment in individuals as risk for PD. However, as these methods are expensive and imply the exposure of yet healthy individuals to radiation, they are not suitable for population based studies to identify persons at risk for PD.

b. Trancranial sonography

More recently, transcranial sonography (TCS) has become an interesting tool for visualizing changes of the SN associated with the development of PD. TCS examinations are performed using a phased-array ultrasound system equipped with a 2.5-MHz transducer with high axial and lateral resolution through the intact skull using a preauricular acoustic bone window (Becker and Berg, 2001). At the mesencephalic scanning plane the SN may be identified within the hypoechogenic butterfly-shaped structure of the mesencephalic brainstem. Normally, the SN is displayed as a small patchy or tie-shaped structure of slighlty increased echogenicity in comparison with the surrounding brainstem tissue. As echogenicity is not qunatifiable the area of SN echogenicity is encircled and measured. Several studies have shown, that PD patients show markedly enlarged areas of SN echogenicity in more than 90% of patients (Becker et al., 1995; Berg et al., 2001a; Walter et al., 2002), reflecting PD specific biochemical alterations like increased iron levels (Berg et al., 1999; Zecca et al., 2005). Although the structure measured is small, reproducibility of findings is high (interrater correlation of $r = 0.8$ in several studies) (Berg et al., 1999, 2001a). Moreover, prospective studies with two independent raters, of whom at least one was completely blinded to the relevant clinical data of patients, indicate a high predictive value of the association of SN echogenicity and nigrostriatal impairment (Berg et al., 1999, 2001b, 2002; Walter et al., 2003). The facts that median SN echogenic size is larger contralateral to the clinically more affected side (Berg et al., 2001a) and that SN echogenicity is enhanced in PD but not in essential tremor (Niehaus et al., 2004) and only very rarely in atypical Parkinsonian syndromes like multiple system atrophy or progressive supranuclear palsy (Walter et al., 2003; Behnke et al., 2005) indicate that SN hyperechogenicity indeed reflects an alteration linked to nigrostriatal impairment.

In 8–10% of healthy adults, independent of age, increased echogenicity of the SN can be detected (Berg et al., 1999, 2002). This percentage is much higher than the expected number of individuals that will develop PD but is in the same range of neuropathologically suspected presymptomatic PD (Fearnly and Lees, 1991). Interestingly, also in these healthy subjects increased SN echogenicity may be associated with a mild functional impairment of the nigrostriatal system, demonstrated by the following observations: (i) Elderly patients without prediagnosed extrapyramidal disorder but with SN hyperechogenicity develop more frequent and more severe signs of motor impairment and in some cases even typical PD than those with normal SN echogenicity (Berg et al., 2001b). (ii) Patients with SN hyperechogenicity but without prediagnosed PD develop more often and more severe extrapyramidal symptoms following neuroleptic therapy for psychiatric disorders (Berg et al., 2001c). (iii) PET studies of clinically healthy subjects with marked SN hyperechogenicity revealed decreased striatal ^{18}F-dopa uptake in 60% of cases, indicating a subclinical impairment of the nigrostriatal system (Berg et al., 1999, 2002). (iv) In asymptomatic *parkin* mutation carriers SN hyperechogenicity is found to be associated with reduced PET values (Walter et al., 2004).

The area of SN echogenicity does not change in the course of the disease (Berg et al., 2005), and is detectable in healthy adults irrespective of age (Berg et al., 1999, 2002). Moreover, first degree relatives of patients with PD display this echofeature in more than 40% (Ruprecht-Dörfler et al., 2003) indicating hereditability of the marker and accordingly of a vulnerability to nigrostriatal dysfunction. SN hyperechogenicity may according to these studies therefore be regarded as a valuable preclinical marker, detectable early in life.

5. Combining features

For application of neuroprotective therapeutic strategies the identification of individuals at risk for nigrostriatal vulnerability is of vital importance. A number of markers seem to be suitable to detect disease related changes often years before disease manifestation. All of these markers have in common, that they are one the one hand typical for PD, but may on the other hand also be found in a small percentage of the healthy population as well as associated with other diseases. None of the markers alone predicts PD with certainty. Olfactory dyfunction, RBD, and depression may occur as own disease entities as well as in combination with a variety of other disorders. Autonomic as well as slight neuropsychological dysfunction, visual impairment and soft motor signs are that unspecific that they only point towards a certain disease entity in combination with other features. Even in monogenetically determined PD it is not entirely clear whether and at to what time point a mutation carrier will become ill of PD. Additionally, a number of possible exo- and endotoxic factors have to be considered.

One possiblity for a better identification of individuals at risk for PD, may be a combination of markers regarded as preclincial so far. For a useful combination, the relation of markers to each other as well as to the possible onset of PD should be known. A number of recent studies have tried to combine some of the presumable preclinical markers:

A large study on first degree relatives of PD patients combined testing for olfactory dysfunction in a 2-year clinical follow-up with $[^{123}I]\beta$-CIT to assess nigrostriatal function at baseline and 2 years later (Ponsen et al., 2004). Two years from baseline, only relatives with "idiopathic" hyposmia, who also had strongly reduced $[^{123}I]\beta$-CIT binding at baseline had developed PD. In the remaining hyposmic relatives a significantly incrased decline in dopamine transporter binding was found in comparison with normosmic relatives. Interstingly, mean SPECT binding ratios at baseline were only slightly different between the groups of hyp- and normosmic relatives. However, two years from baseline mean bilateral striatal and putamen binding ratios were significantly lower in hyposmic compared to normosmic relatives. These findings indicate that "idiopathic" olfactory dysfunction is indeed associated with an increased risk for developing PD and that assessment of olfactory dysfuction may indicate individuals at risk prior to $[^{123}I]\beta$-CIT examinations.

An other study combined "idiopathic" olfactory dysfunction with TCS findings and (123)I-FP-CIT examinations in thirty patients diagnosed with idiopathic olfactory loss (Sommer et al., 2004). Eleven of these patients exhibited an increased echogenicity of the SN on TCS. Ten of these underwent SPECT examinations. In 5 patients median uptake ratios in the basal ganglia were pathological, 2 patients exhibited borderline findings, and only 3 patients had normal results. It may, therefore, be concluded that a subgroup of patients with "idiopathic" olfactory dysfunction, indeed represents a subgroup of the healthy population at risk for nigrostriatal impairment. According to this study this subgroup may be specified by TCS. However, longitudinal follow-up studies are necessary to estimate the ratio of patients with olfactory dysfunction, hyperechogenicity of the SN and dopaminergic cell loss in the basal ganglia who will develop PD in the future.

The value of a combination of "idiopathic" RBD, olfactory dysfunction and (123)I-FP-CIT SPECT as possible preclinical markers for PD was tested in 30 patients with clinical or subclinical RBD (Stiasny-Kolster et al., 2005). The finding that 97% of RBD patients have a pathologically increased olfactory treshold indicates that both symptoms may at least in a large number of cases be related to each other. Moreover, five patients with clinical RBD showed signs of PD, with four of them fulfilling the criteria for the clinical dignosis of PD. In three of these patients (123)I-FP-CIT SPECT revealed a reduced dopamine transporter binding, one showed normal transporter binding and in one the investigation was not performed. (123)I-FP-CIT SPECT results of this study, therefore, also indicate that although early/preclinical changes of the dopaminergic system may be detected by this neuroimaging method, abnormalities may occur later in the neurodegenerative process than other preclinical markers.

Conclusion

A number of markers have been proposed to be valuable in detecting premotor alterations of the nigrostriatal system. In the case of familial PD or first degree relatives of PD patients it may be reasonable to chose non-invasive markers to underline or exclude vulnerability of the nigrostriatal system. In the general population it is more difficult to detect a subgroup at risk. At the moment, it seems that only a combination of possible preclinical signs may be suitable to specify a subroup of individuals at risk for PD. This could mean that any individual with one of the markers listed here as possible preclinical signs may be investigated with another easily applicable, inexpensive, broadly available method. I.e. an individual with RBD, depression or experiencing soft motor signs may be investigated by olfactory testing or TCS. If the investigation reveals an abnormal finding, a further marker could be added. However, it needs to be stressed that a number of future studies are needed to determine the value of each of the proposed markers itself as well as in combination with others for the diagnosis of preclinical PD. Especially longitudinal studies are of vital importance to determine the percentage of individuals with different preclinical markers who will go on to develop PD. Additionally, risk factors that favour the manifestation of the disease in subjects at risk have to be determined.

Moreover, it needs to be stressed, that identification of a subgroup at risk for PD is only of relevance if neuroprotective therapeutic strategies are available. Therefore, the effort of many groups for the development of neuroprotective therapies should even be enhanced. Such therapies need to be harmless, at best side-effect free, as subjects to whom they will be administered will be clinically healthy.

Last but definitely not least: Even if preclinical identification of subjects at risk seems to be within reach we have to consider from the very beginning ethical issues: Careful pretest counseling and informed consent are necessary (McKinnon et al., 1997). As most of the methods adding to the preclinical identification of subjects are quite easy to apply, comprehensive practice guidelines need to be established and considered in each individual case.

References

Ansari KA, Johnson A (1975) Olfactory function in patients with Parkinson's disease. J Chronic Dis 28: 493–497

Antal A, Keri S, Dibo G, Benedek G, Janka Z, Vecsei L, Bodis-Wollner I (2002) Electrophysiological correlates of visual categorization: evidence for cognitive dysfunctions in early Parkinson's disease. Brain Res Cogn Brain Res 13: 153–258

Bandini F, Pierantozzi M, Bodis-Wollner I (2001) Parkinson's disease changes the balance of onset and offset visual responses: an evoked potential study. Clin Neurophysiol 112: 976–983

Beal MF (2001) Experimental models of Parkinson's disease. Nat Rev Neurosci 2: 325–334

Becker G, Berg D, Lesch KP, Becker T (2001) Basal limbic system alteration in major depression: a hypothesis supported by transcranial sonography and MRI findings. Int J Neuropsychopharmacol 4: 21–31

Becker G, Berg D (2001) Neuroimaging in basal ganglia disorders: perspectives for transcranial ultrasound. Mov Disord 16: 23–32

Becker G, Muller A, Braune S, Buttner T, Benecke R, Greulich W, Klein W, Mark G, Rieke J, Thumler R (2002) Early diagnosis of Parkinson's disease. J Neurol 249 [Suppl 3]: 40–48

Becker G, Seufert J, Bogdahn U, Reichmann H, Reiners K (1995) Degeneration of substantia nigra in chronic Parkinson's disease visualized by transcranial color-coded real-time sonography. Neurology 45: 182–184

Becker T, Becker G, Seufert J, Hofmann E, Lange KW, Naumann M, Lindner A, Reichmann H, Riederer P, Beckmann H, Reiners K (1997) Parkinson's disease and depression: evidence for an alteration of the basal limbic system detected by transcranial sonography. J Neurol Neurosurg Psychiatry 63: 590–596

Behnke S, Berg D, Naumann M, Becker G (2005) Differentiation of Parkinson's disease and atypical parkinsonian syndromes by transcranial ultrasound. J Neurol Neurosurg Psychiatry 76: 423–425

Benecke R, Rothwell JC, Dick JP, Day BL, Marsden CD (1987) Disturbance of sequential movements in patients with Parkinson's disease. Brain 110: 361–379

Ben-Sachar D, Eshel G, Finberg JPM, Youdim MB (1991) The iron chelator desferrioxamine (desferal) retards 6-hydroxydopamine induced degeneration of nigro-striatal dopamine neurons. J Neurochem 56: 1441–1444

Berg D, Becker G, Zeiler B, Tucha O, Hofmann E, Preier M, Benz P, Jost W, Reiners K, Lange KW (1999) Vulnerability of the nigrostriatal system as detected by transcranial ultrasound. Neurology 53: 1026–1031

Berg D, Jabs B, Merschdorf U, Beckmann H, Becker G (2001c) Echogenicity of substantia nigra determined by transcranial ultrasound correlates with severity of parkinsonian symptoms induced by neuroleptic therapy. Biol Psychiatry 50: 463–467

Berg D, Merz B, Reiners K, Naumann M, Becker G (2005) Five-year follow-up study of hyperechogenicity of the substantia nigra in Parkinson's disease. Mov Disord 20: 383–385

Berg D, Roggendorf W, Schroder U, Klein R, Tatschner T, Benz P, Tucha O, Preier M, Lange KW, Reiners K, Gerlach M, Becker G (2002) Echogenicity of the substantia nigra: association with increased iron content and marker for susceptibility to nigrostriatal injury. Arch Neurol 59: 999–1005

Berg D, Schweitzer KJ, Leitner P, Zimprich A, Lichtner P, Belcredi P, Brussel T, Schulte C, Maass S, Nagele T, Wszolek ZK, Gasser T (2005) Type and frequency of mutations in the LRRK2 gene in familiar and sporadic Parkinson's disease. Brain Oct 26: [Epub ahead of print]

Berg D, Siefker C, Becker G (2001a) Echogenicity of the substantia nigra in Parkinson's disease and its relation to clinical findings. J Neurol 8: 684–689

Berg D, Siefker C, Ruprecht-Dorfler P, Becker G (2001b) Relationship of substantia nigra echogenicity and motor function in elderly subjects. Neurology 56: 13–17

Berg D, Supprian T, Hofmann E, Zeiler B, Jager A, Lange KW, Reiners K, Becker T, Becker G (1999b) Depression in Parkinson's disease: brainstem midline alteration on transcranial sonography and magnetic resonance imaging. J Neurol 246: 1186–1193

Bernheimer H, Birkmayer W, Hornykiewicz O, Jellinger K, Seitelberger F (1973) Brain dopamine and the syndromes of Parkinson and Huntington: clinical, morphological and neurochemical correlations. J Neurol Sci 20: 415–455

Blum-Degen D, Haas M, Pohli S, et al. (1998) Scavestrogens protect IMR 32 cells from oxidative stress-induced cell death. Toxicol Appl Pharmacol 152: 49–55

Bodis-Wollner I, Marx MS, Mitra S, Bobak P, Mylin L, Yahr M (1987) Visual dysfunction in Parkinson's disease. Loss in spatiotemporal contrast sensitivity. Brain 110: 1675–1698

Bodis-Wollner I, Onofrj M (1987) The visual system in Parkinson's disease. Adv Neurol 45: 323–327

Braak H, Del Tredici K, Bratzke H, Hamm-Clement J, Sandmann-Keil D, Rub U (2002) Staging of the intracerebral inclusion body pathology associated with idiopathic Parkinson's disease (preclinical and clinical stages). J Neurol 249 [Suppl 3]: 1–5

Braak H, Del Tredici K, Rub U, et al. (2003) Staging of brain pathology related to sporadic Parkinson's disease. Neurobiol Aging 24: 197–212

Braune S (2001) The role of cardiac metaiodobenzylguanidine uptake in the differential diagnosis of parkinsonian syndromes. Clin Auton Res 11: 351–355

Brooks DJ (1998) The early diagnosis of Parkinson's disease. Ann Neurol 44 [Suppl 1]: 10–18

Brown RG, Marsden CD (1988) Internal versus external cues and the control of attention in Parkinson's disease. Brain 111: 323–345

Brown RG, Marsden CD (1990) Cognitive function in Parkinson's disease: from description to theory. Trends Neurosci 13: 21–29

Burn DJ, Mark MH, Playford ED, Maraganore DM, Zimmerman TR Jr, Duvoisin RC, Harding AE, Marsden CD, Brooks DJ (1992) Parkinson's disease in twins studied with 18F-dopa and positron emission tomography. Neurology 42: 1894–1900

Buttner T, Kuhn W, Muller T, Patzold T, Heidbrink K, Przuntek H (1995a) Distorted color discrimination in 'de novo' parkinsonian patients. Neurology 45: 386–387

Buttner T, Kuhn W, Patzold T, Przuntek H (1994) L-Dopa improves colour vision in Parkinson's disease. J Neural Transm Park Dis Dement Sect 7: 13–19

Buttner T, Kuhn W, Przuntek H (1995b) Alterations in chromatic contour perception in de novo parkinsonian patients. Eur Neurol 35: 226–229

Chan-Palay V, Asan E (1989) Quantitation of catecholamine neurons in the locus coeruleus in human brains of normal young and older adults and in depression. J Comp Neurol 287: 357–372

Comella CL, Nardine TM, Diederich NJ, Stebbins GT (1998) Sleep-related violence, injury, and REM sleep behavior disorder in Parkinson's disease. Neurology 51: 526–529

Cooper JA, Sagar HJ, Jordan N, Harvey NS, Sullivan EV (1991) Cognitive impairment in early, untreated Parkinson's disease and its relationship to motor disability. Brain 114: 2095–2122

Cummings JL (1992) Depression and Parkinson's disease: a review. Am J Psychiatry 149: 443–454

D'Amato RJ, Zweig RM, Whitehouse PJ, Wenk GL, Singer HS, Mayeux R, Price DL, Snyder SH (1987) Aminergic systems in Alzheimer's disease and Parkinson's disease. Ann Neurol 22: 229–236

Deuschl G (1999) Differential diagnosis of tremor. J Neural Transm 56 [Suppl]: 211–220

Doty RL, Deems DA, Stellar S (1988) Olfactory dysfunction in parkinsonism: a general deficit unrelated to neurologic signs, disease stage, or disease duration. Neurology 38: 1237–1244

Doty RL, Stern MB, Pfeiffer C, Gollomp SM, Hurtig HI (1992) Bilateral olfactory dysfunction in early stage treated and untreated idiopathic Parkinson's disease. J Neurol Neurosurg Psychiatry 55: 138–142

Dubois B, Pillon B (1997) Cognitive deficits in Parkinson's disease. J Neurol 244: 2–8

Dujardin K, Duhamel A, Becquet E, Grunberg C, Defebvre L, Destee A (1999) Neuropsychological abnormalities in first degree relatives of patients with familial Parkinson's disease. J Neurol Neurosurg Psychiatry 67: 323–328

Eisensehr I, Linke R, Noachtar S, Schwarz J, Gildehaus FJ, Tatsch K (2000) Reduced striatal dopamine transporters in idiopathic rapid eye movement sleep behaviour disorder. Comparison with Parkinson's disease and controls. Brain 123: 1155–1160

Eisensehr I, Linke R, Tatsch K, Kharraz B, Gildehaus JF, Wetter CT, Trenkwalder C, Schwarz J, Noachtar S (2003) Increased muscle activity during rapid eye movement sleep correlates with decrease of striatal presynaptic dopamine transporters. IPT and IBZM SPECT imaging in subclinical and clinically manifest idiopathic REM sleep behavior disorder, Parkinson's disease, and controls. Sleep 26: 507–512

Elbaz A, Grigoletto F, Baldereschi M, Breteler MM, Manubens-Bertran JM, Lopez-Pousa S, Dartigues JF, Alperovitch A, Tzourio C, Rocca WA (1999) Familial aggregation of Parkinson's disease: a population-based case-control study in Europe. EUROPARKINSON Study Group. Neurology 52: 1876–1882

Fearnley JM, Lees AJ (1991) Ageing and Parkinson's disease: substantia nigra regional selectivity. Brain 114: 2283–2301

Filippi L, Manni C, Pierantozzi M, Brusa L, Danieli R, Stanzione P, Schillaci O (2005) 123I-FP-CIT semi-quantitative SPECT detects preclinical bilateral dopaminergic deficit in early Parkinson's disease with unilateral symptoms. Nucl Med Commun 26: 421–426

Gagnon JF, Bedard MA, Fantini ML, Petit D, Panisset M, Rompre S, Carrier J, Montplaisir J (2002) REM sleep behavior disorder and REM sleep without atonia in Parkinson's disease. Neurology 59: 585–589

Gal S, Zheng H, Fridkin M, Youdim MB (2005) Novel multifunctional neuroprotective iron chelator-monoamine oxidase inhibitor drugs for neurodegenerative diseases. In vivo selective brain monoamine oxidase inhibition and prevention of MPTP-induced striatal dopamine depletion. J Neurochem Jul 28; [Epub ahead of print]

Gasser T (2005) Genetics of parkinsonism. In: Beal MF, Lang AE, Ludolph A (eds) Neurodegenerative diseases. Cambridge University Press, Cambrigde, pp 586–597

Ghaemi M, Raethjen J, Hilker R, Rudolf J, Sobesky J, Deuschl G, Heiss WD (2002) Monosymptomatic resting tremor and Parkinson's disease: a multitracer positron emission tomographic study. Mov Disord 17: 782–788

Gibb WR, Lees AJ (1988) The relevance of the Lewy body to the pathogenesis of idiopathic Parkinson's disease. J Neurol Neurosurg Psychiatry 51: 745–752

Goetz CG, Lutge W, Tanner CM (1986) Autonomic dysfunction in Parkinson's disease. Neurology 36: 73–75

Hardie RJ (1999) Measuring the rate of progression and estimating the preclinical period of Parkinson's disease with [18F]dopa PET. J Neurol Neurosurg Psychiatry 66: 256

Hawkes CH, Shephard BC, Daniel SE (1997) Olfactory dysfunction in Parkinson's disease. J Neurol Neurosurg Psychiatry 62: 436–446

Hendricks JC, Morrison AR, Mann GL (1982) Different behaviors during paradoxical sleep without atonia depend on pontine lesion site. Brain Res 239: 81–105

Hilker R, Klein C, Hedrich K, Ozelius LJ, Vieregge P, Herholz K, Pramstaller PP, Heiss WD (2002) The striatal dopaminergic deficit is dependent on the number of mutant alleles in a family with mutations in the parkin gene: evidence for enzymatic parkin function in humans. Neurosci Lett 323: 50–54

Hilker R, Schweitzer K, Coburger S, Ghaemi M, Weisenbach S, Jacobs AH, Rudolf J, Herholz K, Heiss WD (2005) Nonlinear progression of Parkinson disease as determined by serial positron emission tomographic imaging of striatal fluorodopa F 18 activity. Arch Neurol 62: 378–382

Hocherman S, Giladi N (1998) Visuomotor control abnormalities in patients with unilateral parkinsonism. Neurology 50: 1648–1654

Holthoff VA, Vieregge P, Kessler J, Pietrzyk U, Herholz K, Bonner J, Wagner R, Wienhard K, Pawlik G, Heiss WD (1994) Discordant twins with Parkinson's disease: positron emission tomography and early signs of impaired cognitive circuits. Ann Neurol 36: 176–182

Hoogendijk WJ, Sommer IE, Tissingh G, Deeg DJ, Wolters EC (1998) Depression in Parkinson's disease. The impact of symptom overlap on prevalence. Psychosomatics 39: 416–421

Kang GA, Bronstein JM, Masterman DL, Redelings M, Crum JA, Ritz B (2005) Clinical characteristics in early Parkinson's disease in a central California population-based study. Mov Disord 20: 1133–1142

Koller WC (1992) When does Parkinson's disease begin? Neurology 42 [Suppl 4]: 27–31

Laihinen A, Ruottinen H, Rinne JO, Haaparanta M, Bergman J, Solin O, Koskenvuo M, Marttila R, Rinne UK (2000) Risk for Parkinson's disease: twin studies for the detection of asymptomatic subjects using [18F]6-fluorodopa PET. J Neurol 247 [Suppl 2]: 110–113

Lees AJ, Smith E (1983) Cognitive deficits in the early stages of Parkinson's disease. Brain 106: 257–270

Lees AJ (1992) When did Ray Kennedy's Parkinson's disease begin? Mov Disord 7: 110–116

Lucking CB, Durr A, Bonifati V, Vaughan J, De Michele G, Gasser T, Harhangi BS, Meco G, Denefle P, Wood NW, Agid Y, Brice A (2000) Association between early-onset Parkinson's disease and mutations in the parkin gene. French Parkinson's Disease Genetics Study Group. N Engl J Med 342: 1560–1567

Maraganore DM, O'Connor MK, Bower JH, Kuntz KM, McDonnell SK, Schaid DJ, Rocca WA (1999) Detection of preclinical Parkinson disease in at-risk family members with use of [123I]beta-CIT and SPECT: an exploratory study. Mayo Clin Proc 74: 681–685

Marder K, Tang MX, Mejia H, Alfaro B, Cote L, Louis E, Groves J, Mayeux R (1996) Risk of Parkinson's disease among first-degree relatives: A community-based study. Neurology 47: 155–160

Markopoulou K, Larsen KW, Wszolek EK, Denson MA, Lang AE, Pfeiffer RF, Wszolek ZK (1997) Olfactory dysfunction in familial parkinsonism. Neurology 49: 1262–1267

Mayeux R, Stern Y, Rosen J, Leventhal J (1981) Depression, intellectual impairment, and Parkinson disease. Neurology 31: 645–650

McKinnon WC, Baty BJ, Bennett RL, Magee M, Neufeld-Kaiser WA, Peters KF, Sawyer JC, Schneider KA (1997) Predisposition genetic testing for late-onset disorders in adults. A position paper of the National Society of Genetic Counselors. JAMA 278: 1217–1220

Mindham RH (1970) Psychiatric symptoms in Parkinsonism. J Neurol Neurosurg Psychiatry 33: 188–191

Montgomery EB Jr, Baker KB, Lyons K, Koller WC (1999) Abnormal performance on the PD test battery by asymptomatic first-degree relatives. Neurology 52: 757–762

Montgomery EB Jr, Koller WC, LaMantia TJ, Newman MC, Swanson-Hyland E, Kaszniak AW, Lyons K (2000a) Early detection of probable idiopathic Parkinson's disease: I. Development of a diagnostic test battery. Mov Disord 15: 467–473

Montgomery EB Jr, Lyons K, Koller WC (2000b) Early detection of probable idiopathic Parkinson's disease: II. A prospective application of a diagnostic test battery. Mov Disord 15: 474–478

Morrish PK, Sawle GV, Brooks DJ (1995) Clinical and [18F] dopa PET findings in early Parkinson's disease. J Neurol Neurosurg Psychiatry 59: 597–600
Morris RG, Downes JJ, Sahakian BJ, Evenden JL, Heald A, Robbins TW (1988) Planning and spatial working memory in Parkinson's disease. J Neurol Neurosurg Psychiatry 51: 757–766
Muller A, Reichmann H, Livermore A, Hummel T (2002) Olfactory function in idiopathic Parkinson's disease (IPD): results from cross-sectional studies in IPD patients and long-term follow-up of de-novo IPD patients. J Neural Transm 109: 805–811
Nagasawa H, Tanji H, Itoyama Y, Saito H, Kimura I, Fujiwara T, Iwata R, Itoh M, Ido T (1996) Brain 6-[18F]fluorodopa metabolism in early and late onset of Parkinson's disease studied by positron emission tomography. J Neurol Sci 144: 70–76
Niehaus L, Savyer N, Weber U, Hertel R, Trottenberg T, Kupsch A (2004) Brain parenchyma sonography in patients with essential tremor and Parkinson's disease. Cerebrovasc Dis 17 [Suppl 4]: 3
Nurmi E, Ruottinen HM, Bergman J, Haaparanta M, Solin O, Sonninen P, Rinne JO (2001) Rate of preogression in Parkisnon's disease. A6-[18F]fluoro-L-dopa PET study. Mov Disord 16: 608–615
Owen AM, Roberts AC, Hodges JR, Summers BA, Polkey CE, Robbins TW (1993) Contrasting mechanisms of impaired attentional set-shifting in patients with frontal lobe damage or Parkinson's disease. Brain 116: 1159–1175
Payami H, Larsen K, Bernard S, Nutt J (1994) Increased risk of Parkinson's disease in parents and siblings of patients. Ann Neurol 36: 659–661
Piccini P, Burn DJ, Ceravolo R, Maraganore D, Brooks DJ (1999) The role of inheritance in sporadic Parkinson's disease: evidence from a longitudinal study of dopaminergic function in twins. Ann Neurol 45: 577–582
Piccini P, Morrish PK, Turjanski N, Sawle GV, Burn DJ, Weeks RA, Mark MH, Maraganore DM, Lees AJ, Brooks DJ (1997) Dopaminergic function in familial Parkinson's disease: a clinical and 18F-dopa positron emission tomography study. Ann Neurol 41: 222–229
Ponsen MM, Stoffers D, Booij J, van Eck-Smit BL, Wolters ECh, Berendse HW (2004) Idiopathic hyposmia as a preclinical sign of Parkinson's disease. Ann Neurol 56: 173–181
Price MJ, Feldman RG, Adelberg D, Kayne H (1992) Abnormalities in color vision and contrast sensitivity in Parkinson's disease. Neurology 42: 887–890
Quinn NP, Rossor MN, Marsden CD (1987) Olfactory threshold in Parkinson's disease. J Neurol Neurosurg Psychiatry 50: 88–89
Riederer P, Wuketich S (1976) Time course of nigrostriatal degeneration in Parkinon's disease: a detailed study of influential factors in human brain amine analogues. J Neural Transm 38: 227–301
Riess O, Krüger R, Hochstrasser H, Soehn AS, Nuber S, Franck T, Berg D. Genetic causes of Parkinson's disease: Extending the pathway. J Neural Transm, in press
Robins AH (1976) Depression in patients with Parkinsonism. Br J Psychiatry 128: 141–145
Ruprecht-Dörfler P, Berg D, Tucha O, Benz P, Meier-Meitinger M, Alders GL, Lange KW, Becker G (2003) Echogenicity of the substantia nigra in relatives of patients with sporadic Parkinson's disease. NeuroImage 18: 416–422
Sanford LD, Morrison AR, Mann GL, Harris JS, Yoo L, Ross RJ (1994) Sleep patterning and behaviour in cats with pontine lesions creating REM without atonia. J Sleep Res 3: 233–240
Santamaria J, Tolosa E, Valles A (1986) Parkinson's disease with depression: a possible subgroup of idiopathic parkinsonism. Neurology 36: 1130–1133
Schenck CH, Bundlie SR, Mahowald MW (1996) Delayed emergence of a parkinsonian disorder in 38% of 29 older men initially diagnosed with idiopathic rapid eye movement sleep behaviour disorder. Neurology 46: 388–393
Schenck CH, Bundlie SR, Mahowald MW (2003) REM behaviour disorder (RBD): delayed emergence of parkinsonism and/or dementia in 65% of older men initially diagnosed with idiopathic RBD, and an analysis of the minimum or phasic electromyographic abnormalities found during REM sleep. Sleep 26 [Suppl]: 0794.M
Schenkel E, Siegel JM (1989) REM sleep without atonia after lesions of the medial medulla. Neurosci Lett 98: 159–165
Schneider JS, Pope-Coleman A (1995) Cognitive deficits precede motor deficits in a slowly progressing model of parkinsonism in the monkey. Neurodegeneration 4: 245–255
Schwarz J, Linke R, Kerner M, Mozley PD, Trenkwalder C, Gasser T, Tatsch K (2002) Striatal dopamine transporter binding assessed by [I-123]IPT and single photon emission computed tomography in patients with early Parkinson's disease: implications for a preclinical diagnosis. Arch Neurol 57: 205–208
Schwarz J, Tatsch K, Linke R, et al. (1997) Measuring the decline of dopamine transporter binding in patients with Parkinson's disease using 123I-IPT and SPECT. Neurology 48: A208
Snow BJ, Tooyama I, McGeer EG, Yamada T, Calne DB, Takahashi H, Kimura H (1993) Human positron emission tomographic [18F]fluorodopa studies correlate with dopamine cell counts and levels. Ann Neurol 34: 324–330
Sommer U, Hummel T, Cormann K, Mueller A, Frasnelli J, Kropp J, Reichmann H (2004) Detection of presymptomatic Parkinson's disease: combining smell tests, transcranial sonography, and SPECT. Mov Disord 19: 1196–1202
Stiasny-Kolster K, Doerr Y, Moller JC, Hoffken H, Behr TM, Oertel WH, Mayer G (2005) Combination of 'idiopathic' REM sleep behaviour disorder and olfactory dysfunction as possible indicator for alpha-synucleinopathy demonstrated by dopamine transporter FP-CIT-SPECT. Brain 128: 126–137
Tissingh G, Berendse HW, Bergmans P, DeWaard R, Drukarch B, Stoof JC, Wolters EC (2001) Loss of olfaction in de novo and treated Parkinson's disease: possible implications for early diagnosis. Mov Disord 16: 41–46
Torack RM, Morris JC (1988) The association of ventral tegmental area histopathology with adult dementia. Arch Neurol 45: 497–501
Turner RS, D'Amato CJ, Chervin RD, Blaivas M (2000) The pathology of REM sleep behavior disorder with comorbid Lewy body dementia. Neurology 55: 1730–1732
Uchiyama M, Isse K, Tanaka K, Yokota N, Hamamoto M, Aida S, Ito Y, Yoshimura M, Okawa M (1995) Incidental Lewy body disease in a patient with REM sleep behavior disorder. Neurology 45: 709–712
Uitti RJ, Shinotoh H, Hayward M, Schulzer M, Mak E, Calne DB (1997) "Familial Parkinson's disease" – a case-control study of families. Can J Neurol Sci 24: 127–132
Walter U, Klein C, Hilker R, Benecke R, Pramstaller PP, Dressler D (2004) Brain parenchyma sonography detects preclinical parkinsonism. Mov Disord 19: 1445–1449
Walter U, Niehaus L, Probst T, Benecke R, Meyer BU, Dressler D (2003) Brain parenchyma sonography discriminates Parkinson's disease and atypical parkinsonian syndromes. Neurology 60: 74–77
Walter U, Wittstock M, Benecke R, Dressler D (2002) Substantia nigra echogenicity is normal in non-extrapyramidal cerebral disorders but increased in Parkinson's disease. J Neural Transm 109: 191–196
Ward CD, Hess WA, Calne DB (1983) Olfactory impairment in Parkinson's disease. Neurology 33: 943–946
Zecca L, Berg D, Arzberger T, Ruprecht P, Rausch WD, Musicco M, Tampellini D, Riederer P, Gerlach M, Becker G (2005) In vivo detection of iron and neuromelanin by transcranial sonography: a new approach for early detection of substantia nigra damage. Mov Disord 20: 1278–1285
Zheng H, Gal S, Weiner LM, Bar-Am O, Warshawsky A, Fridkin M, Youdim MB (2005) Novel multifunctional neuroprotective iron chelator-monoamine oxidase inhibitor drugs for neurodegenerative diseases: in vitro studies on antioxidant activity, prevention of lipid peroxide formation and monoamine oxidase inhibition. J Neurochem Jul 25; [Epub ahead of print]
Zucco GM, Zaglis D, Wambsganss CS (1991) Olfactory deficits in elderly subjects and Parkinson patients. Percept Mot Skills 73: 895–898

J Neural Transm (2006) [Suppl] 71: 133–141

Journal of Neural Transmission
Printed in Austria

Assessing neuroprotection in Parkinson's disease: from the animal models to molecular neuroimaging in vivo

R. Ceravolo, P. Sgadò, D. Frosini, G. U. Corsini

Department of Neuroscience, University of Pisa, Pisa, Italy

Summary An important goal in Parkinson's Disease research is to identify neuroprotective therapy, and the interaction between basic science and clinical research is needed to discover drugs that can slow or halt the disorder progression. At present there is not a perfect animal model of PD to test neuroprotective strategies, however the models that portray the basic characteristics needed are toxin-induced and gene-based models. The first group comprehends 6-OHDA e MPTP and recently rotenone, paraquat and epoxomicin treated animals that shows some of human disease characteristics. Gene-based models are various and, even if with limits, they seem suitable models to test neuroprotection in PD since they present replicable lesions, a predictable pattern of neurodegeneration and a well-characterized behavior, biochemistry and morphology to assist in the understanding of induced changes. In clinical trials researchers have first used as marker of disease progression clinical scores and motor tasks which are limited by the potential symptomatic effect of tested drugs and are not useful in the pre-clinical phases of PD. Recently has emerged the important role of neuroimaging (Dopamine Transporter SPECT, 18FDopa-PET) as surrogate biomarker of PD progression. Even if there are still concerns about the influence of regulatory effects of tested drugs, neuroimaging features could represent a good outcome measure to evaluate PD progression and putative neuroprotective effect of pharmacological and non-pharmacological manipulations.

Introduction

Parkinson's disease (PD) is a progressive neurodegenerative disorder, which affects more than 0.1% of the population older than 40 years of age (Siderowf and Stern, 2003). It is characterized clinically by bradykinesia, rigidity, resting tremor, postural instability, and in a minority of patients cognitive impairment. Loss of dopamine neurons in the substantia nigra pars compacta leads to the major clinical symptoms of PD, but there is widespread neuropathology (Braak et al., 2004). Lewy bodies and dystrophic neuritis are a pathologic hallmark of PD and classically are round eosinophilic inclusions composed of a halo of radiating fibrils and a less defined core (Forno, 1996). Lewy bodies are thought to be a pathognomonic feature of PD, but recent studies suggest that some forms of PD do not have Lewy bodies (Dawson and Dawson, 2003). The etiology of PD is still not fully understood, however genetic analyses, epidemiologic studies, neuropathological investigations, and new experimental models of PD are providing important new insights into the pathogenesis of PD. Although the cause of PD remains unknown, dopaminergic cell loss has been associated with different mechanism of cell damage, including excitotossicity with excess nitric oxide formation (Youdim and Lavie, 1994; Mathew et al., 1997) and glial and inflammatory processes (Hunot et al., 1997), mitocondrial dysfunction (Schapira et al., 1989; Mizuno et al., 1994) and oxidative stress. It is now supposed that the result of these cellular and molecular events is the induction of apoptosis in nigral dopaminergic neurons (Corsini et al., 2002). That there is such selective neuronal vulnerability in the substantia nigra pars compacta in PD is evident from a number of lines of evidence (Prezdborski et al., 1992; Andreassen et al., 2001). The finding of excess iron, decreased GSH, and diffuse oxidative damage in the substantia nigra of PD subjects suggests that the nigra is in a state of oxidant stress and that oxidative damage has occurred. Oxidative stress can directly damage crucial biomolecules and can signal the initiation of apoptosis. The possibility that oxidative stress contributes to cell death in PD offers several therapeutic options to provide neuroprotection, including free radical scavengers, glutathione-enhancing agents, iron chelators and drugs that interfere with the oxidative metabolism of dopamine as well as agents that preserve the mitochondrial membrane potential (Youdim et al., 2005). Recently, the NIH-NINDS-Committee to identify Neuroprotective Agents in Parkinson's

Correspondence: R. Ceravolo, Department of Neuroscience, University of Pisa, Pisa, Italy
e-mail: r.ceravolo@med.unipi.it

(CINAP) published the result of a systematic assessment of currently available pharmacologic neuroprotective agents (Ravina et al., 2003). Specific criteria were drafted for drug evaluation including scientific rationale, blood-brain barrier penetration, evidence of efficacy in animal models or humans, safety and tolerability. In their discussion, CINAP members stated that part of the challenge when comparing neuroprotective agents was that researchers used various animal models and experimental designs for different compounds. The selected agents were: caffeine, coenzyma Q10, estrogen, GM-1 ganglioside, mynociclina, nicotine, GPI-1485, rasagiline/selegiline, ropinirole and pramipexole. At present, however, no studies have definitively illustrated that a therapeutic agent has disease modifying activity in humans by reducing the functional decline of PD patients.

Animal models

Determining neuroprotective effects in clinical trials is rather difficult. The main outcome measures currently used to assess disease progression are clinical evaluations that can be altered by numerous factors (Ahlskog, 2003). Even a small symptomatic effect could be a confounding factor (Ward, 1994). Thus pharmacology and pharmacokinetics of the potential compounds must be fully investigated and elucidated to evaluate potential interactions and wash-out periods. At least some issues can be solved in the laboratory using proper animal models and tests. The proper translation from the laboratory bench to the clinic should require the need of interaction between basic and clinical researchers. An ideal animal model of PD can be described by presenting behavioural signs and pathology that resemble the disease, including its time course. The closer the similarity of a model is to PD, the higher the predictive value for clinical efficacy. However modelling PD is strongly limited by our knowledge of what causes the disease. Also PD models are based on the concept that parkinsonian signs are related to dopaminergic nigral loss: several models exhibit many of the characteristics of the disease, but none mimics the complex chronic neurodegenerative features of human PD (Dawson and Dawson, 2002; Feany and Bender, 2000; Emborg, 2004). There is not a perfect animal model of PD to test neuroprotective strategies, however the models that portray the basic characteristics needed are toxin-induced and gene-based models.

Toxin-induced models for Parkinson's disease

Among the neurotoxins used to induce DA neurodegeneration, 6-hydroxydopamine (6-OHDA), MPTP, and more recently paraquat, rotenone and epoxomicin have received the most attention. Only MPTP is clearly linked to a form of human parkinsonism, and it is thus the most widely studied model. Reserpine and a-methylparatyrosine (AMPT) have been used to discover l-dopa efficacy in the management of PD. Methamphetamine (METH) and substituted amphetamines (MDMA, "ecstasy") have been suggested as risk factors for movement disorders. Administration of these drugs to rodents and non-human primates leads to severe depletion of striatal DA and degeneration of DA nigrostriatal terminals, however the motor behavioral alterations are subtle.

6-OHDA was the first animal model of PD associated with SNc DA neuronal death (Jeon et al., 1995) and it is still extensively used. 6-OHDA-induced toxicity is relatively selective for monoaminergic neurons, resulting from preferential uptake by DA and noradrenergic transporters. 6-OHDA is injected unilaterally in the substantia nigra, median forebrain bundle (MFB), or striatum, with the contralateral side serving as control. A distinctive behavioral feature of this model is rotation, a motor feature that is due to the asymmetry in DA neurotransmission between the lesioned and the intact sides (Perese et al., 1989). Since the unilateral lesion (circling behavior) can be quantitatively assayed, a great advantage of this model is the ability to assess the anti-PD properties of new drugs and the benefit of transplantation or gene therapy to repair the damaged pathways.

Self-administration of MPTP by heroin addicts induces clinical symptoms indistinguishable from idiopathic PD; these findings identified a neurotoxin useful for the development of animal model of PD (Langston et al., 1983; Corsini et al., 2002). MPTP is converted to MPP+, the toxic metabolite, by monoamine oxidase B (MAO-B) in glia and serotoninergic neurons. MPP+ acts as substrate of the dopamine transporter (DAT) leading to the inhibition of mitochondrial complex I, depletion of ATP, and the consequent dopaminergic neuron cell death. Subsequent administration to mice and monkeys showed that MPTP selectively destroys DA neurons in the SNc, and affects, to a lesser extent, neurons of the ventral tegmentum and the locus cruleus (Seniuk et al., 1990).

In addition, DA depletion occurs in putamen and caudate nucleus with a different selectivity depending on the species and mode of administration (Przedborski et al., 2001). Unlike PD, LBs have not been reported in this model; however, eosinophilic inclusions reminiscent of LB have been described in aged nonhuman primates. Injection of MPTP into mice results in subtle behavioral deficits.

However, in humans and monkeys, MPTP produces an irreversible and severe parkinsonian syndrome characterized by all of the features of PD, including tremor, rigidity, slowness of movement, postural instability, and freezing. Also similar to PD, the susceptibility to MPTP increases with age in both monkeys and mice (Ricaurte et al., 1987). This experimental model of PD has given several important insights into the pathogenesis of PD contributing to the development of the current symptomatological therapy for PD. Nevertheless, its neuropathological features have limited the use of this model for the study of compensatory mechanisms and/or the development of new neuroprotective treatments for PD.

The herbicide paraquat also induces a toxic model of PD (Uversky, 2004); it shares structural similarity to MPP+ and is present in the environment. Exposure to paraquat may confer an increased risk for PD. Systemic administration of paraquat to mice leads to SNc dopaminergic neuron degeneration accompanied by α-synuclein containing inclusions, as well as increases in α-synuclein immunostaining in frontal cortex.

Rotenone is the most potent member of the rotenoids, a family of natural cytotoxic compounds extracted from tropical plants; it is widely used as an insecticide and fish poison. Greenamyre and colleagues reported that the administration of low-dose intravenous rotenone to rats produces selective degeneration of nigrostriatal neurons accompanied by α-synuclein-positive LB-like inclusions (Betarbet et al., 2000). This model was the first to link an environmental toxin of possible relevance to PD to the pathologic hallmark of α-synuclein aggregation.

Recently it has been shown that systematically injected subcronic doses of naturally occurring (epoxomicin) or synthetic proteosome inhibitor, into adult rats induce abnormal posture with bradykinesia, rigidity and tremor (McNaught et al., 2004). Post mortem analysis showed striatal DA depletion and signs of apoptotic cell death and inflammation in the SN. In addition, neurodegeneration occurs in the locus cruleus, dorsal motor nucleus of the vagus and the nucleus basalis of Meynert. Neuropathological signs of cytoplasmatic, eosinophilic α-synuclein/ubiquitin-containing inclusions resembling LBs have been reported (McNaught et al., 2004).

Thus, this animal model may contribute to provide valuable insight on the role of the ubiquitin proteosome system in the etiopathogenic mechanisms in hereditary and sporadic forms of PD.

Gene-based models

Recent studies have provided evidence that genetic risk factors are involved in the pathogenesis of the idiopathic form of PD (Vieregge, 1994; Kuopio et al., 2001). A twin study indicates that the concordance rate for PD, including subclinical cases, is approximately three times higher in monozygotic (55%) twins than in dizygotic (18%) twins (Piccini et al., 1999). In addition to sporadic forms of PD, several rare monogenic familial forms of the disease, characterized by early-onset and an autosomal dominant or recessive inheritance have been identified: α-synuclein; parkin, UCH-L1, DJ-1, LRRK2. Polymorphisms at the parkin and synuclein loci may also contribute to the risk of idiopathic PD, and parkin mutations are found in patients without a family history of PD, especially with symptom onset before the age of 30.

α-Synuclein

Rare cases of autosomal dominant familial forms of PD (Contursi and German kindreds) have been linked to point mutations in the gene encoding α-synuclein (Polymeropoulos et al., 1997; Kruger et al., 1998). In addition, certain α-synuclein promoter polymorphisms are associated with sporadic PD and express α-synuclein at higher levels than polymorphisms not associated with the disease (Holzmann et al., 2003). Although no mutant forms of α-synuclein have been identified in idiopathic PD, its localization in LBs has suggested a pathophysiologic link between α-synuclein aggregation and the neurodegenerative disease. To investigate this link several groups have developed mouse models for α-synuclein focusing on altered protein expression using different promoters and gene cassette constructs (Feany and Bender, 2000; Giasson et al., 2002; Lee et al., 2002). However, a striking disappointment has been a complete failure of the mouse models to mimic dopaminergic neurodegeneration (i.e., actual cell death). The models display a variety of neuropathological changes, including neuronal atrophy, dystrophic neurites, and astrocytosis accompanied by α-synuclein-positive LB-like inclusions. However, murine DA neurons appear inexplicably resistant to α-synuclein-induced neurotoxicity, even in the case of marked accumulations of the protein (Giasson et al., 2002; Lee et al., 2002), significantly limiting the utility of these models.

Parkin

Loss-of-function mutations in the gene encoding parkin cause recessively inherited parkinsonism (Kitada et al., 1998). Although this form of parkinsonism was originally termed autosomal recessive juvenile parkinsonism, the clinical phenotype is now known to include older-onset patients. Clinically, parkin mutant patients display the classical signs of parkinsonism, marked improvement of symptoms with sleep, abnormal dystonic movements, and a striking response to levodopa. Heterozygote mutations in parkin may also lead to DA dysfunction and later onset of PD. Pathologically, parkin-related PD is characterized by loss of SNc dopaminergic neurons, but it is not typically associated with LBs. It is uncertain how loss of parkin function leads to DA neuron degeneration, but clues are emerging from the identification of its normal function. Recent biochemical studies indicate that parkin protein may play a critical role in mediating interaction with a number of different proteins involved in the proteasome-mediated degradation pathway. Three parkin-deficient mice have been reported so far (Goldberg et al., 2003; Itier et al., 2003; von Coelln et al., 2004). The first two reports show subtle behavioral deficits, some dysfunctions of dopamine and glutamate neurotransmission but no loss of SNpc or LC catecholaminergic neurons. In contrast, the third parkin knock-out mice show loss of noradrenergic LC neurons and a marked reduction of the norepinephrine dependent startle response (von Coelln et al., 2004).

Ubiquitin C-Terminal Hydrolase-L1

A dominant mutation in Ubiquitin C-Terminal Hydrolase-L1 (UCH-L1) was identified in onefamily with inherited PD (Leroy et al., 1998), but no pathological data were included in this report. The enzyme catalyzes the hydrolysis of C-terminal ubiquityl-esters and is thought to play a role in recycling ubiquitin ligated to misfolded proteins after their degradation by the proteasome. Although the mutation decreases the activity of this deubiquitinating enzyme, mice null for UCH-L1 do not display dopaminergic neurodegeneration. Rather, they develop an axonopathy affecting primary sensory axons in the gracile nucleus of the medulla, whose cell bodies reside in the dorsal root ganglia (Healy et al., 2004).

DJ-1

DJ-1 mutations were identified in two consanguineous pedigrees with autosomal recessive PD (Bonifati et al., 2002). One family carries a deletion predicted to abolish protein function, while the other harboured a missense mutation that results a mutant form of DJ-1 leading to its accumulation in mitochondria (Bonifati et al., 2002).

Dardarin

Linkage of an autosomal dominant form of parkinsonism (PARK8) to chromosome 12 was shown in a Japanese family (Funayama et al., 2002), and later confirmed in two white families. Recently, mutations in a gene termed LRRK2 (leucine-rich repeat kinase 2) were identified in families with PARK8 (Paisan-Ruiz et al., 2004; Zimprich et al., 2004). The ranges of clinical and pathological characteristics associated with LRRK2 mutations are broad, and include typical late-onset Parkinson's disease with Lewy-body pathology, showing that mendelian mutations are associated with the classic form of Parkinson's disease. In other cases, Lewy bodies are absent and unusual inclusions or pathological findings usually associated with different neurodegenerative diseases are present. The LRRK2 gene encodes a large protein of 2527 amino acids and unknown function. The protein, dardarin (Paisan-Ruiz et al., 2004), belongs to a group within the Ras/GTPase superfamily, termed ROCO. Currently there is no available information about mouse models based on this protein.

Transgenic mouse lines have used "knock-out" and "knock-in" strategies that target genes such as superoxide dismutase (SOD), monoamine oxidase (MAO), dopamine receptors, dopamine transporters, caspases, neurotrophic factors, and neurotransmitter receptors. Spontaneous genetic rodent models include weaver, lurcher, reeler, Tshrhyt, tottering, coloboma mice, the ASAGU and circling rats. Several of these spontaneous rodent models display altered dopaminergic functions and neurodegeneration, and have deficits in motor behaviour.

Another interesting model is the Nurr1 heterozygous mouse. Nurr1 is a member of the nuclear receptor superfamily and is required for the induction and the development of the dopaminergic phenotype in the mesencephalon. The homozygous gene knockout (Nurr1$-/-$) mice display at birth a selective and complete loss of DA neurons and dopamine levels in the striatum (Le et al., 1999).

Furthermore, aged Nurr1$+/-$ mice develop slower spontaneous locomotor activity, significantly slower traction reflex, and longer apomorphine-induced climbing behaviour. These behavioural changes are associated with remarkable reduction of striatal DAlevels and nigral DA neurons (Jiang et al., 2005). Furthermore, mutations in the NR4A2 gene, human homologous of the mouse Nurr1 gene, have been associated with DA dysfunction and PD (Le et al., 2003). Nevertheless, this promising animal model shows deficiencies in the DA system not selective for nigral neurons, a feature this that could limit its use (Jiang et al., 2005).

It has been recently demonstrated that the homeobox transcription factors Engrailed 1 and Engrailed 2 (En1, En2) are cell autonomously and in a gene dose dependent manner required for the survival of nigral DA neurons throughout the entire life of these cells (Simon et al., 2001); (Alberi et al., 2004). Most interestingly, in En1$+/-$/En2$-/-$ (EnHT) mice, a progressive degeneration of

DA neurons in the substantia nigra, in the first three postnatal months, results in a selective nigral DA cell loss of more than 70%. The mice develop with the progression of age, motor impairments associated with a reduced storage and release of DA in the caudate nucleus and putamen. In order to evaluate the adaptive response of the striatal output circuits to the DA denervation, expression levels of genes specific to direct (substance P) and indirect pathways (dopamine receptor 2, dynorphin) was measured and found to be significantly reduced in EnHT mice ($54.3 \pm 6.3\%$; $55.2 \pm 8.1\%$; $53.1 \pm 11.8\%$, respectively) (Sgadò et al., submitted).

The slow and progressive degeneration of nigral neurons seen in EnHT mice resembles the features of the human disease and makes it a unique and innovative model compared to the other models in order to study neuroprotection.

Finally all these models, and EnHT mice particularly, represent available models to test neuroprotection in PD since they present replicable lesions, a predictable pattern of neurodegeneration and a well-characterized behavior, biochemistry and morphology to assist in the understanding of induced changes.

Human trials: from clinical end-points to functional imaging measures

The first line approach for testing the efficacy of a putative neuroprotective agent as sort out by the animal models is to longitudinally assess the patients with either clinical rating scales or objective timed motor tasks. The mostly widely accepted rating scale is the Unified Parkinson's disease Rating Scale, that is a sensitive scale with established low-interobserver variability (Martinez-Martin et al., 1994). However its main disadvantages are that it is subjective and emphasizes bradykinesia. As regards objective timed motor tasks, it is not currently clear which of these tasks is the most sensitive for assessing the disease progression and patients can develop later difficulties completing some of these tasks such as the pronation-supination and finger-dexterity tasks (Lang et al., 1995). It should be noted also that one of the biggest problem using clinical rating scales in order to assess the efficacy of a neuroprotective agent in PD, is confounding symptomatic effect due to either the neuroprotective drug itself or dopaminergic agents added over time to maintain patient function. Several evidences have demonstrated that symptoms in PD do not begin until nigral cell loss reaches a certain critical threshold, possibly 50% (Fearnley and Lees, 1991). This implies that clinical measures of disease progression could underestimate the rate of further cell loss and are more likely to provide a measure of the failure of compensatory mechanisms, such as increased dopamine turnover, to maintain motor status in the face of nigral cell loss (Louis et al., 1999). Also the possibility of a preclinical window represents both a challenge, i.e. the detection of individuals during this preclinical period, and an opportunity, i.e. the beginning of preventive therapy during the preclinical period before symptoms appear. On this ground, it has been proposed that in vivo functional imaging might provide a biological marker for early, even pre-symptomatic, diagnosis of PD and for measuring the severity and progression of PD, therefore also providing solutions to the problems confounding clinical trials of neuroprotection. Although functional imaging could be a putative biomarker for progression in PD, a number of caveats must be considered, including reproducibility, reliability, safety and tolerability. The biomarker clearly should reflect a biological process that changes with progression of PD, and the uptake of the imaging tracer used should not be affected by the putative neuroprotective agent or by symptomatic treatments for PD (Brooks, 2003; Brooks et al., 2003). The molecular investigation in vivo of the nigro-striatal pathway by single photon emission computerized tomography (SPECT) and positron emission tomography (PET) is a sensitive method of measuring in vivo PD neurochemistry. Although in general PET cameras have better resolution than SPECT cameras, SPECT studies may be technologically and clinically more feasible, mainly for large clinical studies that require rapid patient accrual. PET studies may benefit from greater flexibility in the range of radiopharmaceuticals that can be tested, but SPECT has the advantage of radiopharmaceuticals with longer half-lives that could be useful in some studies.

18-F-6-fluorodopa (18F-dopa) PET is a marker of presynaptic dopaminergic terminal function, and reflects dopa transport into the terminal, dopa decarboxylase activity, and dopamine storage capacity (Kuwabara et al., 1993). A strong correlation between the 18F-dopa uptake in the striatum and the postmortem nigral cell count has been reported (Snow et al., 1993). Also a 18F-dopa PET study in monkeys unilaterally lesioned with intracarotid injection of MPTP reported significant correlation between striatal tracer uptake and striatal dopamine levels, tyrosine hydroxylase and dopa decarboxylase activity, and nigral cell counts (Pate et al., 1993). 18F-dopa PET is a reasonable measure in vivo of striatal dopamine levels and dopa decarboxylase activity, although it may be less accurate in reflecting nigral dopamine cell counts, mainly in early PD (Deep et al., 1997). Cross-sectional PET studies in PD have demonstrated that putamen 18F-dopa uptake correlates with UPDRS motor scores, in particular with bradykinesia ratings (Morrish et al., 1995; Otsuka et al., 1996), with a good reproducibility (Vingerhoets et al., 1996). The influence of dopaminergic medication on striatal 18F-dopa uptake is still being investigated. Acute oral administration of clinical dose of levodopa appears to have no significant effect on measured striatal 18F-dopa uptake with the percentage change in this value before and after the drug challenge ranging from -7 to $+5\%$ (Ceravolo et al., 2002). Several ligands are available also for SPECT that tag the Dopamine Transporter (DAT), which is the carrier specific to the dopaminergic neurons, responsible for reuptake of dopamine from synaptic cleft. DAT has been reported to be reduced in striatum in postmortem brain from PD patients and in MPTP-treated monkeys; the loss of DAT paralleled the loss of dopamine in the striatum (Niznik et al., 1991; Bezard et al., 2001). In several studies there was a significant correlation between severity of PD, as measured by the UPDRS, and increasing loss of a DAT ligand (123I Beta CIT) binding in the striatum (Seibyl et al., 1995; Asenbaum et al., 1997). Preclinical studies have raised concern that treatment with dopaminergic antagonists, DAT blockers, and monoamine oxidase B inhibitors could affect binding of DAT ligands (Vander Borght et al., 1995). Ahlskog et al. (1999) reported on 12 levodopa-treated PD patients scanned with 123Ibeta- CIT prior to addition of pergolide, after 6 weeks of pergolide therapy, and 4 weeks after pergolide wash-out. The tracer uptake in the putamen and in the caudate did not differ significantly among the three scans, however after 6 weeks of treatment with pergolide there was a non-significant trend for increase in striatal uptake of the tracer. Guttman et al. (2001) by using PET and another DAT ligand (11CRTI-32) reported that patients with early and asymmetric PD had reduced DAT binding in all striatal regions examined by 16 to 22% following treatment for 6 weeks with levodopa, whereas patient treated with pramipexole showed significant reductions only in controlateral caudate and ipsilateral putamen. Innis et al. (1999) conducted a study of the effects of treatment with levodopa and selegiline on 123Ibeta- CIT SPECT in eight drug-naïve patients and found no DAT binding changes after 6 weeks of levodopa or 4 weeks of selegiline. Nurmi et al. (2000) found no effect of levodopa treatment for 3 months in seven de novo PD patients on striatal 11CCFT uptake. In another study 10 weeks of levodopa or pramipexole did not cause any significant changes in striatal 123Ibeta- CIT binding in eight de novo patients (PSD, 2002). Very recently the lack of change induced by levodopa on striatal FP-CIT, another SPECT DAT ligand, uptake has been confirmed (Schillaci et al., 2005). Finally no significative change of striatal FP-CIT uptake was observed in 20 drug-naïve PD patients following 6 weeks of pramipexole or ropinirole or cabergoline (Ceravolo, unpublished data). In conclusion although the available data on the pharmacological potential interference on DAT are not definitive, DAT imaging study could be considered as acceptable biomarker of disease progression in PD. Finally it should be noted however that PET and SPECT studies of dopaminergic presynaptic nigro-striatal pathway provide markers of nerve terminal function rather than cell density and so, like clinical assessments, are potentially influenced by compensatory mechanisms.

Preclinical window

Several lines of evidence strongly suggest that dopaminergic imaging can identify subjects during the preclinical phase of their disease. The most extensive preclinical data are from studies that image patients with hemi-Parkinson's disease. Typically, patients begin disease with PD symptoms on one side of the body and progress to bilateral disease within 3 to 6 years (Hoehn and Yahr, 1967). In several imaging studies there was a significant reduction in putamen DAT uptake, ranging from 25 to 40% in the presymptomatic striatum (controlateral to the side without symptoms), demonstrating preclinical dopaminergic loss in these patients due to progress bilaterally (Marek et al., 1996; Morrish et al., 1995). Other attempts to identify preclinical disease with imaging approach have focused on at-risk populations such as family members or unaffected twins of PD patients. 18F-dopa PET studies have reported that in several well characterized kindreds, 11 of 32 asymptomatic relatives were found to have reduced striatal uptake, and three of these subjects subsequently developed symptomatic PD (Piccini et al., 1997). Several asymptomatic co-twins who also showed a reduction in F-dopa activity later developed symptoms of PD, although the concordance rate for monozygotic and dizygotic twins remains uncertain (Piccini et al., 1999). In kindreds of genetically defined PD families, mild loss of dopaminergic presynaptic tracers has been identified in gene-positive but symptom-negative subjects, suggesting a preclinical period of neurodegeneration (Dekker et al., 2003; Khan et al., 2002). These studies must be confirmed with larger sample size and longer clinical follow-up, however the current evidence strongly suggest that imaging can effectively identify preclinical dopaminergic degeneration thus allowing to test on the humans potential neuroprotective or preventive agents sort out by the experimental models.

Conclusions

At moment no drugs have been proven to be neuroprotective or preventive in PD patients. Putative compound pharmacology and pharmacokinetics must be fully investigated and elucidated in the laboratory using proper animal models and tests. The proper translation from the laboratory bench to the clinic will require the need of interaction between basic and clinical researchers. Determining neuroprotective effects in clinical trials is difficult. Functional imaging studies can offer an objective method of assessing disease progression in PD so avoiding several of the problems associated with clinical studies. However PET and SPECT investigations of the dopaminergic presynaptic nigrostriatal pathway provide markers of nerve terminal function rather than cell density, and for this they are potentially interfered by compensatory mechanisms.

References

Ahlskog J, Uitti R, O'Connor M, et al. (1999) The effect of dopamine agonist therapy on dopamine transporter imaging in Parkinson disease. Mov Disord 14: 940–946

Ahskog JE (2003) Parkinson's disease: is the initial treatment established. Curr Neurol Neurosci Rep 3: 289–295

Alberi L, Sgadò P, Simon HH (2004) Engrailed genes are cell-autonomously required to prevent apoptosis in mesencephalic dopaminergic neurons. Development 131: 3229–3236

Andreassen OA, Ferrante RJ, Dedeoglu DW, et al. (2001) Mice with a partial deficiency of manganese superoxide dismutase show increased vulnerability to the mitochondrial toxins malonate, 3-nitropropionic acid, and MPTP. Exp Neurol 167: 189–195

Asenbaun S, Brucke T, Pirker W, et al. (1997) Imaging of dopamine transporter with iodine-123-βCIT and SPECT in Parkinson's disease. J Nucl Med 38: 1–6

Betarbet R, Sherer TB, MacKenzie G, Garcia-Osuna M, Panov AV, et al. (2000) Chronic systemic pesticide exposure reproduces features of Parkinson's disease. Nat Neurosci 3: 1301–1306

Bezard E, Dovero S, Pruiner C, et al. (2001) Relationship between the appearence of symptoms and the level of nigrostriatal degeneration in a progressive 1-methil-4-phenyl-1,2,3,6-tetrahydropyridine-lesioned macaque model of Parkinson's disease. J Neurosci 21: 6853–6861

Bonifati V, Breedveld GJ, Squitieri F, Vanacore N, Brustenghi P, et al. (2002) Localization of autosomal recessive early-onset parkinsonism to chromosome 1p36 (PARK7) in an independent dataset. Ann Neurol 5: 253–256

Braak H, Ghebremedhin E, Rub U, Bratzke H, Del Tredici K (2004) Stages in the development of Parkinson's disease-related pathology. Cell Tissue Res 318: 121–134

Brooks D (2003) Imaging end points for monitoring neuroprotection in Parkinson's disease. Ann Neurol 53 [Suppl 3]: S110–S119

Brooks DJ, Frey KA, Marek KL, et al. (2003) Assessment of neuroimaging techniques as biomarkers of the progression of Parkinson's disease. Exp Neurol 184: 68–79

Ceravolo R, Piccini P, Bailey DL, et al. (2002) 18F-dopa PET evidence that tolcapone acts as a central COMT inhibitor in Parkinson's disease. Synapse 43: 201–207

Corsini GU, Maggio R, Vaglini F (2002) Molecular and cellular events regulating dopamine neuron survival. In: Chiara GD (ed) Handbook of Experimental Pharmacology. Dopamine in the CNS II. Springer-Verlag, Berlin Heidelberg, pp 321–386

Dawson TM, Dawson VL (2002) Neuroprotective and neurorestorative strategies for Parkinson's disease. Nat Neurosci 5 [Suppl]: 1058–1061

Dawson TM, Dawson VL (2003) Rare genetic mutations shed light on the pathogenesis of Parkinson disease. J Clin Invest 111: 145–151

Deep P, Gjedde A, Cumming P, et al. (1997) On the accuracy of an [^{18}F]FDOPA compartmental model: evidence for vesicular starage of [^{18}F]fluorodopamine in vivo. J Neurosci Methods 76: 157–165

Dekker M, Bonifati V, van Swieten J, Leenders N, Galjaard RJ, Snijders P, Horstink M, Heutink P, Oostra B, van Duijn C (2003) Clinical features and neuroimaging of PARK7-linked parkinsonism. Mov Disord. 18: 751–757

Dunnett SB, Bjorklund A (1999) Prospects for new restorative and neuroprotective treatments in Parkinson's disease. Nature 399: A32–A39

Emborg ME (2004) Evaluation of animal models of Parkinson's disease for neuroprotective strategies. J Neurosci Meth 139: 121–143

Fahn S (2003) Description of Parkinson's disease as a clinical syndrome. Ann N Y Acad Sci 991: 1–14

Feany MB, Bender WW (2000) A Drosophila model of Parkinson's disease. Nature 404: 394–398

Fearnley JM, Lees AJ (1991) Ageing and Parkinson's disease: substantia nigra regional selectivity. Brain 114: 2283–2301

Forno LS (1996) Neuropathology of Parkinson's disease. J Neuropathol Exp Neurol 55: 259–272

Funayama M, Hasegawa K, Kowa H, Saito M, Tsuji S, et al. (2002) A new locus for Parkinson's disease (PARK8) maps to chromosome 12p11.2-q13.1. Ann Neurol 51: 296–301

Giasson BI, Duda JE, Quinn SM, Zhang B, Trojanowski JQ, et al. (2002) Neuronal alpha-synucleinopathy with severe movement disorder in mice expressing A53T human alpha synuclein. Neuron 34: 521–533

Goldberg MS, Fleming SM, Palacino JJ, Cepeda C, Lam HA, et al. (2003) Parkin-deficient mice exhibit nigrostriatal deficits but not loss of dopaminergic neurons. J Biol Chem 278: 43628–43635

Guttman M, Stewart D, Hussey D, et al. (2001) Influence of L-Dopa and pramipexole on striatal dopamine transporter in early PD. Neurology 56: 1559–1564

Healy DG, Abou-Sleiman PM, Wood NW (2004) Genetic causes of Parkinson's disease: UCHL-1. Cell Tissue Res 318: 189–194

Hoehn MM, Yahr MD (1967) Parkinsonism: onset, progression and mortality. Neurology 7: 427–442

Holzmann C, Kruger R, Saecker AM, Schmitt I, Schols L, et al. (2003) Polymorphisms of the alpha-synuclein promoter/expression analyses and association studies in Parkinson's disease. J Neural Transm 110: 67–76

Hunot S, Brugg B, Ricard D, et al. (1997) Nuclear translocation of NF-kappaB is increased in dopaminergic neurons of patients with Parkinson's disease. Proc Natl Acad Sci USA 94: 7531–7536

Innis R, Marek K, Sheff K, et al. (1999) Effect of treatment with Levodopa-Carbidopa or L-Selegiline on striatal dopamine transporter SPECT imaging with I[123]β-CIT. Mov Disord 14: 436–442

Itier JM, Ibanez P, Mena MA, Abbas N, Cohen-Salmon C, et al. (2003) Parkin gene inactivation alters behaviour and dopamine neurotransmission in the mouse. Hum Mol Genet 12: 2277–2291

Jeon BS, Jackson-Lewis V, Burke RE (1995) 6-Hydroxydopamine lesion of the rat substantia nigra/time course and morphology of cell death. Neurodegeneration 4: 131–137

Jiang C, Wan X, He Y, Pan T, Jankovic J, et al. (2005) Age-dependent dopaminergic dysfunction in Nurr1 knockout mice. Exp Neurol 191: 154–162

Khan NL, Valente EM, Bentivoglio AR, Wood NW, Albanese A, Brooks DJ, Piccini P (2002) Clinical and subclinical dopaminergic dysfunction in PARK6-linked parkinsonism: an 18F-dopa PET study. Ann Neurol 52: 849–853

Kitada T, Asakawa S, Hattori N, Matsumine H, Yamamura Y, et al. (1998) Mutations in the parkin gene cause autosomal recessive juvenile parkinsonism. Nature 392: 605–608

Kruger R, Kuhn W, Muller T, Woitalla D, Graeber M, et al. (1998) Ala30Pro mutation in the gene encoding alpha-synuclein in Parkinson's disease. Nat Genet 18: 106–108

Kuopio A, Marttila RJ, Helenius H, Rinne UK (2001) Familial occurrence of Parkinson's disease in a community-based case-control study. Parkinsonism Relat Disord 7: 297–303

Kuwabara H, Cumming P, Reith J, et al. (1993) Human striatal L-Dopa decarboxylase activity estimated in vivo using 6-(^{18}F)fluorodopa and positron emission tomography: error analysis and application to normal subjects. J Cereb Blood Flow Metab 13: 43–56

Lang AE, Benabid AL, Koller WC, et al. (1995) The Core Assessment Program Intracerebral Transplantion. Mov Disord 10: 527–528

Langston JW, Ballard P, Tetrud JW, Irwin I (1983) Chronic Parkinsonism in humans due to a product of meperidine-analog synthesis. Science 219: 979–980

Le W, Conneely OM, Zou L, He Y, Saucedo-Cardenas O, et al. (1999) Selective agenesis of mesencephalic dopaminergic neurons in Nurr1-deficient mice. Exp Neurol 159: 451–458

Le WD, Xu P, Jankovic J, Jiang H, Appel SH, et al. (2003) Mutations in NR4A2 associated with familial Parkinson disease. Nat Genet 33: 85–89

Lee MK, Stirling W, Xu Y, Xu X, Qui D, et al. (2002) Human alpha-synuclein-harboring familial Parkinson's disease-linked Ala-53-> Thr mutation causes neurodegenerative disease with alpha-synuclein aggregation in transgenic mice. Proc Natl Acad Sci USA 99: 8968–8973

Leroy E, Boyer R, Auburger G, Leube B, Ulm G, et al. (1998) The ubiquitin pathway in Parkinson's disease. Nature 395: 451–452

Liu A, Joyner AL (2001) EN and GBX2 play essential roles downstream of FGF8 in patterning the mouse mid/hindbrain region. Development 128: 181–191

Louis ED, Tang MX, Cote L, Alfaro B, Mejia H, Marder K (1999) Progression of parkinsonian signs in Parkinson disease. Arch Neurol 56: 334–347

Marek KL, Seibyl JP, Zoghbi SS, et al. (1996) [123I]β CIT/SPECT imaging demonstrates bilateral loss of dopamine transporter in hemi-Parkinson's disease. Neurology 46: 231–237

Martinez-Martin P, Gil Nagel A, Gracia LM, et al. (1994) Unified Parkinson's disease rating scale: characteristic and structure. Mov Disord 9: 76–83

Mathew RT, Yang L, Beal MF (1997) S-methylthiocitrulline, a neuronal nitric oxidase synthase inhibitor, protects against malonate and MPTP neurotoxicity. Exp Neurol 143: 282–286

McNaught KS, Perl DP, Brownell AL, Olanow CW (2004) Systemic exposure to proteasome inhibitors causes a progressive model of Parkinson's disease. Ann Neurol 56: 149–162

Mizuno Y, Matuda S, Yoshino H, Mori H, Hattori N, Ikebe S (1994) An immunohistochemical study on alfa-ketoglutarate dehydrogenase complex in Parkinson's disease. Ann Neurol 35: 204–210

Morrish PK, Sawle GV, Brooks DJ (1995) Clinical and [18F] dopa PET findings in early Parkinson's disease. J Neurol Neurosurg Psychiatry. 59: 597–600

Niznik HB, Fogel EF, Fassos FF, et al. (1991) The dopamine transporter is absent in parkinsonian putamen and reduced in the caudate nucleus. J Neurochem 56: 192–198

Nurmi E, Bergman J, Eskola O, et al. (2000) Reproducibility and effect of L-dopa on dopamine transporter function measurements: a [18F]CFT PET study. J Cerebr Blood F Met 20: 1604–1609

Otsuka M, Ichiya Y, Kuwabara Y, et al. (1996) Differences in the reduced ^{18}F uptakes of the caudate and the putamen in Parkinson's disease: correlations with the three main symptoms. J Neurol Sci 136: 169–173

Paisan-Ruiz C, Jain S, Evans EW, Gilks WP, Simon J, et al. (2004) Cloning of the gene containing mutations that cause PARK8-linked Parkinson's disease. Neuron 44: 595–600

Pate BD, Kuwamata T, Yamada T, et al. (1993) Correlation of striatal fluorodopa uptake in the MPTP monkey with dopaminergic indices. Ann Neurol 34: 331–338

Perese DA, Ulman J, Viola J, Ewing SE, Bankiewicz KS (1989) A 6-hydroxydopamine-induced selective parkinsonian rat model. Brain Res 494: 285–293

Piccini P, Morrish PK, Turjanski N, Sawle GV, Burn DJ, Weeks RA, Mark MH, Maraganore DM, Lees AJ, Brooks DJ (1997) Dopaminergic function in familial Parkinson's disease: a clinical and 18F-dopa positron emission tomography study. Ann Neurol 41: 222–229

Piccini P, Burn DJ, Ceravolo R, Maraganore D, Brooks DJ (1999) The role of inheritance in sporadic Parkinson's disease/evidence from a longitudinal study of dopaminergic function in twins. Ann Neurol 45: 577–582

Polymeropoulos MH, Lavedan C, Leroy E, Ide SE, Dehejia A, et al. (1997) Mutation in the alpha-synuclein gene identified in families with Parkinson's disease. Science 276: 2045–2047

Prezdborski S, Kostic V, Jackson-Lewis V, et al. (1992) Transgenic mice with increased Cu/Zn superoxide dismutase activity are resistant to MPTP-induced neurotoxicity. J Neurosci 12: 1658–1667

Przedborski S, Jackson-Lewis V, Naini AB, Jakowec M, Petzinger G, et al. (2001) The parkinsonian toxin 1-methyl-4-phenyl-1,2,3,6-tetrahydropyridine (MPTP): a technical review of its utility and safety. J Neurochem 76: 1265–1274

PSD (2002) Dopamine transporter brain imaging to assess the effect of pramipexole vs L-dopa on Parkinson disease progression. JAMA 13: 1653–1661

Ravina BM, Fagan SC, Hart RG, et al. (2003) Neuroprotective agents for clinical trials in Parkinson's disease. A systematic assessment. Neurology 60: 1234–1240

Ricaurte GA, Irwin I, Forno LS, DeLanney LE, Langston E, et al. (1987) Aging and 1-methyl-4-phenyl-1,2,3,6-tetrahydropyridine-induced degeneration of dopaminergic neurons in the substantia nigra. Brain Res 403: 43–51

Schapira AHV, Cooper JM, Dexter D, et al. (1989) Mitochondrial complex I deficiency in Parkinson's disease. Lancet 1: 1269

Schillaci O, Pierantozzi M, Filippi, et al. (2005) The effect of levodopa therapy on dopamine transporter SPECT imaging with (123)I-FP-CIT in patients with Parkinson's disease. Eur J Nucl Med Mol Imaging 19: 169–171

Seibyl JP, Marek KL, Quinland D, et al. (1995) Decreased single-Photon emission tomographic [123 I]β-CIT striatal uptake correlated with symptom severity in Parkinson's disease. Ann Neurol 38: 589–598

Seniuk NA, Tatton WG, Greenwood CE (1990) Dose-dependent destruction of the coeruleus-cortical and nigral-striatal projections by MPTP. Brain Res 527: 7–20

Sgadò P, Albéri L, Galasso SL, Ramakers GMJ, Smidt MP, Dyck RH, Simon HH (2005) Progressive postnatal degeneration of nigral dopaminergic neurons in Engrailed mutant mice. Science (submitted)

Siderowf A, Stern M (2003) Update on Parkinson disease. Ann Intern Med 138: 651–658

Simon HH, Saueressig H, Wurst W, Goulding MD, O'Leary DD (2001) Fate of midbrain dopaminergic neurons controlled by the engrailed genes. J Neurosci 21: 3126–3134

Singleton AB, Farrer M, Johnson J, Singleton A, Hague S, et al. (2003) alpha-Synuclein locus triplication causes Parkinson's disease. Science 302: 841

Snow BJ, Tooyama I, McGeer EG, et al. (1993) Human positron emission tomographic [^{18}F]fluorodopa studies correlate with dopamine cell counts and levels. Ann Neurol 34: 324–330

Ungerstedt U (1968) 6-Hydroxy-dopamine induced degeneration of central monoamine neurons. Eur J Pharmacol 5: 107–110

Uversky VN (2004) Neurotoxicant-induced animal models of Parkinson's disease: understanding the role of rotenone, maneb and paraquat in neurodegeneration. Cell Tissue Res 318: 225–241

Vander Borght T, Killbourn M, Desmond T, Kuhl D, Frey K (1995) The vescicular monoamine transporter is not regulated by dopaminergic drug treatment. Eur J Pharmacol 294: 577–583

Vieregge P (1994) Genetic factors in the etiology of idiopathic Parkinson's disease. J Neural Transm Park Dis Dement Sect 8: 1–37

Vingerhoets FJ, Schulzer M, Ruth TJ, et al. (1996) Reproducibility and discriminating ability of fluorine -18-6-fluoro-L-Dopa PET in Parkinson's disease. J Nucl Med 37: 421–426

Von Coelln R, Dawson VL, Dawson TM (2004) Parkin-associated Parkinson's disease. Cell Tissue Res 318: 175–184

Von Coelln R, Thomas B, Savitt JM, Lim KL, Sasaki M, et al. (2004) Loss of locus coeruleus neurons and reduced startle in parkin null mice. Proc Natl Acad Sci USA 101: 10744–10749

Ward CD (1994) Does selegiline delay the progression of Parkinson's disease? A critical reevaluation of the DATATOP study. J Neurol Neurosurg Psychiatry 57: 217–220

Youdim MBH, Am OB, Yogev-Falach M, et al. (2005) Rasagiline: neurodegeneration, neuroprotection and mitochondrial permeability transition. J Neurosci Res 79: 172–179

Youdim MBH, Lavie L (1994) Selective MAO-A and B inhibitors, radical scavengers and nitric oxide inhibitors in Parkinson's disease. Life Sci 55: 2077–2082

Zimprich A, Biskup S, Leitner P, Lichtner P, Farrer M, et al. (2004) Mutations in LRRK2 cause autosomal-dominant parkinsonism with pleomorphic pathology. Neuron 44: 601–607

J Neural Transm (2006) [Suppl] 71: 143–156

Journal of Neural Transmission
Printed in Austria

Deprenyl: from chemical synthesis to neuroprotection

K. Magyar[1,2], M. Pálfi[2], V. Jenei[3], É. Szökő[1]

[1] Department of Pharmacodynamics, Semmelweis University, Budapest, Hungary
[2] Neurochemical Research Unit, Hungarian Academy of Sciences, Budapest, Hungary
[3] Institute of Biomolecular Chemistry, Chemical Research Center, Hungarian Academy of Sciences, Budapest, Hungary

Summary During the last decades (−)-deprenyl has become the golden standard of MAO-B inhibitors. It possesses dopamine potentiating and antioxidant properties; however, its effects cannot be explained solely by the enzyme inhibitory action. (−)-Deprenyl prevents the toxicity of certain selective neurotoxins and recently it was demonstrated to increase cell-cell adhesion as well. The complexity of its pharmacological effects reflects the action of both the parent compound and the active metabolites. (−)-Deprenyl and related propargylamines (DRPs) show neuroprotective features in a variety of *in vitro* and *in vivo* models that is dependent on the propargyl moiety. The main presumptive targets to date include glyceraldehyde-3-phosphate dehydrogenase, poly(ADP-ribose) polymerase, some kinase cascades, as well as pro- and antiapoptotic proteins, beside the inhibition of MAO-B. The antiapoptotic activity of DRPs converges upon the maintenance of mitochondrial integrity, due to the initiation of a complex transcriptional program, the details of which are yet to be elucidated.

Introduction

If we take a look at the last decades of Hungarian drug research (−)-deprenyl reached the largest success from the scientific point of view. It was synthesized in 1962 as a "psychic energizer", together with many other monoamine oxidase (MAO) inhibitors. Soon became clear, that these compounds were effective antidepressants, but because of their serious side effects, the "cheese reaction", they fell into disrepute and tricyclic compounds became the drugs of choice in the treatment of depression. (−)-Deprenyl fell into the same basket.

Not much later, the outstanding discovery of Johnston in 1968 helped resuscitate (−)-deprenyl (Johnston, 1968). He described that on the basis of substrate specificity and inhibitor sensitivity MAO has two isoforms. The clorgyline sensitive izoenzyme was named MAO-A, while the insensitive MAO-B. The preferred substrate of MAO-A is serotonin (5-HT), whereas that of the B-isoform is β-phenylethylamine (PEA). Regarding inhibitor specificity, (−)-deprenyl preferentially blocks MAO-B, in contrast to clorgyline, the known selective inhibitor of MAO-A. The non-selective and the A-type selective blockers induce "cheese reaction" and are potent antidepressants, whereas the B-type selective inhibitors of MAO neither trigger this serious side effect, nor are in possession of the antidepressive properties. Nevertheless, they potentiate the effect of dopamine (DA) and show antioxidant characteristics. Due to these beneficial actions, (−)-deprenyl has found its therapeutic role in the treatment of Parkinson's disease (PD).

Regarding the milestones of the history of (−)-deprenyl the following events can be highlighted: The first pharmacological paper came out in 1965 (Knoll et al., 1965). In 1967, the (−)-isomer was declared to be responsible for the most part for MAO-B inhibition (Magyar et al., 1967). (−)-Deprenyl was demonstrated to be a selective inhibitor of MAO-B, in contrast to clorgyline (Knoll and Magyar, 1972). The paper dealing with this issue was published in 1972, and became "science citation classic" since then. Based on clinical observations, Birkmayer and his group stated that (−)-deprenyl potentiated the effect of levodopa and improved the quality of life of parkinsonian patients (Birkmayer et al., 1977). The same group was the first to publish that (−)-deprenyl possesses neuroprotective features and delays disease progression in PD patients (Birkmayer et al., 1985).

During the last 25 years more than 2000 papers have been published in the literature dealing primarily with (−)-deprenyl, and it has been registered for treating PD in more than 40 countries. (−)-Deprenyl played an essential role in MAO research, not only due to its clinical effects, but also by facilitating the discovery of MAO inhibitors

Correspondence: K. Magyar, Department of Pharmacodynamics, Semmelweis University, Nagyvárad tér 4., 1089 Budapest, Hungary
e-mail: kalman.magyar@net.sote.hu

with a propargyl group, similarly to (−)-deprenyl. Present research focuses on the elucidation of the effect of (−)-deprenyl and its congeners in neuroprotection and neuronal rescue.

The synthesis of irreversible inhibitors of MAO

During the early sixties more than 200 compounds have been synthesized in the Chinoin Pharmaceutical Company (Budapest, Hungary) – including (−)-deprenyl – with the aim of developing potent and selective MAO inhibitors (Magyar et al., 1980). All of these compounds possessed a propargylamine structure, and in view of their large number some structure-activity relationships (SAR) were possible to be established. (−)-Deprenyl was synthesized by the Chinoin chemist Z. Ecseri, who attached the well known propargyl group of pargyline to methylamphetamine. These compounds were so called mechanism based "suicide inhibitors", which first bind to the target enzyme, where they are converted to an active compound forming a covalent bond with the active center of the enzyme. Because of the irreversible nature of inhibition, the maintenance of selectivity is troublesome during prolonged administration of these drugs. This difficulty may be overcome by the administration of low doses (Ekstedt et al., 1979). The inhibitors usually show stereo selectivity; R-isomers, such as R-(−)-deprenyl or the R-(+)-enantiomer of J-508 proved to be more potent blockers of MAO-B. Valuable pieces of information were obtained from SARs, which could be summarized as follows:

1. Side chain substitution of (−)-deprenyl at α-position with an ethyl, isopropyl or a benzyl group decreased the MAO inhibitory potency of the compounds.
2. Ring substitution (halogenation, methoxy-substitution, saturation) generally diminished inhibitory potency, except in case of p-fluoro-deprenyl, which proved to be an irreversible, potent B-type selective MAO inhibitor, with equal potency and selectivity to (−)-deprenyl.
3. Omitting the methyl group of deprenyl in the α-position of the side chain (TZ-650) did not change the potency and the stereo-selective action of the parent compound.
4. Replacing the phenyl ring by a furan [(−)-U-1424] or an indanyl group [(+)-J-508] gave birth to valuable selective inhibitors of MAO-B. AGN-1135, also known as rasagiline, is the N-desmethyl derivative of AGN-1133 (same as J-508), which was extensively investigated by Youdim and Finberg (Youdim and Finberg, 1986), and is now at the end of clinical studies.
5. Ring alterations led to A-type selective MAO inhibitors in many cases.

R: 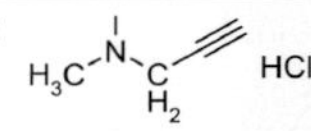	Code No.	Relative efficiency compared to deprenyl in rat brain *in vitro*	
		^{14}C-PEA	^{14}C-5-HT
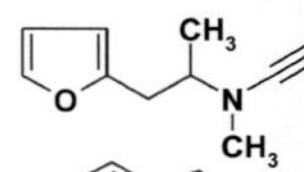	U-1424	0.7	<0.001
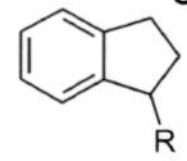	J-508	13	46
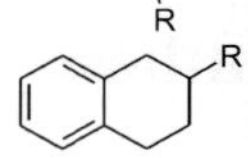	J-518	0.68	45
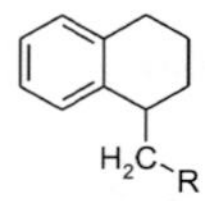	J-517	0.04	75
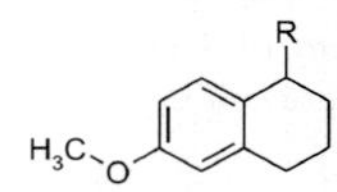	J-519	1.8	163

Fig. 1. Relative efficiency of some selected compounds, compared to (−)-deprenyl, using nuclei free rat brain homogenate and the selective substrates as β-phenylethylamine (^{14}C-PEA) and serotonin (^{14}C-5-HT). The IC_{50} values of the new compounds were divided with that of (−)-deprenyl

The chemical structures of some selected, newly synthesized compounds and their relative potency compared to (−)-deprenyl are depicted in Fig. 1. MAO activity was determined in nuclei free homogenates of rat forebrain, using ^{14}C-labeled β-PEA and 5-HT as selective substrates. The IC_{50} values of the new compounds were compared to that of (−)-deprenyl. (−)-U-1424 and (+)-J-508 are B-type selective MAO inhibitors. The first compound is slightly less potent; however, the efficacy of the latter exceeded that of (−)-deprenyl by one order of magnitude.

(−)-Deprenyl protects against selective neurotoxins

Understanding the mode of action of selective neurotoxins allowed deeper insight into the possible mechanisms of neurodegeneration, thus, facilitating the development of effective neuroprotective substances. Monoamine transmitters are inactivated by means of a membrane-bound high-affinity, energy- and sodium ion-dependent uptake process. Toxins,

Table 1. *Selective neurotoxins*

Dopaminergic	1-methyl-4-phenyl-1,2,3,6-tetrahydropyridine (MPTP) 6-OH-dopamine N-methyl(*R*)salsolinol peroxynitrite N-methyl-isoquinoline (NMIQ)
Noradrenergic	N-[2-chloroethyl]-N-ethyl-2-bromobenzylamine (DSP-4)
Serotonergic	5,6-dihydroxy-serotonin
Cholinergic	ethylcholine aziridinium (AF64A)

being structural analogues to these transmitters, can enter the cell by the same reuptake mechanism, and once inside, they cause selective injury to the neuron. The most widely studied neurotoxins are shown in Table 1.

Selective neurotoxins of Table 1 decrease the transmitter content of the rat brain, which can be prevented by (−)-deprenyl pretreatment. Most of these studies have been carried out with the dopaminergic neurotoxin 1-methyl-4-phenyl-1,2,3,6-tetrahydropyridine (MPTP), whereas our laboratory thoroughly investigated the effect of N-(2-chloroethyl)-N-ethyl-2-bromobenzylamine (DSP-4), a selective noradrenergic neurotoxin as well. In our experiments, DSP-4 was injected i.p., and the noradrenaline (NA) content of the rat hippocampus was determined by an HPLC-EC method, 7 days after DSP-4 treatment. (−)-Deprenyl was administered 1 h before DSP-4 injection. Our recent studies demonstrated that various routes (i.p., oral) and doses (0.25–10 mg/kg) of (−)-deprenyl pretreatment exerted protective effects against DSP-4 induced NA depletion (Fig. 2). Rasagiline, which is a more potent inhibitor of MAO-B than (−)-deprenyl, but lacks uptake inhibitory properties, was not able to prevent DSP-4 induced NA depletion in doses of 1 to 10 mg/kg (for review see: Magyar et al., 2004).

Nevertheless, some contradictory data have also accumulated. Clorgylin, despite its inhibitory action on NA reuptake, does not preclude DSP-4 toxicity. In addition, N-2-hexyl-N-methyl-propargylamine (2-HxMP), a potent selective blocker of MAO-B, without uptake inhibitory features, protects against the NA depleting effect of DSP-4 (for review see: Magyar et al., 2004). It seems possible that the inhibition of uptake cannot fully explain the protection against DSP-4 toxicity, other, yet unknown, mechanisms might also play a role.

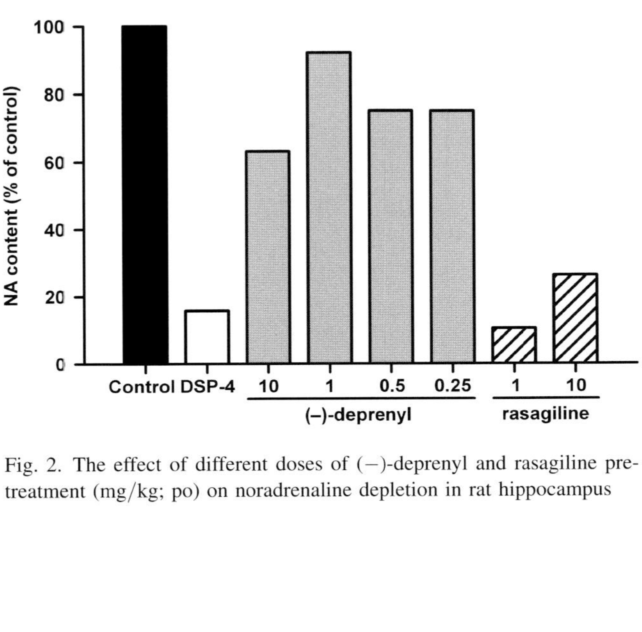

Fig. 2. The effect of different doses of (−)-deprenyl and rasagiline pretreatment (mg/kg; po) on noradrenaline depletion in rat hippocampus

Pharmacokinetics and metabolism of (−)-deprenyl

Therapeutic usage of (−)-deprenyl is based on its DA potentiating effects. The parent compound is established to be responsible for the irreversible inhibition of MAO-B enzyme (for review Magyar et al., 2004). Beside MAO-B inhibition, other mechanisms of action responsible for the therapeutic effects of (−)-deprenyl have also been suggested, and the contribution of the metabolites to its versatile pharmacological profile seems to be essential (Lange et al., 1994; Jenner and Olanow, 1996; Tatton and Chalmers-Redman, 1996; Magyar et al., 1998).

(−)-Deprenyl has considerable first-pass metabolism after oral administration both in humans (Heinonen et al., 1989) and rats (Magyar et al., 1995), and its bioavailability was proved significantly different after various routes of drug administration (Magyar et al., 2004). In humans, rapid oral absorption and low bioavailability was observed (Heinonen et al., 1989; Mahmood, 1997). According to whole body autoradiography and PET studies (Fowler et al., 2001), its maximum brain concentration is reached rapidly, and it is found mainly in brain regions rich in MAO-B enzyme. Reduction of MAO-B activity quickly develops even after a single dose of (−)-deprenyl (Riederer et al., 1978), and is a long-lasting effect because of the irreversible inhibition and slow recovery of the enzyme. The bioavailability was shown to be increased when (−)-deprenyl is administered repeatedly or when taken after food (Barrett et al., 1996a; Laine et al., 2000). Recently, dosage forms providing less first-pass metabolism, such as transdermal patches (Barrett et al., 1996b) or orally disintegrating tablets (Lew, 2005) have been developed, providing higher and more prolonged plasma level of unchanged (−)-deprenyl and lower concentrations of the metabolites compared to those, after oral administration. Because of the considerable metabolic instability of (−)-deprenyl, its plasma and brain concentration is exceeded by some of its metabolites when administered orally (Heinonen et al., 1989; Magyar et al., 1995, 2004).

Desalkylation is recognized as the main metabolic conversion of (−)-deprenyl both in humans and rats: methamphetamine (MA), amphetamine (A) and desmethyldeprenyl (DD) are thus formed (Reynolds et al., 1978; Yoshida et al., 1986; Heinonen et al., 1989). In humans, as well as in rats, MA was proved as the main metabolite of (−)-deprenyl (Reynolds et al., 1978; Heinonen et al., 1989; Shin, 1997; Szökő et al., 1999). In human studies, about 20–60% of a single (−)-deprenyl dose was recovered as MA from the urine within 72 h after treatment (Heinonen et al., 1989; Shin, 1997; Katagi et al., 2002), with considerable interindividual differences. Interestingly, in case of the other enantiomer, (+)-deprenyl, no considerable excess of the formation of MA compared to A was observed. A and MA formed in similar quantities from (+)-deprenyl both in humans and rats (Lengyel et al., 1997; Szökő et al., 1999). In all human studies, very low amount of DD (less than 1.5% of the dose) was detected in the urine (Heinonen et al., 1989; Shin, 1997; Katagi et al., 2002).

During desalkylation, the optical centre on the α-carbon did not change, *R*-(−)-metabolites are formed from *R*-(−)-deprenyl (Szökő and Magyar, 1996; Shin, 1997). The stereochemistry of the metabolites does have importance, because of the differing pharmacological potency of the enantiomers: *R*-(−)-MA is a less potent inhibitor of NA and DA uptake than the *S*-(+)-enantiomer (Tekes and Magyar, 2000). The stereospecific formation of the amphetamine metabolites is in line with the pharmacological differences found between deprenyl enantiomers. (+)-Deprenyl was shown to induce more hyperthermia and possess amphetamine-like psychostimulant effect (Magyar et al., 1967). The different enantiomer forms of the active metabolites should be responsible for these differences. The metabolic studies aimed at the identification of the enantiomeric form of the chiral metabolites of (−)-deprenyl has interest not only to gain information about the stereochemistry of the metabolizing enzymes, but also has forensic importance, because it allows making distinction between (−)-deprenyl and illicit amphetamine users. Cytochrome P450 enzymes are recognized to convert (−)-deprenyl to desalkylated metabolites, although the identification of the isoenzymes involved is equivocal. Based on experiments using various CYP isoform-selective inhibitors, the contribution of CYP2D6 (Grace et al., 1994; Bach et al., 2000), CYP1A2, CYP3A4 (Taavitsainen et al., 2000), and CYP2E1 (Valoti et al., 2000) isoforms to the formation of deprenyl metabolites by desmethylation and despropynylation, has been

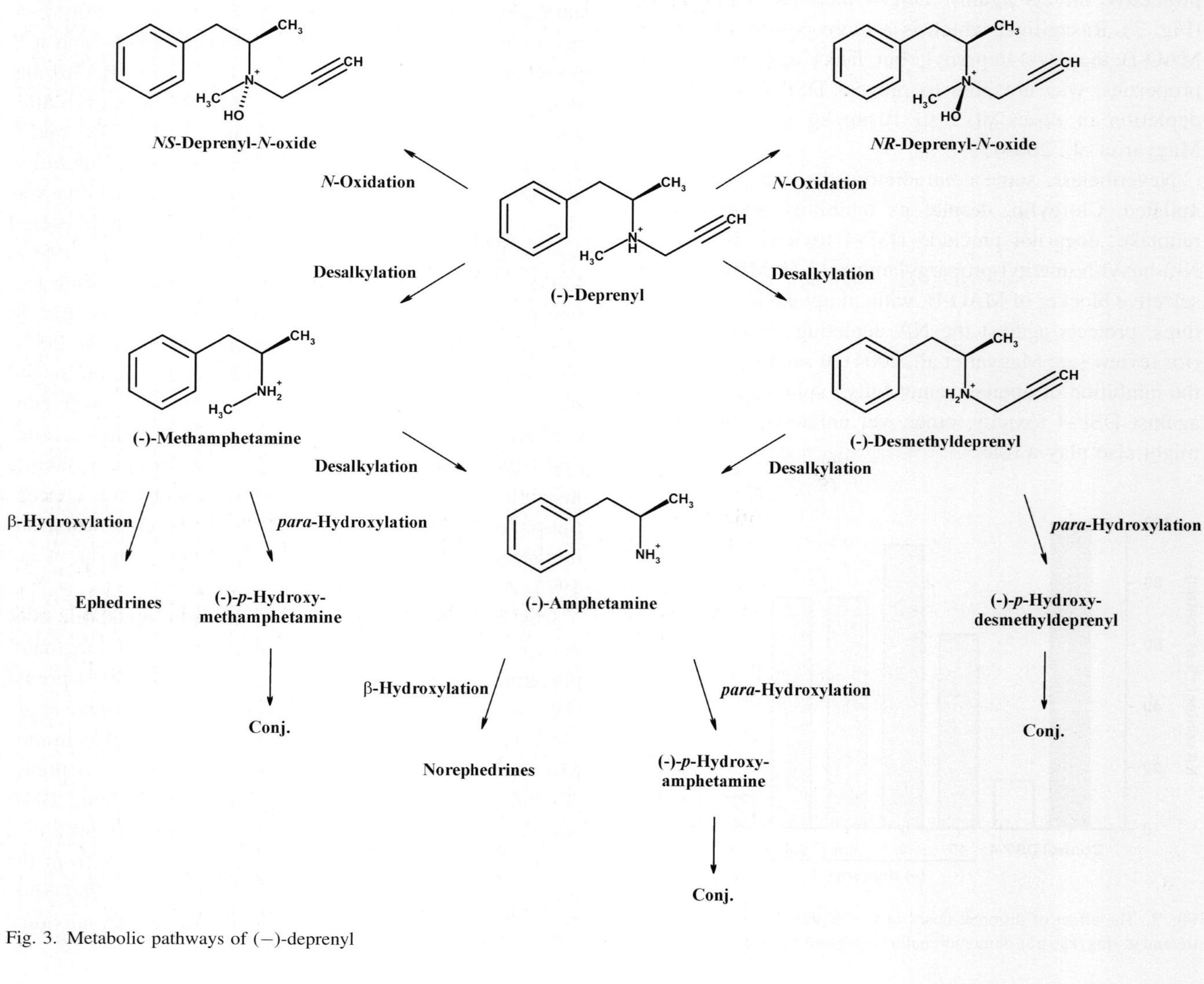

Fig. 3. Metabolic pathways of (−)-deprenyl

suggested. In another type of *in vitro* metabolic study, beside CYP1A2, the involvement of CYP2B6, CYP2C8 and CYP2C19 isoforms in the desalkylation of (−)-deprenyl has been demonstrated (Salonen et al., 2003).

Besides the desalkylated metabolites, formation of other minor metabolites by the hydroxylation of the benzene ring at *para* position (Shin, 1997; Katagi et al., 2002) and by β-hydroxylation (with the formation of ephedrine, pseudoephedrine, norephedrine and norpseudoephedrine) (Shin, 1997) has also been reported in humans. (The scheme of the metabolism is shown in Fig. 3.) Majority of the *para*-hydroxylated metabolites are excreted in the urine as glucuronide conjugates (Shin, 1997; Szökő et al., 2004a), and such, are regarded as inactive metabolites. In humans, about 10% of the dose was recovered as *p*-hydroxy-methamphetamine (*p*-OH-MA) and *p*-hydroxy-amphetamine (*p*-OH-A) in the urine. However, in the rats, they were found as the major metabolites of (−)-deprenyl. The total amount of *p*-hydroxylated compounds; *p*-OH-A, *p*-OH-MA and para-hydroxy-desmethyldeprenyl (*p*-OH-DD) in the urine has reached 50–60% of the dose during 24 h after the last treatment, following a seven-days drug administration, significant proportion (46–64%) of which was excreted as conjugates (Szökő et al., 2004a). Trace amounts of ephedrine-type metabolites were also detected in human urine, although their amount was less than 1% of the dose administered. During β-hydroxylation, the chiral configuration at the α-carbon did not change (Shin, 1997).

Recently, urinary excretion of another deprenyl metabolite, deprenyl-*N*-oxide (DNO) has also been demonstrated (Katagi et al., 2001, 2002). The identification of this metabolite in previous metabolic studies has failed, probably because of the analytical method used. Majority of these studies were performed by gas chromatography after sample derivatization, using acyl reagents (Szebeni et al., 1995; Shin, 1997), and under the derivatization conditions, DNO can degrade to MA and DD. The higher amount of MA metabolites measured in the studies using GC (Reynolds et al., 1978; Heinonen et al., 1989; Shin, 1997) compared to HPLC/MS method (Katagi et al., 2002) can also be explained by the possible conversion of DNO to MA during sample pre-treatment. The oxidation of the tertiary amine resulting in the formation of *N*-oxide was suggested to be catalyzed by the flavin-containing monooxygenase (FMO) enzymes (Tsutsumi et al., 2004). *In vitro* metabolic studies, using liver microsomal preparations, have shown considerable species-differences in the formation of deprenyl-*N*-oxide (Lévai et al., 2005). The oxidation of the tertiary amine, the generation of DNO is accompanied by the creation of a new chiral centre on the quaternary nitrogen atom, *NS*- or *NR*-deprenyl-*N*-oxides thus can be formed. Stereoselective DNO formation in rats has been demonstrated in our laboratory with preferred formation of the *NS* enantiomers; *NS*-DNO was excreted in 3–5 fold excess in urine compared to the *NR*-DNO (Tábi et al., 2003).

Table 2. *Deprenyl-N-oxid enantiomers (% of the parent compound) formed from deprenyl enantiomers during 30 min incubation with recombinant human FMO enzymes*

Compound	Enzyme	*NS*-DNO	*NR*-DNO	S/R ratio
(−)-Deprenyl	FMO1	6.15	0.98	6.28
	FMO3	0.98	1.57	0.62
(+)-Deprenyl	FMO1	4.02	0.30	13.40
	FMO3	0.33	1.09	0.30

Our *in vitro* metabolism studies using human recombinant FMO enzymes have confirmed that *N*-oxidation reaction is catalyzed by both FMO1 and FMO3 isoenzymes (Szökő et al., 2004b). When deprenyl enantiomers were incubated with recombinant human FMO1 and FMO3 preparations, respectively, the metabolic conversion showed considerable product stereoselectivity, which was opposite for the two enzyme isoforms. The preferred configuration after oxidation of nitrogen by FMO3 was *NR*, while it was *NS* in the FMO1 catalyzed reaction (Table 2). More significant product stereoselectivity has been found in case of FMO1. (−)-Deprenyl was more readily oxidized by FMO1, than FMO3. The higher metabolic activity of FMO1, the extrahepatic isoform in humans, toward (−)-deprenyl suggests the importance of extrahepatic organs in the formation of DNO metabolite. Human recombinant FMO1 and FMO3 enzymes have shown not only opposite product stereoselectivity, but their substrate preference was also stereoselective. *N*-oxidation of (−)-deprenyl is preferred compared to that of *S*-(+)-deprenyl. In these studies it was also shown that (−)-MA is a substrate of only the FMO1, but not the FMO3 enzyme. Low amount of (−)-methamphetamine-hydroxylamine was detected in the FMO1 enzyme-catalyzed reaction, which was partly further converted to (−)-amphetamine-hydroxylamine. This product is likely reduced to A, in accordance with findings previously reported by Yoshida (Yoshida et al., 1986). *In vivo* metabolic studies both in humans and rats indicated the rapid urinary excretion of DNO, mainly in the first 6 hours after (−)-deprenyl dosing (Katagi et al., 2002; Szökő et al., 2004a). Its excreted amount is comparable to that of MA during this period after treatment.

Contribution of the metabolites to the complex pharmacological actions of (−)-deprenyl has been suggested by several authors (Tatton and Chalmers-Redman 1996; Magyar et al., 1998). Because of their propargyl structure, DNO and DD are the most probable candidates to possess neuroprotective and/or antiapoptotic activity. Pharmacological studies with DNO performed in our laboratory revealed that it possesses antiapoptotic activity similarly to low dose of (−)-deprenyl, without the proapoptotic activity characteristic of high dose of (−)-deprenyl. The impact of the stereoselectivity of DNO formation, and the potential pharmacological differences between the DNO diastereomers require further studies, as well as the elucidation of the role of the *N*-oxide metabolite in the promising pharmacological effects of (−)-deprenyl.

Neuroprotection by propargylamines: cellular targets in antiapoptotic signalling

Neurodegenerative disorders are characterized by a continuous loss of neurons, that is rather indicative of a slowly progressing apoptotic cell death, than a more drastic and prompt necrotic course. Indeed, apoptosis seems to be more favorable for pharmacologic intervention, because of the broader therapeutic window; necrosis, once begun, is an irreversible process. (−)-Deprenyl was the first propargyl compound that has been shown by Birkmayer's group in a retrospective clinical trial to possess neuroprotective features (Birkmayer et al., 1985; Birkmayer and Birkmayer, 1986), which was later confirmed by Tatton and his colleagues, who demonstrated that (−)-deprenyl interfered with certain apoptotic events in partially differentiated, serum- and NGF-withdrawn PC-12 cells (Tatton et al., 1994). Since then, the neuroprotective and neuronal rescue activities of (−)-deprenyl and ensuing propargylamines (e.g. rasagiline or *N*-propargyl-1-aminoindan; TCH346, also known as CGP 3466B; 2-HMP or 2-heptyl-N-methylpropargylamine) have been justified in a huge variety of *in vitro* and *in vivo* models (for an overview, see Tabakman et al., 2003; Waldmeier and Tatton, 2004); however, their exact mechanism of action still challenges today's scientists.

The antiapoptotic activity of (−)-deprenyl and other related propargylamines (DRPs) is centered upon the protection of mitochondria (Wadia et al., 1998; Naoi et al., 2002). Dissipation of the mitochondrial transmembrane potential ($\Delta\Psi_m$) initiates an apoptotic cascade by opening of the mitochondrial membrane permeability transition pore (PTP), a complex channel through which several proapoptotic factors (e.g. cytochrome-c, apoptosis inducing factor, Smac/DIABLO, etc.) leak to the cytoplasm. In the cytoplasm they assemble into an apoptosome that is able to activate effector caspases, responsible for the execution of the apoptotic program. The role of Bcl-2 protein members in controlling PTP is also of major interest, and their regulation by propargylamines has also been confirmed (Tatton et al., 2002; Mandel et al., 2005). The Bcl-2 protein family is composed of death inhibitors (Bcl-2, Bcl-X_L, Bcl-w), as well as death promoters (Bcl-X_S, Bad, Bax, Bak, Bid), the actual ratio of which is decisive from the point of view of cell survival or death. Bcl-2 proteins can translocate to the mitochondrial membrane, where they enhance or inhibit the increase in membrane permeability (Jayanti et al., 2001). (−)-Deprenyl and rasagiline have been demonstrated to elevate the levels of Bcl-2 and Bcl-X_L and decrease that of Bax and Bad to maintain $\Delta\Psi_m$ and mitochondrial integrity. Mitochondria are a major focus, on which a number of proapoptotic events converge, still, it is not fully understood, whether propargylamines directly influence PTP through binding to MAO-B or a similar structure, located in the mitochondrial membrane, or interfere exclusively with upstream events, thus halting the process before it comes to mitochondria. Surely, both assumptions have a rationale and do not exclude each other. Besides the Bcl-2 proteins, propargylamines upregulate members of antioxidant enzyme systems (e.g. SOD, catalase, heat shock protein 70), while downregulating those of some signal transduction routes favoring apoptosis (c-Jun, c-Fos, glyceraldehyde-3-phosphate dehydrogenase; GAPDH) (Tatton et al., 2002; Mandel et al., 2005).

Propargylamines, originally developed as MAO-B inhibitors, exert their antiapoptotic effect at the transcriptional level, most probably independently of their enzyme inhibitory action, by modulating the expression of a number of genes resulting in new protein synthesis (Tatton et al., 1996; Maruyama et al., 2002). The propargyl moiety seems to be essential for the neuroprotective action. N-propargylamine itself proved to be enough to stabilize mitochondrial membrane potential and protect SH-SY5Y cells and partially NGF-differentiated PC12 cells *in vitro*, though this effect was relatively weak (Yi et al., 2006; Weinreb et al., 2004), while substances lacking the propargyl group failed to prevent apoptosis (e.g. aminoindan, (R)-3-(2-heptylamino)-propionic acid) (Naoi and Maruyama, 2001). Proper stereochemical configuration of the propargylamine residue is of equal importance, since R-enantiomers of deprenyl, rasagiline and 2-HMP proved to be more potent antiapoptotic agents than the S-enantiomers that may even be free of this beneficial activity (Maruyama et al., 2001; Magyar et al., 1996; Szende et al., 2001).

The establishment of structure-activity relationships can be useful to find the active metabolites of propargylamines that may undergo extensive metabolism in the organism. Rasagiline is metabolised to aminoindan that lacks the propargyl moiety, thus, rasagiline itself conveys the antiapoptotic features. In case of (−)-deprenyl, metabolic inhibition was able to eliminate the antiapoptotic character in cell culture, so an active metabolite was proposed to be responsible for preventing cell death (Magyar and Szende, 2000; Szende et al., 2001; Tatton et al., 2002). Deprenyl is metabolized mostly to (−)-DD, (−)-DNO and (−)-MA *in vivo*; the first two are suitable candidates of blocking apoptosis, whereas the third one is supposed to diminish this potency by its neurotoxic character. (−)-MA has been shown to interfere with the neuroprotective activity of (−)-deprenyl in a concentration equal to the parent compound (Abu-Raya et al., 2002; Bar-Am et al., 2004); however, it has never been demonstrated that (−)-MA influences apoptotic cell death in a concentration likely to be present after the metabolic conversion of an antiapoptotic dose of (−)-deprenyl (10^{-9} M). (−)-MA did not alter the survival of trophically withdrawn PC12 cells under 10^{-7} M (Tatton and Chalmers-Redman, 1996), and no amphetamine-like metabolites could be detected after administration of 10^{-6} M (−)-deprenyl in PC12 cell cultures (Abu-Raya et al., 2002). Though the evidence available does not prove unequivocally that the neurotoxic features of (−)-MA negatively influence the antiapoptotic activity of (−)-deprenyl, rasagiline has been synthesized, the metabolite of which, aminoindan, is supposed to be free of neurotoxic effects (Bar-Am et al., 2004).

Propargylamines influence certain signal transduction pathways within the cell. Rasagiline upregulates the phosphorylated α and ε isoforms of protein kinase C (PKC), which are involved in the non-amyloidogenic α-secretase pathway of amyloid precursor protein (APP) processing, an advantageous feature in treating Alzheimer's disease. The propargylamine moiety is a prerequisite for this activity too, and (−)-deprenyl, as well as N-propargylamine also bear this capacity (Yogev-Falach et al., 2003). A downstream event of PKC activation is phosphorylation of MARCKS (myristoilated alanine-rich C-kinase substrate) and upregulation of RACK-1 (receptor for activated C kinase 1), the deficit of which may contribute to Alzheimer's disease and ageing. Rasagiline enhances the phosphorylation and translocation of PKCα and ε to the hippocampal membrane compartment. Phosphorylated PKC activates the MAP kinase (MAPK)/extracellular signal-regulated kinase (Erk) cascade, a known inhibitor of apoptosis, and the α-isoform induces the overexpression of Bcl-2 (Mandel et al., 2005).

Recently, (−)-deprenyl has been shown to protect human SH-SY5Y neuroblastoma cells and mouse primary dopaminergic neurons against MPP^+-toxicity through the upregulation of the redox-active protein, thioredoxin (Andoh et al., 2005). Thioredoxin enhances the DNA binding of some transcription factors (NF-κB, AP-1) and induces Bcl-2 and MnSOD in response to oxidative stress, which promotes cell survival. The mechanism by which (−)-deprenyl upregulates thiredoxin levels is yet unclear, but it may be accomplished via the induction of redox-responsive c-Myc or c-Jun. These transcription factors are activated by protein kinase A mediated phosphorylation of MAPK/Erk1/2, which is translocated to the nucleus to induce c-Myc; or directly through phosphorylation of c-Myc by protein kinase G.

(−)-Deprenyl is antiapoptotic in a dose that is far too low to block MAO-B, thus MAO-B inhibitory action is considered to convey no benefit from the point of view of antiapoptosis. Still, binding to MAO-B or other related NAD- or FAD-containing enzymes, with or without an alteration in enzyme activity, cannot be ruled out as a possible mechanism of action. Recently, a direct link has been established between transcriptional regulation and the metabolic state of the cell, which necessitates the re-evaluation of the role of metabolic enzymes and their cofactors in gene transcription (Shi and Shi, 2004). These metabolism-related transcription factors are homologues of known metabolic enzymes that retain either their enzymatic activity or the ability to bind metabolic cofactors without being enzymatically active. Besides the intrinsic enzymatic activity, cofactors may be required for proper DNA-binding or for stabilizing protein–protein interactions in the final transcription factor complexes. NAD and FAD are the most common representatives of these, often redox-active, cofactors that map and convert changes in the cellular redox state to a complex transcriptional response.

DRPs are most likely inserted into the FAD-pocket of MAO-B, with pargyline shown to be covalently bound to N^5 of the flavin nucleotide (Binda et al., 2002). Propargylamines also bind GAPDH, the NAD-binding site of which is structurally similar to other FAD-containing enzymes, e.g. MAO-B. Therefore, it may not be a far too weird idea to suppose, that DRPs may target other enzymes as well using FAD or NAD as their cofactor. So far, three classical metabolic enzymes have been investigated as a possible target of DRPs (MAO-B, GAPDH and poly(ADP-ribose)-polymerase-1; PARP-1), that function with the above mentioned cofactors. The success in future research may lie in delineating the role of propargylamines as modifiers of transcriptional activity of these enzymes or their related homologues.

DRPs have been demonstrated to bind glyceraldehyde-3-phosphate dehydrogenase (GAPDH), the well known glycolytic enzyme. Besides having central roles in energy metabolism, GAPDH participates in a nuclear apoptotic pathway, via overexpression, aggregate formation and translocation to the nucleus in tetrameric form (Sawa et al., 1997; Ishitani et al., 1998). One of the upstream regulators of GAPDH expression is p53, a critical regulator of cell cycle and apoptosis, which mediates translocation and nuclear accumulation (Chen et al., 1999). Apoptotic cell death may contribute to the progression of neurodegenerative diseases, and GAPDH has been shown to co-immunoprecipitate with the mutant, denaturated proteins accumulating in the nucleus in PD, Alzheimer's (AD), Huntington's and some triplet repeat genetic disorders (Mazzola and Sirover, 2002). Their role in disease progression is still unclear, and we do not know how GAPDH contributes to this process either. Knockdown of GAPDH by antisense oligonucleotides prevents its nuclear translocation and initiation of the apoptotic machinery, thus translocation of the mutant proteins together with GAPDH seems to be more decisive in cell death than nuclear aggregate formation (Fukuhara et al., 2001). GAPDH may function as a molecular carrier or chaperone, stabilizing a given conformation of the mutant proteins in order to be translocated to the nucleus and initiate neuronal apoptosis. Whether these new functions of GAPDH are in connection with energy status or an altered glycolytic capacity is yet to be elucidated.

For all the above mentioned, GAPDH seems to be a suitable target for influencing neurodegenerative processes. Although the precise role of GAPDH in neuronal apoptosis remains to be clarified, this is the first selective target reported in connection with DRPs concerning antiapoptotic action (Kragten et al., 1998; Carlile et al., 2000). GAPDH binds NAD^+ at a site structurally similar to that of the FAD-binding enzymes, and DRP binding site is near the NAD-binding site. DRPs can prevent the overexpression, aggregate formation and nuclear translocation of GAPDH by converting the enzyme to a dimeric state that is less prone to translocation with retained or increased glycolytic capacity (Minton and Wilf, 1981). Glycolytic activity of cells undergoing apoptosis has been shown to be increased, possibly due to overexpression of tetrameric GAPDH, whereas (−)-deprenyl treatment caused a relative decrease in glycolysis, which is the net effect of the elevated glycolytic capacity of the dimer and the prevention of the increase in GAPDH levels (Carlile et al., 2000). Whether altered energy status, or neuron-specific transcriptional control, or some other functions of GAPDH is of primary importance in connection with apoptosis, requires further elucidation.

PARP is a nuclear enzyme that hydrolizes NAD^+ to poly(ADP-ribosyl)ate a number of nuclear targets after DNA damage. Besides, but certainly in connection with, its inevitable role in DNA repair, PARP also regulates transcription either by modifiying chromatin structure or directly participating in enhancer/promoter binding complexes (for review, see Kraus and Lis, 2003; Meyer-Ficca et al., 2005). Histones H1 and H2B are readily ADP-ribosylated by PARP, which induces chromatin decondensation resulting in further exposure of DNA. This phenomenon may be observed in cells not subject to DNA damage as well. Though shorter polymers are generated, it may still be sufficient to induce transcriptional changes. PARP has also been shown to poly(ADP-ribosyl)ate a number of transcription factors *in vitro* (YinYang1, NF-κB, etc.) preventing their DNA-binding. However, PARP may also function as a transcriptional co-activator directly interacting with non-histone proteins e.g. NF-κB, B-Myb, Oct-1, and facilitating the formation of enhancosome-like complexes. In this respect, co-repression also seems feasible. Enzymatic activity may not be a prerequisite for the functional interaction with transcription factors. PARP is considered as the guardian of the genom that maintains its stability through enabling DNA repair (Bouchard et al., 2003). On the other hand, PARP "sentences the cell to death" by overactivation and subsequent depletion of NAD and ATP stores resulting in a failure of energy metabolism and necrosis, when DNA damage is so excessive, that repair enzymes cannot cope with. A transient activity burst of PARP is also dispensible for the initiation of the apoptotic process, but cleavage of the enzyme by caspase 3 and 7, and a consequent loss of activity is required for the appropriate execution of apoptosis.

Hitherto, only one report exists that deals with the interaction of (−)-deprenyl with PARP-1. Recently, (−)-deprenyl has been reported to potentiate the cellular poly(ADP-ribosyl)ation in response to ionizing γ-radiation (Brabeck et al., 2003). A 40-fold increase in poly(ADP-ribose) (PAR) levels could be observed in control irradiated COR4 cells compared to control unirradiated. After (−)-deprenyl pretreatment ranging from 8 h to 7 days an up to 1.8-fold increase was reported in PAR levels, shorter duration of pretreatment did not lead to statistically significant effects. 3 days of (−)-deprenyl treatment without irradiation did not alter PAR levels; however, downregulated PARP-1 protein levels by 40% compared to control. (−)-Deprenyl did not potentiate DNA strand breakage of γ-irradiated cells, and did not influence significantly the activity of human recombinant PARP-1 *in vitro* in a concentration range of 50 nM–5 μM. Poly(ADP-ribosyl)ating capacity has been demonstrated to correlate with the longevity of different species and (−)-deprenyl, accordingly, increased the lifespan of some laboratory animals (Kitani et al., 2002), that may be attributed to the enhancement of the poly(ADP-ribosylation) response to genotoxic stress. Despite of the controversies, the influence of (−)-deprenyl on PARP-1, another NAD-binding enzyme, seems quite conceivable, and offers a brand new field of research from the point of view of transcriptional regulation in connection with neuroprotective potential.

Maintaining genomic stability would further extend (−)-deprenyl's pharmacological profile from neuroprotection to a more general cytoprotective effect. Indeed, (−)-deprenyl and clorgyline (an irreversible inhibitor of MAO-A) have been shown to protect non-tumorigenic cell lines (HaCaT, immortal human keratinocyte) and explant cultures (normal uroepithelium) after γ-irradiation or cisplatin treatment by enhancing Bcl-2 expression (Seymour et al., 2003). Tumorigenic cell lines (HaCaT-ras, HPV-G; tumorigenic human keratinocyte, PC3; human prostate adenocarcinoma) and bladder tumor explants showed no protection; moreover, (−)-deprenyl potentiated delayed reproductive death in case of tumorigenic cell lines. However, Bcl-2 overexpression cannot be the sole reason for the protective effect of MAO inhibitors, but other contributors in this sense are unknown to date. (−)-Deprenyl may also be a potent inhibitor of non-neuronal apoptosis in case of the cardiac and renal tissue (Qin et al., 2003; Toronyi et al., 2002), further demonstrating that the protective effect of (−)-deprenyl cannot be confined to neurons or neuron-like cells.

Adequate trophic support may protect or rescue dying neurons in several *in vitro* and *in vivo* models. (−)-Deprenyl upregulates the mRNA and protein levels of FGF2, NGF, BDNF and GDNF in cultured astrocytes of different species (Semkova et al., 1996; Riva et al., 1997; Mizuta et al., 2000). The mechanism of action, by which (−)-deprenyl alters neurotrophin levels, is not clear, but the activation of astrocytes and the consequent secretion of various cytokines and neurotrophic factors may contribute to the neuroprotective capacity (Biagini et al., 1994). However, it should be kept in mind, that excessive activation of glial cells may exacerbate cell damage through increased production of reactive oxygen species and augmenting the inflammatory response. Rasagiline has also been shown to increase the transcription of GDNF in human neuroblastoma

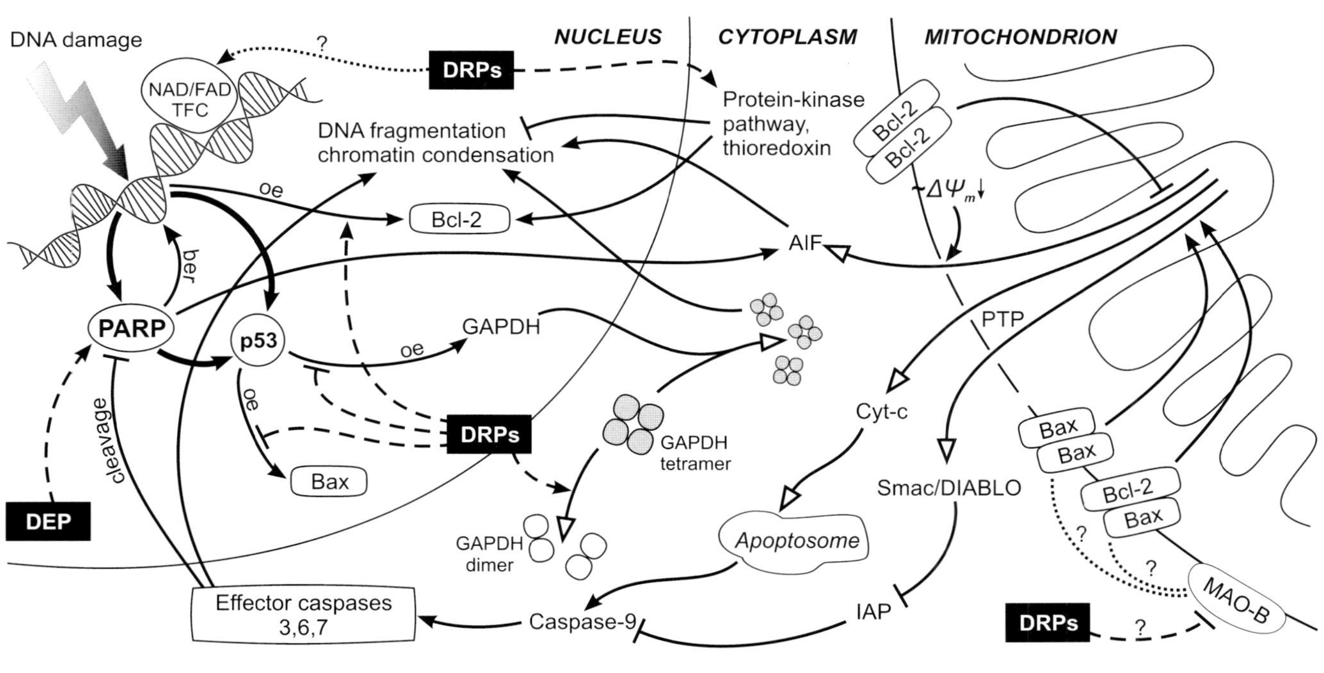

Fig. 4. Possible targets of (−)-deprenyl and related propargylamines in antiapoptotic signalling. DRPs prevent apoptosis by maintaining mitochondrial transmembrane potential through elevated expression of Bcl-2 and decreased expression of Bax. The role of MAO-B, located in the outer mitochondrial membrane, in this process and their blockade by DRPs is still elusive. DRPs convert tetrameric GAPDH to a dimer, thus preventing its overexpression and nuclear translocation that would otherwise initiate an apoptotic program. DRPs also influence protein kinase cascades which further contributes to the neuroprotective potential. Finally, (−)-deprenyl enhances the poly(ADP-ribosyl)ation response to genotoxic stress, promoting repair mechanisms and cell survival. Influencing NAD or FAD binding transcription factor complexes is a hitherto unexplored field in DRP research, which may have a rationale in future. Abbreviations: AIF: apoptosis inducing factor, ber: base excision repair, Cyt c: cytochrome c, DEP: (−)-deprenyl, DRPs: deprenyl related propargylamines, GAPDH: glyceraldehyde-3-phosphate dehydrogenase, IAP: inhibitor of apoptosis, MAO-B: monoamine oxidase B, NAD/FAD TFC: NAD/FAD binding transcription factor complexes, oe: overexpression, PARP: poly(ADP-ribose) polymerase, PTP: permeability transition pore, $\Delta\Psi_m$: mitochondrial transmembrane potential

cell line through an NF-κB-mediated pathway enhancing the phosphorylation of IκB (Maruyama et al., 2004). NF-κB is a two-edged sword in cell death, promoting the transcription of cell survival genes or activating proapoptotic factors depending on the type of cell and conditions of cytotoxic stimuli.

Today, propargylamines presumably interfere with apoptosis, and exert neuroprotective and neurorescue activities by targeting a wide variety of cellular components and influencing multiple pathways of cell death (Fig. 4). The relevance of each of these targets as well as the interdependence of the various routes affected by propargylamines from the point of view of cell survival will be established by future research. Nevertheless, the complex transcriptional changes underlying the effect of these drugs necessitates to reconsider the role of their classical metabolic targets (GAPDH, MAO, PARP) paying more attention to their possible influence of gene expression.

The effect of (−)-deprenyl on cellular functions and signalling

The neuroprotective effect of (−)-deprenyl has been explained by a number of independent theories, including effects on cellular signalling pathways, such as pro- and antiapoptotic pathways, redox signalling or trophic effects of the drug. The pro- and antiapopotic actions of (−)-deprenyl has been described in the previous chapter.

Recently, our research group described a novel, MAO-B independent effect of (−)-deprenyl on cell-cell adhesion, which can also contribute to the protective effect of the drug. We showed that (−)-deprenyl increases cell-cell adhesion of NGF-naïve and NGF-differentiated PC12 cells (originated neuro-ectodermally) and NIH3T3 fibroblasts (non-neuronal) in a concentration-dependent manner (Jenei et al., 2005). Previous results have also shown that (−)-deprenyl is not only neuroprotective, but also protects cells of non-neuronal origin. (−)-Deprenyl can diminish the apoptosis-inducing effect of ischemia-reperfusion in rat kidney (Toronyi et al., 2002), protects the vascular endothelium from the toxic effects of amyloid-beta peptide (Thomas et al., 1998) and reduces myocyte apoptosis *in vivo* (Qin et al., 2003).

We cannot exclude that the cell-cell adhesion-increasing effect of (−)-deprenyl can, to some extent, be attributed to its antiapoptotic effect. Nevertheless, comparison of the antiapoptotic and cell-cell adhesion increasing properties of the drug revealed, that the two functions are most probably, not based on the same mechanism. While both the antiapoptotic and cell-cell adhesion increasing effect of (−)-deprenyl are MAO-B independent, and the (+)-enantiomer of deprenyl was not effective either against apoptosis or in induction of cell-cell adhesion (Magyar and Szende, 2004; Tatton et al., 1994; Jenei et al., 2005), some differences were also found between the two actions of the drug. In case of NIH3T3 cells, the drug was effective in induction of cell-cell adhesion in very low concentrations (10^{-11}–10^{-12} M), however, in PC12 cells the effective concentration range was higher (10^{-7} M in NGF-naïve and 10^{-9} M in NGF-differentiated PC12 cells) than the antiapoptotic concentrations (10^{-11} M in PC12, 10^{-13} M in melanoma) (Tatton et al., 2002; Szende et al., 2001). According to Tatton and his co-workers, (−)-deprenyl prevents apoptotis only of NGF-differentiated PC12 cells, while in our experiments (−)-deprenyl induced cell-cell adhesion of NGF-naïve PC12 cells too, which is another important difference. In several cases, it has been reported that the metabolites of (−)-deprenyl are responsible for the antiapoptotic effects of the drug (Tatton et al., 1996; Szende et al., 2001). In our experiments, SKF525A, an unspecific inhibitor of microsomal drug metabolism, failed to prevent the cell-cell adhesion-inducing effect of (−)-deprenyl, which suggests that this novel action of the drug does not require cytochrome P450-dependent metabolism of (−)-deprenyl. N-oxidation of (−)-deprenyl by flavin containing monooxygenase (FMO) enzymes has also been described (Katagi et al., 2001). Although DNO in a concentration of 10^{-5} M significantly induced cell-cell adhesion of NGF-naïve PC12 cells, this metabolic pathway does not seem to be essential for the effect either, since methimazole (an inhibitor of FMO enzymes) does not appeared to block the effect of (−)-deprenyl on cell-cell adhesion (V. Jenei unpublished results).

The role of cell adhesion has been implicated in a number of processes, which can be involved in the pathogenesis of PD and AD. Cell-matrix and cell-cell adhesion can have regulatory function in cell proliferation and survival by activating signalling cascades *via* integrins and cadherins. This way, adhesion can affect the survival of neurons in neurodegenerative disorders. Although the central nervous system has been considered for a long time to be unable to generate new neurons, by now, a growing number of studies have showed neuroregeneration in certain areas of the adult mammalian brain including the subgranular zone (SGZ) of the hippocampus, or the subvenricular zone (SVZ) of the lateral ventricles. Recent evidences have shown increased neurogenesis in the hippocampus in AD (Jin et al., 2004). Another recent study showed that precursor cell proliferation in the subependymal zone is impaired in PD due to the loss of DA (Höglinger et al., 2004). The existence and importance of neurogenesis in the adult mammalian substantia nigra is not yet clear. It has been shown that progenitor cells exist and can proliferate in this brain region, and some studies have suggested that neurogenesis also occurs in the substantia nigra (Yoshimi et al., 2005; Zhao et al., 2003). Although these findings are still controversial and not all studies could confirm the existence of dopaminergic neurogenesis in this brain region (Frielingsdorf et al., 2004), it cannot be excluded that impaired or insufficient neurogenesis can also contribute to the progression of PD and AD. Cell-cell adhesion is an important process during differentiation and this way neurogenesis as well (Schlett et al., 2000; Hamada-Kanazawa et al., 2004; Laplante et al., 2004), therefore, it is possible that (−)-deprenyl can affect neurogenesis by inducing cell-cell adhesion. Formation of cell–cell contacts is an essential step in synaptogenesis and structural plasticity (the reorganization of synaptic connections) (Garner et al., 2002), which are targets for protective treatments to slow down AD progression and preserve cognitive and functional abilities. Therefore, the positive effect of (−)-deprenyl on cell–cell adhesion could also provide an explanation of the effect of the drug on cognitive functions in AD, which have been shown in some clinical trials (Falsaperla et al., 1990).

It is important to mention here that (−)-deprenyl has been shown to increase the expression of several neurotrophic factors (NGF, BDNF, GDNF, FGF2, IGF1) primarily in astrocytes, which also has the potential to induce survival signals and cell proliferation of progenitor cells in PD and AD (Mizuta et al., 2000; Riva et al., 1997; De la Cruz et al., 1997).

Conclusions

For three decades (−)-deprenyl has been widely used to treat Parkinson's disease, as a consequence of its dopamine-potentiating and antioxidant activity related to MAO-B inhibition. The parent compound itself is primarily responsible for these effects, but the metabolites might also contribute to the complex pharmacological activity of the drug. Usually (−)-deprenyl is administered orally in human therapy, thus, special attention should be paid to the intensive first pass metabolism of the drug (75% of the dose). Increasing the concentration of the parent compound that reaches the systemic circulation might be beneficial; this can be achieved by choosing a more adequate route of administration (nasal spray, transdermal patches). Nevertheless, it has never been noticed, that the (−)-isomers of amphetamin-like metabolites, formed from (−)-deprenyl during metabolism, induce significant amphetaminergic pharmacological activities in doses required for selective MAO-B inhibiton.

Currently, special attention is focused on the effects of (−)-deprenyl in tissue cultures, in concentrations too low to induce MAO-B inhibition. Many laboratories, including ours, investigated the effects of (−)-deprenyl in nanomolar or even lower concentrations *in vitro* and demonstrated that the drug possesses antiapoptotic activity. We have published in 2005 that (−)-deprenyl increases cell adhesion as well. The presence of the propargylamine moiety in the molecule seems indispensable to induce these effects. A good deal of knowledge has accumulated in this field, indicating that an altered complex transcriptional program may be responsible for these activities. *In vitro* studies clearly demonstrate that (−)-deprenyl has a bell-shaped dose-response curve in respect of neuroprotection, which ought to be taken more intensely into consideration during the therapeutic usage of the drug. Finally, it may be concluded that the results obtained in preclinical studies should be considered in human therapy as well, because it could possibly broaden the therapeutic applicability of (−)-deprenyl.

Acknowledgements

This study was supported by the Hungarian National Science Foundation OTKA T-42595 and ETT 141/2003 grants.

References

Abu-Raya S, Tabakman R, Blaugrund E, Trembovler V, Lazarovici P (2002) Neuroprotective and neurotoxic effects of monoamine oxidase-B inhibitors and derived metabolites under ischemia in PC12 cells. Eur J Pharmacol 434: 109–116

Andoh T, Chock PB, Murphy DL, Chiueh CC (2005) Role of the redox protein thioredoxin in cytoprotective mechanism evoked by (−)-deprenyl. Mol Pharmacol 68: 1408–1414

Bach MV, Coutts RT, Baker GB (2000) Metabolism of N,N-dialkylated amphetamines, including deprenyl, by CYP2D6 expressed in human cell line. Xenobiotica 30: 297–306

Bar-Am O, Amit T, Youdim MBH (2004) Contrasting neuroprotective and neurotoxic actions of respective metabolites of anti-Parkinson drugs rasagiline and selegiline. Neurosci Lett 355: 169–172

Barrett JS, Hochadel TJ, Morales RJ, Rohatagi S, DeWitt KE, Watson SK, DiSanto AR (1996b) Pharmacokinetics and safety of a selegiline transdermal system relative to single-dose oral administration in the elderly. Am J Ther 3: 688–698

Barrett JS, Rohatagi S, DeWitt KE, Morales RJ, DiSanto AR (1996a) The effect of dosing regimen and food on the bioavailability of the extensively metabolized, highly variable drug Eldepryl® (selegiline hydrochloride). Am J Ther 3: 298–313

Biagini G, Frasoldati A, Fuxe K, Agnati LF (1994) The concept of astrocyte-kinetic drug in the treatment of neurodegenerative diseases: evidence for L-deprenyl-induced activation of reactive astrocytes. Neurochem Int 25: 17–22

Binda C, Newton-Vinson P, Hubálek F, Edmondson DE, Mattevi A (2002) Structure of human monoamine oxidase B, a drug target for the treatment of neurological disorders. Nat Struct Biol 9: 22–26

Birkmayer W, Birkmayer GD (1986) Effect of (−)-deprenyl in long-term treatment of Parkinson's disease. A 10-years experience. J Neural Transm [Suppl 22]: 219–225

Birkmayer W, Knoll J, Riederer P, Youdim MB, Hars V, Marton J (1985) Increased life expectancy resulting from addition of L-deprenyl to Madopar treatment in Parkinson's disease: a longterm study. J Neural Transm 64: 113–127

Birkmayer W, Riederer P, Ambrozi L, Youdim MB (1977) Implications of combined treatment with 'Madopar' and L-deprenil in Parkinson's disease. A long-term study. Lancet 309: 439–443

Bouchard VJ, Rouleau M, Poirier GG (2003) PARP-1, a determinant of cell survival in response to DNA damage. Exp Hematol 31: 446–454

Brabeck C, Pfeiffer R, Leake A, Beneke S, Meyer R, Bürkle A (2003) L-Selegiline potentiates the cellular poly(ADP-ribosyl)ation to ionizing radiation. J Pharmacol Exp Ther 306: 973–979

Carlile GW, Chalmers-Redman RME, Tatton NA, Pong A, Borden KE, Tatton WG (2000) Reduced apoptosis after nerve growth factor and serum withdrawal: conversion of tetrameric glyceradehyde-3-phosphate dehydrogenase to a dimer. Mol Pharmacol 57: 2–12

Chen R-W, Saunders PA, Wei H, Li Z, Seth P, Chuang DM (1999) Involvement of glyceraldehyde-3-phosphate dehydrogenase (GAPDH) and p53 in neuronal apoptosis: Evidence that GAPDH is upregulated by p53. J Neurosci 19: 9654–9662

De la Cruz CP, Revilla E, Rodriguez-Gomez JA, Vizuete ML, Cano J, Machado A (1997) (−)-Deprenyl treatment restores serum insulin-like growth factor-I (IGF-I) levels in aged rats to young rat level. Eur J Pharmacol 53: 593–604

Ekstedt B, Magyar K, Knoll J (1979) Does the B form selective monoamine oxidase inhibitor lose selectivity by long term treatment? Biochem Pharmacol 28: 919–923

Falsaperla A, Monici Preti PA, Oliani C (1990) Selegiline versus oxiracetam in patients with Alzheimer-type dementia. Clin Ther 12: 376–384

Fowler JS, Volkow ND, Logan J, Franceschi D, Wang GJ, MacGregor R, Shea C, Garza V, Pappas N, Carter P, Netusil N, Bridge P, Liederman D, Elkashef A, Rotrosen J, Hitzemann R (2001) Evidence that L-deprenyl treatment for one week does not inhibit MAO A or the dopamine transporter in the human brain. Life Sci 68: 2759–2768

Frielingsdorf H, Schwarz K, Brundin P, Mohapel P (2004) No evidence for new dopaminergic neurons in the adult mammalian substantia nigra. P Natl Acad Sci USA 101: 10177–10182

Fukuhara Y, Takeshima T, Kashiwaya Y, Shimoda K, Ishitani R, Nakashima K (2001) GAPDH knockdown rescues mesencephalic dopaminergic neurons from MPP^+-induced apoptosis. Neuroreport 12: 2049–2052

Garner CC, Zhai RG, Gundelfinger D, Ziv NE (2002) Molecular mechanisms of CNS synaptogenesis. Trends Neurosci 25: 243–250

Grace JM, Kinter MT, Macdonald TL (1994) Atypical metabolism of deprenyl and its enantiomer, (S)-(+)-N-alpha-dimethyl-N-propynylphenethylamine, by cytochrome P450 2D6. Chem Res Toxicol 7: 286–290

Hamada-Kanazawa M, Ishikawa K, Nomoto K, Uozumi T, Kawai Y, Narahara M, Miyake M (2004) Sox6 overexpression causes cellular aggregation and the neuronal differentiation of P19 embryonic carcinoma cells in the absence of retinoic acid. FEBS Lett 560: 192–198

Heinonen EH, Myllyla V, Sotaniemi K, Lammintausta R, Salonen JS, Anttila M, Savijarvi M, Kottila M, Rinne UK (1989) Pharmacokinetics and metabolism of selegiline. Acta Neurol Scand 126: 93–99

Höglinger GU, Rizk P, Muriel MP, Duyckaerts C, Oertel WH, Caille I, Hirsch EC (2004) Dopamine depletion impairs precursor cell proliferation in Parkinson disease. Nat Neurosci 7: 726–735

Ishitani R, Tanaka M, Sunaga K, Katsube N, Chuang D-M (1998) Nuclear localization of overexpressed glyceraldehyde-3-phosphate dehydrogenase in cultured cerebellar neurons undergoing apoptosis. Mol Pharmacol 53: 701–707

Jayanthi S, Deng X, Bordelon M, McCoy MC, Cadet JL (2001) Methamphetamine causes differential regulation of pro-death and anti-death Bcl-2 genes in the mouse neocortex. FASEB J 15: 1745–1752

Jenei V, Zor K, Magyar K, Jakus J (2005) Increased cell-cell adhesion, a novel effect of R-(−)-deprenyl. J Neural Transm 112: 1433–1445

Jenner P, Olanow CW (1996) Oxidative stress and the pathogenesis of Parkinson's disease. Neurology 47: S161–S170

Jin K, Peel AL, Mao XO, Xie L, Cottrell BA, Henshall DC, Greenberg DA (2004) Increased hippocampal neurogenesis in Alzheimer's disease. P Natl Acad Sci USA 101: 343–347

Johnston JP (1968) Some observations upon a new inhibitor of monoamine oxidase in brain tissue. Biochem Pharmacol 17: 1285–1297

Katagi M, Tatsuno M, Miki A, Nishikawa M, Nakajima K, Tsuchihashi H (2001) Simultaneous determination of selegiline-N-oxide, a new indicator for selegiline administration, and other metabolites in urine by high-performance liquid chromatography-electrospray ionization mass spectrometry. J Chromatogr B 759: 125–133

Katagi M, Tatsuno M, Tsutsumi H, Miki A, Kamata T, Nishioka H, Nakajima K, Nishikawa M, Tsuchihashi H (2002) Urinary excretion of selegiline N-oxide, a new indicator for selegiline administration in man. Xenobiotica 32: 823–831

Kitani K, Minami C, Isobe K, Maehara K, Kanai S, Ivy GO, Carillo M-C (2002) Why (−)-deprenyl prolongs survival of experimental animals: Increase of anti-oxidant enzymes in brain and other body tissues as well as mobilization of various humoral factors may lead to systemic anti-aging effects. Mech Ageing Dev 123: 1087–1100

Knoll J, Ecseri Z, Kelemen K, Nievel J, Knoll B (1965) Phenylisopropylmethylpropinyl-amine (E-250), and new spectrum psychic energizer. Arch Int Pharmacodyn Ther 155: 154–164

Knoll J, Magyar K (1972) Some puzzling pharmacological effects of monoamine oxidase inhibitors. Adv Biochem Psychopharmacol 5: 393–408

Kragten E, Lalande I, Zimmermann K, Roggo S, Schindler P, Müller D, Van Oostrum J, Waldmeier P, Fürst P (1998) Glyceraldehyde-3-phosphate dehydrogenase, the putative target of the anti-apoptotic compounds CGP 3466 and R-(−)-deprenyl. J Biol Chem 273: 5821–5828

Kraus WL, Lis JT (2003) PARP goes transcription. Cell 113: 677–683

Laine K, Anttila M, Huupponen R, Maki-Ikola O, Heinonen E (2000) Multiple-dose pharmacokinetics of selegiline and desmethylselegiline suggest saturable tissue binding. Clin Neuropharmacology 23: 22–27

Lange KW, Riederer P, Youdim MB (1994) Biochemical actions of l-deprenyl (selegiline). Clin Pharmacol Ther 56: 734–741

Laplante I, Beliveau R, Paquin J (2004) RhoA/ROCK and Cdc42 regulate cell–cell contact and N-cadherin protein level during neurodetermination of P19 embryonal stem cells. J Neurobiol 60: 289–307

Lengyel J, Magyar K, Hollósi I, Bartók T, Báthori M, Kalász H, Fürst S (1997) Urinary excretion of deprenyl metabolites. J Chromatogr A 762: 321–326

Levai F, Fejer E, Szeleczky G, Szabo A, Eros Takacsy T, Hajdu F, Szebeni G, Szatmari I, Hermecz I (2005) In vitro formation of selegiline-N-oxide as a metabolite of selegiline in human, hamster, mouse, rat, guinea-pig, rabbit and dog. Eur J Drug Metab Ph 29: 169–178

Lew MF (2005) Selegiline orally disintegrating tablets for the treatment of Parkinson's disease. Expert Rev Neurother 5: 705–712

Magyar K, Ecseri Z, Bernáth G, Sátory É, Knoll J (1980) Structure-activity relationship of selective inhibitors of MAO-B. In: Magyar K (ed) Monoamines oxidases and their selective inhibition. Third Congress of the Hungarian Pharmacological Society, Pergamon Press, Budapest, pp 11–21

Magyar K, Lengyel J, Szatmari I, Gaal J (1995) The distribution of orally administered (−)-deprenyl-propynyl-14C and (−)-deprenyl-phenyl-3H in rat brain. Prog Brain Res 106: 143–153

Magyar K, Pálfi M, Tábi T, Kalász H, Szende B, Szökő É (2004) Pharmacological aspects of (−)-deprenyl. Curr Med Chem 11: 2017–2031

Magyar K, Szende B (2000) In: Cameron EG, Feuer G (eds) Handbook of experimental pharmacology. Apoptosis and its modulation by drugs. Springer-Verlag, Berlin-Heidelberg, Vol 142, pp 457–472

Magyar K, Szende B (2004) (−)-Deprenyl, a selective MAO-B inhibitor, with apoptotic and antiapoptotic properties. Neurotoxicology 25: 233–242

Magyar K, Szende B, Lengyel J, Tekes K (1996) The pharmacology of B-type selective monoamine oxidase inhibitors; milestones in (−)-deprenyl research. J Neural Transm [Suppl 48]: 29–43

Magyar K, Szende B, Lengyel J, Tarczali J, Szatmary I (1998) The neuroprotective and neuronal rescue effects of (−)-deprenyl. J Neural Transm [Suppl 52]: 109–123

Magyar K, Vízi ES, Ecseri Z, Knoll J (1967) Comparative pharmacological analysis of the optical isomers of phenyl-isopropyl-methyl-propinylamine (E-250). Acta Physiol Hung 32: 377–387

Mahmood I (1997) Clinical pharmacokinetics and pharmacodynamics of selegiline. An update. Clin Pharmacokinet 33: 91–102

Mandel S, Weinreb O, Amit T, Youdim MB (2005) Mechanism of neuroprotective action of the anti-Parkinson drug rasagiline and its derivatives. Brain Res Rev 48: 379–387

Maruyama W, Akao Y, Carillo MC, Kitani K, Youdim MBH, Naoi M (2002) Neuroprotection by propargylamines in Parkinson's disease. Suppression of apoptosis and induction of prosurvival genes. Neurotoxicol Teratol 24: 675–682

Maruyama W, Nitta A, Shamoto-Nagai M, Hirata Y, Akao Y, Youdim M, Furukawa S, Nabeshima T, Naoi M (2004) *N*-propargyl-1(*R*)-aminoindan, rasagiline, increases glial cell line-derived neurotrophic factor (GDNF) in neuroblastoma SH-SY5Y cells through activation of NF-κB transcription factor. Neurochem Int 44: 393–400

Maruyama W, Youdim MBH, Naoi M (2001) Antiapoptotic properties of rasagiline, *N*-propargylamine-1(*R*)-aminoindan, and its optical (*S*)-isomer TV1022. Ann NY Acad Sci 939: 320–329

Mazzola JL, Sirover MA (2002) Alteration of intracellular structure and function of glyceraldehydes-3-phosphate dehydrogenase: a common phenotype of neurodegenerative disorders? Neurotoxicology 23: 603–609

Meyer-Ficca ML, Meyer RG, Jacobson EL, Jacobson MK (2005) Poly(ADP-ribose) polymerases: managing genome stability. Int J Biochem Cell B 37: 920–926

Minton AP, Wilf J (1981) Effect of macromolecular crowding upon the structure and function of an enzyme: glyceraldehyde-3-phosphate dehydrogenase. Biochemistry 20: 4821–4826

Mizuta I, Ohta M, Ohta K, Nishimura M, Mizuta E, Hayashi K, Kuno S (2000) Selegiline and desmethylselegiline stimulate NGF, BDNF, and GDNF synthesis in cultured mouse astrocytes. Biochem Bioph Res Co 279: 751–755

Naoi M, Maruyama W (2001) Future of neuroprotection in Parkinson's disease. Parkinsonism Relat D 8: 139–145

Naoi M, Maruyama W, Akao Y, Yi H (2002) Mitochondria determine the survival and death in apoptosis by an endogenous neurotoxin, N-methyl(R)salsolinol, and neuroprotection by propargylamines. J Neural Transm 109: 607–621

Qin F, Shite J, Mao W, Liang CS (2003) Selegiline attenuates cardiac oxidative stress and apoptosis in heart failure: association with improvement of cardiac function. Eur J Pharmacol 461: 149–158

Reynolds GP, Elsworth JD, Blau K, Sandler M, Lees AJ, Stern GM (1978) Deprenyl is metabolized to methamphetamine and amphetamine in man. Brit J Clin Pharmaco 6: 542–544

Riederer P, Youdim MB, Rausch WD, Birkmayer W, Jellinger K, Seeman D (1978) On the mode of L-Deprenyl in the human central nervous system. J Neural Transm 43: 217–226

Riva MA, Molteni R, Racagni G (1997) L-deprenyl potentiates cAMP-induced elevation of FGF-2 mRNA levels in rat cortical astrocytes. Neuroreport 8: 2165–2168

Salonen JS, Nyman L, Boobis AR, Edwards RJ, Watts P, Lake BG, Price RJ, Renwick AB, Gómez-Lechón M-J, Castell JV, Ingelman-Sundberg M, Hidestrand M, Guillouzo A, Corcos L, Goldfarb PS, Lewis DFV, Taavitsainen P, Pelkonen O (2003) Comparative studies on the cytochrome P450-associated metabolism and interaction potential of selegiline between human liver-derived in vitro systems. Drug Metab Dispos 31: 1093–1102

Sawa A, Khan AA, Hester LD, Snyder SH (1997) Glyceraldehyde-3-phosphate dehydrogenase: Nuclear translocation participates in neuronal and nonneuronal cell death. P Natl Acad Sci USA 94: 11669–11674

Schlett K, Czirók A, Tárnok K, Vicsek T, Madarász E (2000) Dynamics of cell aggregation during in vitro neurogenesis by immortalized neuroectodermal progenitors. J Neurosci Res 60: 184–194

Semkova I, Wolz P, Schilling M, Krieglstein J (1996) Selegiline enhances NGF synthesis and protects central nervous system neurons from excitotoxic and ischemic damage. Eur J Pharmacol 315: 19–30

Seymour CB, Mothersill C, Mooney R, Moriarty M, Tipton KF (2003) Monoamine oxidase inhibitors *l*-deprenyl and clorgyline protect non-malignant human cells from ionizing radiation and chemotherapy toxicity. Brit J Cancer 89: 1979–1986

Shi Y, Shi Y (2004) Metabolic enzymes and coenzymes in transcription – a direct link between metabolism and transcription? Trends Genet 20: 445–452

Shin H-S (1997) Metabolism of selegiline in humans. Identification, excretion, and stereochemistry of urine metabolites. Drug Metab Dispos 25: 657–662

Szebeni G, Lengyel J, Székács G, Magyar K, Gaál J, Szatmári I (1995) Gas chromatographic procedure for simultaneous determination of selegiline metabolites, amphetamine, methamphetamine and desmethyl-deprenyl in pig plasma. Acta Physiol Hung 83: 135–141

Szende B, Bökönyi J, Bocsi J, Kéri Gy, Timár F, Magyar K (2001) Anti-apoptotic and apoptotic action of (−)-deprenyl and its metabolites. J Neural Transm 108: 25–33

Szökő É, Kalász H, Magyar K (1999) Biotransformation of deprenyl enantiomers. Eur J Drug Metab Ph 24: 315–319

Szökő É, Magyar K (1996) Enantiomer identification of the major metabolites of (−)-deprenyl in rat urine by capillary electrophoresis. Int J Pharm Adv 1: 320–328

Szökő É, Tábi T, Halász AS, Pálfi M, Kalász H, Magyar K (2004a) Chiral characterization and quantification of deprenyl-N-oxide and other deprenyl metabolites in rat urine by capillary electrophoresis. Chromatographia 60: S245–S251

Szökő É, Tábi T, Borbás T, Dalmadi B, Tihanyi K, Magyar K (2004b) Assessment of the N-oxidation of deprenyl, methamphetamine, and amphetamine enantiomers by chiral capillary electrophoresis: an in vitro metabolism study. Electrophoresis 25: 2866–2875

Taavitsainen P, Anttila M, Nyman L, Karnani H, Salonen JS, Pelkonen O (2000) Selegiline metabolism and cytochrome P450 enzymes: in vitro study in human liver microsomes. Pharmacol Toxicol 86: 215–221

Tabakman R, Lecht S, Lazarovici P (2003) Neuroprotection by monoamine oxidase inhibitors: a therapeutic strategy for Parkinson's disease? Bioessays 26: 80–90

Tábi T, Magyar K, Szökő É (2003) Chiral characterization of deprenyl-N-oxide and other deprenyl metabolites by capillary electrophoresis using dual cyclodextrin system in rat urine. Electrophoresis 24: 2665–2673

Tatton WG, Chalmers-Redman RME (1996) Modulation of gene expression rather than monoamine oxidase inhibition: (−)-Deprenyl-related compounds in controlling neurodegeneration. Neurology 47 [Suppl 3]: S171–S183

Tatton WG, Chalmers-Redman RME, Ju WJH, Mammen M, Carlile GW, Pong AW, Tatton NA (2002) Propargylamines induce antiapoptotic new protein synthesis in serum- and nerve growth factor (NGF)-

withdrawn, NGF-differentiated PC-12 cells. J Pharmacol Exp Ther 301: 753–764

Tatton WG, Ju WYL, Holland DP, Tai C, Kwan M (1994) Deprenyl reduces PC12 cell apoptosis by inducing new protein synthesis. J Neurochem 63: 1572–1575

Tekes K, Magyar K (2000) Effect of MAO inhibitors on the hjgh-affinity reuptake of biogenic amines in rat subcortical regions. Neurobiology (Bp.) 8: 257–264

Thomas T, McLendon C, Thomas G (1998) L-deprenyl: nitric oxide production and dilation of cerebral blood vessels. Neuroreport 9: 2595–2600

Toronyi E, Hamar J, Magyar K, Szende B (2002) Antiapoptotic effect of (−)-deprenyl in rat kidney after ischemia reperfusion. Med Sci Monitor 8: BR65–68

Tsutsumi H, Katagi M, Nishikawa M, Tsuchihashi H, Kasuya F, Igarashi K (2004) In vitro confirmation of selegiline N-oxidation by flavin-containing monooxygenase in rat microsome using LC-ESI MS. Biol Pharm Bull 27: 1572–1575

Valoti M, Fusi F, Frosini M, Pessina F, Tipton KF, Sgaragli GP (2000) Eur J Pharmacol 391: 199–206

Wadia JS, Chalmers-Redman RME, Ju WJH, Carlile GW, Phillips JL, Fraser AD, Tatton WG (1998) Mitochondrial membrane potential and nuclear changes in apoptosis caused by serum and nerve growth factor withdrawal: time course and modification by (−)-deprenyl. J Neurosci 18: 932–947

Waldmeier PC, Tatton WG (2004) Interrupting apoptosis in neurodegenerative disease: potential for effective therapy? Drug Discov Today 9: 210–218

Weinreb O, Bar-Am O, Amit T, Chillag-Talmor O, Youdim MBH (2004) Neuroprotection via pro-survival PKC isoforms associated with Bcl-2 family members. FASEB J 18: 2033–2043

Yi H, Maruyama W, Akao Y, Takahashi T, Iwasa K, Youdim MBH, Naoi M (2006) *N*-Propargylamine protects SH-SY5Y cells from apoptosis induced by an endogenous neurotoxin, *N*-methyl(*R*)salsolinol, through stabilization of mitochondrial membrane and induction of anti-apoptotic Bcl-2. J Neural Transm 113: 21–32

Yogev-Falach M, Amit T, Bar-Am O, Youdim MBH (2003) The importance of propargylamine moiety in the anti-Parkinson drug rasagiline and its derivatives for MAPK-dependent amyloid preursor protein processing. FASEB J 17: 2325–2327

Yoshida T, Yamada Y, Yamamoto T, Kuroiwa Y (1986) Metabolism of deprenyl, a selective monoamine oxidase (MAO) B inhibitor in rat: relationship of metabolism to MAO-B inhibitory potency. Xenobiotica 16: 129–136

Yoshimi K, Ren YR, Seki T, Yamada M, Ooizumi H, Onodera M, Saito Y, Murayama S, Okano H, Mizuno Y, Mochizuki H (2005) Possibility for neurogenesis in substantia nigra of parkinsonian brain. Ann Neurol 58: 31–40

Youdim MBH, Finberg JPM (1986) MAO type B inhibitors as adjunct to L-dopa therapy. In: Yahr MD, Bergmann KJ (eds) Advances in Neurology Vol. 45, pp 127–136

Zhao M, Momma S, Delfani K, Carlen M, Cassidy RM, Johansson CB, Brismar H, Shupliakov O, Frisen J, Janson AM (2003) Evidence for neurogenesis in the adult mammalian substantia nigra. P Natl Acad Sci USA 100: 7925–7930

J Neural Transm (2006) [Suppl] 71: 157–161

Journal of Neural Transmission
Printed in Austria

The use of rasagiline in Parkinson's disease

A. H. V. Schapira

University Department of Clinical Neurosciences, Royal Free and University College Medical School, University College London, London, UK, and
Institute of Neurology, University College London, Queen Square, London, UK

Summary Rasagiline is a novel, potent, irreversible inhibitor of monoamine oxidative B developed for the symptomatic treatment of Parkinson's disease. The drug has shown efficacy in improving motor features in both early and advanced Parkinson's disease patients. The drug appears to be well tolerated and its once daily fixed dose formulation should make for excellent compliance. Rasagiline has also demonstrated important neuroprotective properties in both in vitro and in vivo laboratory studies. A provisional study of neuroprotection in a delayed start clinical trial of early PD patients has also suggested that this benefit may be translated to the clinic. Additional clinical trials are underway to confirm this.

Introduction

Parkinson's disease (PD) is the second most common neurodegenerative disease after Alzheimer disease. It involves the loss of neurones and the development of Lewy body inclusions in multiple areas of the central nervous system including the substantia nigra pars compacta (SNc), the dorsal vagal nucleus, locus coeruleus and cerebral cortex. The characteristic clinical features of PD are the asymmetric onset of bradykinesia rigidity and tremor and these emerge when there is significant cell loss of the dopaminergic neurons in the SNc. The consequent deficiency of dopamine in the nigrostriatal pathway is the basis for the symptomatic treatment of PD by dopaminergic drugs. The first of these to be used was levodopa, now combined with a DOPA-decarboxylase inhibitor. Levodopa remains the most potent drug to improve the motor features of PD, but its use is complicated by the development of 'wearing off' (shortening of its duration of action) and dyskinesias (involuntary movements) at a rate of approximately 10% per annum, although this is much greater in young onset (age <50 years) PD.

A number of other drugs have been introduced for the treatment of PD including the dopamine agonists and monoamine oxidase (MAO)-B inhibitors. Dopamine agonists interact directly with the post-synaptic dopamine receptors of the striatum and can significantly improve motor symptoms. They have the added advantage of a substantially lower risk for the development of motor complications. MAO-B inhibitors reduce the metabolism of synaptic dopamine and therefore increase the duration of action and preservation of dopamine. The first MAO-B inhibitor used in PD was selegiline and this demonstrated an improvement in symptom control in combination with a good tolerance and safety profile. This review focuses on a new MAO-B inhibitor, rasagiline, which has recently received a licence for use in early and advanced PD.

Correspondence: Prof. A. Schapira, University Department of Clinical Neurosciences, Royal Free and University College Medical School, Rowland Hill Street, NW3 2PF London,
e-mail: a.schapira@medsch.ucl.ac.uk

Rasagiline structure and mechanism of action

Selegiline and rasagiline, both propargylamine derivatives but with different base chemical structures, are irreversible selective MAO-B inhibitors. The two drugs have a propargylamine group in common but give rise to different metabolites with distinct pharmacologic properties and structures. Selegiline undergoes metabolism in the liver to L-methamphetamine and desmethylselegiline, which is then converted into L-amphetamine. Like selegiline, desmethylselegiline is an irreversible and selective inhibitor of MAO-B, but the end metabolites of selegiline, L-methamphetamine and L-amphetamine, have no effects on MAO-B. These amphetamine compounds may actually be neurotoxic and inhibit the beneficial effects of selegiline (Mandel et al., 2005; Bar et al., 2004).

Rasagiline is up to 15 times more potent than selegiline in animal models in vivo and in vitro (Bar et al., 2004; Youdim et al., 2001c). In vivo, after either acute or chronic administration, rasagiline is significantly more potent than selegiline in inhibiting rat brain or liver MAO-B (Youdim et al., 2001c). Rasagiline is metabolized to aminoindan via the hepatic cytochrome P450 (CYP) isozyme CYP1A2 (Chen and Swope, 2005), while selegiline, a sympathomimetic amine associated with increases in blood pressure and heart rate, is primarily metabolized to L-methamphetamine via CYP2B6 (Kamada et al., 2002). While some reports suggest that the aminoindan metabolite of rasagiline has neuroprotective activity, L-methamphetamine has neurotoxic activity in vitro and blocks the neuroprotective action of selegiline and rasagiline (Bar et al., 2004). These differences between rasagiline and selegiline have enabled development of the basic moiety of rasagiline in new drugs with potential utility in other neurodegenerative diseases (Youdim et al., 2003).

Neuroprotective properties

The neuroprotective activity of rasagiline has been demonstrated in vitro against a variety of neurotoxins, including the nitric oxide donor 3-morpholinosydnonimine hydrochloride (SIN-1), as well as glutamate, 6-hydroxydopamine (6-OHDA), 1-methyl-4-phenyl-1,2,3,6-tetrahydropyridine (MPTP), β-amyloid, tetrahydroisoquinoline, and serum and growth factor deprivation (Mandel et al., 2005).

In cultures of neonatal rat cerebellar granule cells, the increase in cell death by glutamate-induced excitotoxicity was significantly reduced by the presence of rasagiline in a wide range of concentrations (1 mM to 1 nM) (Bonneh-Barkay et al., 2005). The neuroprotective properties of rasagiline was evaluated in cultured rat adrenal pheochromocytoma PC-12 cells and dopaminergic human neuroblastoma SH-SY5Y cells subjected to serum and nerve growth factor (NGF) withdrawal (Bar et al., 2004). In the absence of serum or NGF, these cells die via an apoptotic process, with significant loss of cell viability within 24 hours. Pretreatment of cells with rasagiline or selegiline significantly reduced cell death, with rasagiline showing a greater efficacy than selegiline. The neuroprotective activity of both rasagiline and selegiline was blocked by the addition of the selegiline metabolite, methamphetamine, but not by the rasagiline metabolite, aminoindan.

Embryonic rat mesencephalic neurons cultured in serum-containing medium for 12 hours showed a substantial reduction in cell survival after being switched to serum-free, defined medium (Finberg, 1998). The addition of rasagiline (1 or 10 μM) but not selegiline (1 or 10 μM) to the cultures significantly improved survival of dopaminergic neurons and increased total neuronal survival. Rasagiline was more effective as a neuronal survival factor than selegiline, increasing total neuronal survival as well as selectively increasing the survival of dopaminergic neurons in rat mesencephalic cultures (Goggi et al., 2000). Both 6-OHDA or SIN-1 induced apoptosis in SH-SY5Y cells and treatment with rasagiline stabilized mitochondrial membrane potential and suppressed the apoptotic cascade (Naoi and Maruyama, 2001).

In the rodent 6-OHDA model of PD treatment with rasagiline produced a considerable reduction in dopaminergic TH-positive cell loss (33 to 39%) and a significant reduction in the area encompassed by the lesion (Blandini et al., 2004). Control animals showed stereotypical rotational behavior following systemic administration of apomorphine, which was significantly reduced in animals treated with a low dose of rasagiline (0.8 mg/kg). This study showed that chronic administration of rasagiline counteracts the progressive degeneration of nigrostriatal dopaminergic neurons caused by 6-OHDA injection.

Molecular mechanisms of neuroprotection

In vitro studies suggest that the antiapoptotic, neuroprotective activity of rasagiline resides in the propargyl moiety and is not related to MAO inhibition. TVP1022, the S-enantiomer of rasagiline, has 1000-fold weaker MAO inhibitory activity but exhibits similar neuroprotective effects in vitro (Youdim and Weinstock, 2001a; Youdim et al., 2001b; Maruyama et al., 2003). Some of the neuroprotective effects of rasagiline have been seen in cell lines and primary neurons that express only the MAO-A isoenzyme. Furthermore, the S-enantiomer of rasagiline, which lacks MAO-inhibitory activity, has also shown protective effects in vitro and in vivo. Thus, the neuroprotective effects of rasagiline cannot be attributed in the main to its inhibition of MAO-B.

By activating antiapoptotic molecules like Bcl-2 and Bcl-xL and the protein kinase C/mitogen-activated protein kinase (PKC/MAPK) pathway, and down-regulating proapoptotic molecules such as Bax and Bad, the propargylamine moiety protects mitochondrial viability and prevents opening of the mitochondrial PTP, caspase activation, and the apoptotic cascade (Mandel et al., 2005; Youdim et al., 2005).

Rasagiline's neuroprotective activity was blocked by an inhibitor of the PKC/MAPK pathway in cultured PC-12 and SH-SY5Y cells subjected to serum and NGF withdrawal (Bar et al., 2004). Rasagiline reduced cell death in PC12 cells following serum deprivation, and prevented the appearance of cleaved forms of caspase-3 and the caspase substrate poly(ADP-ribose) polymerase (PARP) (Weinreb et al., 2004). Results showed that GF109203X, a broad-spectrum PKC inhibitor, markedly reversed rasagiline's suppressive effect on the cleavage and activation of caspase-3 and PARP, suggesting the PKC pathway mediates neuroprotection by rasagiline. Reverse transcriptase-polymerase chain reaction analysis showed that treatment of PC12 cells with rasagiline for 24 hours significantly increased expression of the PKC isoenzymes PKC-α and PKC-ε and antiapoptotic Bcl-2 family members Bcl-xL and Bcl-w, while decreasing the proapoptotic Bcl-2 family member, Bad. These observations suggest that the activation of PKC in association with the Bcl-2 protein family mediates the neuroprotective activity of rasagiline.

Glial cell line-derived neurotrophic factor (GDNF) is known to promote the survival of dopaminergic neurons in vivo and in vitro. Treatment of SH-SY5Y cells with rasagiline (100 nM) produced a marked (6-fold) increase in GDNF protein (Maruyama et al., 2004). This study also showed that rasagiline activated nuclear factor κB (NF-κB), a common transcription factor for GDNF as well as for brain-derived neurotrophic factor, SOD, and Bcl-2. These authors suggested that part of the pharmacological activity of rasagiline and related propargylamines may be due to induction of prosurvival genes such as GDNF and Bcl-2 through NF-κB activation.

Clinical use: early PD

Two studies have been published on the use of rasagiline in patients with early PD (Parkinson Study Group, 2002, 2004). Four hundred and four patients with typical PD and Hoehn and Yahr stage no greater than stage III who had not received dopaminergic drug therapy were enrolled and randomised to placebo or rasagiline (1 or 2 mg/day). In the placebo and rasagiline 1 mg and 2 mg groups, 81%, 83% and 80% respectively were still on 'monotherapy', there were no statistical differences in the rates for either levodopa supplementation or withdrawal. At the end of the six month period, the 1 mg rasagiline group had an improved unified PD rating scale (UPDRS) score compared to placebo of 4.2 units ($p<0.001$), and this was 3.56 ($p<0.001$) for the 2 mg group. Better quality of life scores in the rasagiline arms also accompanied the improvement in motor features. The degree of motor improvement over the six month period was comparable to that seen for selegiline in the DATATOP study (Parkinson Study Group, 1993), but not as great as that seen for dopamine agonists (Adler et al., 1997; Shannon et al., 1997). There were no significant differences in the adverse event profile between the treatment arms and placebo. At six months, the two treatment arms were almost back to their respective baseline UPDRS scores.

The six month study was extended by a further six months with 380 of the original 404 patients entering the treatment phase (Parkinson Study Group, 2004). Patients were continued on their original dose of rasagiline or if on placebo, were given rasagiline 2 mg/day. Patients requiring additional dopaminergic therapy were prescribed either levodopa or a dopamine agonist. The UPDRS was assessed at baseline and various time points up to 52 weeks from initiation. The primary endpoint was the change in total UPDRS from baseline to week 52. Of those in the original placebo, 1 mg or 2 mg rasagiline arms, 68%, 71% and 65% respectively were still on 'monotherapy' at the end of the study.

For the whole 12-month period, improvement from baseline scores was 3.0, 2.0 and 4.1 UPDRS units for the 1 mg, 2 mg and delayed 2 mg cohorts. Those given rasagiline 1 mg/day for 12 months compared to those on the 2 mg dose for only the last 6 months maintained a total UPDRS improvement of 1.82 UPDRS units ($p=0.05$). The 12-month rasagiline 2 mg group had a 2.29 unit ($p=0.01$) improvement over the 2 mg 6-month group.

This long-term study provides several important clinical insights into the potential for rasagiline use in early PD. Rasagiline is well tolerated. There was no significant excess of adverse events in the rasagiline arms compared to the placebo. Specifically, there was no increase in nausea, somnolence or hallucinations, features that occur with other dopaminergic drugs, particularly the dopamine agonists. The symptomatic benefits of rasagiline are maintained over 12 months. In the two rasagiline groups, 52.5% and 63.8% of patients were considered responders respectively. There are also some interesting implications for a potential disease modifying effect in PD, which is discussed in more detail below.

Clinical use: adjunctive therapy

Two studies have been published on the efficacy of rasagiline in PD patients already taking levodopa. The PRESTO trial investigated a total of 472 patients, mean age approximately 63 years, on stable levodopa with at least 2.5 hours of 'off' i.e. poor motor state (Parkinson Study Group, 2005). Patients could also be taking other drugs for PD including a dopamine agonist. The primary end point was a change in mean total daily 'off' time. Placebo decreased 'off' time by 0.9 hours (15% of 'off' time). Rasagiline 0.5 mg/day reduced 'off' time by a mean of 1.4 hours ($p = 0.02$ vs placebo), and 1 mg/day by 1.9 hours ($p < 0.001$ vs placebo), equating to 23% and 29% of 'off' time respectively. Benefits were seen within 6 weeks of randomisation and maintained throughout the 26 week study period. The 1 mg rasagiline dose also resulted in significant improvements in the UPDRS score. Balance difficulty, weight loss, anorexia and weight loss occurred more commonly in the rasagiline groups, but there was no increase in hallucinations, confusion or somnolence. Depression was slightly less common in the 0.5 mg rasagiline group.

The LARGO study investigated the effect of 1 mg/day rasagiline compared to entacapone or placebo in 687 PD patients on stable levodopa but with at least 1 hour of motor fluctuations per day (Rascol et al., 2005). Entacapone is a catechol-O-methyl transferase inhibitor and its administration increases levodopa absorption and prolongs its half-life. Its use with levodopa has been demonstrated to increase 'on' time and reduce 'off' time (Parkinson Study Group, 1997). Placebo reduced 'off' time by 0.4 hours, both rasagiline and entacapone decreased 'off' time by 1.2 hours ($p < 0.0001$ vs placebo). There was a comparable and significant increase in 'on' time without dyskinesias of 0.8 hours with both drugs. Secondary end points including UPDRS and clinical global impression were significantly improved in the treatment groups. Similar benefits were seen in patients above (approximately 28% of subjects) or below age 70 years of age. There was no significant difference in adverse event rates between the placebo and treatment arms, 2% of patients in the rasagiline and entacapone arms had postural hypotension.

These two studies demonstrate that once a day rasagiline (1 mg) significantly improves PD control in patients optimised on levodopa with or without additional therapy e.g. dopamine agonist. It is well tolerated and is effective in younger (<70 years) and older (>70 years) patients. It efficacy is comparable to entacapone, but probably less than that of dopamine agonists which induce a 1–2 hour improvement in PD control (Lieberman et al., 1997, 1998).

Disease modification

The ability to slow or prevent the progression is the most important goal of future therapies for PD. Several compounds have shown promise in the laboratory and some have even shown positive signals in clinical trials. However, no drug has yet demonstrated unequivocally that it has neuroprotective properties (Schapira, 2004).

MAO-B inhibitors were one of the first drugs to be assessed for neuroprotective action. The DATATOP study was a prospective double blind, placebo-controlled, trial that investigated the effect of selegiline 5 mg twice daily and/or 2000iu vitamin E as putative neuroprotective therapies (Parkinson Disease Study Group, 1993). Selegiline significantly delayed the need for levodopa compared to placebo, an effect consistent with slowing of disease progression. However, selegiline was also found to exert a mild symptomatic effect that confounded interpretation of the study. In a long term follow up study of the DATATOP cohort, levodopa patients who had been taking selegiline for seven years compared to those who were changed to placebo after five years, had a significantly slower decline, less wearing off, on-off and freezing, but more dyskinesias in those on deprenyl (Shoulson et al., 2002).

Rasagiline has demonstrated neuroprotective effects in the laboratory (see above). At the end of the TEMPO study, the change in UPDRS motor score between baseline and final visit was greater in patients who were randomised to the placebo group and received only 6 months of rasagiline in comparison to those who had received rasagiline for the entire 12 month period. These results cannot be explained by a symptomatic effect alone as patients in all groups were receiving the drug at the end of the study. At face value, they represent an early disease modifying effect whereby 12 months of rasagiline had a greater effect than 6 months. However, there are potential confounding effects, including the possibility that earlier treatment of PD has a long lasting beneficial effect. Nevertheless, these early results with rasagiline are promising and offer a tempting clinical correlate to the pre-clinical studies.

Conclusions

Rasagiline has proven efficacy in both early and more advanced disease, it is easy to give, well tolerated and compliance should be high in clinical practice. It has an acceptable side effect profile that appears to be better than other drugs for PD. It has shown some early signals for a disease modifying effect but needs further study in this respect.

References

Adler CH, Sethi KD, Hauser RA, Davis TL, Hammerstad JP, Bertoni J (1997) Ropinirole for the treatment of early Parkinson's disease. The Ropinirole Study Group. Neurology 49: 393–399

Bar Am O, Amit T, Youdim M (2004) Contrasting neuroprotective and neurotoxic actions of respective metabolites of anti-Parkinson drugs rasagiline and selegiline. Neurosci Lett 355: 169–172

Blandini F, Armentero MT, Fancellu R, Blaugrund E, Nappi G (2004) Neuroprotective effects of rasagiline in a rodent model of Parkinson's disease. Exp Neurol 187: 455–459

Bonneh-Barkay D, Ziv N, Finberg JPM (2005) Characterization of the neuroprotective activity of rasagiline in cerebellar granule cells. Neuropharm 48: 406–416

Chen J, Swope D (2005) Clinical pharmacology of rasagiline: a novel, second-generation propargylamine for the treatment of Parkinson's disease. J Clin Pharm 45: 878–894

Finberg JP, Takeshima T, Johnston JM, Commissiong JW (1998) Increased survival of dopaminergic neurons by rasagiline, a monoamine oxidase-B inhibitor. Neuroreport 9: 703–707

Goggi J, Theofilipoulos S, Riaz SS, Jauniaux E, Stern GM, Bradford HF (2000) The neuronal survival effects of rasagiline and deprenyl on fetal human and rat ventral mesencephalic neurons in culture. Neuroreport 11: 3937–3941

Kamada T, Chow T, Hiroi T (2002) Metabolism of selegiline hydrochloride, a selective monoamine B-type inhibitor, in human liver microsomes. Drug Metab Pharmacokinet 17: 199–206

Lieberman A, Ranhosky A, Korts D (1997) Clinical evaluation of pramipexole in advanced Parkinson's disease: results of a double-blind, placebo-controlled, parallel-group study. Neurology 49: 162–168

Lieberman A, Olanow CW, Sethi K, Swanson P, Waters CH, Fahn S (1998) A multicenter trial of ropinirole as adjunct treatment for Parkinson's disease. Ropinirole Study Group. Neurology 51: 1057–1062

Mandel S, Weinreb O, Amit T, Youdim MBH (2005) Mechanism of neuroprotection of the anti-Parkinson drug rasagiline and its derivatives. Brain Res Brain Res Rev 48: 379–387

Maruyama W, Weinstock M, Youdim MBH, Nagai M, Naoi M (2003) Anti-apoptotic action of anti-Alzheimer drug, TV3326 [(N-propargyl)-(3R)-aminoindan-5-yl]-ethyl methyl carbamate, a novel cholinesterase-monoamine oxidase inhibitor. Neurosci Lett 341: 233–236

Maruyama W, Nitta A, Shamoto-Nagai M (2004) N-propargyl-1(R)-aminoindan, rasagiline, increases glial cell line-derived neurotrophic factor (GDNF) in neuroblastoma SH-SY5Y cells through activation of NF-κ B transcription factor. Neurochem Intl 44: 393–400

Naoi M, Maruyama W (2001) Future of neuroprotection in Parkinson's disease. Parkinsonism Relat Disord 8: 139–145

Parkinson Study Group (1993) Effects of tocopherol and deprenyl on the progression of disability in early Parkinson's disease. The Parkinson Study Group. N Engl J Med 328: 176–183

Parkinson Study Group (1997) Entacapone improves motor fluctuations in levodopa-treated Parkinson's disease patients. Parkinson Study Group. Ann Neurol 42: 747–755

Parkinson Study Group (2002) A controlled trial of rasagiline in early Parkinson disease: the TEMPO study. Arch Neurol 59: 1937–1943

Parkinson Study Group (2004) A controlled, randomized, delayed-start study of rasagiline in early Parkinson disease. Arch Neurol 61: 561–566

Parkinson Study Group (2005) A randomized placebo-controlled trial of rasagiline in levodopa-treated patients with Parkinson disease and motor fluctuations: the PRESTO Study. Arch Neurol 62: 241–248

Rascol O, Brooks DJ, Melamed E (2005) for the LARGO study group. Rasagiline as an adjunct to levodopa in patients with Parkinson's disease and motor fluctuations (LARGO, Lasting effect in Adjunct therapy with Rasagiline Given Once daily, study): a randomised, double-blind, parallel-group trial. Lancet 365: 947–954

Schapira AH (2004) Disease modification in Parkinson's disease. Lancet Neurol 3: 362–368

Shannon KM, Bennett JP Jr, Friedman JH (1997) Efficacy of pramipexole, a novel dopamine agonist, as monotherapy in mild to moderate Parkinson's disease. The Pramipexole Study Group. Neurology 49: 724–728

Shoulson I, Oakes D, Fahn S, Lang A, Langston JW, LeWitt P (2002) Impact of sustained deprenyl (selegiline) in levodopa-treated Parkinson's disease: a randomized placebo-controlled extension of the deprenyl and tocopherol antioxidative therapy of parkinsonism trial. Ann Neurol 51: 604–612

Weinreb O, Bar-Am O, Amit T, Chillag-Talmor O, Youdim MBH (2004) Neuroprotection via pro-survival protein kinase C isoforms associated with Bcl-2 family members. FASEB J 18: 1471–1473

Youdim MBH, Weinstock M (2001a) Molecular basis of neuroprotective activities of rasagiline and the anti-Alzheimer drug TV3326 [(N-propargyl)-(3R)-aminoindan-5-yl]-ethyl methyl carbamate]. Cell Mol Neurobiol 21: 555–573

Youdim MBH, Wadia A, Tatton W, Weinstock M (2001b) The anti-parkinson drug rasagiline and its cholinesterase inhibitor derivatives exert neuroprotection unrelated to MAO inhibition in cell culture and in vivo. Ann N Y Acad Sci 939: 450–458

Youdim MD, Gross A, Finberg JP (2001c) Rasagiline [N-propargyl-1R(+)-aminoindan], a selective and potent inhibitor of mitochondrial monoamine oxidase B. Br J Pharmacol 132: 500–506

Youdim MBH, Amit T, Bar-Am O, Weinstock M, Yogev-Falach M (2003) Amyloid processing and signal transduction properties of antiparkinson-antialzheimer neuroprotective drugs rasagiline and TV3326. Ann N Y Acad Sci 993: 378–386

Youdim MBH, Bar-Am O, Yogev-Falach M (2005) Rasagiline: neurodegeneration, neuroprotection, and mitochondrial permeability transition. J Neurosci Res 79: 172–179

J Neural Transm (2006) [Suppl] 71: 163–172

Journal of
Neural
Transmission
Printed in Austria

Novel neuroprotective neurotrophic NAP analogs targeting metal toxicity and oxidative stress: potential candidates for the control of neurodegenerative diseases

H. Zheng, D. Blat, M. Fridkin

Department of Organic Chemistry, The Weizmann Institute of Science, Rehovot, Israel

Summary A large body of data indicates that a cascade of events contributes to the neurodegeneration in Alzheimer's disease (AD) and Parkinson's disease (PD). Metal (Fe, Cu, Zn) dyshomeostasis and oxidative stress are believed to play a pivotal role in the pathogenesis of these diseases. Accordingly, multifunctional compounds combining metal chelating and antioxidative activity hold a great promise as potential drugs for treating AD and PD. In this study, two novel NAPVSIPQ (NAP) analogs (M98 and M99) with potential antioxidant-metal chelating ability were designed and investigated, aiming to improve the poor metal chelating and antioxidative activity of NAP. Our studies showed that both M98 and M99 formed stable metal (Fe, Cu, Zn) complexes in water and demonstrated good metal (Fe, Cu, Zn) chelating properties as opposed to the poor metal (Fe, Cu, Zn) chelating properties of their parent peptide NAP. M98 and M99 exhibited significant inhibition of iron-induced lipid peroxidation in rat brain homogenates at concentrations of $\geq$30 μM, while NAP failed to show any inhibition even at 100 μM. In human neuroblastoma cell (SH-SY5Y) culture, M98 and M99 at 1 μM completely protected against 6-hydroxydopamine (6OHDA) toxicity with potency similar to NAP and desferal (DFO), a strong iron chelator and a highly potent radical scavenger. In PC12 cell culture, M98 at the range of 0.001–1 μM displayed potent protection against 6-OHDA toxicity, comparable to NAP and DFO. These results suggest that M98 and M99 deserve further investigation as potential drug candidates for neuroprotection.

Introduction

Alzheimer's disease (AD) and Parkinson's disease (PD) are the most common human neurodegenerative diseases, affecting at least 5% of the population above the age of 65 years. AD is a progressive disease characterized by two types of brain deposits: neurofibrillary tangles and senile plaques. PD is also a progressive syndrome characterized at the cellular level mainly by degeneration of dopamine (DA)-containing neurons within the substantia nigra (McDowell, 2001; Drukarch and van Muiswinkel, 2000). However, despite many decades of research, the etiology of these disorders remains unclear. The complex process of neurodegeneration in these diseases is believed to be attributed to a number of factors (Mandel et al., 2003). In recent years, several lines of evidence indicate that metal ion (Fe^{3+}, Cu^{2+}, Zn^{2+}) dyshomeostasis and oxidative stress may play a pivotal role in the pathogenesis of PD, AD, and other neurodegenerative diseases (Zecca et al., 2004; Reiderer et al., 1989; Jellinger, 1999). First, in PD there is selective increase of iron in the substantia nigra pars compacta (SNPC) (Takanashi et al., 2001) and within the melanized dopamine neurons (Jellinger, 1999); in AD, Fe, Cu, and Zn accumulate within plaques and tangle-bearing neurons (Lovellm et al., 1998). Second, iron and/or copper interact with H_2O_2 (released through normal metabolism in the brain), to yield the highly toxic $^{\bullet}OH$ radical via Fenton reaction, which induces and exacerbates oxidative stress leading to neuronal death (Desport et al., 2002; Huang et al., 2000). Third, the high level of iron in the brain is closely linked to the proliferation of the reactive microglia and the inflammatory responses, as observed in neurotoxin-induced neurodegeneration and neurodegenerative diseases (Shoham et al., 2000). Fourth, amyloid-β (Aβ) aggregation, the hallmark of amyloid deposits in AD brain, occurs even at low physiological concentrations (submicromolar) of Zn^{2+} (Bush et al., 1994). Cu^{2+} and Fe^{3+} also induce marked Aβ aggregation (Christa et al., 2005). Hence, antioxidants and/or metal (Fe, Cu, Zn) chelators are considered

Correspondence: Prof. M. Fridkin, Department of Organic Chemistry, Weizmann Institute of Science, 76100 Rehovot, Israel
e-mail: mati.fridkin@weizmann.ac.il

to have great potential for treating PD, AD, and other neurodegenerative diseases.

In the past decade, a large number of antioxidants such as Vitamin E, ebselen, carotenoids, flavonoids, lipoic acid and lazaroid have been investigated as potential therapeutic agents to control oxidative stress in neurodegenerative disorders (Sen, 1998; Gilgun-Sherki et al., 2002). A few metal chelators such as desferal (DFO), VK28, clioquinol, and M10 have also been shown to possess neuroprotective activity in cell cultures and/or in animal models (Lan and Jiang, 1997; Ben-Shachar et al., 2004; Kaur et al., 2003; Zheng et al., 2005a). However, none of these antioxidants and metal chelators has been successfully introduced for clinical use.

In view of the complexity of neurodegenerative diseases in which a cascade of events contributes to neuronal death (Grunblatt et al., 2004; Zecca et al., 2004), it has become apparent that a single drug therapy may not suffice to significantly modify the course of the disease and offer complete and lasting benefit to patients. It is more likely that syndromes such as AD and PD require the use of multifunctional drugs with several pharmacological traits to target multiple brain systems. Indeed, many bifunctional compounds have improved efficacy as cognitive enhancing agents and/or offer potential for neuroprotection and disease modification. (Youdim and Buccafusco, 2005a, b).

Recently, we have developed multifunctional drugs possessing MAO inhibitory-neuroprotective and iron chelating moieties based on our prototype neuroprotective iron chelator, VK-28 (Ben-Shachar et al., 1990). M30, a representative of this novel class of iron chelators, has been shown to have neuroprotective activity in cell culture and in animal MPTP model of PD. Besides acting as an antioxidant and iron chelator, M30 is also a highly potent brain selective (striatum, hippocampus) MAO-A and -B inhibitor in vivo with little effects on enzyme activities of the liver and small intestine (Zheng et al., 2005b, c; Gal et al., 2005).

Neuropeptides and their analogs as neuroprotective agents may represent another potential therapeutic strategy in neurodegenerative diseases (Gozes et al., 1997). Some neuropeptides and their analogs, such as VIP and its analog [stearyl-norleucine^{17}]-VIP, have been reported to possess neuroprotective activity in cell cultures and in animal models (Offen et al., 1995; Gozes et al., 1997). Neuropeptides are widely distributed in the central nervous system (CNS), exhibiting neurotransmitter and/or neuromodulator functions in the brain. These peptides are associated with specific neuronal receptors in the brain (Gozes et al., 1997). Thus, antioxidant metal (Fe, Cu, Zn) chelators conjugated to neuropeptides may be directed toward their respective loci where they may exert significant therapeutic activity in various neurodegenerative diseases. This effect may be augmented by the intrinsic capacity of the peptide carrier. Recently, we have designed and synthesized a number of peptidic metal chelators. Preliminary studies have shown that three of them, M7, M27, and M28 (derivatives of VIP and substance-P, respectively) are potent neuroprotective agents in vitro with multifunctional properties: metal ions (Fe^{3+}, Cu^{2+}, Zn^{2+}) chelation, $^{\bullet}OH$ radical scavenging, and lipid peroxidation (LPO) inhibition (Zheng et al., 2005d).

An eight-amino-acid peptide, NAPVSIPQ (NAP), has been identified as the smallest active element of activity-dependent neuroprotective protein (ADNP), a glial cell mediator of VIP-induced neuroprotection. NAP was reported to possess potent neuroprotective action in cell cultures and animal models (Gozes et al., 2003). Various NAP analogs were synthesized and investigated, some of which have been shown to possess, in vitro and/or in vivo, neuroprotective activities comparable to their parent peptide NAP (Wilkemeyer et al., 2003; Brenneman et al., 2004). However, NAP and all its known analogs appear to have poor affinity for metal ions (Fe^{3+}, Cu^{2+}, Zn^{2+}).

In the present study, two NAP analogs with potential metal (Fe, Cu, Zn) binding affinity were designed and synthesized. Their metal binding ability, antioxidative activity and in vitro neuroprotective effects were investigated and compared with their parent peptide NAP and a prototype iron chelator DFO.

Materials and methods

General

Unless otherwise stated, all chemicals and reagents were of analytical grade and were purchased from Sigma-Aldrich (St Louis, MO, USA), Merck (Darmstadt, Germany), or Fluka (Buchs, Switzerland). Trifluoroacetic acid (TFA) for high performance liquid chromatography (HPLC) was obtained from Merck (Darmstadt, Germany). N-α-9-fluorenylmethoxycarbonyl (Fmoc)-protected amino acid derivatives and Rink amide resin were purchased from Novabiochem (Laufelfingen, Switzerland). Crude peptides were subjected to preparative HPLC purification, performed on a Waters system composed of two model 510 pumps: model 680 automated gradient controller and model 441 absorbance detector (Waters, Milford, MA). The column effluents were monitored by UV absorbance at 220 nm. HPLC pre-packed columns were Vydac RP-18 or RP-4 columns (250 × 22 mm; 10 μm bead size, Merck, Darmstadt, Germany) for preparative purifications and Vydac RP-4 (250 × 3.2 mm; 5 μm bead size) or Lichrospher100 RP-8 (250 × 4 mm; 5 μm bead size, Merck, Darmstadt, Germany) for analytical purposes. HPLC purification was achieved by using a linear gradient established between 0.1% TFA in water as solvent A and 0.1% TFA in 75% acetonitrile in water (v/v) as solvent B. Solutions containing purified peptides were lyophilized overnight. Molecular weights of all peptides were confirmed by mass spectrometry. Mass spectra (DI, EI-MS) were measured on a VG-platform-II electrospray single quadropole mass spectrometry (Micro Mass, UK). Unless otherwise specified, spectrophotometric studies were performed with an Ultrospec 2100 Pro UV/visible spectrophotometer (Biochrom, UK).

Synthesis of NAP (Asn-Ala-Pro-Val-Ser-Ile-Pro-Gln) and [Cys⁴]NAP

NAP (Asn-Ala-Pro-Val-Ser-Ile-Pro-Gln) and $[Cys^4]$NAP (Asn-Ala-Pro-Cys-Ser-Ile-Pro-Gln) were synthesized via the Fmoc strategy by automatic procedure with an APEX 396 synthesizer (Advanced Chemtech, Louisville, KY, USA), using commercially available protocols. Benzotriazol-1-yloxy-tris-pyrrolidino-phosphonium hexafluorophosphate (PyBOP) and, when necessary, a combination of N,N′-dicyclohexylcarbodiimide (DCC) and 1-hydroxybenzotriazole (HOBT) were utilized as coupling agents. N-methyl pyrrolidone (NMP) and N,N′-di-methylformamide (DMF) were used as solvents. Before each coupling, deprotection of the α-amino group was achieved by reaction with 20% piperidine in DMF. All synthesized peptides were deprotected and cleaved from the resin using a solution of TFA: triethylsilane (TES): anisole: water (85:5:5:5 v/v). The cleavage mixtures were filtered and the peptides were precipitated from the solution with peroxide-free dry ether at 0°C. Precipitated peptides were washed with cold dry ether, dissolved in water or water/acetonitrile solution, and lyophilized. Since the purity of the crude peptides was usually >90%, they were used for the next conjugation stage without further purification.

Synthesis of M98: Asn-Ala-Pro-Val-Ser-Ile-Pro-Glu(NHOH)-OH

To 2-chlorotrityl chloride resin (17.9 mg, 25 μmole) was added a mixture of Fmoc-Glu(ODmab)-OH (17.0 mg, 25 μM), N, N-diisopropylethylamine (DIPEA, 13.0 mg, 100 μM), and dry CH_2Cl_2 (179 μl). After 120 min shaking, the solution was drained and the resin was washed with 3 × DCM/MeOH/DIPEA (17:2:1), 2 × DCM, 2 × DMF, 2 × DCM, and dried in vacuum over KOH. The attachment of the other amino acids to the resin was carried out via the Fmoc strategy as described above in the synthesis of NAP. To remove the protective group Dmab, the synthesized peptide on the resin was treated with 2% hydrazine · H_2O in DMF for 7 min and washed with 5% DIPEA in DMF. To the peptide-resin was added O-tert-butyl-hydroxylamine hydrochloride (Me_3CONH_2 · HCl, 6.3 mg, 50 μmol) and PyBOP (26 mg, 50 μM) in 0.5 ml DMF, and NMM (10 mg 100 μmol). The resulting mixture was shaken for 1 h. The liquid was drained and a second coupling was performed with equal amounts of Me_3CONH_2 · HC, PyBOP and NMM. A third coupling was performed via DCC/HOBT activation: a mixture of Me_3CONH_2 (9.5 mg, 75 μmol), HOBT (20.3 mg, 150 μmol), and DCC (31 mg, 150 μmol) in 1 ml DMF was added to the resin followed by shaking for 18 h. The solution was drained and the resin was washed (DMF × 3, DCM × 3). The resulting peptide was cleaved from the resin using a solution of TFA: H_2O: TES: Thioanisole (85: 5: 5: 5 v/v) and precipitated with ether. The crude modified peptide was purified to homogeneity by semi-preparative HPLC, as described above. MS: m/z 841.44 $(M+H^+)$ calculated 841.92.

Synthesis of M99: [Cys⁴(HQ)]NAP or Asn-Ala-Pro-Cys[HQ]-Ser-Ile-Pro-Gln

The peptide $[Cys^4]$NAP (6.9 mg, 8.2 μmol) was dissolved in DMF (200 μl), and NMM (13 mg, 7.6 μl, 123 μmol) was added. After 1 h stirring at room temperature (*RT*), a solution of 5-chloromethyl-8-hydroxyquinoline hydrochloride (2 mg, 8.6 μmol) in 150 μl mixed solvent (DMF: DMSO: CH_3CN 3: 3: 1 v/v) was added dropwise. The reaction mixture was stirred overnight at *RT*. Upon completion of the reaction, the crude peptide was precipitated with peroxide-free ice-cold *tert*-butyl methyl ether, collected by centrifugation, and then purified by preparative HPLC. HPLC purification was achieved using a linear gradient established between 0.1% TFA in water as solvent A and 0.1% TFA in 75% acetonitrile in water (v/v) as solvent B. MS: m/z 986.84 $(M+H^+)$ calculated 987.10.

Measurement of Fe (II)-binding potency

Fe (II)-binding capacity of drugs was determined by assessing their ability to compete with ferrozine for ferrous ions, resulting in decrease in the absorbance at 562 nm.

Briefly, the reacted mixture containing ferrozine (50 μM) and various concentrations of the tested compounds was initiated by the addition of $FeSO_4$ (20 μM). After 20 min incubation at RT, the absorbance (at 562 nm) of the resulting solutions was read. Fe (II)-binding capacity was calculated as follows: Fe (II)-binding potency (%) = [1-(Δ absorbance of sample at 562 nm)/(Δ absorbance of control at 562 nm)] × 100.

Lipid peroxidation assay

Lipid peroxidation (LPO) was measured in rat brain mitochondrial membrane homogenates as previously described [36]. This method is based on the oxidation of polyunsaturated fatty acids in biologic membranes, giving rise to a variety of lipid breakdown products such as malondialdehyde (MDA). By reacting MDA with thiobarbituric acid (TBA) a pink pigment is formed, which can be detected by UV-vis spectroscopy. LPO was induced by 50 μM ascorbic acid and 1.5 μM $FeSO_4$. The absorption of thiobarbituric acid derivatives (TBARS) was measured spectrophotometrically at 532 nm.

Cell cultures and treatments

Rat PC12 cells, originating from rat pheochromocytoma, were grown at 37°C in a humid 5% CO_2, 95% air environment in a growth medium containing Dulbecco's modified Eagle's medium (DMEM, Invitrogen, Groningen, the Netherlands) supplemented with glucose (1 mg/1 ml), 5% FCS (fetal calf serum, Bet Haemek, Israel), 10% horse serum and a 1% mixture of penicillin/streptomycin. Human SH-SY5Y neuroblastoma cells were plated in 100-mm culture dishes and cultured in DMEM (4,500 mg/l glucose), containing 10% FCS and 1% of a mixture of penicillin/streptomycin/nystatin. When cells reached the required confluence, the culture medium was removed and the cells were detached by vigorous washing followed by centrifugation at 200 *g* for 5 min. PC12 cells (3×10^3 cells/well) in DMEM with one-third full serum content, or SH-SY5Y cells (1.5×10^4 cells/well) in DMEM with 2% of fetal calf serum, were placed in microtiter plates (96 wells) precoated with collagen (10 mg/cm^2) and allowed to attach for 24 h before treatment. Drugs were added to cells 30 min before insults with 6-hydroxydopamine (200 μM for PC12 or 25 μM for SH-SY5Y). The cells were incubated at 37°C for 24 h before being assayed with MTT.

MTT test for cell viability

The MTT test is based on the conversion of MTT to blue formasan crystals by viable cells. Briefly, 24 h after treatment, the medium was removed and replaced with a medium (100 ml/well) lacking serum. To each well, 10 ml of a 5 mg/ml MTT solution in PBS was added. After incubation at 37°C for 2 h, 100 ml of 10% SDS in 0.01N HCl was added and the solution was mixed thoroughly and incubated for additional 24 h. Absorption was determined in a Perkin-Elmer Dual Wave-length Eliza-Reader at 570 nm/650 nm after automatic subtraction of background readings. Cell viability was expressed as a percentage of cells untreated with 6-hydroxydopamine, which served as the control group and was designated as 100%. The results are expressed as percentage of the control.

Statistical analysis

All assays were performed at least in triplicate and the data were expressed as mean ± SEM. Data were analyzed by Student's *t* test. Variations were considered to be statistically significant at a p value of ≤ 0.05.

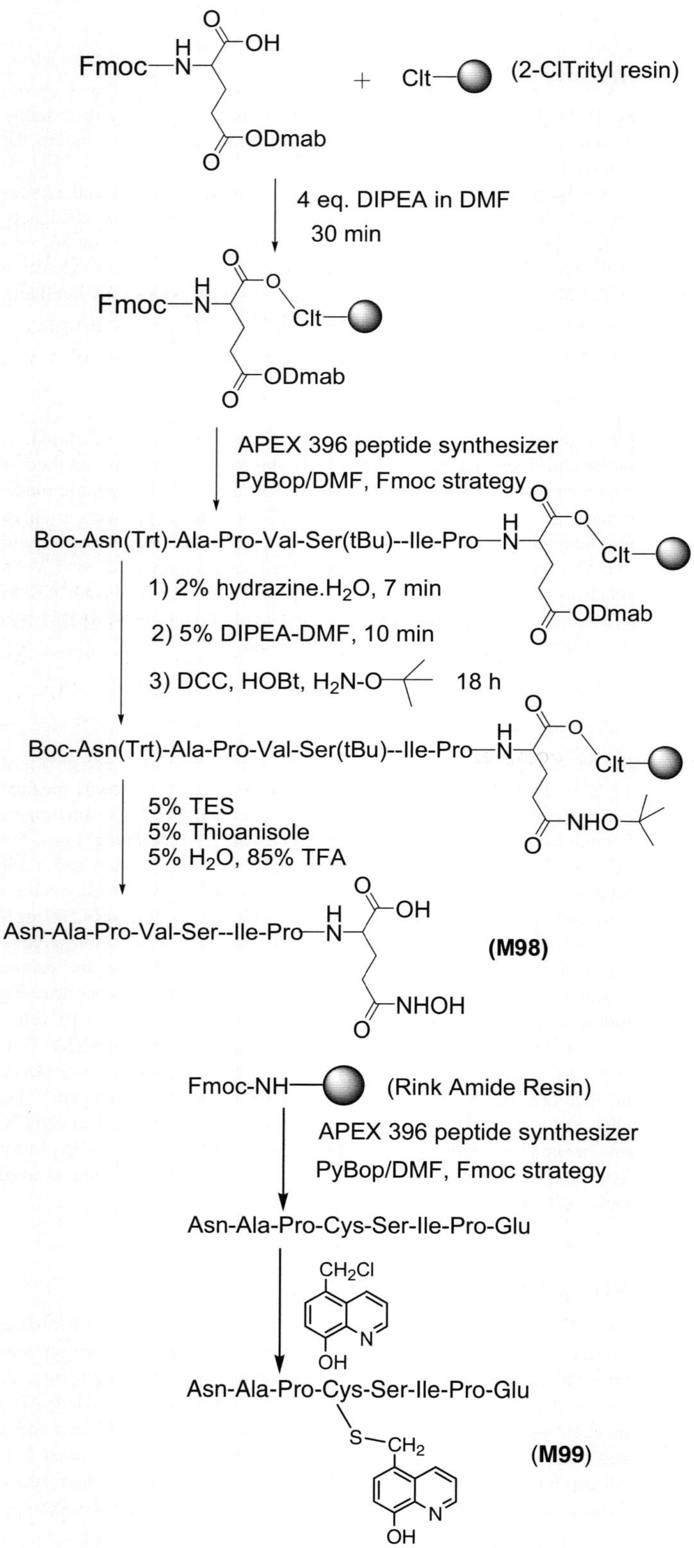

Fig. 1. Strategy for the synthesis of two novel NAP analogs, M98 and M99

Results

Design and synthesis of novel NAP analogs

To obtain novel NAP analogs with potential metal ion (Fe^{3+}, Cu^{2+}, Zn^{2+}) binding affinity, we selected to modify Val^4 and Glu^8 in NAP (Asn-Ala-Pro-Val-Ser-Ile-Pro-Glu). This modification was based on a series of previous observations: (a) The Ser-Ile-Pro region of NAP is crucial for NAP neuroprotection. Ala substitution for either Ser-5 or Pro-7 or Ile-6 abolished NAP neuroprotection or caused a decrease in potency (Wilkemeyer et al., 2003). (b) Ala substitution at Asn^1, Val^4, or Glu^8 in NAP did not reduce neuroprotective efficacy (Wilkemeyer et al., 2003). (c) Hydrophobic amino acids, including the two prolines, are important in preventing beta sheet conformation in order to inhibit or prevent Aβ aggregation (Soto, 1999). The synthetic manipulations yielded two novel NAP analogs, one with an 8-hydroxyquiniline (HQ) moiety, the other with a hydroxamate moiety (RCONHOH). Here we selected HQ and RCONHOH as the metal-chelating moieties because of several attributes: (i) 8-hydroxyquiniline and hydroxamates such as desferal are strong Fe chelators with moderate Cu and Zn binding affinity (Turnquist and Sandell, 1968; Anderegg et al., 1963). (ii) 8-hydroxyquiniline and desferal possess antioxidant properties (Kayyali et al., 1998). (iii) More importantly, neuroprotective activity of desferal and HQ derivatives such as clioquinol and M30 in preventing MPTP neurotoxicity in mice has been reported (Kaur et al., 2003; Zheng et al., 2005b, c; Gal et al., 2005).

The synthesis strategy of the two novel NAP analogs (M98 and M99) is outlined in Fig. 1.

Spectrophotometric study of the formation of metal ion ($Fe^{3+/2+}$, Cu^{2+}, Zn^{2+}) complexes

UV-vis spectroscopy was employed to study the formation of metal ion ($Fe^{3+/2+}$, Cu^{2+}, Zn^{2+}) complexes. The formation of complexes of organic ligands with transition metal ions affects the ligand absorption spectrum, resulting in shift and/or disappearance of bands and appearance of new ones. Our experiments suggested that both M98 and M99 formed stable complexes with Fe(III)/(II), Cu(II) and Zn(II) in water at RT. The absorption spectra of M99 and NAP in the absence and presence of metal ions in water are reported here. As shown in Fig. 2, there were no significant changes in absorption upon the addition of $CuSO_4$ or $FeSO_4$ or $ZnCl_2$ solution to NAP in water. In contrast, substantial absorbance changes were observed when the above metal salt solutions were added to M99 solution. Addition of $FeCl_3$ to either NAP or M99 resulted in absorbance changes, with more substantial changes in the M99 solution. The maximal absorbance changes in the NAP and M99 solutions after the addition of metal salt solutions are shown in Fig. 3. Notably, no significant changes in absorbance of M99-metal complex solutions were observed after 24 h incubation, implying the stability of these complexes in water (not shown).

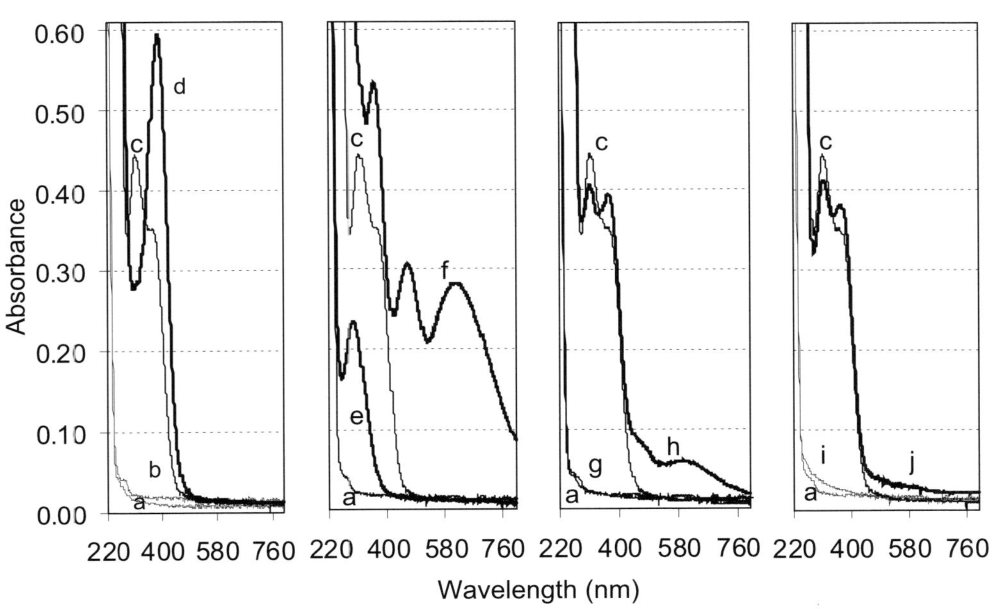

Fig. 2. Absorption spectra of NAP and M99 (both at 0.3 mM in water, pH = 5–7) in the absence and presence of metal salts (0.1 mM): (a) NAP, (b) NAP + $CuSO_4$, (c) M99, (d) M99 + $CuSO_4$, (e) NAP + $FeCl_3$, (f) M99 + $FeCl_3$, (g) NAP + $FeSO_4$, (h) M99 + $FeSO_4$, (i) NAP + $ZnCl_2$, (j) M99 + $ZnCl_2$

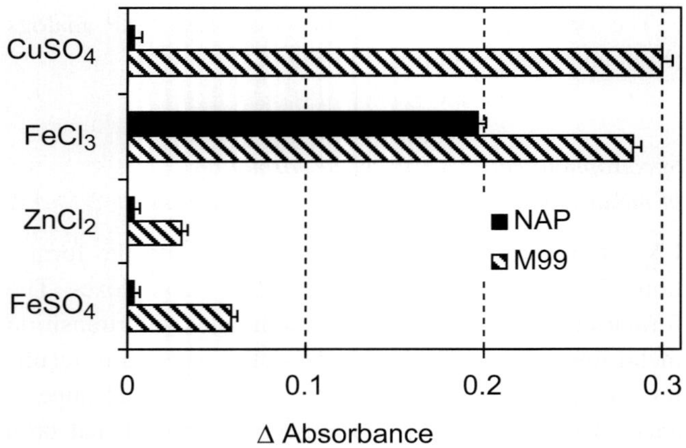

Fig. 3. Maximal spectral increases in NAP and M99 (both at 0.3 mM in water, pH = 5–7) upon the addition of metal salts (0.1 mM): M99 + $CuSO_4$ at 390 nm; M99 + $FeCl_3$ or $FeSO_4$ at 470 nm; M99 + $ZnCl_2$ at 370 nm; NAP + $FeCl_3$ at 300 nm; NAP + $CuSO_4$ or $FeSO_4$ or $ZnCl_2$ showed no significant changes in absorbance at 200–800 nm. Data ± SEM, $n = 2$ in duplicate

Iron-binding potency

The iron-binding capacity of NAP and M99 was measured by the ferrozine method. In this method, iron-binding capacity of drugs is determined by assessing their ability to compete with ferrozine for Fe(II) ions, resulting in decreased absorbance at 562 nm (Carter, 1971). Since high-affinity iron(III) chelators chelate iron(II) cations and rapidly autoxidize them to the corresponding stable Fe(III)-complex under aerobic conditions (Harris et al., 1973), this method actually reflects the Fe (II)/(III)-binding potency. As expected, DFO, a very strong Fe(III) chelator [log $\beta = 30.6$ for Fe (III), 7.2 for Fe(II)] (Anderegg et al., 1963), showed very high iron-binding capacity (Fig. 4). NAP did not exhibit any significant iron-binding capacity, while its analog M99 displayed strong iron-binding capacity with an IC_{50} of 0.1 mM (Fig. 4).

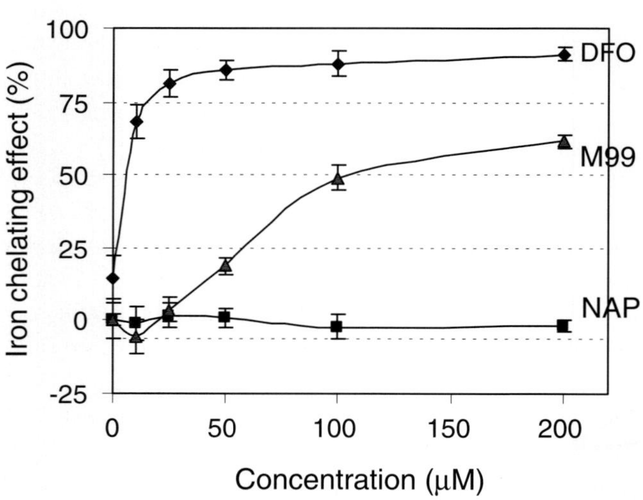

Fig. 4. Effects of the novel iron chelator M99, NAP and DFO on Fe(II)-ferrozine formation as expressed by iron-binding capacity (%). Values represent the means ± SEM, $n = 2$ in duplicate

Effects on lipid peroxidation in rat brain homogenates

As shown in Fig. 5, the parent peptide NAP did not show any significant inhibitory activity on iron (II)-induced lipid

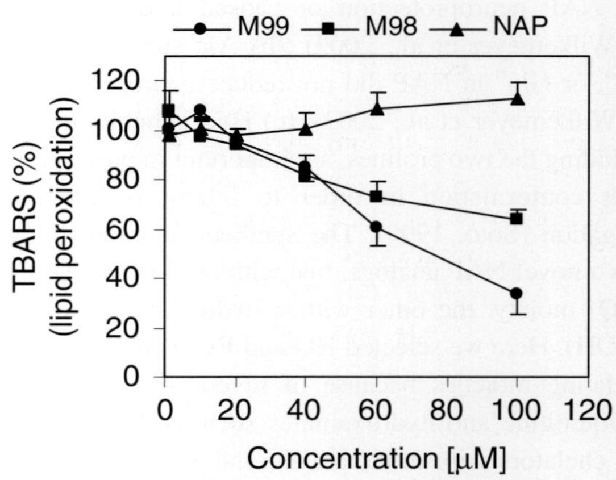

Fig. 5. Effects of NAP, M98 and M99 on lipid peroxidation in rat brain homogenates. TBARS formation was induced by 1.5 μM FeSO4/50 μM ascorbic acid. The results represent the means ± SEM, $n = 3$, $p < 0.05$

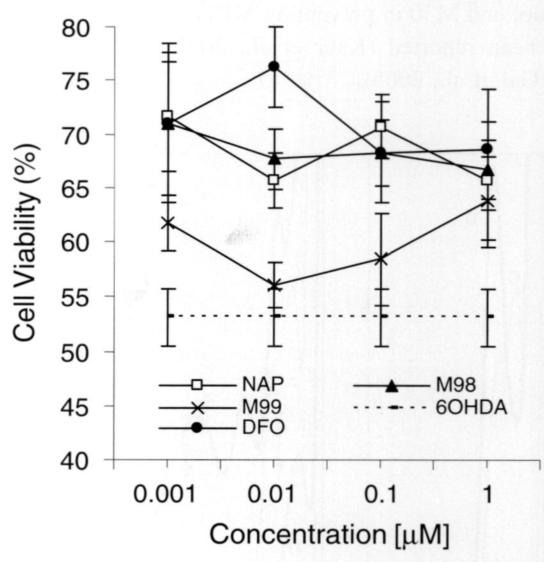

Fig. 6. Protective effects of NAP, M98, M99 and DFO against 6-OHDA-induced toxicity in PC12 cells. PC12 cells (3×10^3 cells/well) in medium containing one third of full serum content were incubated for 24 h and then pretreated with the indicated concentrations of the tested compounds, 30 min before the addition of 6-OHDA (200 μM). Cell viability was assayed with MTT after 24 h incubation. Data are means ± SEM of the percent of untreated control, $n = 5$. $p < 0.05$, compared with 6-OHDA-only treated cultures

peroxidation at the range of 1–100 μM. In contrast, both its analogs M98 and M99 exhibited significant inhibition of LPO at concentrations of ≥30 μM.

Effects on 6-OHDA toxicity in PC12 cells

The protective effects of M98 and M99 against 6-OHDA-induced apoptosis in PC12 cells are shown in Fig. 6. For comparison, this figure also presents the protection exerted by their parent peptide NAP and DFO. DFO is a strong iron chelator and a highly potent radical scavenger with neuroprotective activity in both cell cultures and animal models (Lan and Jiang, 1997). As shown in Fig. 6, M98 and NAP had similar potency in preventing PC12 cell death induced by 6OHDA. The maximum efficacies produced by each peptide were not significantly different from each other, and both afforded protection against cell death with approximately the same potency as DFO. M99 was less potent than NAP, M98 and DFO in protecting against cell death.

Effects on 6-OHDA toxicity in NB SH-SY5Y cells

The neuroprotective action of M98 and M99 was further investigated and validated in NB SH-SY5Y cells. As demonstrated in Fig. 7, exposure of SH-SY5Y cells to 25 μM 6-OHDA resulted in cell death by about 25%. Preincubation with NAP, M98, M99 or DFO (all at 1 μM) before the addition of 6-OHDA almost completely blocked cell death, increasing the cell viability to approximately control levels. In these experiments, the two novel NAP analogs (M98 and M99) showed similar effects to their parent peptide NAP and DFO in protecting the cells against 6-OHDA toxicity. In addition, treatment with only NAP, M98, M99 or DFO (all at 1 μM) did not affect significantly cell death (Fig. 7), suggesting that NAP, M98, M99 or DFO were not toxic to SH-SY5Y cells at the tested concentration (1 μM).

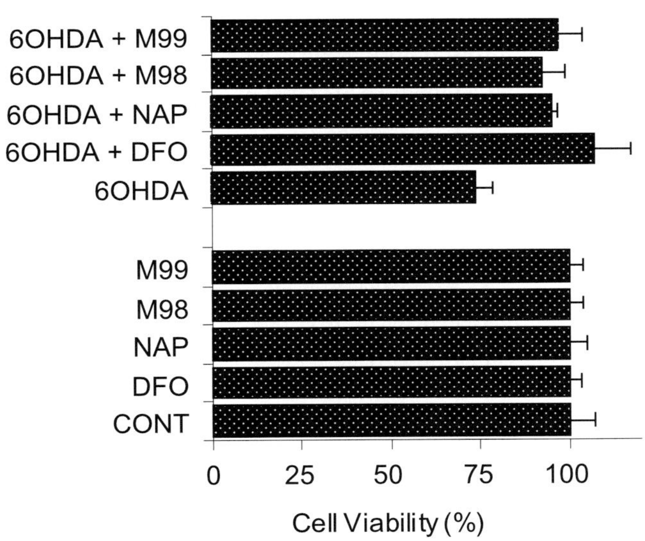

Fig. 7. Protection against 6-OHDA-induced toxicity in SH-SY5Y cells by NAP, M98, M99 and DFO at 1 μM. Cells (1.5×10^4 cells/well) in 2% fetal calf serum were incubated for 24 h and then pretreated with the tested compounds 30 min before the addition of 6-OHDA (25 μM). Cell viability was assayed with MTT after 24 h incubation. Data are means ± SEM of the percent of untreated control, $n = 5$. $p < 0.05$, compared with 6-OHDA-only treated cultures

Discussion

Oxidative stress in the brain has long been implicated in the pathogenesis of a number of neurodegenerative diseases, including AD and PD (Moreira et al., 2005). However, until now, the use of antioxidants to reduce oxidative stress has offered very limited neuroprotection in the clinic (Casetta et al., 2005). The brain is known to contain high levels of polyunsaturated lipids and transition metals such as iron and copper, and to utilize large quantities of oxygen. Transition metals (Fe and Cu) present in the brain, which catalyze the continual production of free radicals through the Fenton or the Haber-Weiss reactions, could undermine the efficacy of antioxidants to reduce oxidative damage (Halliwell, 1992; Zecca et al., 2004). This may explain, at least in part, the failure of many antioxidants to provide neuroprotection in the clinic although they all show neuroprotective activity in animal models. We have adopted a more sophisticated strategy to fight oxidative stress by developing multifunctional antioxidant-metal chelators that can scavenge free radicals and, more importantly, block their production. During our search for multifunctional antioxidant-metal chelators as neuroprotective agents, a number of new compounds have been investigated, and a few of them hold great promise as multifunctional neuroprotective agents (Zheng et al., 2005a, b, c, d; Gal et al., 2005; Youdim and Buccafusco, 2005). In the present study, two novel NAPVSIPQ (NAP) analogs with potential metal chelating ability were investigated. Our studies have shown that M98 and M99 form stable metal ion ($Fe^{3+/2+}$, Cu^{2+}, Zn^{2+}) complexes in water (pH 5–7) while their parent peptide NAP has no binding affinity to Fe^{2+}, Cu^{2+}, or Zn^{2+} (Figs. 2 and 3). NAP may have some binding to Fe^{3+} in water as shown in Figs. 2 and 3. However, Fig. 4 clearly demonstrates that NAP has no significant iron(II)/(III)-binding capacity. These results imply that NAP has some Fe(III)-binding ability, but it is not strong enough to compete with ferrozine, as no significant iron(II)/(III)-binding capacity was observed in the ferrozine method. Figure 4 also suggests that M99 is a strong iron chelator but its iron binding capacity is lower than that of DFO. The high affinity of DFO for iron precludes its use for prolonged period of time in situations unrelated to iron overload due to serious cytotoxicity. The serious cytotoxicity of DFO is very likely attributed to its interaction with iron containing enzymes and proteins, resulting in the mobilization of iron from these enzymes and proteins (Singh et al., 1996). The fact that M99 and M98 form a stable metal ion ($Fe^{3+/2+}$, Cu^{2+}, Zn^{2+}) complexes in water are of importance in biological systems since these metal ions are reported to be associated with oxidative stress, Aβ toxicity, and Aβ aggregation in the brain (Maynard et al., 2005). Previous studies have shown that Fe, Cu and Zn are accumulated in and around insoluble Aβ amyloid plaques in post-mortem AD brain (Lovell et al., 1998). It is also known that the production of free radicals is a normal consequence of metabolic activity. However, high levels of Fe and Cu exacerbate free radical related oxidative stress in the brain by catalyzing the formation of highly toxic $^{\bullet}OH$ radicals through the Fenton or the Haber-Weiss reactions. Aβ toxicity is mediated by the interaction of the Aβ peptide with Cu^{2+} or Fe^{3+}. Also, Aβ, when bound to Cu^{2+} or Fe^{3+}, reduces the metal ions to Cu^{+} or Fe^{2+} and produces H_2O_2, which further reacts with Cu^{+} or Fe^{2+} to generate the highly toxic hydroxyl ($^{\bullet}OH$) radicals leading directly to widespread oxidative stress (Huang et al., 2000). In vitro, Aβ, a central element in the neuropathology of AD, possesses selective high and low affinity Cu^{2+}- and Zn^{2+}-binding sites that mediate its aggregation via interaction with Cu^{2+}, Zn^{2+} and, to a lesser extent, Fe^{3+}. In vivo, zinc is more powerful in inducing Aβ aggregation than Cu or any other metal (Atwood et al., 1998; Atwood et al., 2000b). At neutral pH, Zn^{2+} binds to Aβ resulting in insoluble aggregates, while Cu^{2+} binding induces a soluble conformation (Clements et al., 1996; Miura et al., 2000). At mildly acidic pH, however, which occurs in an aged brain and in response to inflammation, Cu^{2+}also causes Aβ aggregation (Atwood et al., 1998).

As demonstrated in Fig. 5, NAP showed no significant inhibitory activity on iron-induced lipid peroxidation (LPO) even at the concentration of 100 μM. In contrast, both M98 and M99 exhibited significant inhibition on iron-induced LPO at concentrations of $\geq$30 μM. LPO is an important factor involved in neurodegenerative disorders such as AD and PD (Pratico et al., 2004; Mattson, 2004). For example, the brains of AD patients contain high levels of LPO products such as 4-hydroxy-2-nonenal or acrolein, and increased LPO can be detected in the cerebrospinal fluid and plasma of such patients (Pratico et al., 2001). The interplay between transition metals (Fe, Cu, and Zn), amyloid-β peptide, and lipid peroxidation is believed to be responsible for increased oxidative stress and cell damage in AD (Maynard et al., 2005). Fe plays a key role in both the initiation and propagation of oxygen free radicals and the lipid peroxidation process in the brain (O'Brien, 1969; Pipette et al., 1993). Thus, compounds that chelate Fe, inhibit Fe-induced LPO, and prevent free radical-mediated neuronal damage could be of great therapeutic importance.

The neuroprotective activity of M98 and M99 was investigated using PC12 and SH-SY5Y cell models (Glinka et al., 1997; Walkinshaw and Waters, 1994; Seitz et al., 2000; Sachs and Jonsson, 1975). Here we showed that both M98 and M99 display potent protection, similar to their parent peptide NAP and DFO, against 6-OHDA toxicity in SH-SY5Y cell culture at 1 μM. In PC12 cell culture, M98 affords protection against 6-OHDA toxicity, comparable to NAP and DFO at the range of 0.001–1 μM. As for M99, significant protective effects were observed either at 0.001 or 1 μM. These effects are in agreement with its parent peptide NAP, which also exhibits two peaks of neuroprotective activity as shown in previous studies (Gozes et al., 2003). The mechanism of protective effects of M98 and M99 remain to be determined. It is known that neurotoxin 6-OHDA at neutral pH is readily autooxidized and oxidatively deaminated by monoamine oxidase (MAO), resulting in considerable amounts of reactive oxygen species (ROS), among them H_2O_2. It also potently inhibits mitochondrial respiratory chain complex I and IV activity, generating intracellular ROS. The redox iron released from ferritin due to ROS-related oxidative stress, via the Fenton reaction, exacerbates formation of the highly toxic hydroxyl radical, which in turn causes DNA strand breaks, damages protein residues, and initiates lipid peroxidation associated with neuronal death (Glinka et al., 1997). DFO was reported to protect cell death induced by 6-OHDA, apparently mediated by its iron chelating and free radical scavenging capabilities (Lan and Jiang, 1997). The potential mechanism of NAP activity was reported to be associated with decreased activity of the proapoptotic protein P53, a key regulator of cellular apoptosis (Gozes et al., 2004).

In conclusion, we have designed and synthesized two novel NAP analogs, M98 and M99. Both possess good metal ion ($Fe^{3+/2+}$, Cu^{2+}, Zn^{2+}) chelating properties as opposed to the poor metal chelating properties of their parent peptide NAP. M98 and M99 exhibited significant inhibition of iron-induced lipid peroxidation in rat brain homogenates at concentrations of $\geq$30 μM, while NAP did not show any inhibition even at 100 μM. In cell (PC12 and NB SH-SY5Y) cultures, M98 and M99 showed potent protection against 6-OHDA toxicity, comparable to NAP and DFO. These results suggest that M98 and M99 deserve further investigation as potential drug candidates for neuroprotection.

Acknowledgements

We thank Ms Aviva Kapitkowsky and Ms Sarah Rubinraut for synthesizing neuropepetide analogs. We are grateful to Ms Orit Bar-Am, Shunit Gal and Tamar Amit for technical assistance. M.F. is a Lester Pearson Professor of Protein Chemistry. We are grateful to Technion-Research and Development (Haifa, Israel) National Parkinson Foundation (Miami, USA) and Michael J. Fox Foundation (New York, USA) for supporting this work. We also thank Mr. Yigal Avivi for editing the manuscript.

References

Anderegg G, L'Eplattenier F, Schwarzenbach G (1963) Hydroxamate complexes: Application of the pH method. Helvetica Chimica Acta 46: 1400–1408

Atwood CS, Moir RD, Huang X, Scarpa RC, Bacarra NM, Romano DM, Hartshorn MA, Tanzi RE, Bush AI (1998) Dramatic aggregation of Alzheimer abeta by Cu(II) is induced by conditions representing physiological acidosis. J Biol Chem 273: 12817–12826

Ben-Shachar D, Nava Kahana N, Kampel V, Warshawsky A, Youdim MHB (2004) Neuroprotection by a novel brain permeable iron chelator, VK-28, against 6-hydroxy-dopamine lession in rats. Neuropharmacol 46: 254–263

Brenneman DE, Spong CY, Hauser JM, Abebe D, Pinhasov A, Golian T, Gozes I (2004) Protective peptides that are orally active and mechanistically nonchiral. J Pharmacol Expl Therapeutics 309: 1190–1197

Bush AI, Pettingell WH, Multhaup G, Paradis MD, Vonsattel J-P, Beyreuther K, Masters CL, Tanzi RE (1994) Rapid induction of Alzheimer A b amyloid formation by zinc. Science 265: 1464–1467

Carter P (1971) Spectrophotometric determination of serum iron at the submicrogram level with a new reagent (ferrozine). Anal biochem 40: 450–458

Casetta I, Govoni V, Granieri E (2005) Oxidative stress, antioxidants and neurodegenerative diseases. Current Pharmaceutical Design 11: 2033–2052

Clements A, Allsop D, Walsh DM, Williams CH (1996) Aggregation and metal-binding properties of mutant forms of the amyloid A beta peptide of Alzheimer's disease. J Neurochem 66: 740–747

Desport JC, Couratier P (2002) Oxidative stress in neurodegenerative diseases. Nutr Clin Metab 16: 253–259

Drukarch B, van Muiswinkel FL (2000) Drug treatment of Parkinson's disease. Time for phase II. Biochem Pharmacol 59: 1023–1031

Gal S, Zheng H, Fridkin M, Youdim MBH (2005) Novel multifunctional neuroprotective iron chelator-monoamine oxidase inhibitor drugs for neurodegenerative diseases: In vivo selective brain monoamine oxidase inhibition and neuro-protective activity. J Neurochem 95: 79–88

Gilgun-Sherki Y, Melamed E, Offen D (2001) Oxidative stress induced-neurodegenerative diseases: the need for antioxidants that penetrate the blood–brain barrier. Neuropharmacol the blood–brain barrier. Neuropharmacol 40: 959–975

Glinka Y, Gassen M, Youdim MBH (1997) Mechanism of 6-hydroxydopamine neurotoxicity. Adv Res Neurodegen 5: 55–66

Gozes I, Lilling G, Glazer R, Ticher A, Ashkenazi IE, Davidson A, Rubinraut S, Fridkin M, Brenneman DE (1995) Superactive lipophilic peptides discriminate multiple vasoactive intestinal peptide receptors. J Pharmacol Exp Ther 273: 161–167

Gozes I, Bardea A, Bechar M, Pearl O, Reshef A, Zamostiano R, Davidson A, Rubinraut S, Giladi E, Fridkin M, Brenneman DE (1997) Neuropeptides and neuronal survival: neuroprotective strategy for Alzheimer's disease. Ann NY Acad Sci 814: 161–166

Gozes I, Divinsky I, Pilzer I, Fridkin M, Brenneman DE, Spier AD (2003) From vasoactive intestinal peptide (VIP) through activity-dependent neuroprotective protein (ADNP) to NAP: A view of neuroprotection and cell division. J Mol Neurosci 20: 315–322

Gozes I, Steingart RA, Spier AD (2004) NAP mechanisms of neuroprotection. J Mol Neurosci 24: 67–72

Grunblatt E, Mandel S, Jacob-Hirsch J, Zeligson S, Amariglo N, Rechavi G, Li J, Ravid R, Roggendorf W, Riederer P, Youdim MBH (2004) Gene expression profiling of parkinsonian substantia nigra pars compacta; alterations in ubiquitin-proteasome, heat shock protein, iron and oxidative stress regulated proteins, cell adhesion/cellular matrix and vesicle trafficking genes. J Neural Transm 111: 1543–1573

Halliwell B (1992) Reactive oxygen species and the central nervous system. J Neurochem 59: 1609–1623

Harris DC, Aisen P (1973) Facilitation of Fe(II) autoxidation by Fe(III) complexing agents. Biochimica et biophysica acta 329: 156–158

Huang X, Cuajungco MP, Atwood CS, Moir RD, Tanzi RE, Bush AI (2000) Alzheimer's disease, b-amyloid protein and zinc. J Nutr 130: 1488S–1492S

Jellinger KA (1999) The role of iron in neurodegeneration: prospects for pharmacotherapy of Parkinson's disease. Drugs Aging 14: 115–140

Kaur D, Yantiri F, Rajagopalan S, Kumar J, Mo JQ, Boonplueang R, Viswanath V, Jacobs R, Yang L, Beal MF, DiMonte D, Volitaskis I, Ellerby L, Cherny RA, Bush AI, Andersen JK (2003) Genetic or pharmacological iron chelation prevents MPTP-induced neurotoxicity in vivo: a novel therapy for Parkinson's disease. Neuron 37: 899–909

Kayyali R, Pannala AS, Khodr H, Hider RC (1998) Comparative radical scavenging ability of bidentate iron(III) chelators. Biochem Pharmacol 55: 1327–1332

Lan J, Jiang DH (1997) Desferrioxamine and Vitamin E protect against iron and MPTP-induced neurodegeneration in mice. J Neural Transm 104: 469–481

Lovell MA, Robertson JD, Teesdale WJ, Campbell JL, Mandel S, Grunblatt E, Riederer P, Gerlach M, Levites Y, Youdim MBH (2003) Neuroprotective strategies in Parkinson's disease: an update on progress. CNS Drugs 17: 729–762

Markesbery WR (1998) Copper, iron and zinc in Alzheimer's disease senile plaques. J Neurol Sci 158: 47–52

Mattson MP (2004) Metal-catalyzed disruption of membrane protein and lipid signaling in the pathogenesis of neurodegenerative disorders. Ann NY Acad Sci 1012: 37–50

Maynard CJ, Bush AI, Masters CL, Cappaiand R, Li QX (2005) Metals and amyloid-β in Alzheimer's disease. Int J Exp Path 86: 147–159

McDowell I (2001) Alzheimer's disease: insights from epidemiology. Aging 13: 143–162

Miura T, Suzuki K, Kohata N, Takeuchi H (2000) Metal binding modes of Alzheimer's amyloid beta-peptide in insoluble aggregates and soluble complexes. Biochemistry 39: 7024–7031

Moreira PI, Siedlak SL, Aliev G, Zhu X, Cash AD, Smith MA, Perry G (2005) Oxidative stress mechanisms and potential therapeutics in Alzheimer disease. J Neural Transm 112: 921–932

Munoz-Patino AM, Labandeira-Garcia JL (2000) Autoxidation and neurotoxicity of 6-hydroxy-dopamine in the presence of some antioxidants: potential implication in relation to the pathogenesis of Parkinson's disease. J Neurochem 74: 1605–1612

Obrien PJ (1969) Intracellular mechaniims for the decomposition of a lipid peroxide: decomposition of a lipid peroxide by metal ions, nerve compounds, and nucleophiles. Can J Biochem 47: 485–492

Offen D, Sherki Y, Melamed E, Fridkin M, Brenneman DE, Gozes I (2000) Vasoactive intestinal peptide (VIP) prevents neurotoxicity in neuronal cultures: relevance to neuroprotection in Parkinson's disease. Brain Res 854: 257–262

Pipette LH, Baxely LH, Grover TA, Harwood PJ (1983) A Comparative Kinetic Study of the Initiation of Lipid Peroxidation with OH Radicals and Ferrous Ion. In: Bors W, Saran M, Tait D (eds) Oxygen Radicals in Chemistry and Biology. Walter de Gruyter & Co., Berlin, p 137

Pratico D, Uryu K, Leight S, Trojanoswki JQ, Lee VM (2001) Increased lipid peroxidation precedes amyloid plaque formation in an animal model of Alzheimer amyloidosis. J Neurosci 21: 4183–4187

Pratico D, Sung S (2004) Lipid peroxidation and oxidative imbalance: Early functional events in Alzheimer's disease. J Alzheimer's Disease 6: 171–175

Riederer P, Sofic E, Rausch WD, Schmidt B, Reynolds GP, Jellinger K, Youdim MB (1989) Transition metals, ferritin, glutathione, and ascorbic acid in parkinsonian brains. J Neurochem 52: 515–520

Sachs C, Jonsson G (1975) Mechanism of action of 6-hydroxydopamine. Brain Res 99: 277–291

Seitz G, Stegmann HB, Jager HH, Schlide HM, Wolburg H, Roginsky VA, Niethammer D, Bruchelt G, Shoham S, Youdim MBH (2000) Iron involvement in neural damage and microgliosis in models of neurodegenerative diseases. Cell Mol Biol 46: 743–760

Sen CK (1998) Redox signaling and the emerging therapeutic potential of thiol antioxidants. Biochem Pharmacol 55: 1747–1758

Singh S, Khodr H, Taylor MI, Hider RC (1996) Therapeutic iron chelators and their potential side effects. Biochem Soc Symp 61: 127–137

Soto C (1999) Plaque busters: strategies to inhibit amyloid formation in Alzheimer's disease. Mol Med Today 5: 343–350

Soto-Otero R, Mendez-Alvarez E, Hermida-Ameijeiras A, Turnquist TD, Sandell EB (1968) Stability constants of iron(III)-8-hydroxylquinolinecomplexes. Anal Chim Acta 42: 239–245

Takanashi M, Mochizuki H, Yokomizo K, Hattori N, Mori H, Yamamura Y, Mizuno Y (2001) Iron accumulation in the substantia nigra of autosomal recessive juvenile parkinsonism (ARJP). Parkinson's Relat Disord 7: 311–314

Walkinshaw G, Waters CM (1994) Neurotoxin-induced cell death in neuronal PC12 cells is mediated by induction of apoptosis. Neurosci 63: 975–987

Wilkemeyer MF, Chen S, Menkari CE, Brenneman DE, Sulik KK, Charness ME (2003) Differential effects of ethanol antagonism and neuroprotection in peptide fragment NAPVSIPQ prevention of ethanol-induced developmental toxicity. Proc Nati Acad Sci USA 100: 8543–8548

Youdim MBH, Buccafusco JJ (2005a) CNS Targets for multi-functional drugs in the treatment of Alzheimer's and Parkinson's diseases. J Neural Transm 112: 519–537

Youdim MBH, Buccafusco JJ (2005b) Multi-functional drugs for various CNS targets in the treatment of neurodegenerative disorders. Trends Pharmacol Sci 26: 27–35

Zecca L, Youdim MBH, Riedrere P, Connor JR, Crichton RR (2004) Iron, brain, ageing and neurodegenerative disorders. Nat Rev Neurosci 5: 863–873

Zheng H, Youdim MBH, Weiner LM, Fridkin M (2005a) Novel potential neuroprotective agent with both iron chelating and amino acid-based derivatives targeting the central nervous system neurons. Biochem Pharmacol 70: 1642–1652

Zheng H, Gal S, Weiner LM, Bar-Am O, Warshawsky A, Fridkin M, Youdim MBH (2005b) Novel multifunctional neuroprotective iron chelator-monoamine oxidase inhibitor drugs for neurodegenerative diseases: in vitro studies on antioxidant activity, prevention of lipid peroxide formation and monoamine oxidase inhibition. J Neurochem 95: 68–78

Zheng H, Weiner LM, Bar-Am O, Epsztejn M, Cabantchik I, Warshawsky A, Youdim MBH, Fridkin M (2005c) Design, synthesis and evaluation of novel bifunctional iron-chelators as potential agents for neuroprotection in neurodegenerative diseases. Bioorg Med Chem 13: 773–783

Zheng H, Youdim MBH, Weiner LM, Fridkin M (2005d) Synthesis and Evaluation of Peptidic Metal Chelators for Neuroprotection in Neurodegenerative Diseases. J Pept Res 66: 190–203

J Neural Transm (2006) [Suppl] 71: 173–196

Journal of Neural Transmission
Printed in Austria

Acute and chronic effects of developmental iron deficiency on mRNA expression patterns in the brain

S. L. Clardy[1], X. Wang[1], W. Zhao[2], W. Liu[2], G. A. Chase[2], J. L. Beard[3], B. True Felt[4], J. R. Connor[1]

[1] Department of Neurosurgery, M.S. Hershey Medical Center, Hershey, USA
[2] Department of Health Evaluation Sciences, M.S. Hershey Medical Center, Hershey, USA
[3] Department of Nutrition, Pennsylvania State University, College Park, USA
[4] Department of Pediatrics and Communicable Diseases, University of Michigan, Ann Arbor, USA

Summary Because of the multiple biochemical pathways that require iron, iron deficiency can impact brain metabolism in many ways. The goal of this study was to identify a molecular footprint associated with ongoing versus long term consequences of iron deficiency using microarray analysis. Rats were born to iron-deficient mothers, and were analyzed at two different ages: 21 days, while weaning and iron-deficient; and six months, after a five month iron-sufficient recovery period. Overall, the data indicate that ongoing iron deficiency impacts multiple pathways, whereas the long term consequences of iron deficiency on gene expression are more limited. These data suggest that the gene array profiles obtained at postnatal day 21 reflect a brain under development in a metabolically compromised setting that given appropriate intervention is mostly correctable. There are, however, long term consequences to the developmental iron deficiency that could underlie the neurological deficits reported for iron deficiency.

Introduction

Insufficient amounts of body iron affect up to one billion people worldwide (Andrews, 2000). Iron is especially crucial during development, as it is required for proper myelination, and is also a cofactor for enzymes in neurotransmitter synthesis (Larkin, 1990; Beard and Connor, 2003; Beard et al., 2003). Studies in animals dating back over three decades have documented the damage resulting from iron deficiency. Dallman et al. demonstrated that even after iron-deficient rats were returned to a normal iron diet for several days, non-heme iron remained depressed, as did ferritin in brain (Dallman et al., 1975). Weinberg et al. also noted that rats exposed to iron deficiency for the first 28 days of life never recovered, exhibiting a persistent deficit in brain non-heme iron, as well as changes in behavior and physiological responsiveness (Weinberg et al., 1979). Decreased motor activity and reversed circadian rhythms of thermoregulation and motor activity were found in another study of rats that were iron-deprived for 28 days postnatally, indicating the major role iron plays in the normal function of the dopaminergic system in the brain (Youdim et al., 1981). More recent animal studies have distinguished differences between pre- and post-natal recovery from iron deficiency. If the iron deficiency occurs during neonatal and post-weaning periods, and an iron sufficient diet is given two-to four weeks postnatally, recovery occurs upon iron repletion (Chen et al., 1995; Erikson et al., 1997; Pinero et al., 2000), but the effects of iron deficiency *in utero* appear irreversible, even after iron repletion (Felt and Lozoff, 1996; Kwik-Uribe, Gietzen et al., 2000; Kwik-Uribe et al., 2000).

In humans, a study of second grade children who were anemic in infancy revealed that the learning achievement score and the positive task orientation was significantly lower in the anemic group than in the non-anemic control group. Data were controlled for maternal education and sex of child (Palti et al., 1985). A more recent study by Lozoff et al. found that children who had iron deficiency in infancy scored lower on tests of mental and motor functioning as teens (greater than ten years later) than those infants who were not iron-deficient as infants. Additionally, more of the previously iron-deficient infants had repeated a grade, had been referred for special services, and/or was the object of parental and teacher concern regarding anxiety, depression, social difficulties, or attention problems (Lozoff et al., 2000). A study of iron deficiency anemia in young South African anemic mothers of full-term infants found

Correspondence: J. R. Connor, 500 University Drive, Department of Neurosurgery, H110, Hershey, PA 17033, USA
e-mail: jconnor@psu.edu

that the infants of anemic mothers were developmentally delayed at 10 weeks. At nine months, despite normalization of iron status in some mothers, the developmental delays were not diminished in the infants. The iron deficiency also affected the mothers, and even nine months post-partum, anemic mothers were more negative, less engaged, and less responsive toward their babies than were control mothers. Mothers treated for iron deficiency exhibited behaviors similar to controls (Perez et al., 2005). A study of South African women by Beard et al. (2005) found that iron treatment of anemic mothers up to nine months postpartum resulted in 25% improvement of depression, stress, and cognitive function, further suggesting the importance of maternal iron status on infant development (Beard et al., 2005). These studies highlight the need to study iron deficiency over time, from infancy onward, and hint at the differences between ID at different stages in life (birth, infancy, and motherhood).

It is now accepted that dietary iron deficiency lowers brain iron and interferes with protein synthesis in the brain (Beard and Connor, 2003). There is, however, a notable lack of research into the effects of such early iron deficiency in later, adult life. In these studies, we obtained a gene expression profile of rat brain to identify the molecular footprint of the iron-deficient brain. This information may point to the specific pathways causing the underlying pathophysiology of both acute iron deficiency and its long-term, chronic effects. A benefit of microarrays in the analysis of iron-deficient brain is the ability to investigate global gene changes without the bias of *a priori* hypotheses. We also wanted to examine as broad a range of systems as possible in this first pass analysis in the iron-deficient brains, and thus we tested the entire brain in our analysis to gain an understanding of the most dramatic and global changes caused by iron deficiency.

Methods and materials

Animal characteristics

The studies reported here were performed in compliance with the animal procedures approved by the University of Michigan institutional animal use committee (protocols 2002-129 and 7623). Pregnant Sprague-Dawley dams were fed an iron-deficient diet (4–10 mg/kg iron) or an iron-sufficient diet (40 mg/kg iron) beginning at gestational day 5. Diets were prepared by Harlan Teklad Nutritionals (Madison, WI). Mothers and litters were maintained on their diets through gestation and lactation. After postnatal day 20, all animals were fed the iron-sufficient diet. The first experimental group was sacrificed at 21 days of age. For the second group of animals, pups were weaned at postnatal day 23 and maintained on the iron-sufficient diet until they were killed at six months of age. There were 4 animals per group for the 21-day analyses and 4 animals per group for the six-month analyses.

RNA preparation and microarray analysis

Frozen brain tissue was homogenized and extracted with TRIzol reagent (Gibco BRL Life Technologies, Baltimore, MD, USA) and further purified with the Qiagen RNeasy kit (Qiagen, Valencia, CA) utilizing the clean-up step according to the manufacturer's instructions. RNA quality was evaluated by A260/A280 ratio. Randomly selected samples were further analyzed for RNA integrity using an Agilent 2100 Bioanalyzer (Agilent Technologies, Palo Alto, CA, USA); all samples analyzed demonstrated acceptable quality. Synthesis of double-stranded DNA and biotinylated cRNA from total RNA, and its subsequent hybridization to the chips, were performed according to Affymetrix (Santa Clara, CA) recommendations. Streptavidin-phycoerythrin staining of arrays after hybridization also followed Affymetrix recommendations. Biotin-labeled and fragmented RNA was hybridized to Rat Genome U34A Gene Chips containing approximately 7000 full-length sequences and 1000 expressed sequence tag (EST) clusters. The microarrays were scanned by the Affymetrix gene array system (http://www.affymetrix.com). Preliminary data analyses were performed with the Affymetrix GCOS software package and the Affymetrix Data Mining Tool.

Real-time PCR

Total RNA was prepared for qualitative real-time PCR using Invitrogen's SuperScript(tm) III First-Strand Synthesis System for RT-PCR (Invitrogen Corporation, Carlsbad, CA). PCR was performed using TaqMan detection probe and primers either purchased from inventory or designed with the online software Custom TaqMan® Gene Expression Assay File Builder (Applied Biosystems, Foster City, CA). Real-time PCR amplification of cDNA was performed using TaqMan Universal PCR Master Mix (Applied Biosystems). Values were normalized to those obtained for ribosomal 18s mRNA.

Statistical analysis

Before testing significant changes in gene expression, expression signals were normalized by using the R-Affy package from Bioconductor (version 1.2, Irizarry et al., 2003) to remove background noise and non-biological variations among arrays. The background noise was removed from the PM (perfect match) probe intensities using the "RMA" method (Irizarry, 2003), which assumes a global model for the distribution of probe intensities and models the PM probe intensities as the sum of a normal noise component and an exponential signal component. Normalization was performed according to the quantile normalization method (Bolstad, 2003). Quantile normalization assumes that the expression of majority of genes on the arrays does not change in different treatments, and that the distribution of probe intensities for each array in the dataset is the same. For each probe set, the logs of the background corrected, normalized PM intensities were fitted with an additive multi-chip linear model, which had a chip-wise abundance term and a probe-wise affinity term. The robust median polish procedure was utilized for fitting (Tukey, 1977). Estimates were reported on the log2 scale. Because approximately thirty percent of the probes were found with MM (mismatch) > PM, and there existed a high correlation between PM and MM intensities, the use of MM as internal control was questionable. Therefore, expression values were obtained based on PM intensities not PM-MM intensities.

Significant gene expression alterations were identified using Significance Analysis of Microarrays (SAM) computer software (Tusher et al., 2001). SAM assigns a score to each gene on the basis of gene expression change relative to the standard deviation of repeated measurements and identifies genes with statistically significant changes in expression using a permutation procedure. SAM controls the false positives resulting from multiple comparisons through controlling the false discovery rate (FDR) (Benjamini, 1995). FDR is defined as the expected proportion of false positive genes among all genes that are considered significant. The FDR

Table 1. *This table lists the 50 most significantly changed genes – 25 up-regulated and 25 down-regulated – from over 300 significantly genes in the 21-day rat group. Both the fold change and the q-value are listed, as the combination of these two values was considered in determining significance*

	Gene name	Symbol	Fold change	q-value (%)
Up-regulated				
L06040_s_at	arachidonate 12-lipoxygenase	Alox12	3.38871	0.83181
rc_AI237007_at	electron-transferring-flavoprotein dehydrogenase	Etfdh	2.51510	0.83181
M58040_at	transferrin receptor	Tfrc	2.39091	0.83181
AF102853_at	membrane-associated guanylate kinase-interacting protein	LOC59322	1.87739	0.83181
AB011679_at	tubulin, beta 5	Tubb5	1.87635	0.83181
rc_AA900769_s_at	smooth muscle alpha-actin	Acta2	1.84847	1.37095
rc_AA926149_g_at	catalase	Cat	1.84026	0.83181
X60767mRNA_s_at	cell division cycle 2 homolog A (S. pombe)	Cdc2a	1.67649	0.83181
rc_AI008836_s_at	high mobility group box 2	Hmgb2	1.66875	0.83181
AF022083_s_at	guanine nucleotide binding protein, beta 1	Gnb1	1.61726	0.83181
X03369_s_at	Rat mRNA for beta-tubulin T beta15	–	1.58431	0.83181
rc_AA899854_at	topoisomerase (DNA) 2 alpha	Top2a	1.57366	3.94082
rc_AA892390_s_at	solute carrier family 11 member 2	Slc11a2	1.56078	0.83181
D86642_at	FK506 binding protein 1b	Fkbp1b	1.55962	0.83181
rc_AA925762_at	Rattus norvegicus similar to Myristoylated alanine-rich C-kinase substrate (MARCKS), mRNA	–	1.55113	0.83181
rc_AI639294_at	Rattus norvegicus similar to protein ref (H.sapiens) KIAA0275 gene product	–	1.54511	2.90318
U75405UTR#1_f_at	collagen, type 1, alpha 1	Col1a1	1.54275	4.87630
rc_AA997865_at	thymosin beta-like protein	LOC286978	1.52727	0.83181
X13016_at	CD48 antigen	Cd48	1.51357	0.83181
M58364_at	GTP cyclohydrolase 1	Gch	1.50412	0.83181
rc_AI145680_s_at	solute carrier family 16, member 1	Slc16a1	1.50408	2.00860
D86297_at	aminolevulinic acid synthase 2	Alas2	1.49073	0.83181
U93306_at	kinase insert domain protein receptor	Kdr	1.48794	2.90318
AB000362_at	cold inducible RNA-binding protein	Cirbp	1.45745	4.87630
M64755_at	cysteine-sulfinate decarboxylase	Csad	1.45583	2.90318
Down-regulated				
K01934mRNA#2_at	thyroid hormone responsive protein	Thrsp	0.39906	0.83181
U31866_g_at	Rattus norvegicus Nclone10 mRNA	–	0.47015	0.83181
D38380_g_at	Transferrin	Tf	0.49119	0.83181
U31367_at	myelin and lymphocyte protein	Mal	0.51875	0.83181
AF016269_at	kallikrein 6	Klk6	0.53451	0.83181
AB003726_at	homer, neuronal immediate early gene, 1	Homer1	0.53698	0.83181
D28111_at	myelin-associated oligodendrocytic basic protein	Mobp	0.53918	0.83181
X55572_at	apolipoprotein D	Apod	0.54264	0.83181
rc_AI639532_at	Rat troponin-c mRNA	–	0.55172	0.83181
L21995_s_at	myelin oligodendrocyte glycoprotein	Mog	0.61224	0.83181
X60351cds_s_at	crystallin, alpha B	Cryab	0.61292	0.83181
D90401_at	afadin	Af6	0.63107	1.37095
U48828_g_at	Rattus norvegicus retroviral-like ovarian specific transcript 30-1 mRNA	–	0.63803	1.37095
X15512_at	apolipoprotein C-I	Apoc1	0.64339	0.83181
X58294_at	carbonic anhydrase 2	Ca2	0.64519	0.83181
AF081196_at	RAS guanyl releasing protein 1	Rasgrp1	0.64721	1.37095
AF026529_s_at	stathmin-like 4	Stmn4	0.64929	0.83181
rc_AI639465_r_at	ring finger protein 28	Rnf28	0.65888	0.83181
rc_AA892775_at	lysozyme	Lyz	0.65940	1.37095
AF091563_r_at	olfactory receptor	LOC309574	0.66307	0.83181
H32189_s_at	glutathione S-transferase, mu 1	Gstm1	0.66508	0.83181
L03201_at	cathepsin S	Ctss	0.66680	0.83181
L33894_at	deoxycytidine kinase	Dck	0.67197	3.94082
rc_AI228548_g_at	Rattus norvegicus similar to S-100 protein, alpha chain (LOC295214), mRNA	–	0.67279	0.83181
D84479_at	Rat PMSG-induced ovarian mRNA, 3'sequence, N1	–	0.67470	3.78031

was set at 0.05 for the 21-day animals and 0.063 for the six-month animals. Computer software dChip (Li and Wong, 2001; Li, 2003) version 1.3 was used to cluster samples and genes, and to identify functionally significant gene clusters. Normalized chip intensity data were imported into dChip. Gene information file for Affymetrix rat genome RG U34A array was obtained from dChip's website at www.dChip.org. After hierarchical clustering of genes, dChip systematically assesses the significance of all functional categories in all branches of the hierarchical clustering tree. Finite sampling and hypergeometric distribution was used to measure the significance. p-value is the probability of seeing $\times$ genes of a certain function occurring in a cluster of k genes at random, given n annotated genes on the array or of a list of genes, of which m genes have a certain function. Clusters with p-values <0.005 were considered significant and were reported. The less than 0.005 rule was suggested by the dChip program. The p-values were unadjusted for multiple comparisons. Therefore, a more stringent rule (less than 0.005) need to be used instead of the usual less than 0.05 rule.

For statistical analysis of the real time PCR data, the Sequence Detection Software (ver. 1.2.3) provided by Applied Biosystems was used to export the raw data for each 96-well plate. Each plate had 6 sets of 12 numbers: 1 set for Gene 1 control, 1 set for Gene 1 target (iron-deficiency), 1 set for Gene 2 control, 1 set for Gene 2 target, 1 set for 18S control, and 1 set for 18S target. For each set, an outlier was identified if it was not in the range of mean-2 X standard deviation and mean + 2 X standard deviation. Outliers were then omitted manually using the Sequence Detection Software. The RQ value was then recalculated using the software. Results were exported from the software for each of the 12 plates. Most sets did not have any outliers (the use of ± 3 times standard deviation as the limits did not yield any outliers).

Results

The statistical analysis revealed 334 significantly changed genes in the 21-day rats. These genes are listed in the Supplemental Table. To meet significance, the genes had an FDR of <0.05 (the expected proportion of false positive genes among all genes that are considered significant). The 50 most dramatically changed genes from the 334 significantly changed genes – the 25 most up-regulated and the 25 most down-regulated – are shown in Table 1. Several significant gene clusters were identified from the 334 significantly changed genes, including: myelin-related, signal transduction, channel/pore class transporter and alpha-type channel activity, ion channel activity, DNA binding, transitional metal binding, and solute carrier family members (Fig. 1). Clusters with p-values <0.005 were considered significant. The identity of the genes in each cluster is displayed in Table 2.

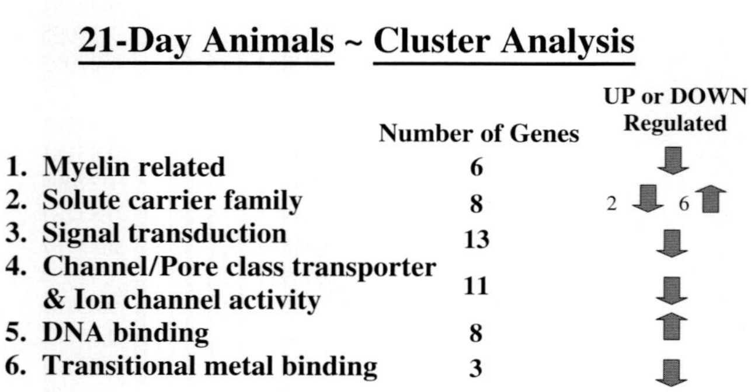

Fig. 1. Gene clusters from 21-day-old animals. Several significant gene clusters were identified, including: myelin-related, signal transduction, channel/pore class transporter and alpha-type channel activity & ion channel activity, DNA binding, transitional metal binding, and solute carrier family members. This figure illustrates these clusters, the number of genes in each, and the direction of change

From the over 300 genes identified in the 21-day animals, twelve genes were selected for verification by real-time PCR. These twelve genes were chosen based on several criteria. The genes tested for verification were not only those genes with the most the dramatic fold change and q values, but also included genes considered to be less significantly changed according to the fold change and q-value. Some of the genes were selected as possible candidates for iron-related disorders, including possible relationship to iron deficiency based on QTL analyses (for example, see (Jones et al., 2003)). Of the twelve genes selected for PCR analyses, six were up-regulated on the microarray studies and six were down-regulated. The verification results are shown in Fig. 2A. The expression of the genes was consistent between the microarray study and the real-time PCR study: all twelve genes changed in the same direction, and nine of the twelve changes were significant.

In the six-month-old animals, twelve genes were identified as significantly changed. Of the twelve genes found, all were down-regulated, and seven were expressed sequence tags or transcribed sequences, leaving five genes for further investigation. Of the five genes, two of the protein products are cytoplasmic, two are nuclear, and one is found in both the nucleus and cytoplasm. The results of the real-time PCR verification of all five genes are shown in Fig. 2B. The expression of the genes in the real-time PCR study was consistent with the microarray analysis, with all five genes showing down-regulation. The down-regulation was significant in four out of five genes.

Real-time PCR was additionally performed on biological replicates of the 21-day-old animals, and the results are displayed in Fig. 3. Brains from eight different animals (four control, four iron-deficient) were used to verify the changes in each gene. The ID animals underwent the same iron deficient diet regimen as the animals examined in the microarray analysis. Six of the twelve genes investigated in the original PCR analysis were randomly selected for verification, of which four were up-regulated and two were down-regulated. The direction of change for these genes was consistent with the initial set of animals.

Table 2. *Cluster analysis. Each gene, symbol, and biological process is displayed within each of 6 clusters*

Symbol	Name	Biological process
Signal transduction – 13 genes		
Mal	myelin and lymphocyte protein	ionic insulation of neurons by glial cells, intracellular protein transport
Mog	Myelin oligodendrocyte glycoprotein	ionic insulation of neurons by glial cells
Af6	afadin	neuropeptide signaling pathway
Mbp	Myelin basic protein	ionic insulation of neurons by glial cells
Drd1a	dopamine receptor 1A	G-protein coupled receptor protein signaling pathway
Chn2	chimerin (chimaerin) 2	intracellular signaling cascade
Pik4cb	phosphatidylinositol 4-kinase	signal transduction
Gabrd	gamma-aminobutyric acid A receptor, delta	synaptic transmission; gamma-aminobutyric acid signaling pathway; chloride transport
Gal	galanin	neuropeptide signaling pathway
–	gamma-aminobutyric acid A receptor, alpha 6	–
Dlgh1	discs, large homolog 1 (Drosophila)	intracellular signaling cascade
Pmp22	peripheral myelin protein 22	ionic insulation of neurons by glial cells; cell cycle arrest
Fgf9	fibroblast growth factor 9	signal transduction
Channel/pore class transporter & ion channel activity – 11 genes		
P2rx4	purinergic receptor P2X, ligand-gated ion channel, 4	ion transport
Clcn4-2	putative chloride channel (similar to Mm Clcn4-2)	–
Kcnab1	potassium voltage gated channel, shaker related subfamily, beta member 1	potassium ion transport
Fxyd1	FXYD domain-containing ion transport regulator 1	muscle contraction; calcium ion homeostasis
Scn1a	sodium channel, voltage-gated, type 1, alpha polypeptide	–
Gabrd	gamma-aminobutyric acid A receptor, delta	synaptic transmission; gamma-aminobutyric acid signaling pathway; chloride transport
Kv8.1	neuronal potassium channel alpha subunit	–
Cacna2d1	calcium channel, voltage-dependent, alpha2/delta subunit 1	ion transport
–	gamma-aminobutyric acid A receptor, alpha 6	–
Kcnd3	potassium voltage gated channel, Shal-related family, member 3	potassium ion transport
Gjb1	gap junction membrane channel protein beta 1	cell-cell signaling
DNA binding – 8 genes		
Hmgb2	high mobility group box 2	–
Nsep1	nuclease sensitive element binding protein 1	regulation of transcription, DNA-dependent
Nfib	nuclear factor I/B	regulation of transcription, DNA-dependent; DNA replication
Pou3f1	POU domain, class 3, transcription factor 1	regulation of transcription
Pcna	Proliferating cell nuclear antigen	–
Hmgb1	high mobility group box 1	regulation of transcription, DNA-dependent; DNA packaging; chromosome organization and biogenesis (sensu Eukarya)
Pax6	Paired box homeotic gene 6	development; regulation of transcription, DNA-dependent; eye morphogenesis (sensu Drosophila)
Hes1	hairy and enhancer of split 1 (Drosophila)	regulation of transcription, DNA-dependent
Transition metal ion binding – 3 genes		
Tf	Transferrin	–
Ca2	carbonic anhydrase 2	–
Ca4	carbonic anhydrase 4	one-carbon compound metabolism
Myelin related – 6 genes		
Mobp	myelin-associated oligodendrocytic basic protein	–
Mal	myelin and lymphocyte protein	ionic insulation of neurons by glial cells; intracellular protein transport
Mog	Myelin oligodendrocyte glycoprotein	ionic insulation of neurons by glial cells
Mbp	Myelin basic protein	ionic insulation of neurons by glial cells
Plp	proteolipid protein	nerve ensheathment
Pmp22	peripheral myelin protein 22	ionic insulation of neurons by glial cells; cell cycle arrest

(*continued*)

Table 2 (*continued*)

Symbol	Name	Biological process
Solute carrier family – 8 genes		
Slc11a2	solute carrier family 11, member 2	–
Slc16a1	solute carrier family 16, member 1	transport
Slc18a2	solute carrier family 18, member 2	transport
Slc6a6	solute carrier family 6, member 6	neurotransmitter transport; neurotransmitter secretion
Slc7a1	solute carrier family 7, member 1	transport; amino acid transport
Slc6a4	solute carrier family 6, member 4	neurotransmitter transport; neurotransmitter secretion
Slc21a5	solute carrier family 21, member 5	organic anion transporter
Slc25a10	solute carrier family 25, member 10	mitochondrial carrier; dicarboxylate transporter

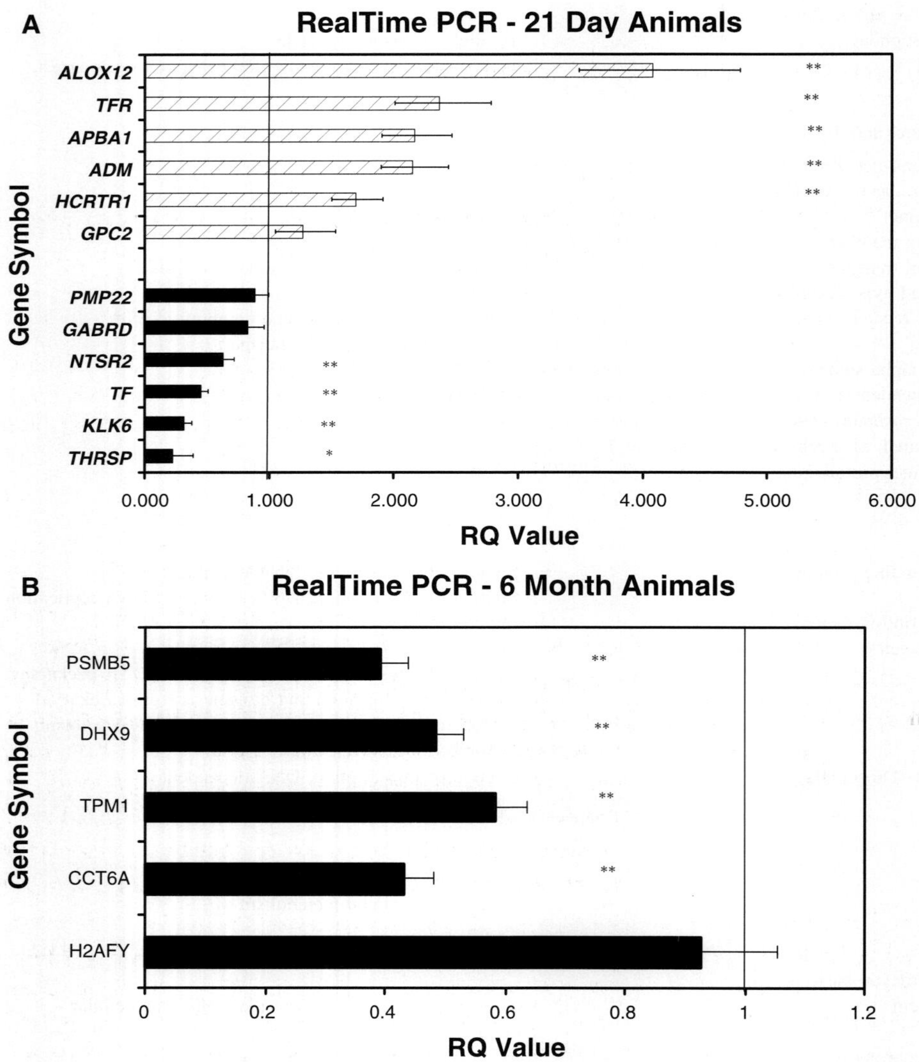

Fig. 2. Real-time PCR verification of gene changes from animals both 21 days of age and six months of age. From the over 300 genes identified in the 21-day animals, twelve genes were selected for verification by real-time PCR using brains from the same animals studied in the microarray analysis. Four iron-deficient animals and four control animals were tested in each real-time PCR experiment. Of the twelve genes, six were up-regulated and six were down-regulated. The verification results are displayed as mean RQ value for each gene. Values are normalized to a control value of one (A). In the six-month animals, a total of twelve genes were identified as significantly changed. Of the twelve genes found, all were down-regulated, and seven were either estimated sequence tags or transcribed sequences, leaving five genes for further investigation. The RQ values of the real-time PCR verification of all five genes are shown in (B). Error bars display the standard error of the mean ($^*p<0.05$ and $^{**}p<0.005$)

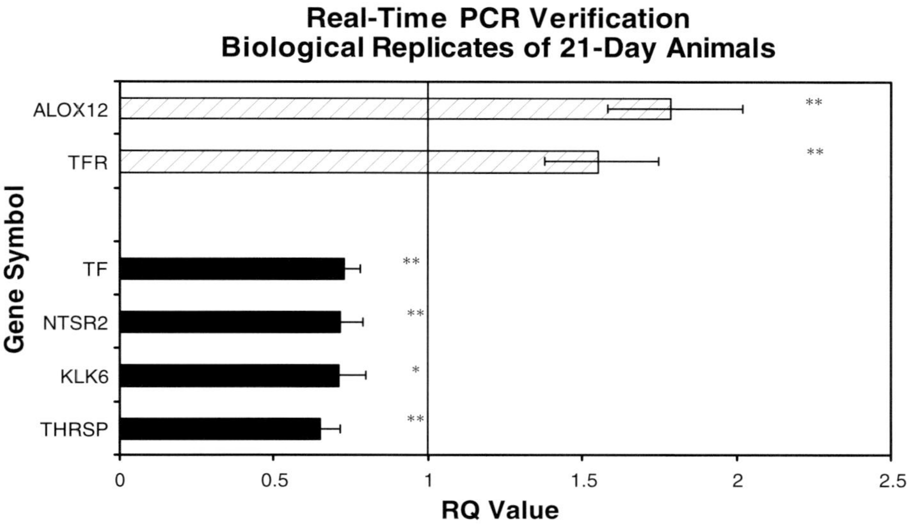

Fig. 3. Real-time PCR verification of gene changes from biological replicates of 21 day old animals. This figure displays the results of real-time PCR on biological replicates of the 21 day old animals; brains from eight different animals (four control, four iron-deficient) were used to verify the change in each gene. The ID animals underwent the same 21-day iron deficient diet as the animals examined in the microarray analysis. Six of the twelve genes were randomly selected for verification, of which four were up-regulated and two were down-regulated. The direction of change of the six genes is in agreement with the PCR verification for the brains of the original animals. Error bars display the standard error of the mean ($^{*}p<0.05$ and $^{**}p<0.005$)

Discussion

Microarray analysis provides the opportunity to study a broad spectrum of changes that occur in iron deficiency. In this study, two experimental groups of rats were investigated. One group, 21-day-old rats represented a state of brain development during which iron availability was compromised. This group permitted evaluation of on-going responses in the brain which could be adaptive (i.e. limiting processes because of the limited iron) or compensatory (i.e. increase in expression in an attempt to acquire more iron or other nutrients). The arrays in the six-month-old animals provided the opportunity to identify any long term consequences of the early developmental iron deficiency. We observed changes in the expression of over 300 genes in the 21-day-old animals. The mRNA expression patterns in the 21-day animals indicate that multiple pathways throughout the brain are affected during iron deficiency. Because the array studies were performed during iron deficiency in the 21-day-old rats, these changes both reflect deficits directly due to the iron deficiency and possibly short-term adaptive changes to metabolic insufficiencies related to compromised iron availability. Contrastingly, the six-month animals demonstrate the long-term, apparently irreversible changes resulting from the pre- and post-natal iron deficiency that are present even after five months of iron repletion. The changes in gene expression in the six-month animals were not identified at the 21-day time period, suggesting that the gene changes at six months represent the chronic impact of iron deficiency that develops subsequent to iron repletion and as a result of the insufficient adaptive responses during iron deficiency.

Known iron transport proteins, 21-day-old animals

Transferrin receptor was among the most significantly up-regulated genes in the 21-day-old rats. TfR up-regulation at the protein level is a consistent finding in models of iron deficiency for numerous cell types (Pinero et al., 2000; Han et al., 2003; Siddappa et al., 2003) but the mRNA expression is not always altered. An increase in TfR mRNA in our animals is an indication that the brains of these animals were iron-deficient (personal communication, JL Beard). Neurons express TfR during development (Bartlett et al., 1991; Roskams and Connor, 1992), and gestationally iron-deficient Sprague Dawley rats have increased neuronal expression of TfR protein in the hippocampus and the cerebral cortex (Siddappa et al., 2003). Moos et al. did not find an increase in Tf mRNA in medial habenular neurons in a rat iron-deficient model, which may be due to the specific nuclei investigated (Moos et al., 1999). On the other hand, Han et al. measured TfR RNA levels in rat brain, and found a regional increase in TfR RNA in iron deficiency all areas examined, but the increase was significant only in striatum and the CA2 and CA3 regions of hippocampus (Han et al., 2003). Additionally, the Han et al., study utilized a model of iron deficiency wherein the animals were iron sufficient until placed on an iron-deficient diet at postnatal day 21 for the next 6 weeks. The animal model in our study was significantly different, as the animals were iron-deficient prenatally through postnatal day 21. The timing of the iron deficiency in animal models suggests that the increase in Tf receptor mRNA is a typical response to brain iron deficiency. The inborn mechanism(s) governing the level and priority of regional brain iron requirements in early prenatal life are unclear, but certainly crucial, and the expression pattern of TfR mRNA may help elucidate the impact of these various models on iron status and hence metabolism.

Transferrin mRNA expression was significantly down-regulated in this study. In an acquired systemic iron deficiency, generally there is an increase in the level of Tf mRNA in the liver (Fleming et al., 2000; Han et al., 2003). The contrast between the liver Tf mRNA response and brain Tf mRNA response in iron deficiency is not unique to this study. Han et al. (2003) examined both Tf mRNA and protein regionally throughout the brain in a different rat model of iron deficiency (Han et al., 2003). In agreement with our studies, they found that Tf mRNA content was decreased in iron-deficient animals in most brain regions. Contrastingly, levels of Tf protein increased throughout the brain in iron-deficient animals, demonstrating an inverse correlation between Tf and its mRNA in iron deficiency, and suggesting that the translation efficiency of Tf mRNA is increased in the brain or that Tf protein may be derived from tissue outside the brain. An increase in Tf transport into the brain in conditions of iron deficiency has been demonstrated (Crowe and Morgan, 1992). Additionally, the Han study also measured liver Tf mRNA and found the levels to be increased in the iron-deficient animals arguing against an increase in Tf translation efficiency within the brain to account for the increased Tf levels.

Cluster analysis, 21-day-old animals

Myelin-related genes

The importance of myelin in development is underscored by its involvement in an array of neurological diseases, including leukodystrophies and multiple sclerosis. In the brain, the oligodendrocyte is the primary cell responsible for the formation of myelin and the cell that stains most robustly for iron in the brain (LeVine and Goldman, 1988; LeVine and Macklin, 1990; Connor et al., 1992). Hypomyelination is a consistent finding in iron deficiency (Larkin, 1990; Beard et al., 2003; Ortiz et al., 2004). Transferrin mRNA, which is down-regulated in our model, is normally found in oligodendrocytes and the choroid plexus (Aldred et al., 1987; Espinosa de los Monteros et al., 1990; Roskams and Connor, 1992). Tf mRNA production and oligodendrocyte maturation are tightly coupled (Bartlett et al., 1991). Therefore the decrease in Tf mRNA in the brain suggests a delay in maturation of oligodendrocytes.

In addition to Tf mRNA, several genes related to myelin were found to be down-regulated. Those genes include myelin and lymphocyte protein, myelin oligodendrocyte glycoprotein, myelin basic protein, myelin-associated oligodendrocytic basic protein, proteolipid protein, and peripheral myelin protein 22. Tf mRNA is, as mentioned, associated with oligodendrocyte maturation, and the myelin genes affected in our study impact on a number of myelin processes. Myelin-associated oligodendrocytic basic protein (MOBP) mediates the later steps of myelin formation, possibly myelin compaction and myelin sheath maintenance (Holz et al., 1996). Myelin and lymphocyte protein (MAL) is an integral membrane protein that appears to be involved in myelin biogenesis and function and is critical in the maintenance of CNS paranodes, likely as a component in vesicular trafficking cycling between the Golgi complex and the apical plasma membrane (Schaeren-Wiemers et al., 2004). Myelin-oligodendrocyte glycoprotein (MOG) is also an integral membrane protein, and is a component of the compact myelin of the CNS, and is implicated in myelin stability, likely in completion and maintenance of the myelin sheath and in cell-cell communication. Reduced concentrations of MOG are observed in *jimpy* and *quaking* dysmyelinating mutant mice (Pham-Dinh et al., 1993). Found exclusively in the CNS, MOG is localized on the surface of myelin and oligodendrocyte cytoplasmic membranes.

Myelin basic protein (MBP) also stabilizes the myelin membrane in the CNS. There are several isoforms of MBP; isoforms 4–13 are among the most abundant protein components of the myelin membrane in the CNS and they have a role in both its formation and integrity. The non-classic group of MBP isoforms (isoforms 1–3) may have a role in the developing brain before myelination, possibly as components of transcriptional complexes and/or in signaling pathways in neural cells (Pedraza et al., 1997). The expression of MBP isoforms is developmentally regulated, with expression of the classic isoforms (isoforms 4–14, missing the first 134 amino acids) occurring later, likely as the oligodendrocytes approach terminal differentiation.

Defects in MBP cause dysmyelinating diseases, as seen in *shiverer* (*shi*) and myelin-deficient (*mld*) mice. Both types of mice have decreased myelination in the CNS, tremors, and progressive convulsions. The *shiverer* mice express only isoform 2, while the *mld* mice have a reduction in MBP (Shiota et al., 1991). The consequences of these defective MBP animal models highlight the potential risks of decreased MBP expression. Our finding of reduced MBP mRNA expression supports work by Beard et al. (2003) that found reduced MBP in hindbrain in both pre-weaning and post-weaning rats iron-deficient rat models (Beard et al., 2003).

Peripheral myelin protein 22 (PMP22) is an integral membrane protein found in the Schwann cells that mediates growth and peripheral myelin compaction. The human homolog gene duplication causes Charcot-Marie-Tooth 1A (CMT1A) neuropathy. A defect in PMP-22 is the cause of *trembler* (*tr*) phenotype in mice, which show a Schwann cell defect characterized by severe hypomyelination and Schwann cell proliferation throughout life.

One final myelin-related gene, proteolipid protein (PLP), is found in myelin but its cellular function remains obscure. Mutations of the X-chromosome-linked PLP gene can be lethal, as shown in the *jimpy* mouse and later in patients with Pelizaeus-Merzbacher disease. Phenotypically, these mutations include degeneration of oligodendrocytes and associated hypomyelination (Schneider et al., 1992).

Given the diverse and essential roles of all these genes in all stages of myelination, these data are highly suggestive of myelin deficiencies in the 21-day animals. The decrease in myelin related genes and Tf mRNA could reflect an adaptive response to the lack of a key nutrient that is required for metabolic support to maintain myelin. Given the neurological deficits associated with defective myelin, there may be an advantage to the system to delay myelination until nutrients become available. The signaling mechanism for inducing myelin onset may include iron release from microglia (Cheepsunthorn et al., 2001) which would be consistent with delayed myelination and iron deficiency. The decreased expression of myelin genes may also reflect a decreased number of oligodendrocytes. A decrease in the number or maturation of oligodendrocytes would be consistent with the decrease in Tf mRNA and mRNAs for carbonic anhydrases (see Transition Metal Cluster in Table 2) seen in our study and the decrease in CNPase activity (a marker of oligodendrocyte metabolic activity) in iron deficiency reported by Beard et al. (Larkin, 1990; Beard and Connor, 2003; Beard et al., 2003). Morath and Mayer-Proschel (2002) found that iron deficiency during pregnancy disrupts fetal glial precursor cell proliferation and oligodendrocyte generation, yielding an increased number of oligodendrocytes in the corpus callosum, but a decreased number of oligodendrocytes in the spinal cord. Based on previous *in vitro* studies comparing embryonic and postnantal precursor cells, they suggest that it may be possible for precursor cells to generate more or less mature subpopulations, and thus affect the timing of myelination (Morath and Mayer-Proschel, 2002). At this time the data do not allow us to rule out whether the decrease in myelin genes is related to fewer oligodendrocytes or altered metabolic activity of a normal number of oligodendrocytes, but clearly further research is warranted in this area.

In our six-month-old rats using the same prenatal iron deficiency paradigm, the myelin genes were no longer altered, but there was a decrease in myelin and in PLP and MBP protein (Ortiz et al., 2004) using this model despite normal levels of iron in the myelin fraction. These data suggest that the iron supplementation at weaning was sufficient to support normal gene expression, but that critical timing events between axons and oligodendrocytes may have been disrupted or metabolic compromises occurred that could not be completely corrected.

Solute carrier family

Members of the solute carrier family can be involved both in uptake and efflux in transcellular transport and include, for example, transporters for glutamate, glucose, bicarbonate, sodium, chloride, and amino acids (Hediger et al., 2004). Several members of the solute carrier family were identified among the significantly changed genes. Because of their diversity and importance in nutrient transport, solute carrier (SLC) proteins are studied extensively as a mechanism to increase drug absorption (Zhang et al., 2002). In our study, six genes in this cluster were up-regulated and two genes were down-regulated in the iron-deficient rats. Slc11a2 (DMT1) was up-regulated, as noted in the discussion of known iron transport proteins. DMT1 is a transmembrane proton symporter not only for ferrous iron, but also for Mn^{2+}, Co^{2+}, and Cu^{2}. In rat brain, DMT1 is expressed in the striatal neurons, the thalamus, the cerebellum, and the ependyma, and it likely mediates iron export from the endosome to the cytosol. Our gene findings support the work of Erikson and colleagues, who found increased DMT1 protein in all iron-deficient rat brain regions examined (Erikson et al., 2004). This study extends the investigation of DMT1 in iron deficiency to the gene level. The versatility of DMT1 and the other up-regulated solute carrier family members is significant in the context of metal transport in the iron-deficient state and signals a compensatory response to increase iron uptake. A side-effect of the increase in DMT1, however, may be to increase uptake of other metals that are not deficient in these animals (Erikson et al., 2004). For example, manganese uptake into the brain is elevated in iron deficiency and the increased uptake may be via DMT1 (Erikson et al., 2004).

The up-regulated gene Slc16a1 (MCT1) codes for the proton-linked monocarboxylic acid transporter that catalyzes the transport across the plasma membrane of many monocarboxylates, including lactate, pyruvate, valine and isoleucine, as well as ketone bodies. Baud et al. (2003) studied the expression of the monocarboxylate transporters MCT1 in the rat brain and found that during the first postnatal week, MCT1 immunoreactivity extended to the vessel walls and to the developing astrocytes in the cortex. They proposed that the transient pattern of expression of MCTs throughout the perinatal period suggests a potential relationship with the maturation of the blood-brain barrier (BBB). In addition, Vannucci and Simpson (2003) suggest that the normal peak in MCT1 mRNA in the BBB during suckling and its later decline with maturation is directly related to a switch from a combination of glucose and ketone bodies to glucose as the predominant cerebral fuel. Glia, however, maintain constant MCT1 levels, implying a major role for these proteins in transferring glycolytic intermediates during cerebral metabolism (Vannucci and Simpson, 2003). MCT1 is up-regulated in our study at PND 21, which could suggest perturbed development of the BBB (Baud et al., 2003) and altered timing of the switch from ketone bodies to glucose during development for metabolic support.

Another solute carrier, that is expressed in the BBB (and also the choroid plexus) is Slc21a5 (Reichel et al., 1999; Gao et al., 2000). The expression of this gene was decreased in iron deficiency. It transports digoxin and accepts the cyclic opioid pentapeptide [D-penicillamine2,5]enkephalin (DPDPE) as a substrate (Noe et al., 1997; Kakyo et al., 1999; Reichel et al., 1999), and may be involved in the transport of opioid peptides across the BBB in humans. The other gene in this cluster that was also down-regulated was Slc21a10 which was though to be a liver-specific. This gene is a sodium-independent transporter that mediates transport of a variety of compounds (Li et al., 2002). Our findings suggest that there are significant alterations in transport mechanisms in the BBB as a result of iron deficiency that may significantly alter metabolic processes and homeostatic mechanisms for metal regulation.

Three solute carrier genes whose proteins are involved in neurotransmitter regulation were up-regulated. Slc18a2 (SVAT) is involved in the ATP-dependent vesicular transport of biogenic amine neurotransmitters, and was up-regulated by iron deficiency. SVAT pumps cytosolic monoamines (dopamine, norepinephrine, serotonin, and histamine) into synaptic vesicles. It can also transport N-methyl-4-phenylpyridinium (MPP+), a neurotoxin metabolite associated with Parkinson's disease that utilizes iron to induce apoptosis (Gerlach et al., 1991; Kalivendi et al., 2003; Shang et al., 2004). Slc6a4 (5HTT, 5HT transporter, Sert) is directly involved with serotonin, as it terminates the action of serotonin by reuptake into presynaptic terminals. Kaladhar and Narasinga (1982) found that in both moderate and severe forms of iron deficiency, 5-HT uptake by brain synaptic vesicles is decreased (Kaladhar and Narasinga Rao, 1982). Burhans et al. (2005) found that iron-deficient adult male rats had reduced 5-HT transporter binding in some brain regions, but females demonstrated increased 5-HT transporter binding. In our study, we included only males (Burhans et al., 2005). These results indicate that iron deficiency disrupts serotonin homeostasis, but also indicates a disconnect between the mRNA expression and protein expression. Therefore, the serotoninergic system could be impacted by metabolic compromises due to iron deficiency that affect protein translation. The third up-regulated transporter in this group effecting neurotransmitters is Slc6a6, a sodium and chloride dependent taurine transporter that plays a role in neurotransmitter metabolism.

Finally, Slc7a1, a high-affinity, low capacity amino acid transporter involved in the transport of the cationic amino acids (arginine, lysine and ornithine) is up-regulated. The importance of this discussion on the effects of iron on these solute carriers is that the solute carrier (SLC) proteins have critical physiological roles in nutrient transport. The significant alterations shown here in their levels demonstrate how loss of iron availability can broadly impact nutrient transport (Zhang et al., 2002). The gene array data strongly suggest that movement of ions and molecules between cells is compromised in the 21-day-old iron-deficient animals.

Signal transduction

In the signal transduction cluster, some of the myelin-related genes appear because of their role in ionic insulation of neurons by glial cells. These are myelin and lymphocyte protein, myelin oligodendrocyte glycoprotein, myelin basic protein, and peripheral myelin protein 22. Chimerin 2 was down-regulated by iron deficiency. Mizuno et al. (2004)

report that chimerin transcription is up-regulated after exposure to neurotrophins in cerebellar neurons (Mizuno et al., 2004). Chimerin 2 is important to regulating neurite outgrowth in relation to myelin signals (Mizuno et al., 2004). Fibroblast growth factor (FGF9), also known as glia-activating factor, is also down-regulated in this cluster. FGF9 is produced mainly by neurons and can act on FGF receptors (FGFR) and the major myelin proteins. In developing rat brain oligodendrocytes, for example, Cohen et al. found that FGF-9 decreased levels of myelin proteins (Cohen and Chandross, 2000). This down-regulation of both chimerin 2 and FGF9 suggests a mechanism for disrupting the timing of myelin-axon relationships which may be associated with the myelin deficits seen at the protein level in the six-month-old rats using this iron deficiency model (Ortiz et al. (2004)). Furthermore, phosphatidylinositol 4-kinase, which is also involved in cell signaling and cytoskeleton function (Zambrzycka and Kacprzak, 2003) is also down-regulated and may relate to the genes involved in the cytoskeleton that are underexpressed in the six-month-old rats.

Three neurotransmitter receptors in the signal transduction cluster: dopamine receptor 1A, gamma-aminobutyric acid A receptor delta, and gamma-aminobutyric acid A receptor alpha 6 are down-regulated in the cluster. These data support research suggesting that early iron-deficiency can affect GABA and dopamine neurotransmitter metabolism (Taneja et al., 1986; Youdim et al., 1989; Erikson, 2000). The neurotransmitter/neuromodulator, Galanin is also down-regulated in this cluster. The inhibitory effects of galanin on several forms of synaptic plasticity, including long-term potentiation, have been demonstrated in normal and transgenic animals (Xu et al., 2005). A decrease in galanin thus represents less inhibition of synaptic plasticity, and coupled with the decreased expression of receptors involved in inhibition, suggests an overall state of decreased inhibition in the 21-day ID brain.

Two genes in this cluster that influence cytoskeletal function, afadin and phosphatidylinositol 4-kinase, are down-regulated. Afadin is a nectin- and actin-filament-binding protein, and several of the nectins that afadin binds are involved in formation of synapses (Kakunaga et al., 2005), so a decrease in this gene expression could be consistent with the aforementioned loss of synaptic plasticity.

Channel/pore class transporter & alpha-type channel activity

This cluster contains several important types of transport channels, and reflects a broad-ranging down-regulation of ionic transport. Of the eleven genes in this cluster, nine are calcium, potassium, and chloride, or GABA channel subunits. Also down-regulated are the FXYD domain-containing ion transport regulator 1, the purinergic receptor P2X ligand-gated ion channel 4, and gap junction membrane channel protein beta 1 (gjb1), defects in which can cause the demyelinating form of X-linked Charcot-Marie-Tooth disease. These data further support the concept that cell to cell communication is compromised by iron deficiency.

DNA binding

All members of the DNA binding cluster were up-regulated in the iron-deficient rats.

These genes included high mobility group box 1, high mobility group box 2, nuclease sensitive element binding protein 1 (Y-box binding protein 1 – inhibits protein synthesis), nuclear factor I/B, POU domain class 3 transcription factor 1, proliferating cell nuclear antigen, and paired box homeotic gene 6. The function of several of these genes is just beginning to be intensively investigated. Paired box homeotic gene 6 (PAX6), for example, has been shown to have an anti-proliferation function in cortical cell development by *in vivo* mouse studies (Estivill-Torrus et al., 2002). In the case of the gene nuclear factor I/B, recent studies have defined a role for the NFI proteins as neuronal transcriptional regulators that participate in directing the differentiation of cerebellar granule neurons via GABRA6; NFI proteins are required by GABRA6 for promoter activity and expression in neurons (Wang et al., 2004). As discussed earlier in the context of signal transduction, GABRA6 mRNA is down-regulated in iron deficiency, and up-regulation of Nfib mRNA expression may be a compensatory response to improve the efficiency of the NFI/GABRA6 directed neuronal differentiation. Nfib, specifically, is essential for brain development, and Nfib-deficient mice exhibit forebrain defects as well as defects in basilar pons and hippocampus formation (Steele-Perkins et al., 2005). Based on current evidence, the up-regulation of at least the majority of these genes suggests slower replication of cells in the iron-deficient brain.

The up-regulation of some of these DNA binding genes also occurs in the setting of cell stress, particularly injury or inflammation. The identification of these genes therefore suggests that the iron-deficient brain is likely under stress. The up-regulated high-mobility group box 1 protein (HMGB1), for example, was recently discovered to be a crucial cytokine in mediating the response to injury and inflammation (Lotze and Tracey, 2005; Tsung et al., 2005). Inhibition of HMGB1 activity with antibody decreased liver damage, and addition of recombinant HMGB1 worsened damage. Proliferating cell nuclear antigen (PCNA) mediates recruitment of DNA methyltransferase (Dnmt1), which plays a direct role in the restoration of epigenetic information during DNA repair (Mortusewicz et al., 2005) is also up-regulated by iron deficiency. The up-regulation of the DNA binding genes associated with cell stress supports the idea that impaired energy metabolism and transmitter synthesis makes iron-deficient neurons more vulnerable (Youdim and Ben-Shachar, 1987; de Deungria et al., 2000). These data may be relevant to the cell stress markers seen in H-ferritin-deficient mice that have compromised iron storage capacity and show increased evidence of stress (Thompson et al., 2003).

Additional genes identified as significantly changing expression in the 21-day old animals

The human kallikrein 6 gene (KLK6) encodes for a secreted serine protease, hK6, which is highly expressed in brain. Kallikrein was down-regulated in the 21-day iron-deficient animals. Previous reports have associated KLK6 with the pathogenesis of Alzheimer's disease. Zarghooni et al. (2002) found that the brain of Alzheimer's disease (AD) patients contains significantly less KLK6 than the brain of non-affected individuals (Zarghooni et al., 2002). KLK6 (also known as neurosin) may be an aging-related protease, and a decreased concentration of neurosin may be a risk factor for developing AD in older humans. KLK6 has not been studied in the context of iron, but these data suggest a direct relationship. It is possible that the KLK6 findings in humans may be related to the iron deposition found in Alzheimer's disease (Jellinger et al., 1990; Connor et al., 1992).

Arachindonate 12-lipoxygenase (Alox12, 12-LOX) is significantly up-regulated in the 21-day animals. 12-LOX has been identified as a facilitator of glutamate-induced cell death in neurons, and Khanna et al. (2003) demonstrated that glutamate-induced 12-LOX activity can be blocked by nanomolar concentrations of α-tocotrienol (generically known as Vitamin E) (Khanna et al., 2003). In addition, they showed that 12-LOX-deficient primary cortical neurons are resistant to glutamate challenge, further supporting the role of 12-LOX in executing glutamate-induced neuronal death. Up-regulation of this gene suggests the potential for increased cell death, and supports the concept that iron deficiency results in an environment of increased stress.

Membrane-associated guanylate kinase-interacting protein (MAGUIN) is expressed in neurons and is significantly up-regulated in the 21-day animals. MAGUIN co-immunoprecipitates with the synaptic scaffolding proteins PSD-95/SAP90 and S-SCAM from rat crude synaptosome (Yao et al., 1999), suggesting that MAGUIN-1 may play an important role (with PSD-95/SAP90 and S-SCAM) in the assembly of synaptic junctions. Up-regulation of MAGUIN could be reflective of an effort to increase the number and/or stability of synaptic junctions.

Thyroid hormone responsive protein (THRSP) was the most significantly down-regulated gene from the 21-day animals. Iron deficiency impairs thyroid hormone synthesis by reducing activity of heme-dependent thyroid peroxidase (Zimmermann and Kohrle, 2002), and THRSP is known to be responsive to thyroid hormone. Iron deficiency is known to be associated with decreased thyroid hormone levels (Beard et al., 1989). It is possible, therefore, that the decreased expression of THRSP mRNA is an adaptive response that will slow development under the current metabolic limitations imposed by decreased iron availability. A function of thyroid hormones in the developing brain is to provide a timing signal for the induction of differentiation and maturation programs, and inappropriate initiation of these timing events leads to asynchrony in developmental processes and a deleterious outcome (Anderson et al., 2003). Studies have historically suggested deficient development of the central nervous system in the absence of thyroid hormone – most notably reduced myelination (Balazs et al., 1969; Balazs, 1971; Rosman et al., 1972). In brain, THRSP is localized to neurons (Shah et al., 1997). THRSP and thyroid hormone are likely involved in synaptic plasticity in hippocampal neurons (Tang et al., 2001). It is also relevant to note that Faivre et al. (1984) reported a dramatic decrease in microtubule numbers in Purkinje cells in thyroid hormone-deficient states (Faivre, 1984), and Aniello et al. (1991) also demonstrated a delay in the developmental expression patterns of various tubulin isotype mRNAs (Aniello et al., 1991). The decrease in THRSP could be associated with the loss of synaptic plasticity discussed earlier, the decrease in myelin, and the decrease in cytoskeletal genes and myelin-axon interaction. The decrease in THRSP are perhaps also related to the down-regulation of CCT6A and TPM1 – and their resultant effects on tubulin and microtubules – observed in the six-month animals, discussed in detail below. In the context of intervention strategies, a mechanism to increase THRSP may be essential before such strategies can be completely effective.

Six-month animals

Data from the six-month-old developmental iron-deficient rats is a striking contrast to the 21-day data: there are only five genes whose expression was changed and all are down-regulated. The significantly fewer gene changes at this later time point indicate that the adaptive and compensatory changes that occurred during the iron-deficient period were adequate in many areas but that iron repletion was not capable of overcoming all the development perturbations. The down-regulation of these genes that were still altered after five months of iron repletion represents decreased cytoskeletal stability, decreased nucleic acid translation, and decreased responsiveness to oxidative stress.

Two genes, DHX9 and H2AFY, are involved in nucleic acid translation. DHX9, or DEAD box polypeptide 9, is a putative RNA helicase. It is localized to the nucleus and is implicated in a number of cellular processes involving the alteration of RNA secondary structure, including translation initiation, nuclear and mitochondrial splicing, and ribosome and spliceosome assembly (Zhang and Grosse 1994). It unwinds double-stranded DNA and RNA in a 3′ to 5′ direction and creates secondary structures capable of influencing RNA-binding proteins. H2A histone family, member Y (H2AFY) is a ubiquitous nuclear gene involved in DNA metabolism. Histones are responsible for the nucleosome structure of the chromosomal fiber in eukaryotes. Nucleosomes consist of approximately 146 bp of DNA wrapped around a histone octamer comprised of a pair of each of the four core histones (H2A, H2B, H3, and H4). Down-regulated expression of the DHXP and H2AFY genes suggests broad-ranging decreases in the efficiency of translation in the brain.

Two of the other genes identified in this array analysis, CCT6A and TPM1, are involved in cytoskeletal functioning and cell structure and stability. CCT6A encodes a cytoplasmic molecular chaperone that is member of the chaperonin containing TCP1 complex (CCT). This complex consists of two identical stacked rings, each containing eight different proteins, which fold in an ATP-dependent manner. The complex folds various proteins, including actin and tubulin – both of which are in turn also crucial to muscular and cytoskeletal stability. Tubulin is a component of the centrosome. Before microtubules can be nucleated, the tubulin must first be folded; this is achieved by the cytoplasmic chaperone complex TCP-1. A disruption in tubulin folding would have a negative impact on cell division and axonal transport. Actin, a protein abundant in many cells, especially muscle cells, significantly contributes to the cell's structure and motility. Actin can assemble microfilaments, interact with myosin to permit movement of the cell, or pinch the cell into two during cell division. Actin is found in neuronal growth cones and in synaptic complexes in the brain, specifically at the base of dendritic spines. Thus a disruption in actin could result in fewer branches on neurons and a decrease in synaptic efficacy associated with changes in dendritic spine configuration.

A common mechanism is likely involved in both the formation of dendritic spines and the structural plasticity at mature synapses, and that common mechanism is centered on dynamic actin filaments (Matus, 2000). Fernandez-Valle et al. (1997) found that disrupting actin polymerization with cytochalasin D inhibited myelination of Schwann cell/Neuron co-cultures, suggesting that filamentous actin is needed during SC differentiation for both cell shapes changes as well as expression of myelin-specific mRNAs (Fernandez-Valle et al., 1997). Dendritic spines are comprised of two major structural elements: postsynaptic densities (PSD) and actin cytoskeletons. Takahashi et al. (2003) demonstrated that synaptic clustering of drebrin, an actin-binding protein, regulates spine morphogenesis. Further, suppression of drebrin up-regulation by antisense nucleotides attenuated synaptic clustering of PSD-95 and clustering of drebrin and filamentous actin (Takahashi et al., 2003). Learning and memory deficits associated with early iron deficiency persist beyond development despite iron repletion (Felt and Lozoff, 1996; Kwik-Uribe et al., 2000; Youdim and Yehuda, 2000). A possible mechanism for the long-term deficits is provided by dendritic analysis of the hippocampus in iron-deficient rats (Rao et al., 1999, 2003) that show decreased dendritic branching in the iron-deficient rats. Additionally, Georgieff and colleagues specifically found that severe perinatal iron deficiency disrupted hippocampal apical dendritic growth and branching patterns as indexed by microtubule associated protein-2 (MAP-2) when examined early in life (Jorgenson et al., 2003). These data are consistent with our gene array studies that predict a loss of dendritic profiles could be found in iron-deficient brains. Cytoskeleton actin filaments are stabilized by the ubiquitous protein Tropomyosin 1 (TPM1). TPM1 binds to actin filaments in muscle and non-muscle cells and plays a role in the regulation of striated muscle contraction (along with the troponin complex). The observed decreases in CCT6A and TPM1 in the brains of the six-month animals is suggestive of long-term damage to the cytoskeletal infrastructure of neurons and possibly the glial cells – a particularly devastating finding in the brain, where such proteins (and the affected downstream proteins) are necessary to form interneuronal connections. Again, these findings provide further support and potential precipitating mechanisms for the long-term deficits of iron deficiency.

Tropomyosins (TMs) are actin binding proteins that can be made more diverse by alternative RNA splicing. TMBr-1 and TMBr-3, for example, are two brain-specific isoforms of TPM1 in rat generated by alternative splicing. TMBr-3 appears embryonically at 16 days of gestation throughout the brain, while TMBr-1 does not appear until 20 days after birth and is expressed only in areas primarily derived from the prosencephalon (Stamm et al., 1993). TMBr-1 and TMBr-3 are expressed relatively late in development, with their levels remaining at a constant level in the normal adult. Further, TMBr-1 has been shown to have the strongest expression in areas of the brain thought to have the greatest plasticity after birth. Such patterns suggest a specialized role of these isoforms in nervous system development and plasticity. The function of TMs in non-muscle cells is not yet clear, but is certainly distinct from their function in muscle cells, where TMs function in association with the troponin complex to regulate calcium-sensitive actin and myosin interaction. Interestingly, TM expression is changed in some neurodegenerative diseases, including Parkinson's and Alzheimer's diseases (Galloway et al., 1990; Galloway and Perry, 1991). Stamm et al. (1993) suggest that TMBr-1 and TMBr-3 may play a role in process outgrowth and the formation of dendritic spines and synapses, as TMs have been shown to be present in all of these structures (Stamm et al., 1993). Additionally, the likely weaker binding properties of the two isoforms may allow for the dynamic cytoskeletal changes necessary for adult plasticity. The gene array data, both at the six-month and 21-day-old groups suggest plasticity is compromised in the iron-deficient brain.

The fifth down-regulated gene, proteasome subunit beta type 5 (PSMB5), is a member of the proteasome B-type family that is a 20S core subunit in the proteasome. Proteasomes degrade oxidized, damaged, or misfolded proteins, thus promoting cell survival. Proteasomes are both cytoplasmic and nuclear and are distributed throughout eukaryotic cells. They cleave peptides in an ATP/ubiquitin-dependent process in a non-lysosomal pathway. Some neurodegenerative diseases and age-related disorders are associated with reduced proteasome activity. Kwak et al. (2003) showed that the expression of most subunits of the 20S proteasome were enhanced up to threefold in the livers of mice following treatment with dithiolethiones, which act as indirect antioxidants (Kwak et al., 2003). A gene known as Nrf2 is a central molecular target of indirect antioxidants, and they demonstrated that the genes forming the 26S proteasome complex (of which PSMB5 and the 20s proteasome are a part) are regulated by Nrf2. Promoter activity of PSMB5 increased with either Nrf2 over-expression or treatment with antioxidants in mouse embryonic fibroblasts, and they identified antioxidant response elements in the promoter of PSMB5 that controlled these responses. Induction of this protective pathway provides a means for cells to survive conditions of stress. We observe down-regulation of the PSMB5 gene in our six-month animals, suggesting less effective protein degradation compared to those animals who did not suffer the iron-deficient insult early in life.

Kabashi et al. (2004) found that the level of 20S proteasome was reduced in lumbar spine motor neurons of transgenic SOD-1 mice relative to the surrounding neuropil, suggesting that impaired proteasomal function is an early event in amyotrophic lateral sclerosis (ALS) contributing to its pathology (Kabashi et al., 2004). Studies of the *trembler* mouse model of Charcot-Marie-Tooth disease Type 1A also suggested a role for impaired proteasome activity (Fortun et al., 2005). Aggregates containing ubiquitin and peripheral myelin protein 22 (PMP22) were found in neuropathy nerves, suggesting a mechanism by which defective degradation of Schwann cell proteins could contribute to PMP22 neuropathies.

Alternatively, the down-regulation of PSMB5 could reflect an attempt to delay or prevent degradation in a stressful environment. MacInnis and Campenot (2005) suggest that the proteasome does not function as an effector of protein degradation during axonal degeneration, but rather it regulates the signaling pathways that control axonal survival or degeneration (MacInnis and Campenot, 2005). They treated transected distal axons from rat sympathetic neurons with an inhibitor of proteasome activity, and found that it preserved axonal mitochondrial function over the tested 24 hours. The protected axons demonstrated persistent Erk1/2 phosphorylation, which, upon inhibition of MEK activity, restored axonal degeneration. Regardless of the exact role of PSMB5 in the six-month animals, decreased proteasomal function could increase cell vulnerability.

Conclusion

The inability of normal iron in the diet beginning at weaning to reverse changes in the brain that affect cytoskeletal stability and synaptic function reinforces the importance of early intervention in iron deficiency. The gene arrays in the 21-day-old rats identified a set of responses that could be characterized as adaptive to the existing state of iron deficiency and another set of responses that could be characterized as compensatory. The compensatory response (defined as changes in gene expression that would be aimed at normalizing iron status) consists of elevated Tf receptor mRNA and increase in DMT1. The adaptive responses, such as decreased replication of cells, decreased myelin gene expression, decreased signal transduction pathway genes etc. indicate changes in gene expression that were caused by the altered iron status. These adaptive responses could be returned to normal if iron repletion occurs in a sufficient and timely manner. The purpose of the adaptive responses may be to limit the metabolic demands of a brain in a metabolically compromised setting. The gene array suggests that the brain "makes choices" in the nutrient compromised setting. The gene array data from the six-month-old animals suggests that most of the adaptive responses were effective. Some long term changes in gene expression where identified that could be related to the adaptive responses in the 21-day-old rats. For example, the cytoskeletal and synaptic plasticity deficits in the adult brain suggested by down-regulation of tropomyosins and CCT6A could be related to the altered gene expression patterns associated with signal transduction and myelin proteins. In addition, a decrease in the integrity of this relationship may account for the myelin deficits seen in the six-month-old animals (Ortiz et al., 2004) despite the absence of changes in myelin gene profiles.

Embedded in the interpretation of our data is that the adaptive responses are likely to be dependent upon the developmental age at which the iron deficiency is encountered and the length of time that the animals are exposed to iron deficiency. At some point, if the adaptive responses are allowed to persist, the brain develops under the influence of these responses which should result in compromised function. The long term goal of this project is to identify the adaptive responses and the time frame in which they do not negatively impact outcome. Arguably, the adaptive response in the 21-day-old rats coupled with iron rescue in this model was effective, given that so few genes remain changed at six months. The specific implications of the down-regulated genes, however, must be considered: metabolically, there is slowed translation and slowed degradation; structurally, there is cytoskeletal insufficiency. Despite normal iron availability for five months, these genes which underlie multiple processes (e.g. axonal transport, cell repair) were still altered. Such findings are remarkable in the context of such a long recovery time, and are suggestive of the long term implications and irreversibility of an early iron insult. These data provide novel evidence for the behavioral and neurological deficits that are associated with developmental iron deficiency and identify key areas in the early development iron deficiency model that can be targeted to minimize the long term consequences.

Acknowledgements

This work was supported in part by a program project grant from the National Institutes of Health (NICHD 39386 to Betsy Lozoff, M.D.) awarded to the group in Brain and Behavior in Early Iron Deficiency and by tobacco settlement funds from the Pennsylvania State Department of Health. We would like to thank Dr. David Drubin, Dr. Willard Freeman, Kruti Patel, and Robert Brucklacher for their expert technical advice.

References

Aldred AR, Dickson PW, et al. (1987) Distribution of transferrin synthesis in brain and other tissues in the rat. J Biol Chem 262: 5293–5297

Anderson GW, Schoonover CM, et al. (2003) Control of thyroid hormone action in the developing rat brain. Thyroid 13: 1039–1056

Andrews NC (2000) Iron metabolism: iron deficiency and iron overload. Annu Rev Genomics Hum Genet 1: 75–98

Aniello F, Couchie D, et al. (1991) Regulation of five tubulin isotypes by thyroid hormone during brain development. J Neurochem 57: 1781–1786

Balazs R (1971) Biochemical effects of thyroid hormones in the developing brain. UCLA Forum Med Sci 14: 273–320

Balazs R, Brooksbank BW, et al. (1969) The effect of thyroid deficiency on myelination in the rat brain. J Physiol 201: 28–29

Bartlett WP, Li X-S, et al. (1991) Expression of transferrin mRNA in the CNS of normal and jimpy mice. J Neurochem 57: 318–322

Baud O, Fayol L, et al. (2003) Perinatal and early postnatal changes in the expression of monocarboxylate transporters MCT1 and MCT2 in the rat forebrain. J Comp Neurol 465: 445–454

Beard J, Tobin B, et al. (1989) Evidence for thyroid hormone deficiency in iron-deficient anemic rats. J Nutr 119: 772–778

Beard JL, Connor JR (2003) Iron status and neural functioning. Annu Rev Nutr 23: 41–58

Beard JL, Hendricks MK, et al. (2005) Maternal iron deficiency anemia affects postpartum emotions and cognition. J Nutr 135: 267–272

Beard JL, Wiesinger JA, et al. (2003) Pre- and postweaning iron deficiency alters myelination in Sprague-Dawley rats. Dev Neurosci 25: 308–315

Benjamini Y, Hochberg Y (1995) Controlling the false discovery rate: a practical and powerful approach to multiple testing. J Roy Statist Soc Series B: 289–300

Bolstad B, Irizarry RA, Astrand M, Speed TP (2003) A comparison of normalization methods for high density oligonucleotide array data based on variance and bias. Bioinformatics 19: 185–193

Burhans MS, Dailey C, et al. (2005) Iron deficiency: differential effects on monoamine transporters. Nutr Neurosci 8: 31–38

Cheepsunthorn P, Radov L, et al. (2001) Characterization of a novel brain-derived microglial cell line isolated from neonatal rat brain. Glia 35: 53–62

Chen Q, Connor JR, et al. (1995) Brain iron, transferrin and ferritin concentrations are altered in developing iron-deficient rats. J Nutr 125: 1529–1535

Cohen RI, Chandross KJ (2000) Fibroblast growth factor-9 modulates the expression of myelin related proteins and multiple fibroblast growth factor receptors in developing oligodendrocytes. J Neurosci Res 61: 273–287

Connor JR, Menzies SL, et al. (1992) A histochemical study of iron, transferrin, and ferritin in Alzheimer's diseased brains. J Neurosci Res 31: 75–83

Crowe A, Morgan EH (1992) Iron and transferrin uptake by brain and cerebrospinal fluid in the rat. Brain Res 592: 8–16

Dallman PR, Siimes MA, et al. (1975) Brain iron: persistent deficiency following short term iron deprivation in the young rat. Br J Heamatol 31: 209–215 de Deungria M, Rao R, et al. (2000) Perinatal iron deficiency decreases cytochrome c oxidase (CytOx) activity in selected regions of neonatal rat brain. Pediatr Res 48: 169–176

Erikson K, Jones BC, Beard JL (2000) Dopamine reuptake is altered in iron deficiency anemia. J Nutr 130: 2831–2837

Erikson KM, Pinero DJ, et al. (1997) Regional brain iron, ferritin and transferrin concentrations during iron deficiency and iron repletion in developing rats. J Nutr 127: 2030–2038

Erikson KM, Syversen T, et al. (2004) Globus pallidus: a target brain region for divalent metal accumulation associated with dietary iron deficiency. J Nutr Biochem 15: 335–341

Espinosa de los Monteros A, Kumar S, et al. (1990) Transferrin gene expression and secretion by rat brain cells in vitro. J Neurosci Res 25: 576–580

Estivill-Torrus G, Pearson H, et al. (2002) Pax6 is required to regulate the cell cycle and the rate of progression from symmetrical to asymmetrical division in mammalian cortical progenitors. Development 129: 455–466

Faivre C, Legrand C, Rabie A (1984) In Purkinje cell dendrites of the young rat, thyroid hormone controls the resistance of microtubules to fixation at low temperature. Int J Dev Neurosci 2: 427–436

Felt BT, Lozoff B (1996) Brain iron and behavior of rats are not normalized by treatment of iron deficiency anemia during early development. J Nutr 126: 693–701

Fernandez-Valle C, Gorman D, et al. (1997) Actin plays a role in both changes in cell shape and gene-expression associated with Schwann cell myelination. J Neurosci 17: 241–250

Fleming RE, Migas MC, et al. (2000) Transferrin receptor 2: continued expression in mouse liver in the face of iron overload and in hereditary hemochromatosis. Proc Natl Acad Sci USA 97: 2214–2219

Fortun J, Li J, et al. (2005) Impaired proteasome activity and accumulation of ubiquitinated substrates in a hereditary neuropathy model. J Neurochem 92: 1531–1541

Galloway PG, Mulvihill P, et al. (1990) Immunochemical demonstration of tropomyosin in the neurofibrillary pathology of Alzheimer's disease. Am J Pathol 137: 291–300

Galloway PG, Perry G (1991) Tropomyosin distinguishes Lewy bodies of Parkinson disease from other neurofibrillary pathology. Brain Res 541: 347–349

Gao B, Hagenbuch B, et al. (2000) Organic anion-transporting polypeptides mediate transport of opioid peptides across blood-brain barrier. J Pharmacol Exp Ther 294: 73–79

Gerlach M, Riederer P, et al. (1991) MPTP mechanisms of neurotoxicity and their implications for Parkinson's disease. Eur J Pharmacol 208: 273–286

Han J, Day JR, et al. (2003) Gene expression of transferrin and transferrin receptor in brains of control vs. iron-deficient rats. Nutr Neurosci 6: 1–10

Hediger MA, Romero MF, et al. (2004) The ABCs of solute carriers: physiological, pathological and therapeutic implications of human membrane transport proteins introduction. Pflugers Arch 447: 465–468

Holz A, Schaeren-Wiemers N, et al. (1996) Molecular and developmental characterization of novel cDNAs of the myelin-associated/oligodendrocytic basic protein. J Neurosci 16: 467–477

Irizarry R, Hobbs B, Collin F, Beazer-Barclay YD, Antonellis KJ, Scherf U, Speed TP (2003) Exploration, normalization, and summaries of high density oligonucleotide array probe level data. Biostatistics 4: 249–264

Jellinger K, Paulus W, et al. (1990) Brain iron and ferritin in Parkinson's and Alzheimer's diseases. J Neural Transm Park Dis Dement Sect 2: 327–340

Jones BC, Reed CL, et al. (2003) Quantitative genetic analysis of ventral midbrain and liver iron in BXD recombinant inbred mice. Nutr Neurosci 6: 369–377

Jorgenson LA, Wobken JD, et al. (2003) Perinatal iron deficiency alters apical dendritic growth in hippocampal CA1 pyramidal neurons. Dev Neurosci 25: 412–420

Kabashi E, Agar JN, et al. (2004) Focal dysfunction of the proteasome: a pathogenic factor in a mouse model of amyotrophic lateral sclerosis. J Neurochem 89: 1325–1335

Kakunaga S, Ikeda W, et al. (2005) Nectin-like molecule-1/TSLL1/SynCAM3: a neural tissue-specific immunoglobulin-like cell-cell adhesion molecule localizing at non-junctional contact sites of presynaptic nerve terminals, axons and glia cell processes. J Cell Sci 118: 1267–1277

Kakyo M, Sakagami H, et al. (1999) Immunohistochemical distribution and functional characterization of an organic anion transporting polypeptide 2 (oatp2). FEBS Lett 445: 343–346

Kaladhar M, Narasinga Rao BS (1982) Effects of iron deficiency on serotonin uptake in vitro by rat brain synaptic vesicles. J Neurochem 38: 1576–1581

Kalivendi SV, Kotamraju S, et al. (2003) 1-Methyl-4-phenylpyridinium (MPP+)-induced apoptosis and mitochondrial oxidant generation: role of transferrin-receptor-dependent iron and hydrogen peroxide. Biochem J 371: 151–164

Khanna S, Roy S, et al. (2003) Molecular basis of vitamin E action: tocotrienol modulates 12-lipoxygenase, a key mediator of glutamate-induced neurodegeneration. J Biol Chem 278: 43508–43515

Kwak MK, Wakabayashi N, et al. (2003) Antioxidants enhance mammalian proteasome expression through the Keap1-Nrf2 signaling pathway. Mol Cell Biol 23: 8786–8794

Kwik-Uribe CL, Gietzen D, et al. (2000) Chronic marginal iron intakes during early development in mice result in persistent changes in dopamine metabolism and myelin composition. J Nutr 130: 2821–2830

Kwik-Uribe CL, Golub MS, et al. (2000) Chronic marginal iron intakes during early development in mice alter brain iron concentrations and behavior despite postnatal iron supplementation. J Nutr 130: 2040–2048

Larkin E, Rao GA (1990) Importance of fetal and neonatal iron: Adequacy for normal development of central nervouse system. Brain, Behavior and Iron in the Infant Diet. J. Dobbing. London, UK, Springer-Verlag: 43–63

LeVine SM, Goldman JE (1988) Spatial and temporal patterns of oligodendrocyte differentiation in rat cerebrum and cerebellum. J Comp Neurol 277: 441–455

LeVine SM, Macklin WB (1990) Iron-enriched oligodendrocytes: a reexamination of their spatial distribution. J Neurosci Res 26: 508–512

Li C, Wong WH (2001) Model-based analysis of oligonucleotide arrays: expression index computation and outlier detection. Proc Natl Acad Sci USA 98: 31–36

Li C, Wong WH (2003) DNA-Chip Analyzer (dChip) The analysis of gene expression data: methods and software. G. Parmigiani, Garrett, ES, Irizarry, R and Zeger, SL., Springer

Li N, Hartley DP, et al. (2002) Tissue expression, ontogeny, and inducibility of rat organic anion transporting polypeptide 4. J Pharmacol Exp Ther 301: 551–560

Lotze MT, Tracey KJ (2005) High-mobility group box 1 protein (HMGB1): nuclear weapon in the immune arsenal. Nat Rev Immunol 5: 331–342

Lozoff B, Jimenez E, et al. (2000) Poorer behavioral and developmental outcome more than 10 years after treatment for iron deficiency in infancy. Pediatrics 105: E51

MacInnis BL, Campenot RB (2005) Regulation of Wallerian degeneration and nerve growth factor withdrawal-induced pruning of axons of sympathetic neurons by the proteasome and the MEK/Erk pathway. Mol Cell Neurosci 28: 430–439

Matus A (2000) Actin-based plasticity in dendritic spines. Science 290: 754–758

Mizuno T, Yamashita T, et al. (2004) Chimaerins act downstream from neurotrophins in overcoming the inhibition of neurite outgrowth produced by myelin-associated glycoprotein. J Neurochem 91: 395–403

Moos T, Oates PS, et al. (1999) Iron-independent neuronal expression of transferrin receptor mRNA in the rat. Brain Res Mol Brain Res 72: 231–234

Morath DJ, Mayer-Proschel M (2002) Iron deficiency during embryogenesis and consequences for oligodendrocyte generation in vivo. Dev Neurosci 24: 197–207

Mortusewicz O, Schermelleh L, et al. (2005) Recruitment of DNA methyltransferase I to DNA repair sites. Proc Natl Acad Sci USA

Noe B, Hagenbuch B, et al. (1997) Isolation of a multispecific organic anion and cardiac glycoside transporter from rat brain. Proc Natl Acad Sci USA 94: 10346–10350

Ortiz E, Pasquini JM, et al. (2004) Effect of manipulation of iron storage, transport, or availability on myelin composition and brain iron content in three different animal models. J Neurosci Res 77: 681–689

Palti H, Meijer A, et al. (1985) Learning achievement and behavior at school of anemic and non-anemic infants. Early Hum Dev 10: 217–223

Pedraza L, Fidler L, et al. (1997) The active transport of myelin basic protein into the nucleus suggests a regulatory role in myelination. Neuron 18: 579–589

Perez EM, Hendricks MK, et al. (2005) Mother-infant interactions and infant development are altered by maternal iron deficiency anemia. J Nutr 135: 850–855

Pham-Dinh D, Mattei MG, et al. (1993) Myelin/oligodendrocyte glycoprotein is a member of a subset of the immunoglobulin superfamily encoded within the major histocompatibility complex. Proc Natl Acad Sci USA 90: 7990–7994

Pinero DJ, Hu J, et al. (2000) Alterations in the interaction between iron regulatory proteins and their iron responsive element in normal and Alzheimer's diseased brains. Cell Mol Biol (Noisy-le-grand) 46: 761–776

Pinero DJ, Li NQ, et al. (2000) Variations in dietary iron alter brain iron metabolism in developing rats. J Nutr 130: 254–263

Rao R, de Ungria M, et al. (1999) Perinatal brain iron deficiency increases the vulnerability of rat hippocampus to hypoxic ischemic insult. J Nutr 129: 199–206

Rao R, Tkac I, et al. (2003) Perinatal iron deficiency alters the neurochemical profile of the developing rat hippocampus. J Nutr 133: 3215–3221

Reichel C, Gao B, et al. (1999) Localization and function of the organic anion-transporting polypeptide Oatp2 in rat liver. Gastroenterology 117: 688–695

Roskams AJ, Connor JR (1992) Transferrin receptor expression in myelin deficient (md) rats. J Neurosci Res 31: 421–427

Rosman NP, Malone MJ, et al. (1972) The effect of thyroid deficiency on myelination of brain. A morphological and biochemical study. Neurology 22: 99–106

Schaeren-Wiemers N, Bonnet A, et al. (2004) The raft-associated protein MAL is required for maintenance of proper axon-glia interactions in the central nervous system. J Cell Biol 166: 731–742

Schneider A, Montague P, et al. (1992) Uncoupling of hypomyelination and glial cell death by a mutation in the proteolipid protein gene. Nature 358: 758–761

Shah GN, Li J, et al. (1997) Cloning and characterization of a complementary DNA for a thyroid hormone-responsive protein in mature rat cerebral tissue. Biochem J 327: 617–623

Shang T, Kotamraju S, et al. (2004) 1-Methyl-4-phenylpyridinium-induced apoptosis in cerebellar granule neurons is mediated by transferrin receptor iron-dependent depletion of tetrahydrobiopterin and neuronal nitric-oxide synthase-derived superoxide. J Biol Chem 279: 19099–19112

Shiota C, Ikenaka K, et al. (1991) Developmental expression of myelin protein genes in dysmyelinating mutant mice: analysis by nuclear run-off transcription assay, in situ hybridization, and immunohistochemistry. J Neurochem 56: 818–826

Siddappa AJ, Rao RB, et al. (2003) Iron deficiency alters iron regulatory protein and iron transport protein expression in the perinatal rat brain. Pediatr Res 53: 800–807

Stamm S, Casper D, et al. (1993) Brain-specific tropomyosins TMBr-1 and TMBr-3 have distinct patterns of expression during development and in adult brain. Proc Natl Acad Sci USA 90: 9857–9861

Steele-Perkins G, Plachez C, et al. (2005) The transcription factor gene Nfib is essential for both lung maturation and brain development. Mol Cell Biol 25: 685–698

Takahashi H, Sekino Y, et al. (2003) Drebrin-dependent actin clustering in dendritic filopodia governs synaptic targeting of postsynaptic density-95 and dendritic spine morphogenesis. J Neurosci 23: 6586–6595

Taneja V, Mishra K, et al. (1986) Effect of early iron deficiency in rat on the gamma-aminobutyric acid shunt in brain. J Neurochem 46: 1670–1674

Tang YP, Ma YL, et al. (2001) mRNA differential display identification of thyroid hormone-responsive protein (THRP) gene in association with early phase of long-term potentiation. Hippocampus 11: 637–646

Thompson K, Menzies S, et al. (2003) Mouse brains deficient in H-ferritin have normal iron concentration but a protein profile of iron deficiency and increased evidence of oxidative stress. J Neurosci Res 71: 46–63

Tsung A, Sahai R, et al. (2005) The nuclear factor HMGB1 mediates hepatic injury after murine liver ischemia-reperfusion. J Exp Med 201: 1135–1143

Tukey J (1977) Exploratory Data Analysis. Reading, MA, Addison-Wesley

Tusher VG, Tibshirani R, et al. (2001) Significance analysis of microarrays applied to the ionizing radiation response. Proc Natl Acad Sci USA 98: 5116–5121

Vannucci SJ, Simpson IA (2003) Developmental switch in brain nutrient transporter expression in the rat. Am J Physiol Endocrinol Metab 285: E1127–E1134

Wang W, Stock RE, et al. (2004) A role for nuclear factor I in the intrinsic control of cerebellar granule neuron gene expression. J Biol Chem 279: 53491–53497

Weinberg J, Levine S, et al. (1979) Long-term consequences of early iron deficiency in the rat. Pharmacol Biochem Behav 11: 631–638

Xu ZQ, Zheng K, et al. (2005) Electrophysiological studies on galanin effects in brain – progress during the last six years. Neuropeptides 39: 267–273

Yao I, Hata Y, et al. (1999) MAGUIN, a novel neuronal membrane-associated guanylate kinase-interacting protein. J Biol Chem 274: 11889–11896

Youdim MB, Ben-Shachar D (1987) Minimal brain damage induced by early iron deficiency: modified dopaminergic neurotransmission. Isr J Med Sci 23: 19–25

Youdim MB, Ben-Shachar D, et al. (1989) Putative biological mechanisms of the effect of iron deficiency on brain biochemistry and behavior. Am J Clin Nutr 50 [Suppl 3]: 607–615; discussion 615–617

Youdim MB, Yehuda S (2000) The neurochemical basis of cognitive deficits induced by brain iron deficiency: involvement of dopamine-opiate system. Cell Mol Biol (Noisy-le-grand) 46: 491–500

Youdim MB, Yehuda S, et al. (1981) Iron deficiency-induced circadian rhythm reversal of dopaminergic-mediated behaviours and thermoregulation in rats. Eur J Pharmacol 74: 295–301

Zambrzycka A, Kacprzak M (2003) Apolipoprotein E4 and A beta peptide 1-42 inhibit polyphosphoinositide biosynthesis in rat brain cortex. Pol J Pharmacol 55: 911–913

Zarghooni M, Soosaipillai A, et al. (2002) Decreased concentration of human kallikrein 6 in brain extracts of Alzheimer's disease patients. Clin Biochem 35: 225–231

Zhang EY, Knipp GT, et al. (2002) Structural biology and function of solute transporters: implications for identifying and designing substrates. Drug Metab Rev 34: 709–750

Zhang S, Grosse F (1994) Nuclear DNA helicase II unwinds both DNA and RNA. Biochemistry 33: 3906–3912

Zimmermann MB, Kohrle J (2002) The impact of iron and selenium deficiencies on iodine and thyroid metabolism: biochemistry and relevance to public health. Thyroid 12: 867–878

Supplemental Table. *All significantly changed genes in the 21-day animals. This table lists the 334 significantly changed genes in the 21-day rats. All genes have an FDR of <0.05 (the expected proportion of false positive genes among all genes that are considered significant). Each gene title, name, symbol, and ID is listed, as well as the fold change and q-value*

Title	Symbol	Gene name	Accession number	Fold change	q-value (%)
UP-REGULATED GENES					
arachidonate 12-lipoxygenase	Alox12	L06040_s_at	NM_031010	3.38871	0.831810561
arachidonate 12-lipoxygenase	Alox12	S69383_at	NM_031010	3.11209	0.831810561
Rattus norvegicus transcribed sequences	–	rc_AA866443_at	–	2.71356	0.831810561
electron-transferring-flavoprotein dehydrogenase	Etfdh	rc_AI237007_at	–	2.51510	0.831810561
transferrin receptor	Tfrc	M58040_at	–	2.39091	0.831810561
Rattus norvegicus transcribed sequences	–	rc_AA893172_at	–	2.14911	0.831810561
–	–	M93257_s_at	–	1.88482	3.940821135
membrane-associated guanylate kinase-interacting protein	LOC59322	AF102853_at	NM_021686	1.87739	0.831810561
tubulin, beta 5	Tubb5	AB011679_at	NM_173102	1.87635	0.831810561
smooth muscle alpha-actin	Acta2	rc_AA900769_s_at	–	1.84847	1.370947035
catalase	Cat	rc_AA926149_g_at	NM_012520	1.84026	0.831810561
cell division cycle 2 homolog A (S. pombe)	Cdc2a	X60767mRNA_s_at	NM_019296	1.67649	0.831810561
high mobility group box 2	Hmgb2	rc_AI008836_s_at	NM_017187	1.66875	0.831810561
guanine nucleotide binding protein, beta 1	Gnb1	AF022083_s_at	NM_030987	1.61726	0.831810561
Rat mRNA for beta-tubulin T beta15	–	X03369_s_at	–	1.58431	0.831810561
topoisomerase (DNA) 2 alpha	Top2a	rc_AA899854_at	–	1.57366	3.940821135
–	–	X62951mRNA_s_at	–	1.57265	0.831810561
solute carrier family 11 member 2	Slc11a2	rc_AA892390_s_at	NM_013173	1.56078	0.831810561
FK506 binding protein 1b	Fkbp1b	D86642_at	NM_022675	1.55962	0.831810561
Rattus norvegicus similar to Myristoylated alanine-rich C-kinase substrate (MARCKS) (LOC294446), mRNA	–	rc_AA925762_at	–	1.55113	0.831810561
Rattus norvegicus transcribed sequence with weak similarity to protein ref:NP_055582.1 (H.sapiens) KIAA0275 gene product [Homo sapiens]	–	rc_AI639294_at	–	1.54511	2.903181957
collagen, type 1, alpha 1	Col1a1	U75405UTR#1_f_at	–	1.54275	4.876302628
thymosin beta-like protein	LOC286978	rc_AA997865_at	NM_173313	1.52727	0.831810561
–	–	AF034899_r_at	–	1.52307	1.370947035
CD48 antigen	Cd48	X13016_at	NM_139103	1.51357	0.831810561
GTP cyclohydrolase 1	Gch	M58364_at	NM_024356	1.50412	0.831810561
solute carrier family 16, member 1	Slc16a1	rc_AI145680_s_at	NM_012716	1.50408	2.008596819
aminolevulinic acid synthase 2	Alas2	D86297_at	NM_013197	1.49073	0.831810561
collagen, type 1, alpha 1	Col1a1	M27207mRNA_s_at	–	1.48835	4.876302628
kinase insert domain protein receptor	Kdr	U93306_at	NM_013062	1.48794	2.903181957
Rattus norvegicus transcribed sequence with moderate similarity to protein pir:I37421 (H.sapiens) I37421 glutaminyl-peptide cyclotransferase (EC 2.3.2.5) – human	–	rc_AA859661_at	–	1.46779	0.831810561
Rattus norvegicus transcribed sequences	–	rc_AA875126_g_at	–	1.46017	0.831810561
cold inducible RNA-binding protein	Cirbp	AB000362_at	NM_031147	1.45745	4.876302628
cysteine-sulfinate decarboxylase	Csad	M64755_at	NM_021750	1.45583	2.903181957
fatty acid Coenzyme A ligase, long chain 4	Facl4	D85189_at	NM_053623	1.45503	1.370947035
high mobility group box 2	Hmgb2	rc_AA996401_s_at	NM_017187	1.44818	0.831810561
guanine nucleotide binding protein gamma subunit 11	Gng11	rc_AA860043_at	NM_022396	1.44635	2.008596819
cyclin-dependent kinase 4	Cdk4	L11007_at	NM_053593	1.42897	2.008596819
tissue factor pathway inhibitor	Tfpi	D10926_s_at	NM_017200	1.42397	0.831810561
Rattus norvegicus transcribed sequence with moderate similarity to protein pdb:1LBG (E. coli) B Chain B, Lactose Operon Repressor Bound To 21-Base Pair Symmetric Operator Dna, Alpha Carbons Only	–	rc_AI639203_at	–	1.42285	0.831810561
cd36 antigen	Cd36	AF072411_g_at	NM_031561	1.41508	2.903181957
lipocalin 2	Lcn2	rc_AA946503_at	NM_130741	1.41052	0.831810561
–	–	S83025_s_at	–	1.40337	0.831810561
carnitine O-octanoyltransferase	Crot	U26033_at	NM_031987	1.40241	0.831810561
Rattus norvegicus clone D920 intestinal epithelium proliferating cell-associated mRNA sequence	–	U21719mRNA_s_at	–	1.40037	3.940821135

(*continued*)

Supplemental Table (*continued*)

Title	Symbol	Gene name	Accession number	Fold change	q-value (%)
TGFB inducible early growth response	Tieg	rc_AI172476_at	NM_031135	1.39376	3.780313527
Kruppel-like factor 4 (gut)	Klf4	L26292_g_at	NM_053713	1.38722	2.435234865
topoisomerase (DNA) 2 alpha	Top2a	D14045_s_at	–	1.38641	0.831810561
v-ets erythroblastosis virus E26 oncogene homolog 1 (avian)	Ets1	L20681_at	NM_012555	1.38250	4.876302628
Rattus norvegicus transcribed sequence with moderate similarity to protein sp:P00722 (E. coli) BGAL_ECOLI Beta-galactosidase (Lactase)	–	rc_AA799751_at	–	1.37841	0.831810561
Rattus norvegicus similar to replication protein A3 (LOC288727), mRNA	–	rc_AI171243_at	–	1.37818	4.876302628
high mobility group box 2	Hmgb2	D84418_s_at	NM_017187	1.37812	0.831810561
nuclease sensitive element binding protein 1	Nsep1	D13309_s_at	NM_031563	1.37323	0.831810561
solute carrier family 18, member 2	Slc18a2	L00603_at	NM_013031	1.37097	4.266201283
Rattus norvegicus transcribed sequence with weak similarity to protein sp:Q99536 (H.sapiens) VAT1_HUMAN Synaptic vesicle membrane protein VAT-1 homolog	–	rc_AA875639_at	–	1.37095	2.435234865
histamine N-methyltransferase	Hnmt	S82579_s_at	NM_031044	1.37068	3.940821135
high mobility group box 2	Hmgb2	D84418_r_at	NM_017187	1.36975	1.370947035
ribosomal protein L27	Rpl27	rc_AI176589_at	NM_022514	1.36464	0.831810561
Rattus norvegicus transcribed sequence with strong similarity to protein ref:NP_004042.1 (H.sapiens) 3-hydroxybutyrate dehydrogenase precursor; (R)-3-hydroxybutyrate dehydrogenase [Homo sapiens]	–	rc_AA817846_at	–	1.35981	4.876302628
nitric oxide synthase 3, endothelial cell	Nos3	AJ011116_at	–	1.35870	2.903181957
dihydropyrimidinase-like 3	Crmp4	U52104_at	NM_012934	1.35597	2.435234865
parathyroid hormone receptor 1	Pthr1	M77184_i_at	NM_020073	1.34793	2.903181957
Rattus norvegicus transcribed sequences	–	rc_AA894210_at	–	1.34657	4.266201283
neuronatin	Nnat	U08290_at	NM_053601	1.34477	2.008596819
solute carrier family 6, member 6	Slc6a6	M96601_at	NM_017206	1.34394	3.940821135
POU domain, class 3, transcription factor 1	Pou3f1	M72711_at	NM_138838	1.34375	2.903181957
solute carrier family 16, member 1	Slc16a1	D63834_at	NM_012716	1.33983	0.831810561
proline-rich proteoglycan 2	Prpg2	L17318_at	NM_172065	1.33929	2.903181957
RAB11a, member RAS oncogene family	Rab11a	M75153_g_at	NM_031152	1.33755	3.940821135
cell division cycle 42 homolog (S. cerevisiae)	Cdc42	rc_AA925473_at	NM_171994	1.33461	3.940821135
nuclear factor I/B	Nfib	rc_AI176488_at	–	1.33438	2.435234865
nuclear factor I/X	Nfix	AB012235_at	–	1.33244	3.780313527
fatty acid binding protein 7	Fabp7	U02096_at	NM_030832	1.33049	2.008596819
methionine aminopeptidase 2	Metap2	L10652_g_at	NM_022539	1.32941	2.903181957
Rattus norvegicus similar to Tde1 protein (LOC296350), mRNA	–	rc_AA799641_g_at	–	1.32728	2.903181957
hypocretin receptor 1	Hcrtr1	AF041244_at	NM_013064	1.32437	2.435234865
myristoylated alanine rich protein kinase C substrate	Marcks	rc_AA899253_at	–	1.32349	2.903181957
amyloid beta (A4) precursor protein-binding, family A, APBA1: amyloid beta (A4) precursor protein-binding, family A, member 1 (X11)	Apba1	AF029105_at	NM_031779	1.32122	3.940821135
myosin regulatory light chain	Mrlcb	X54617mRNA_s_at	NM_017343	1.31934	2.435234865
paired box gene 6	Pax6	S74393_s_at	NM_013001	1.31871	4.876302628
solute carrier family 11 member 2	Slc11a2	AF008439_g_at	NM_013173	1.31643	2.008596819
rabphilin 3A-like (without C2 domains)	Rph3al	AF022774_g_at	NM_133591	1.31547	2.903181957
cyclin B1	Ccnb1	rc_AA998164_s_at	NM_171991	1.31417	2.903181957
Rattus norvegicus transcribed sequences	–	rc_AA799764_at	–	1.31083	4.876302628
agrin	Agrn	M64780_at	NM_175754	1.31033	2.435234865
integrin alpha M	Itgam	U59801_at	NM_012711	1.30846	2.435234865
agrin	Agrn	M64780_g_at	NM_175754	1.30844	3.940821135
thymosin, beta 10	Tmsb10	M58404_at	NM_021261	1.30837	2.903181957
Rattus norvegicus transcribed sequences	–	rc_AA893663_at	–	1.30783	2.903181957
tyrosine 3-monooxgenase/tryptophan 5-monooxgenase activation protein, gamma polypeptide	Ywhag	S55305_s_at	NM_019376	1.30555	0.831810561

(*continued*)

Supplemental Table (*continued*)

Title	Symbol	Gene name	Accession number	Fold change	q-value (%)
TGFB inducible early growth response	Tieg	rc_AI071299_at	NM_031135	1.30535	3.940821135
high mobility group box 1	Hmgb1	M64986_at	NM_012963	1.30395	3.940821135
neurotrophin-3 (HDNF/NT-3)	Ntf3	M34643_at	NM_031073	1.30317	2.903181957
nuclear protein E3-3	LOC56769	U95162_at	NM_020080	1.30064	4.876302628
high mobility group box 2	Hmgb2	rc_AI044390_s_at	NM_017187	1.29966	2.903181957
ras-related protein rab10	Rab10	rc_AI230406_at	NM_017359	1.29807	3.940821135
Rattus norvegicus transcribed sequences	–	rc_AI639359_at	–	1.29613	2.008596819
cytochrome P450, subfamily 2G, polypeptide 1	Cyp2g1	M31931cds_s_at	–	1.29574	2.903181957
mitogen activated protein kinase kinase kinase 1	Map3k1	U48596_at	NM_053887	1.29104	2.903181957
–	–	K00750exon#2-3_g_at	–	1.28964	2.435234865
–	–	X65190mRNA_s_at	–	1.28905	2.903181957
solute carrier family 7, member 1	Slc7a1	rc_AA957917_s_at	NM_013111	1.28611	4.266201283
Rattus norvegicus similar to dimethylarginine dimethylaminohydrolase 1; NG,NG dimethylarginine dimethylaminohydrolase (LOC365956), mRNA	–	rc_AI058941_s_at	–	1.28423	3.940821135
phosphodiesterase 7A	Pde7a	U77880_at	–	1.28365	3.940821135
solute carrier family 6, member 4	Slc6a4	X63253cds_s_at	NM_013034	1.28237	3.940821135
collapsin response mediator protein 1	Crmp1	U52102_at	NM_012932	1.28073	2.903181957
Rattus norvegicus transcribed sequences	–	rc_AI639142_at	–	1.27885	3.780313527
Olf-1/EBF associated Zn finger protein Roaz	Roaz	U92564_g_at	NM_053583	1.27619	3.940821135
glycine receptor, alpha 2 subunit	Glra2	X57281_at	NM_012568	1.27507	3.780313527
Rattus norvegicus transcribed sequences	–	rc_AI639521_at	–	1.27328	2.903181957
ribosome associated membrane protein 4	RAMP4	AF100470_at	NM_030835	1.27136	4.266201283
platelet-activating factor acetylhydrolase beta subunit (PAF-AH beta)	Pafah1b1	rc_AI234730_at	NM_031763	1.27109	3.940821135
proliferating cell nuclear antigen	Pcna	M24604_at	NM_022381	1.26833	3.780313527
calcitonin receptor	Calcr	L13040_s_at	NM_053816	1.26802	3.780313527
hairy and enhancer of split 1 (Drosophila)	Hes1	D13417_g_at	NM_024360	1.26743	4.876302628
pancreatic lipase	Pnlip	D88534_s_at	NM_013161	1.26675	3.780313527
Rattus norvegicus transcribed sequences	–	rc_AA799964_at	–	1.26464	3.780313527
cytochrome P450, IVA1	Cyp4a1	M14972_i_at	NM_175837	1.26340	4.876302628
carnitine palmitoyltransferase 1, liver	Cpt1a	L07736_at	NM_031559	1.26231	4.876302628
brain acidic membrane protein	Basp1	D14441_at	NM_022300	1.26001	3.780313527
S-100 related protein, clone 42C	S100a10	J03627_at	NM_031114	1.25712	4.266201283
Rattus norvegicus transcribed sequences	–	rc_AA893743_g_at	–	1.25544	3.780313527
cysteine rich protein 2	Csrp2	U44948_at	NM_177425	1.25498	4.266201283
–	–	X07944exon#1-12_s_at	–	1.25495	2.903181957
cyclin L	Ccnl	AF030091UTR#1_g_at	NM_053662	1.25233	4.876302628
solute carrier family 11 member 2	Slc11a2	AF008439_at	NM_013173	1.25224	2.903181957
acyl-coenzyme A:cholesterol acyltransferase	Soat1	D86373_s_at	NM_031118	1.25218	3.940821135
glutamate receptor, ionotropic, N-methyl-D-aspartate 3A	Grin3a	AF061945_g_at	–	1.24936	3.780313527
cerebroglycan	Gpc2	L20468_at	NM_138511	1.24907	4.266201283
topoisomerase II beta	Top2b	D14046_at	–	1.24804	4.876302628
chondroitin sulfate proteoglycan 3	Cspg3	AF060879_s_at	NM_031653	1.24717	4.266201283
cellular retinoic acid binding protein I	Crabp1	rc_AA875025_at	–	1.24457	4.876302628
adrenomedullin	Adm	D15069_s_at	NM_012715	1.24032	4.876302628
Bcl2-associated X protein	Bax	U59184_at	NM_017059	1.23951	4.876302628
Rattus norvegicus transcribed sequence with moderate similarity to protein ref:NP_002485.1 (H.sapiens) NADH dehydrogenase (ubiquinone) 1, subcomplex unknown, 1 (6kD, KFYI) [Homo sapiens]	–	rc_AI104679_s_at	–	1.23711	4.266201283
Rattus norvegicus transcribed sequences	–	rc_AA859536_at	–	1.23592	3.940821135
Rattus norvegicus transcribed sequences	–	rc_AA860029_at	–	1.23586	3.940821135
cytochrome P450 2c22	Cyp2c22	M58041_s_at	NM_138512	1.23401	4.876302628
Rattus norvegicus transcribed sequence with strong similarity to protein sp:P00722 (E. coli) BGAL_ECOLI Beta-galactosidase (Lactase)	–	rc_AA859994_at	–	1.23342	4.876302628
Chorionic somatomammotropin hormone 1 variant; Placental lactogen-1	Csh1v	rc_AI179075_i_at	NM_033233	1.23287	4.266201283

(*continued*)

Supplemental Table (*continued*)

Title	Symbol	Gene name	Accession number	Fold change	q-value (%)
cyclin B1	Ccnb1	X64589_at	NM_171991	1.23239	3.940821135
Rattus norvegicus similar to dimethylarginine dimethylaminohydrolase 1; NG, NG dimethylarginine dimethylaminohydrolase (LOC365956), mRNA	–	D86041_at	–	1.23180	4.876302628
fatty acid binding protein 5, epidermal	Fabp5	S69874_s_at	NM_145878	1.22974	3.940821135
variable coding sequence A1	Vcsa1	A07543cds_s_at	NM_012634	1.22931	4.266201283
protease (prosome, macropain) 28 subunit, alpha	Psme1	D45249_g_at	NM_017264	1.22924	4.266201283
–	–	X77117exon#1-3_at	–	1.22895	4.876302628
cyclin D1	Ccnd1	D14014_at	NM_171992	1.22667	2.435234865
microtubule-associated protein 6	Mtap6	AJ002556_s_at	NM_017204	1.22297	3.940821135
–	–	X57529cds_s_at	–	1.21046	4.876302628
ribosomal protein S4, X-linked	Rps4x	X14210cds_at	–	1.18362	3.940821135
DOWN-REGULATED GENES					
thyroid hormone responsive protein	Thrsp	K01934mRNA#2_at	NM_012703	0.39906	0.831810561
Rattus norvegicus Nclone10 mRNA	–	U31866_g_at	–	0.47015	0.831810561
Transferrin	Tf	D38380_g_at	NM_017055	0.49119	0.831810561
myelin and lymphocyte protein	Mal	U31367_at	NM_012798	0.51875	0.831810561
Transferrin	Tf	D38380_at	NM_017055	0.53227	0.831810561
kallikrein 6	Klk6	AF016269_at	NM_019175	0.53451	0.831810561
homer, neuronal immediate early gene, 1	Homer1	AB003726_at	NM_031707	0.53698	0.831810561
myelin-associated oligodendrocytic basic protein	Mobp	D28111_at	NM_012720	0.53918	0.831810561
apolipoprotein D	Apod	X55572_at	NM_012777	0.54264	0.831810561
Rat troponin-c mRNA	–	rc_AI639532_at	–	0.55172	0.831810561
–	–	rc_AA892551_f_at	–	0.57617	0.831810561
myelin-associated oligodendrocytic basic protein	Mobp	D28111_g_at	NM_012720	0.59637	0.831810561
–	–	rc_AA874877_r_at	–	0.60311	0.831810561
myelin oligodendrocyte glycoprotein	Mog	L21995_s_at	NM_022668	0.61224	0.831810561
crystallin, alpha B	Cryab	X60351cds_s_at	NM_012935	0.61292	0.831810561
myelin-associated oligodendrocytic basic protein	Mobp	D28110_g_at	NM_012720	0.61885	0.831810561
afadin	Af6	D90401_at	NM_013217	0.63107	1.370947035
Rattus norvegicus retroviral-like ovarian specific transcript 30-1 mRNA	–	U48828_g_at	–	0.63803	1.370947035
apolipoprotein C-I	Apoc1	X15512_at	NM_012824	0.64339	0.831810561
carbonic anhydrase 2	Ca2	X58294_at	NM_019291	0.64519	0.831810561
RAS guanyl releasing protein 1	Rasgrp1	AF081196_at	NM_019211	0.64721	1.370947035
stathmin-like 4	Stmn4	AF026529_s_at	–	0.64929	0.831810561
–	–	rc_AA799594_at	–	0.65539	2.008596819
–	–	rc_AI102044_at	–	0.65630	0.831810561
ring finger protein 28	Rnf28	rc_AI639465_r_at	NM_080903	0.65888	0.831810561
lysozyme	Lyz	rc_AA892775_at	NM_012771	0.65940	1.370947035
myelin oligodendrocyte glycoprotein	Mog	M99485_at	NM_022668	0.66050	0.831810561
–	–	X70141_r_at	–	0.66242	0.831810561
olfactory receptor	LOC309574	AF091563_r_at	–	0.66307	0.831810561
carbonic anhydrase 2	Ca2	U60578cds_s_at	NM_019291	0.66321	0.831810561
glutathione S-transferase, mu 1	Gstm1	H32189_s_at	NM_017014	0.66508	0.831810561
afadin	Af6	D90401_g_at	NM_013217	0.66667	0.831810561
cathepsin S	Ctss	L03201_at	NM_017320	0.66680	0.831810561
Rattus norvegicus transcribed sequences	–	rc_AI007824_g_at	–	0.66928	0.831810561
Rattus norvegicus transcribed sequences	–	rc_AA891690_g_at	–	0.67005	2.435234865
deoxycytidine kinase	Dck	L33894_at	NM_024158	0.67197	3.940821135
Rattus norvegicus similar to S-100 protein, alpha chain (LOC295214), mRNA	–	rc_AI228548_g_at	–	0.67279	0.831810561
Rat PMSG-induced ovarian mRNA, 3′sequence, N1	–	D84479_at	–	0.67470	3.780313527
–	–	AF028784cds#1_s_at	–	0.67531	0.831810561
purinergic receptor P2X, ligand-gated ion channel, 4	P2rx4	U47031_at	NM_031594	0.67637	0.831810561
MEGF1	Fat2	AB011527_at	NM_022954	0.67692	0.831810561
avian erythroblastosis oncogene B 3	Erbb3	U29339_at	NM_017218	0.68155	1.370947035
neurotensin receptor 2	Ntsr2	X97121_at	NM_022695	0.68834	0.831810561
cytochrome P450, family 27, subfamily a, polypeptide 1	Cyp27	M38566mRNA_s_at	NM_178847	0.69094	0.831810561
Rattus norvegicus transcribed sequences	–	rc_AI639170_at	–	0.69337	2.903181957

(*continued*)

Supplemental Table (*continued*)

Title	Symbol	Gene name	Accession number	Fold change	q-value (%)
stearoyl-Coenzyme A desaturase 2	Scd2	M15114_at	NM_031841	0.69670	3.780313527
Rattus norvegicus transcribed sequences	–	rc_AA874805_at	–	0.69783	2.903181957
heat-responsive protein 12	Hrsp12	D49363_s_at	NM_031714	0.69849	1.370947035
ectonucleotide pyrophosphatase/phosphodiesterase 2	Enpp2	D28560_at	NM_057104	0.69910	0.831810561
crystallin, alpha B	Cryab	M55534mRNA_s_at	NM_012935	0.69912	0.831810561
Rattus norvegicus transcribed sequences	–	rc_AA891690_at	–	0.70103	2.903181957
secreted phosphoprotein 1	Spp1	M14656_at	NM_012881	0.70182	1.370947035
–	–	X83671cds_r_at	–	0.70462	0.831810561
myelin basic protein	Mbp	K00512_at	NM_017026	0.70604	0.831810561
–	–	K03045cds_s_at	–	0.70996	3.780313527
serum/glucocorticoid regulated kinase	Sgk	L01624_at	NM_019232	0.71101	2.435234865
Rattus norvegicus hypothetical gene supported by NM_053936 (LOC360403), mRNA	–	rc_AA848831_at	–	0.71152	0.831810561
cytochrome P450CMF1b	Cyp2d5	J02869mRNA_s_at	NM_173304	0.71157	0.831810561
Eph receptor A7	Epha7	U21954_at	NM_134331	0.71186	2.903181957
Rattus norvegicus transcribed sequence	–	rc_AI639471_r_at	–	0.71198	2.435234865
parvalbumin	Pva	rc_AI175539_at	NM_022499	0.71353	0.831810561
chemokine (C-X-C motif) ligand 2	Cxcl2	U45965_at	NM_053647	0.71378	4.876302628
–	–	L08495cds_s_at	–	0.71522	3.780313527
potassium voltage-gated channel, subfamily H (eag-related), member 1	Kcnh1	Z34264_at	NM_031742	0.71633	2.008596819
tropomodulin 1	Tmod1	U59241_at	NM_013044	0.71899	0.831810561
carbonic anhydrase 4	Ca4	S68245_g_at	NM_019174	0.71970	0.831810561
–	–	D37934_at	–	0.71982	2.008596819
Rattus norvegicus transcribed sequences	–	rc_AA866432_at	–	0.72186	0.831810561
–	–	rc_AA799671_at	–	0.72235	2.008596819
chimerin (chimaerin) 2	Chn2	rc_AI232194_at	NM_032084	0.72322	1.370947035
glycerol 3-phosphate dehydrogenase	Gpd3	AB002558_at	NM_022215	0.72603	0.831810561
proteasome (prosome, macropain) subunit, beta type 4	Psmb4	rc_AI172162_at	NM_031629	0.72621	0.831810561
Rattus norvegicus transcribed sequences	–	rc_AA800853_at	–	0.72883	3.780313527
–	–	X51531cds_g_at	–	0.72920	2.903181957
protein disulfide isomerase related protein (calcium-binding protein, intestinal-related)	Erp70	M86870_at	NM_053849	0.73317	1.370947035
fumarylacetoacetate hydrolase	Fah	M77694_at	NM_017181	0.73325	2.435234865
neuronal potassium channel alpha subunit	Kv8.1	X98564cds_at	NM_021697	0.73511	2.903181957
Rattus norvegicus transcribed sequence with strong similarity to protein sp:O43236 (H.sapiens) SEP4_HUMAN Septin 4 (Peanut-like protein 2) (Brain protein H5) (Cell division control-related protein 2) (hCDCREL-2) (Bradeion beta) (CE5B3 beta)	–	rc_AA800004_at	–	0.73664	0.831810561
solute carrier family 21 (organic anion transporter), member 5	Slc21a5	U88036_at	NM_131906	0.74072	1.370947035
–	–	U26356mRNA_s_at	–	0.74099	2.008596819
proteolipid protein	Plp	rc_AI072770_s_at	NM_030990	0.74110	0.831810561
cAMP responsive element modulator	Crem	S66024_at	NM_013086	0.74164	2.008596819
Rattus norvegicus transcribed sequence	–	rc_AI639098_at	–	0.74270	2.008596819
kangai 1	Kai1	rc_AI231213_g_at	NM_031797	0.74471	2.008596819
Mg87 protein	Mg87	AF095741_at	NM_134410	0.74517	4.266201283
aldehyde dehydrogenase family 1, member A1	Aldh1a1	AF001898_at	NM_022407	0.74614	2.903181957
myosin, heavy polypeptide 3	Myh3	K03467_s_at	NM_012604	0.74628	4.266201283
Rattus norvegicus transcribed sequence with moderate similarity to protein ref:NP_060369.1 (H.sapiens) hypothetical protein FLJ20607; tescalcin; likely ortholog of mouse tescalcin [Homo sapiens]	–	rc_AA892511_at	–	0.74700	1.370947035
retinoblastoma-like 2	Rbl2	rc_AI230602_at	NM_031094	0.74707	4.876302628
adenylyl cyclase-associated protein 2	Cap2	rc_AI145367_at	NM_053874	0.74797	0.831810561
Rattus norvegicus similar to kIAA0367 (LOC293823), mRNA	–	rc_AA894264_at	–	0.75082	3.780313527
Rattus norvegicus transcribed sequence with moderate similarity to protein sp:P07902 (H.sapiens) GAL7_HUMAN Galactose-1-phosphate uridylyltransferase	–	L05541_at	–	0.75139	1.370947035

(*continued*)

Supplemental Table (*continued*)

Title	Symbol	Gene name	Accession number	Fold change	q-value (%)
Potassium voltage gated channel, shaker related subfamily, beta member 1	Kcnab1	X70662_at	NM_017303	0.75175	2.435234865
–	–	M64733mRNA_s_at	–	0.75290	1.370947035
B-cell translocation gene 1	Btg1	L26268_at	NM_017258	0.75291	0.831810561
–	–	AF028784mRNA#1_s_at	–	0.75373	2.435234865
–	–	X62327cds_r_at	–	0.75497	2.008596819
Rattus norvegicus transcribed sequence with strong similarity to protein ref:NP_060904.1 (H.sapiens) goliath protein; likely ortholog of mouse g1-related zinc finger protein [Homo sapiens]	–	rc_AA891810_at	–	0.75520	2.435234865
Inhibitor of DNA binding 3, dominant negative helix-loop-helix protein	Id3	rc_AI171268_at	NM_013058	0.75603	4.876302628
FXYD domain-containing ion transport regulator 1	Fxyd1	rc_AA799645_g_at	NM_031648	0.75604	2.903181957
CD9 antigen	Cd9	X76489cds_at	–	0.75604	4.266201283
S100 protein, beta polypeptide	S100b	S53527mRNA_s_at	NM_013191	0.75796	4.266201283
gamma-aminobutyric acid A receptor, delta	Gabrd	L08496cds_s_at	NM_017289	0.75881	4.876302628
muscle glycogen phosphorylase	Pygm	L10669_g_at	–	0.75899	2.903181957
Cys2/His2 zinc finger protein (rKr1)	rKr1	U41164_at	NM_144757	0.76013	2.008596819
sterol-C4-methyl oxidase-like	Sc4mol	E12625cds_at	NM_080886	0.76023	2.903181957
liver mitochondrial glutaminase	Ga	J05499_at	NM_138904	0.76200	2.435234865
dopamine receptor 1A	Drd1a	S46131mRNA_r_at	NM_012546	0.76203	0.831810561
Mg87 protein	Mg87	AF095741_g_at	NM_134410	0.76213	3.780313527
potassium voltage gated channel, Shal-related family, member 3	Kcnd3	rc_AI230211_s_at	NM_031739	0.76244	4.266201283
Rattus norvegicus transcribed sequence with moderate similarity to protein pir:T50629 (H.sapiens) T50629 hypothetical protein DKFZp762L1710.1 – human (fragment)	–	rc_AA800258_at	–	0.76337	2.903181957
xanthine dehydrogenase	Xdh	rc_AI172247_at	NM_017154	0.76447	2.435234865
Rattus norvegicus transcribed sequences	–	rc_AA799534_at	–	0.76458	2.903181957
gamma-aminobutyric acid A receptor, delta	Gabrd	M35162_at	NM_017289	0.76509	2.903181957
peroxiredoxin 6	Prdx6	AF014009_at	NM_053576	0.76517	0.831810561
glycine methyltransferase	Gnmt	X06150cds_at	NM_017084	0.76603	3.940821135
calpain, small subunit 1	Capns1	U53859_at	–	0.76690	2.008596819
Rattus norvegicus transcribed sequence with strong similarity to protein ref:NP_060904.1 (H.sapiens) goliath protein; likely ortholog of mouse g1-related zinc finger protein [Homo sapiens]	–	rc_AA891810_g_at	–	0.76880	2.008596819
galectin-related inter-fiber protein	Grifin	AF082160_at	NM_057187	0.76896	3.780313527
Rattus norvegicus similar to glyoxylate reductase/hydroxypyruvate reductase (LOC298085), mRNA	–	rc_AA892799_s_at	–	0.76962	3.780313527
–	–	rc_AA859928_at	–	0.77063	2.903181957
D site albumin promoter binding protein	Dbp	J03179_at	NM_012543	0.77116	2.903181957
Rattus norvegicus transcribed sequence	–	rc_AI639471_f_at	–	0.77150	4.876302628
pyruvate dehydrogenase kinase 2	Pdk2	U10357_g_at	NM_030872	0.77193	3.780313527
proprotein convertase subtilisin/kexin type 4	Pcsk4	L14937cds#1_s_at	NM_133559	0.77248	2.903181957
Rattus norvegicus similar to APC-binding protein EB1 homolog (LOC300647), mRNA	–	rc_AA891727_at	–	0.77260	2.903181957
Rattus norvegicus transcribed sequences	–	rc_AA800549_at	–	0.77312	3.780313527
FXYD domain-containing ion transport regulator 1	Fxyd1	rc_AA799645_at	NM_031648	0.77347	2.903181957
glutathione S-transferase, mu 1	Gstm1	J02810mRNA_s_at	NM_017014	0.77369	2.435234865
cellular retinoic acid binding protein 2	Crabp2	U23407_at	NM_017244	0.77538	4.876302628
–	–	M90660exon_at	–	0.77647	4.266201283
lifeguard	Lfg	AF044201_at	NM_144756	0.77706	2.903181957
pregnancy upregulated non-ubiquitously expressed CaM kinase	Pnck	D86556_i_at	NM_017275	0.77814	3.780313527
phosphatidylinositol 4-kinase	Pik4cb	rc_AI102103_g_at	NM_031083	0.77839	2.903181957
Rattus norvegicus similar to RING-finger protein MURF (LOC362708), mRNA	–	rc_AA800245_at	–	0.77950	2.903181957

(*continued*)

Supplemental Table (*continued*)

Title	Symbol	Gene name	Accession number	Fold change	q-value (%)
Rattus norvegicus transcribed sequences	–	rc_AA894297_at	–	0.77963	3.780313527
Rab3B protein	Rab3b	AA799389_g_at	NM_031091	0.78252	2.903181957
complement component 3	C3	rc_AA894304_at	NM_016994	0.78284	4.266201283
proteolipid protein	Plp	rc_AI070277_s_at	NM_030990	0.78385	1.370947035
plasmolipin	Z49858	Z49858_at	NM_022533	0.78418	2.903181957
discs, large homolog 1 (Drosophila)	Dlgh1	rc_AI144926_s_at	NM_012788	0.78422	4.266201283
short stature homeobox 2	Shox2	AJ002259_g_at	NM_013028	0.78546	4.266201283
Rattus norvegicus Tclone4 mRNA	–	U30788_at	–	0.78569	4.876302628
peripheral myelin protein 22	Pmp22	S55427_s_at	NM_017037	0.78677	4.266201283
galanin	Gal	J03624_at	NM_033237	0.78824	3.780313527
–	–	U75927UTR#1_at	–	0.78992	2.435234865
Glucose-dependent insulinotropic peptide	Gludins	L08831_i_at	NM_019630	0.79211	4.266201283
guanidinoacetate methyltransferase	Gamt	J03588_at	NM_012793	0.79233	2.903181957
Rattus norvegicus transcribed sequences	–	rc_H31859_at	–	0.79395	4.266201283
gap junction membrane channel protein beta 1	Gjb1	X04070_at	NM_017251	0.79543	4.876302628
Rattus norvegicus transcribed sequences	–	rc_AA892541_at	–	0.79598	1.370947035
–	–	S87522_g_at	–	0.79600	4.266201283
calcium channel, voltage-dependent, alpha2/delta subunit 1	Cacna2d1	M86621_at	NM_012919	0.79639	3.780313527
sodium channel, voltage-gated, type 1, alpha polypeptide	Scn1a	M22253_at	NM_030875	0.79685	2.903181957
v-jun sarcoma virus 17 oncogene homolog (avian)	Jun	X17163cds_s_at	NM_021835	0.79742	2.903181957
proteolipid protein	Plp	M25888_at	NM_030990	0.79874	2.435234865
hydroxy-delta-5-steroid dehydrogenase, 3 beta- and steroid delta-isomerase 1	Hsd3b1	rc_AI235576_s_at	NM_017265	0.80152	3.780313527
putative chloride channel (similar to Mm Clcn4-2)	Clcn4-2	Z36944cds_at	NM_022198	0.80158	2.008596819
CD9 antigen	Cd9	X76489cds_g_at	–	0.80167	3.780313527
3-hydroxy-3-methylglutaryl CoA lyase	Hmgcl	rc_AI171090_at	NM_024386	0.80230	4.266201283
cytochrome P450 monooxygenase	Cyp2J3	U40004_s_at	NM_175766	0.80317	4.266201283
myosin heavy chain, polypeptide 6	Myh6	rc_AI104924_f_at	NM_017239	0.80320	4.876302628
ubiquitin conjugating enzyme	LOC81816	rc_AA799612_at	NM_031138	0.80326	4.266201283
fibroblast growth factor 9	Fgf9	D14839_at	NM_012952	0.80525	4.876302628
stearoyl-Coenzyme A desaturase 2	Scd2	U67995_s_at	NM_031841	0.80532	3.940821135
CaM-kinase II inhibitor alpha	LOC287005	rc_AA858621_at	NM_173337	0.80569	4.876302628
cAMP responsive element modulator	Crem	U04835_at	NM_013086	0.80586	2.008596819
Max interacting protein 1	Mxi1	AF003008_at	NM_013160	0.80629	4.266201283
ephrin A1	Efna1	D38056_at	NM_053599	0.80672	4.266201283
pyridoxine 5-phosphate oxidase	U91561	rc_AA800211_at	NM_022601	0.80743	4.266201283
protease, serine, 8 (prostasin)	Prss8	rc_AA892468_g_at	NM_138836	0.80859	3.780313527
Rattus norvegicus transcribed sequences	–	rc_AA875362_at	–	0.80903	3.940821135
Rattus norvegicus cDNA clone MGC:72479 IMAGE:5600078, complete cds	–	rc_AA891877_at	–	0.80944	4.876302628
calpain, small subunit 1	Capns1	U53859_g_at	–	0.80973	4.876302628
glutamine synthetase 1	Glns	rc_AI232783_s_at	NM_017073	0.80992	4.266201283
Rattus norvegicus transcribed sequence with strong similarity to protein ref:NP_076424.1 (H.sapiens) chromosome 20 open reading frame 116 [Homo sapiens]	–	rc_AI638949_s_at	–	0.81126	4.876302628
Rattus norvegicus transcribed sequence with strong similarity to protein pir:T08783 (H.sapiens) T08783 hypothetical protein DKFZp586O0120.1 – human (fragment)	–	rc_AA892310_at	–	0.81420	2.903181957
solute carrier family 25 (mitochondrial carrier; dicarboxylate transporter), member 10	Slc25a10	rc_AA859666_i_at	NM_133418	0.81457	3.780313527
Rattus norvegicus transcribed sequence	–	rc_AA866259_at	–	0.81529	2.435234865
–	–	E12275cds_s_at	–	0.81713	4.876302628
protein tyrosine kinase 2 beta	Ptk2b	AF063890_s_at	NM_017318	0.81777	2.903181957
potassium channel erg3	erg3	AF016191_at	NM_131912	0.82728	3.780313527
secretory granule neuroendocrine protein 1	Sgne1	M63901_g_at	NM_013175	0.83321	4.876302628
interleukin 1 receptor accessory protein	Il1rap	U48592_g_at	NM_012968	0.84996	4.876302628

J Neural Transm (2006) [Suppl] 71: 197–200

Journal of Neural Transmission
Printed in Austria

Long lasting effects of infancy iron deficiency – Preliminary results

S. Yehuda[1], **M. Yehuda**[2]

[1] Psychopharmacology Laboratory, Department of Psychology and Brain Research Institute, Bar Ilan University, Ramat Gan, Israel
[2] Department of Otolaryngology, Head and Neck surgery, Kaplan Medical Center, Rehovot, Israel

Summary The long-term effects of rehabilitated infancy (1 year old) iron deficiency (ID) were examined at age 10. The children were examined for the following variables: auditory system function, the level of morning cortisol, I.Q. score (WISC-R), and behavioral profile. The results indicate that while the former ID children's hearing system appears to function well, there was a delay in brain stem processing of the auditory signals. In addition, the level of morning cortisol was reduced, the general I.Q. scores were lower than the normal group (mainly in the performed subtest), and more sleep disturbances and fatigue during day were reported. These outcomes are consistent with established reports on the effect of iron deficiency on the rate of myelination in selected brain areas during critical period of 1 year olds. The findings of increased sleep disturbances and lower I.Q. tests require further study.

Introduction

Despite some successful intervention programs, iron deficiency (ID) and anemia remain the most common nutritional disorders in the world. Numerous behavioral manifestations can be observed among ID children and adults, such as lethargy, irritability, apathy, restlessness, fatigue, lack of concentration, paropghia (pathological craving for ice) and pica (pervert craving for substances unfit for food), inattention, hypoactivity (or hyperactivity) and sleep disturbances. However, the most disturbing functional hallmark of ID is a decrease in mental performances (Youdim and Yehuda, 2000).

While the frequency of ID is greater among children in the Third World, many cases of ID can be found at all ages, even among people in wealthy countries (Scrimshaw, 1991, 1998). Recently the population of healthy elderly people, living in Old Age Homes was identified as a high ID risk group (Buzina et al., 1998). In addition, pregnant women and children were identified as two other high-risk groups.

Many ID effects are mediated via brain biochemistry, with prominent modification in the level and the activity of brain neurotransmitters (mainly the dopaminegic system and DA D2 receptors). In addition, iron plays a major role in fatty acid and lipid metabolism via the family of cytochrome P-450. There is an important link between iron and lipids that affects myelin and all its processes, especially myelin formation and myelin disintegration. An adequate supply of iron and essential fatty acids during the developing period is a requirement for the normal rate of myelination (Youdim and Yehuda, 2000). Using Luxol fast blue stain, Yu et al. (1986) confirmed earlier findings by Youdim and Yehuda, that the degree of myelination is decreased in pups of pregnant ID rats.

It seems that the ID also affects the sensory system. For example, ID rats are much more sensitive to strong noise. Hearing loss is induced in low amplitude noise in ID rats compared to normal rats (Sun et al., 1991). This finding was explained as due to ID induced changes in the inner ear. Similarly, a delay in maturation of the auditory brain stem responses was found in ID infants (Roncagliolo et al., 1998). The explanation was based on a delay in brain and auditory system myelination. In addition, some endocrinological changes were found in ID rats. Lower levels of thyroid hormone concentration were found in ID humans and rats (Beard et al., 1997), along with lower levels of cortisol in ID humans and rats (Weinberg et al., 1981; Saad et al., 1991).

In general the infancy period is a "critical period" for proper development of several sensory systems. Animal studies have shown that cognitive deficits induced by iron deficiency are very difficult to rehabilitate (Ben-Shachar et al., 1986; Youdim et al., 1989; Lozoff et al., 1996).

The aim of this study was to examine the long lasting effects of infancy ID. While many studies have investigated

Correspondence: S. Yehuda, Psychopharmacology Laboratory, Department of Psychology and Brain Research Institute, Bar Ilan University, Ramat Gan 52900, Israel
e-mail: yehudas@mail.biu.ac.il

the effect of an iron deficient diet, this study took advantage of a group of children in the age of 8–10 years old, who were ID at age 1 year and now are considered rehabilitated with respect to normal values of iron and hemoglobin. We tested their I.Q., auditory system, and basic cortisol levels, in order to find which parameters were not fully rehabilitated after so many years.

Methods

Subjects

The participants of this study were rehabilitating non-anemic children who were healthy full-term infants (birth weights ≥3.0 kg, with no perinatal complications, nor acute or chronic illnesses. As infants they were identified as having (Iron deficiency anemia) IDA at 12 mo. Anemia was defined as venous Hb <110 g/L at 12 mo. Iron deficiency was defined as two of three iron measures in the iron-deficient range [mean cell volume <70 fL, erythrocyte protoporphyrin >100 μg/dL red blood cells (1.77 μM), serum ferritin <12 μg/L) and/or an increase in Hb ≥10 g/L after 6 mo of iron therapy. Very strict exclusion criteria were used (e.g., chronic disease, head injury, jaundice, syphilis, toxoplasma, rubella, frequent ear infections, ototoxic medication, etc). A matched group of children, who were non-anemic during infancy served as a control group. 17 children, (13 boys and 4 girls, age 5.8 ± 1 year) tested in the audiometric test, 27 children (20 boys and 7 girls, age 10.2 ± 1 year) were tested in all other studies.

The ethics committees of Kaplan Hospital and Bar Ilan University approved the study.

Audiometric tests

All audiometric measures were obtained and processed without knowledge of whether a given child had been diagnosed as IDA or control. The children were studied while awake during the daytime. Audiometric tests included air and bone thresholds, in each ear, in frequencies of 250, 500, 1000, 2000, 4000, and 8000 Hertz, and SRT (Speech Reception Threshold). ABR (Auditory Brainstem Response) recordings were carried out in a quiet, dimly lit, and electrically shielded room using an integrated instrument (Bio Logic). ABR recorded using silver-silver chloride disk electrodes placed according to the 10–20 International. Interelectrode impedance was kept below 5 kilo ohms.

Using the same procedures as for infants, ABR were performed with the child in the supine position, elicited monaurally, stimulating the ipsilateral ear with a series of square wave rarefaction clicks (0.1 ms) through TDH-39 headphones at 80 dB nHL. The ABR were recorded twice to insure reproducibility. Results were stored for off-line analyses. The following parameters were determined for every response: absolute latency and amplitude for waves I, III, and V, and inter-peak latencies I–III, III–V, and I–V.

Cortisol

Morning salivary cortisol samples were collected at 08:00 PM, while the subjects were still at home. No food intake was allowed 30 min. before taking the sample. Samples were collected using cotton swabs chewed for 2 min. and inserted into a plastic test tube and then to a commercially available double-chamber device Salivette® (Sarstedt, Nümbrecht, Germany). After centrifuging and cooling to 4°C and storage at −20°C, the cortisol level was measured by radioimmunoassay.

WISC

Intelligence was tested using the Wechsler Intelligence Scale for Children-Revised (WISC) that included Verbal, Performance, and Full-Scale IQ derived from 12 subtests of different facets of cognitive functioning.

Behavior

After completion of the WISC, all subjects were asked to complete a 5-point rating scale for each of the following six dimensions (with 5 meaning "very good" and 1 meaning "very bad"):

1. *Appetite*.
2. Overall mood state.
3. *Concentration* during the school day.
4. *Fatigue* experienced during the day.
5. Ability to *organize* materials for home work.
6. *Quality* of sleep.

Results

Hemoglobin

The mean Hb level of the experimental group at the time of diagnosis (12.4 months) was 9.68 gr/DL ± 0.70, and 11.80 ± 0.70 at the time of the test (9.6 ± 1.1 years old). The Hb level of control group was 12.01 ± 0.90.

Audiometric test

Seventeen subjects completed the auditory test. All subjects exhibited normal hearing of pure tunes (250–8000 Hz) threshold, and normal SRT threshold. Both were less than 20 dB in both ears.

In the ABR test, (Tables 1 and 2) there was a slight (0.09–0.20 ms), yet statistically significant, prolongation of waves I, III, and V, and I–III and III–V latencies were

Table 1. *Left ear ABR (milliseconds)*

	ABR wave I	ABR III	ABR wave V	ABR IPL I–III	ABR IPL III–V	ABR IPL I–V
Population mean	1.63	3.86	5.74	2.15	1.93	4.08
Population SD	0.13	0.32	0.19	0.15	0.13	0.19
Normal value	1.54	3.69	5.54	2.14	1.86	4
Normal value SD	0.12	0.1	0.19	0.23	0.14	0.2
T-test p-value	$p=0.013$*	$p=0.044$*	$p=0.006$*	$p=0.79$	$p=0.046$*	$p=0.11$

* Statistical significant difference, $p=0.05$

Table 2. *Right ear ABR (milliseconds)*

	ABR wave I	ABR III	ABR wave V	ABR IPL I–III	ABR IPL III–V	ABR IPL I–V
Population mean	1.64	3.75	5.68	2.13	1.92	3.93
Population SD	0.15	0.18	0.22	0.18	0.19	0.22
Normal value	1.54	3.67	5.52	2.13	1.85	3.98
Normal value SD	0.11	0.12	0.22	0.14	0.17	0.19
T-test P-value	$p=0.015^*$	$p=0.08$	$p=0.001^*$	$p=1$	$p=0.15$	$p=0.37$

* Statistical significant difference, $p=0.05$

similar to the normal group. Increased I–V latency was found only in the left ear.

Cortisol

The mean level of saliva cortisol of the 27 experimental group children was 2.8 ± 0.4 nmol/L, while the level of 27-matched control group was 2.5 ± 0.7 nmol/L ($p=0.001$).

WISC

The I.Q. test revealed some cognitive deficiencies in the experimental group. While all subjects were in the normal range of I.Q., some statistical differences between the experimental and control group were found. The experimental group scored lower mainly in the performance subtests and the serial learning subtest (Table 3).

Behavior

The analysis of the results showed that in general the members of the experimental group self-rated themselves lower than the members of the control groups in all 6 tested variables. In two variables, the differences were statistically significant viz. more fatigue experienced during day and more reported sleep disturbances (Table 4).

Table 3. *Results of WISC*

	Experimental group ($n=27$)	Control group ($n=27$)
Full Scale I.Q.	$96.7 \pm 2.1^{**}$	105.1 ± 1.3
Verbal I.Q.	$99.1 \pm 2.4^{*}$	104.5 ± 1.8
Performance I.Q.	$95.9 \pm 2.2^{**}$	104.9 ± 2.4

Statistical significant, $^*p=0.05$; $^{**}p=0.001$

Table 4. *Behavioral variables*

	Former ID	Control
Appetite	3.5 ± 0.6	4.9 ± 0.7
Good mood	3.8 ± 0.8	4.8 ± 0.8
Ability to concentrate	3.5 ± 0.6	4.7 ± 0.5
Fatigue during day	$3.0 \pm 0.5^*$	4.5 ± 0.8
Organizing academic materials	$4.0 \pm 0.0.6$	4.8 ± 4.6
Quality of sleep	$3.1 \pm 1.3^*$	4.8 ± 1.0

*Statistical significant difference, $p=0.05$

Discussion

The results of this study showed that despite rehabilitation of the hematological profile of infant ID as a group, those children still carried some deficiencies at age 10. Those deficiencies are not pathological, but they are at the lower range of the normal values. All subjects had normal hearing, however they had a delay in processing auditory signals. They exhibited lower morning cortisol values, lower scores in the WISC test, mainly in the performance subtests, and they reported more sleep disturbances and fatigue during daytime. They also rated themselves low on other behavioral variables.

Some of the results of this study confirm earlier results obtained by Lozoff's group. They found that former ID infants exhibited modifications in the auditory and visual systems at age 5 (Algarin et al., 2003), despite normal values of blood iron and hemoglobin. When similar groups were tested at age 10, changes in behavioral and cognitive variables were similar to those found in our study (Lozoff et al., 2000). They explained their results by delay in the myelination process in the brain stem attributable to an insult during a critical developmental period.

Reduced cortisol secretion in ID patients has been reported earlier (Saad et al., 1991), similar to the decreased level of cortisol that we found in former ID children. The significance of this finding is still not clear, however, many confirmed Attention-Deficit Hyperactivity Disorder (ADHD) children were found to be ID. It is not clear to us if ID is a part of the ADHD syndrome, or whether the ID is due to very poor eating habits. It is noteworthy that a lower level of cortisol, and a modified response to stress was found among ID children (King et al., 1998; Kariyawasam et al., 2002).

In terms of behavioral variables, the experimental group rated itself much lower (but not statistically significant) with respect to appetite, general mood, ability to concentrate and organization of school materials. The somewhat surprising finding was their report (statistically significant) about their sleep disturbances (mainly insomnia) and fatigue during day. It was reported that sleep disturbances are correlated with decreased morning awakening salivary cortisol (Backhaus et al., 2004).

The WSIC scores showed that the experimental group archived lower scores than the control group. While the scores are within the normal range, the scores in the performance subtests were even lower. This interesting finding (which had been found also by Lozoff's group) might indicate that ID has preferential effects on spatial learning and memory, more than on serial learning and memory. Animal studies showed similar effects in that the spatial learning and memory of ID rats (as measured by Morris Water Maze) were substantially poorer than serial learning (Youdim et al., 2000).

We would suggest that all deficits found in this study share the same basic cause i.e., the long term effects of infant ID.

This study also demonstrates the significance of critical periods during development. A delay in myelanation of several brain areas in the critical period modifies physiological, endocrinological and cognitive variables that persist for a number of years.

The main conclusion from this study is that despite rehabilitation of the hematological profile of infant ID, there are some physiological and cognitive functions that do not rehabilitate even after 10 years. The new findings of this study, e.g., reduced morning cortisol and sleep disturbances, indicate that this group of former ID infants, should be under close observation, and may need special care and intervention. More studies are needed to establish those effects and to devise methods to overcome those deficits.

Acknowledgments

We would like to thank the William Farber Center for Alzheimer Research and the Ginsburg Chair for Research into Alzheimer Disease for their support. Anat Yashfe performed the cognitive preliminary studies.

We would also like to thank Pnina Yakir, Clinical Audiologist, Audiology Department, Kaplan Medical Center, Rehovot, Israel.

References

Algarin C, Peirano P, Garrido M, Pizarro F, Lozoff B (2003) Iron deficiency anemia in infancy: long-lasting effects on auditory and visual system functioning. Pediatr Res 51: 1–7

Backhaus J, Junghanns K, Hohagen F (2004) Sleep disturbances are correlated with decreased morning awakening salivary cortisol. Psychoendocrinology 29: 1184–1191

BeardJ, Borel M, Peterson FJ (1997) Changes in iron status during weight loss with very-slow-energy diets. Am J Clin Nutr 66: 104–110

Ben-Shachar D, Ashkenazi R, Youdim MB (1986) Long-term consequence of early iron-deficiency on dopaminergic neurotransmission in rats. Int J Dev Neurosci 4: 81–88

Buzina SK, Buzina R, Stavljenic A, Farley TM, Haller J, Bergman M, Gorajscan M (1998) Aging, nutritional status and immune response. Int Vitm Nutr Res 68: 133–141

Kariyawasam SH, Zaw F, Handley SL (2002) Reduced salivary cortisol in children with comorbid attention deficit hyperactivity disorder and oppositional defiant disorder. Neuro Endocrinol Lett 23: 45–48

King JA, Barkley RA, Barrett S (1997) Attention-deficit hyperactivity disorder and the stress response. Biol Psychiatry 44: 72–74

Lozoff B, Jimenez E, Hagen J, Mollen E, Wolf AW (2000) Poorer behavioral and developmental outcome more than 10 years after treatment for iron deficiency in infancy. Pediatrics 105: E51–E84

Lozoff B, Wolf AW, Jimenez E (1996) Effects of extended oral iron therapy. J Pediatr 129: 382–389

Roncagliolo M, Garrido M, Walter T, Peirano P, Lozoff B (1998) Evidence of altered central nervous system development in infants with iron deficiency anemia at 6 months. Delayed maturation of auditory brainstem responses. Am J Clin Nutr 68: 683–690

Saad MJ, Morais SL, Saad ST (1991) Reduced cortisol secretion in patients with iron deficiency. Ann Nutr Metabol 35: 111–115

Scrimshaw NS (1991) Iron deficiency. Sci Am 265: 24–30

Scrimshaw NS (1998) Malnutrition, brain development learning and behavior. Nutr Res 18: 351–379

Scrimshaw NS, SanGiovanni JP (1997) Synergism of nutrition, infection and immunity. Am J Clin Nutr 66: 464S–477S

Sun AH, Wang ZM, Xiao SZ, Li ZJ, Liang ZF, Hu GY, Ye XT (1991) Noise-induced hearing loss in iron-deficient rats. Acta Otolaryngol 111: 684–690

Weinberg J, Brett LP, Levine S, Dallman PR (1981) Long-term effects of early iron deficiency on consummately behavior in the rat. Pharmacol Biochem Behav 14: 447–453

Youdim MB, Yehuda S (2000) The neurochemical basis of cognitive deficits induced by brain iron deficiency: involvement of dopamine-opiate system. Cell Mol Biol 46: 491–500

Youdim MBH, Ben-Shachar D, Yehuda S (1989) Putative biological mechanisms of the effect of iron deficiency on brain biochemistry and behavior. Am J Clin Nutr 50: 607–617

Youdim MBH, Yehuda S (2000) The neurochemical basis of cognitive deficits induced by brain iron deficiency: involvement of dopamine-opiate system. Cell Mol Biol 46: 491–500

J Neural Transm (2006) [Suppl] 71: 201–204

Journal of Neural Transmission
Printed in Austria

Altered regulation of iron transport and storage in Parkinson's disease

E. C. Hirsch

INSERM, UMR679, Experimental Neurology and Therapeutics, Hôpital de la Salpêtrière; Université Pierre & Marie Curie – Paris 6, Paris, France

Summary Parkinson's disease (PD) is characterized by the death of dopaminergic neurons in the substantia nigra. This neuronal degeneration is associated with a strong microglial activation and iron accumulation in the affected brain structures. The increased iron content may result from an increased iron penetration into the brain parenchyma due to a higher expression of lactoferrin and lactoferrin receptors at the level of the blood vessels and dopaminergic neurons in the substantia nigra in PD. Iron may also accumulate in microglial cells after phagocytosis of dopaminergic neurons. These effects may be reinforced by a lack of up-regulation of the iron storage protein ferritin, as suggested by an absence of change in iron regulatory protein 1 (IRP-1) control of ferritin mRNA translation in PD. Thus, a dysregulation of the labile iron pool may participate in the degenerative process affecting dopaminergic neurons in PD.

Introduction

Parkinson's disease (PD) is characterized by a preferential vulnerability of dopaminergic neurons in the substantia nigra. Yet evidence suggests that the loss of these neurons is heterogeneous across different catecholaminergic cell groups (Hirsch et al., 1988). Despite the recent identification of genes involved in inherited forms of the disease, the exact mechanism by which dopaminergic neurons degenerate in idiopathic Parkinson's disease is still poorly understood. Several molecular and cellular alterations may, however, contribute to cellular dysfunction and ultimately cell death. Among these factors, protein accumulation, proteasome dysfunction, mitochondrial complex-1 deficiency, and oxidative stress are believed to participate in the cascade of events leading to neuronal death. In line with this, the research groups headed by Youdim and Riederer were among the first to report an increase in the content of iron (III) and total iron in the postmortem substantia nigra of patients with PD (Sofic et al., 1988). These results, which were confirmed by several other studies, raised several questions, which have been addressed during the last fifteen years: is there a dysregulation of iron entry into the substantia nigra? Is there a dysregulation of iron storage in the substantia nigra? Where is iron increased within the substantia nigra? What is the consequence of increased iron content in the parkinsonian substantia nigra?

Correspondence: E. C. Hirsch, INSERM U679 – Experimental Neurology and Therapeutics, Hôpital de la Salpêtrière, 47 Boulevard de l'Hôpital, 75651 Paris Cedex 13, France
e-mail: hirsch@ccr.jussieu.fr

Altered iron penetration into the parkinsonian nigrostriatal pathway

The mechanism by which iron accumulates in the substantia nigra pars compacta in Parkinson's disease is poorly understood. A possible pathway for iron to penetrate into brain parenchyma involves the binding of diferric transferrin to a high affinity receptor (Aisen, 1992). To address this question, we performed a quantitative analysis of iodotransferrin binding in the mesencephalon of patients with PD and matched control subjects (Faucheux et al., 1993). We found a low level of binding of transferrin in the substantia nigra pars compacta of healthy control subjects and no change in PD. These data suggest that transferrin and its receptor are unlikely to be involved in the increased iron content in the substantia nigra of patients with PD. Nevertheless, this does not exclude a retrograde transport of iron taken up in the dopaminergic terminals at the striatal level. In human control subjects, iodotransferrin binding was highest in the putamen and caudate nucleus and lowest in the globus pallidus (Faucheux et al., 1995). In parkinsonian patients, mean density values of transferrin binding were increased in the putamen and caudate nucleus as compared to control subjects. These data suggest transferrin receptors may be located in the putamen and caudate nucleus and iron could be retrogradely transported to perikarya of melanized dopaminergic neurons (Arvidson, 1994). Furthermore, despite the small number of patients studied in this report, PD patients with the highest density of transferrin binding were those in whom the severity of the disease was the highest, in agreement with data published by Riederer et al. (1989). Yet, using film autoradiography, it is difficult to precisely localize transferrin binding sites. Thus, a higher density at the level of blood vessels or glial cells could also explain the increased binding found in PD. Studies at the cellular level are the only means of determining the exact contribution of transferrin receptors to the increased iron content seen in the parkinsonian substantia nigra. To address this issue, we measured the density of transferrin receptors on perikarya of melanized neurons using micro-autoradiography. The mean transferrin receptor density on melanized perikarya was decreased by 50% in the ventral part of the substantia nigra where dopaminergic neuronal loss is the most severe. These data are thus in apparent contradiction with our results obtained microscopically. Yet the absence of decrease observed macroscopically is very likely explained by the presence of transferrin receptors on blood vessels, astrocytes and reactive microglial cells, since the density of these receptors is known to increase in PD (Sofic et al., 1991; Faucheux et al., 1997). In sum, it is unlikely that transferrin receptors are involved in the increased iron content found in melanized dopaminergic neurons in PD.

Lactoferrin receptors could represent another way of iron entry into neurons. Indeed, lactoferrin is another protein binding iron that is also involved in iron transport into the brain via specific receptors called lactoferrin receptors (Mazurier et al., 1989). Using immunohistochemistry, we demonstrated the presence of lactoferrin receptors at the level of blood vessels and nigral dopaminergic neurons (Faucheux et al., 1995). This suggests that these receptors may be involved in iron penetration into brain parenchyma from the blood circulation and from the parenchyma to the cytoplasm of melanized neurons. Moreover, in the substantia nigra, we found lactoferrin receptor immunoreactivity to be increased on both melanized dopaminergic neurons and microvasculature in patients with PD as compared to healthy control subjects (Faucheux et al., 1995). Interestingly, this increase was highest in the most severely affected dopaminergic cell groups, suggesting a relationship between lactoferrin receptor increase and dopaminergic degeneration. The involvement of lactoferrin and its receptor is further supported by an increase in lactoferrin staining within nigral neurons in PD cases. Thus, the concomitant increase of lactoferrin and its receptor on dopaminergic neurons in PD may be responsible for the excessive accumulation of iron in vulnerable neuronal populations. This concept is further supported by the fact that lactoferrin expression is increased in MPTP-intoxicated mice (Fillebeen et al., 2001). Yet, the involvement of lactoferrin and its receptor is not selective for neuronal degeneration in PD but merely represents a common pathway of neuronal degeneration, as similar changes have been described in several neurodegenerative disorders including Alzheimer's disease (AD), Down syndrome, Pick's disease, sporadic amyotrophic lateral sclerosis, and amyotrophic lateral sclerosis/parkinsonism-dementia complex of Guam (Kawamata et al., 1993; Leveugle et al., 1994; Osmand et al., 1991; Rebeck et al., 1995). The identification of lactoferrin changes in other neurodegenerative disorders raises the question as to whether these changes play a primary role in the neurodegenerative process or are merely a consequence of neuronal degeneration.

The exact mechanism by which iron concentration increases in the substantia nigra of patients with PD is not fully understood. Yet the data reviewed here suggest that it is unlikely that transferrin and its receptor participate in this increase in iron content. Other iron transporters such as lactoferrin and its receptor may therefore be particularly relevant to this increased iron concentration. Further studies on the expression level of lactoferrin and/or its receptor are now needed to determine whether these changes are really involved in neuronal degeneration. Likewise, studies on other iron transport proteins such as DMT1 and ferroportin are also needed. Furthermore, a better knowledge of the regulation of iron transport and buffering mechanisms may also help to address this question.

Altered regulation of iron homeostasis in Parkinson's disease

Well regulated iron homeostasis is necessary for cell survival because this metal is a co-factor of numerous biochemical reactions. In contrast, an increased iron concentration is deleterious given the ability of iron to react with hydrogen peroxide and catalyze the formation of the highly reactive hydroxyl radical. Thus, intracellular iron concentrations are controlled by ferritin and transferrin, the level of which depends on both transcriptional control and a post-transcriptional regulatory system (Harrison and Arosio, 1996; Hentze and Künh, 1996). Two cytoplasmic proteins, iron regulatory proteins 1 and 2 (IRP1 and 2) are involved in the control of ferritin synthesis by binding to a stem-loop structure located in the 5′ untranslated region of ferritin mRNA and known as the iron responsive element (IRE). When the concentration of cellular iron is low, IRP binds to IRE, thus inhibiting translation of ferritin. In contrast, if iron concentration increases, IRP does not bind to IRE, allowing translation of ferritin mRNA. Similarly, IRP binds to the 3′ non-coding region of the transferrin receptor mRNA and, when cellular iron levels are low, it stabilizes the transferrin receptor message by preventing its endonuclease cleavage. In contrast, when the iron level increases, this stabilization of the transferrin receptor mRNA is reduced, leading to a decreased transferrin receptor expression and consequently a reduced iron penetration in the cell. Given the high iron concentration observed in the substantia nigra of patients in PD, one may thus expect IRP to be bound to the iron responsive element of ferritin mRNA in the substantia nigra. To test this hypothesis we performed electrophoretic mobility shift assays on post-mortem samples from patients with PD and control subjects (Faucheux et al., 2002). We observed no change in the binding activity of IRP to an IRE-ferritin mRNA probe, indicating the absence of any substantial change in post-transcriptional regulation in the substantia nigra in PD. In agreement with these data, we found no change in ferritin mRNA transcript, thus confirming our previous results and other studies performed both in parkinsonian patients and MPTP-intoxicated monkeys (Dexter et al., 1991; Mann et al., 1994; Connor et al., 1995; Goto et al., 1996). Furthermore, using the supershift technique, we showed that one of the IRPs, IRP1 but not IRP2, bound to ferritin mRNA in these samples. This indicates that the increased iron content found in the substantia nigra of patients with PD is not-associated with an up-regulation of ferritin at the translational level. The reason for such an absence of regulation is not known but may be explained by several non-exclusive mechanisms. First, a cellular dysfunction associated with the disease may prevent ferritin up-regulation. In line with this, the mRNA coding for tyrosine hydroxylase has also been shown to be decreased in the surviving dopaminergic neurons in the substantia nigra of patients with PD (Javoy-Agid et al., 1990). Alternatively, it has been reported that nitric oxide increases the binding activity of IRP1 to IRE-ferritin mRNA and blocks ferritin mRNA translation (Mulero and Brock, 1999). In line with this, astroglial and microglial cells expressing the inducible form of nitric synthase have been found in the vicinity of dopaminergic neurons in the substantia nigra of patients with PD and animal models of the disease (Hunot et al., 1996, 1999; Liberatore et al., 1999; Dehmer et al., 2000). Thus, the production of nitric oxide could interfere with the binding of IRP1 to IRE and may contribute to a deficiency in ferritin subunit synthesis in the substantia nigra of patients with PD.

Another explanation for the absence of ferritin up-regulation could be related to the fact that the pool of iron resulting in an increased concentration may not be located in the cytoplasm where ferritin mRNA is localized. Indeed, intra-cellular analysis of iron has shown that it is also localized on the melanin granules (Good et al., 1992; Jellinger et al., 1992) and in Lewy bodies (Hirsch et al., 1991). Thus, neuromelanin may be involved in intra-neuronal iron homeostasis as a result of its strong chelating ability for iron (Zecca et al., 2001). In line with this, the level of redox activity detected in neuromelanin aggregates was significantly increased in parkinsonian patients and was highest in patients with the most severe neuronal loss (Faucheux et al., 2003). A possible consequence of an overloading of neuromelanin with redox element may thus be an increased contribution to oxidative stress and intra-neuronal damage in patients with PD. The increase in iron concentration may also take place in non-dopaminergic neurons. Indeed, histochemical identification of iron within the parkinsonian substantia nigra evidenced strong staining in microglial cells. Thus, a part of the iron contributing to its increase concentration as measured on brain homogenates may be localized in microglial cells. This may result in an indirect involvement in the neurodegenerative process by inducing glial activation and neuroinflammatory processes.

Conclusion

In summary, while it has been well established that iron concentration increases in the substantia nigra of patients with PD, its exact role in neurodegeneration has yet to be determined. The mechanisms potentially involved in such an increase include the possible release of iron from neuromelanin aggregates and an increased penetration by lactoferrin and its receptor. Furthermore, the absence of ferritin and transferrin regulation, possibly due to the presence of nitric oxide, may facilitate iron entry into dopaminergic neurons. The consequence of this increase may be oxidative stress, protein alteration including alpha-synuclein aggregation and ultimately cell death. Thus, therapies aimed at regulating iron concentration within dopaminergic neurons may be useful in helping to reduce neuronal degeneration in PD.

References

Aisen P (1992) Entry of iron into cells: a new role for the transferrin receptor in modulating iron release from transferrin. Ann Neurol 32 [Suppl]: S62–S68

Arvidson B (1994) A review of axonal transport of metals. Toxicology 88: 1–14

Connor JR, Snyder BS, Arosio P, Loeffler DA, LeWitt P (1995) A quantitative analysis of isoferritins in select regions of aged, parkinsonian, and Alzheimer's diseased brains. J Neurochem 65: 717–724

Dehmer T, Lindenau J, Haid S, Dichgans J, Schulz JB (2000) Deficiency of inducible nitric oxide synthase protects against MPTP toxicity *in vivo*. J Neurochem 74: 2213–2216

Dexter DT, Carayon A, Javoy-Agid F, Agid Y, Wells FR, Daniel SE, Lees AJ, Jenner P, Marsden CD (1991) Alterations in the levels of iron, ferritin and other trace metals in Parkinson's disease and other neurodegenerative diseases affecting the basal ganglia. Brain 114: 1953–1975

Faucheux BA, Hauw JJ, Agid Y, Hirsch EC (1997) The density of [^{125}I]-transferrin binding sites on perikarya of melanized neurons of the substantia nigra is decreased in Parkinson's disease. Brain Res 749: 170–174

Faucheux BA, Herrero MT, Villares J, Levy R, Obeso JA, Hauw JJ, Agid Y, Hirsch EC (1995) Autoradiographic localization and density of [125I]-Ferrotransferrin binding sites in the striatum of control subjects, patients with Parkinson's disease and MPTP-lesioned monkeys. Brain Res 691: 115–124

Faucheux BA, Hirsch EC, Villares J, Selimi F, Mouatt-Prigent A, Javoy-Agid F, Hauw JJ, Agid Y (1993) Distribution of 125I-Ferrotransferrin binding sites in the mesencephalon of control subjects and patients with Parkinson's disease. J Neurochem 60: 2338–2341

Faucheux BA, Martin ME, Beaumont C, Hauw JJ, Agid Y, Hirsch EC (2003) Neuromelanin associated redox-active iron is increased in the substantia nigra of patients with Parkinson's disease. J Neurochem 86: 1142–1148

Faucheux BA, Martin ME, Beaumont C, Hunot S, Hauw JJ, Agid Y, Hirsch EC (2002) Lack of up-regulation of ferritin is associated with sustained iron regulatory protein-1 binding activity in the substantia nigra of patients with Parkinson's disease. J Neurochem 83: 320–330

Faucheux BA, Nillesse N, Damier P, Spik G, Mouatt-Prigent A, Pierce A, Leveugle B, Kubis N, Hauw JJ, Agid Y, Hirsch EC (1995) Expression of lactoferrin receptors is increased in the mesencephalon of patients with Parkinson's disease. Proc Natl Acad Sci 92: 9603–9607

Fillebeen C, Ruchoux MM, Mitchell V, Vincent S, Benaissa M, Pierce A (2001) Lactoferrin is synthesized by activated microglia in the human substantia nigra and its synthesis by the human microglial CHME cell line is upregulated by tumor necrosis factor alpha or 1-methyl-4-phenylpyridinium treatment. Brain Res Mol Brain Res 96: 103–113

Good PF, Olanow CW, Perl DP (1992) Neuromelanin-containing neurons of the substantia nigra accumulate iron and aluminum in Parkinson's disease: a LAMMA study. Brain Res 593: 343–346

Goto K, Mochizuki H, Imai H, Akiyama H, Mizuno Y (1996) An immunohistochemical study of ferritin in 1-methyl-4-phenyl-1,2,3,6-tetrahydropyridine (MPTP)-induced hemiparkinsonian monkeys. Brain Res 724: 125–128

Harrison PM, Arosi P (1996) The ferritins: molecular properties, iron storage function and cellular regulation. Biochim Biophys Acta 1275: 161–203 Review

Hentze MW, Kuhn LC (1996) Molecular control of vertebrate iron metabolism: mRNA-based regulatory circuits operated by iron, nitric oxide, and oxidative stress. Proc Natl Acad Sci USA 93: 8175–8182 Review

Hirsch EC, Brandel JP, Galle P, Javoy-Agid F, Agid Y (1991) Iron and aluminum increase in the substantia nigra of patients with Parkinson's disease: an X-ray microanalysis. J Neurochem 56: 446–451

Hirsch EC, Graybiel AM, Agid Y (1988) Melanized dopaminergic neurons are differentially susceptible to degeneration in Parkinson's disease. Nature 334: 345–348

Hunot S, Boissiere F, Faucheux B, Brugg B, Mouatt-Prigent A, Agid Y, Hirsch EC (1996) Nitric oxide synthase and neuronal vulnerability in Parkinson's disease. Neuroscience 72: 355–363

Hunot S, Dugas N, Faucheux BA, Hartmann A, Tardieu M, Debre P, Agid Y, Dugas B, Hirsch EC (1999) Fc(epsilon)RII/CD23 is expressed in Parkinson's disease and induces, in vitro, production of nitric oxide and tumor necrosis factor-a in glial cells. J Neurosci 19: 3440–3447

Javoy-Agid F, Hirsch EC, Dumas S, Duyckaerts C, Mallet J, Agid Y (1990) Decreased tyrosine hydroxylase messenger mRNA in the surviving dopamine neurons in Parkinson's disease: an in situ hybridization study. Neuroscience 38: 245–253

Jellinger K, Kienzl E, Rumpelmair G, Riederer P, Stachelberger H, Ben-Shachar D, Youdim MB (1992) Iron-melanin complex in substantia nigra of parkinsonian brains: an x-ray microanalysis. J Neurochem 59: 1168–1171

Kawamata T, Tooyama I, Yamada T, Walker DG, McGeer PL (1993) Lactotransferrin immunocytochemistry in Alzheimer and normal human brain. Am J Pathol 142: 1574–1585

Leveugle B, Spik G, Perl DP, Bouras C, Fillit HM, Hof PR (1994) The iron-binding protein lactotransferrin is present in pathologic lesions in a variety of neurodegenerative disorders: a comparative immunohistochemical analysis. Brain Res 650: 20–31

Liberatore GT, Jackson-Lewis V, Vukosavic S, Mandir AS, Vila M, McAuliffe WG, Dawson VL, Dawson TM, Przedborski S (1999) Inducible nitric oxide synthase stimulates dopaminergic neurodegeneration in the MPTP model of Parkinson disease. Nature Med 5: 1403–1409

Mann VM, Cooper JM, Daniel SE, Srai K, Jenner P, Marsden CD, Schapira AH (1994) Complex I, iron, and ferritin in Parkinson's disease substantia nigra. Ann Neurol 36: 876–881

Mazurier J, Legrand D, Hu WL, Montreuil J, Spik G (1989) Expression of human lactotransferrin receptors in phytohemagglutinin-stimulated human peripheral blood lymphocytes. Isolation of the receptors by antiligand-affinity chromatography. Eur J Biochem 179: 481–487

Mulero V, Brock JH (1999) Regulation of iron metabolism in murine J774 macrophages: role of nitric oxide-dependent and -independent pathways following activation with gamma interferon and lipopolysaccharide. Blood 94: 2383–2389

Osmand AP, Switzer III RC (1991) Differential distribution of lactoferrin and Alz-50 immunoreactivities in neuritic plaques and neurofibrillary tangles in Alzheimer's disease. In: Iqbal K, McLachlan RC, Winblad B, Wisniewski HM (eds) Alzheimer's disease: basic mechanism, diagnosis and therapeutic strategies. Wiley, New York, pp 219–227

Rebeck GW, Harr SD, Strickland DK, Hyman BT (1995) Multiple, diverse senile plaque-associated proteins are ligands of an apolipoprotein E receptor, the alpha 2-macroglobulin receptor/low-density-lipoprotein receptor-related protein. Ann Neurol 37: 211–217

Riederer P, Sofic E, Rausch WD, Schmidt B, Reynolds GP, Jellinger K, Youdim MB (1989) Transition metals, ferritin, glutathione, and ascorbic acid in parkinsonian brains. J Neurochem 52: 515–520

Sofic E, Paulus W, Jellinger K, Riederer P, Youdim MB (1991) Selective increase of iron in substantia nigra zona compacta of parkinsonian brains. J Neurochem 56: 978–982

Sofic E, Riederer P, Heinsen H, Beckmann H, Reynolds GP, Hebenstreit G, Youdim MB (1988) Increased iron (III) and total iron content in post mortem substantia nigra of parkinsonian brain. J Neural Transm 74: 199–205

Zecca L, Gallorini M, Schunemann V, Trautwein AX, Gerlach M, Riederer P, Vezzoni P, Tampellini D (2001) Iron, neuromelanin and ferritin content in the substantia nigra of normal subjects at different ages: consequences for iron storage and neurodegenerative processes. J Neurochem 76: 1766–1773

J Neural Transm (2006) [Suppl] 71: 205–213

Journal of Neural Transmission
Printed in Austria

Iron dyshomeostasis in Parkinson's disease

J. Salazar[1,2], **N. Mena**[1], **M. T. Núñez**[1]

[1] Department of Biology, and Cell Dynamic and Biotechnology Research Center, Faculty of Sciences, University of Chile, Santiago, Chile
[2] INSERM U679, Hopital de la Salpetriere, Paris, France

Summary Owing to its ability to undergo one-electron reactions, iron transforms the mild oxidant hydrogen peroxide into hydroxyl radical, one of the most reactive species in nature. Deleterious effects of iron accumulation are dramatically evidenced in several neurodegenerative diseases. The work of Youdim and collaborators has been fundamental in describing the accumulation of iron confined to the substantia nigra (SN) in Parkinson's disease (PD) and to clarify iron toxicity pathways and oxidative damage in dopaminergic neurons. Nevertheless, how the mechanisms involved in normal neuronal iron homeostasis are surpassed, remain largely undetermined. How nigral neurons survive or succumb to iron-induced oxidative stress are relevant questions both to know about the etiology of the disease and to design neuroprotective strategies. In this work, we review the components of neural iron homeostasis and we summarize evidence from recent studies aimed to unravel the molecular basis of iron accumulation and dyshomeostasis in PD.

In vertebrates, numerous physiological processes including oxygen transport, respiration, DNA synthesis, formation of some neurotransmitters and hormones, xenobiotic metabolism, and certain aspects of host defense use iron-containing proteins (Gutteridge and Halliwell, 2000). However, because of its ability to undergo one-electron reactions, Fe^{2+} transforms the mild oxidant hydrogen peroxide into hydroxyl radical ($HO^{\bullet}$), one of the most reactive species in nature (Symons and Gutteridge, 1998). The Fenton reaction, as this reaction is known, follows mass action law, so $HO^{\bullet}$ production is proportional to reactive Fe^{2+} concentration. There are no known specific mechanisms to detoxify $HO^{\bullet}$, so this species quickly reacts and modifies lipids, proteins, lipids and DNA (Gutteridge and Halliwell, 2000; Haupmann and Cadenas, 1997). To maintain iron inside a concentration window that allows for physiological functions, and impedes the formation of highly reactive oxygen species (ROS), cells display transcriptional and post-transcriptional mechanism of regulation.

Correspondence: Dr. Marco T. Núñez, Department of Biology, Faculty of Sciences, University of Chile, Las Palmeras 3425, Ñuñoa, Santiago, Chile
e-mail: mnunez@uchile.cl

Neuronal iron homeostasis

Components of cell iron homeostasis

The components of cell iron homeostasis are shown in Fig. 1. The scheme includes the inflow and efflux iron transporters, DMT1 and Ireg1, respectively; the iron storage protein ferritin; the ferrireductase Dcytb, responsible for the reduction of Fe^{3+} prior to transport by DMT1 (McKie et al., 2001); and the ferroxidase ceruloplasmin, responsible for the oxidation of Fe^{2+} after transport by Ireg1 and prior to the binding by apoTf (Hellman and Gitlin, 2002). The cell uptake system includes the endocytosis of the iron-binding protein transferrin (Tf) mediated by transferrin receptors (TfR) located in the cell surface.

The labile iron pool (LIP)

The LIP is defined as a pool of weakly bound iron. When determined by calcein fluorescence quenching, the affinity constant of LIP complexes is operationally defined as $<10^6$ (Epsztejn et al., 1997). Because of the reductive environment of the cell, iron in the LIP is predominantly in the Fe^{+2} state, although transient Fe^{+3} is expected because of cellular oxidations. The nature of the LIP binding counterpart is unknown, but has been ascribed to diverse low-molecular weight substances as phosphate, nucleotides, hydroxyl, amino and sulphydryl groups (Kakhlon and Cabantchik, 2002; Petrat et al., 2002). Normally, the LIP represents 3–5% of the total cellular iron, but this proportion changes with the iron status of the cell. Neuroblastoma

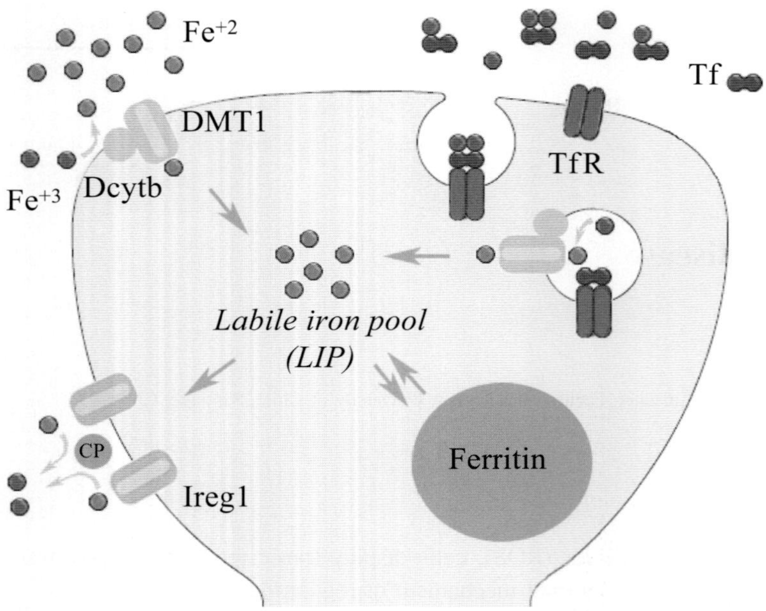

Fig. 1. Neuronal Iron Homeostasis. Neurons may acquire iron from two sources, Tf-bound iron and non-Tf-bound iron (NTBI). The total iron content and Tf concentration in CSF (about 0.7 and 0.24 μM, respectively) ensures that both sources of iron are readily available to brain cells. Tf- bound Fe is taken up via a TfR-mediated process. This process involves the binding of diferric Tf to TfR, the internalization of the complex into an acidic endosomal compartment, which promotes the dissociation of iron from Tf. Dissociation is followed by the reduction of released Fe^{3+} to Fe^{2+} and the transport into the cytosol through DMT1. NTBI uptake involves the reduction of Fe^{3+} to Fe^{2+} by Dcytb and the transport by DMT1. The high content of ascorbate in CSF (about 150 μM) ensures that CSF iron will be mainly in the Fe^{2+}, readily transportable state. Once in the cytosol, Fe^{2+} incorporates in to the labile iron pool, where it establishes multiple equilibriums with other iron-containing compartment in the cell, the quantitatively most important of them being ferritin. Recent reports indicate that iron exit loaded neurons (Aguirre et al., 2005). Iron transporter Ireg1 is the most probable candidate to mediate this transport, since its increased expression due to iron loading closely correlates with the rate of iron efflux (Aguirre et al., 2005). After Ireg1 transport, and prior to the binding with Tf, Fe^{2+} is oxidized to Fe^{3+}. The oxidation is mediated by ceruloplasmin present in CSF. Abbreviations: DMT1, divalent metal transporter 1; Ireg1, iron-regulated transporter 1; Dcytb, duodenal cytochrome b ferrireductase; CP, ceruloplasmin; Tf, transferrin; TfR, transferrin receptor; FN, ferritin

cells cultured with high iron media contain 3-4-fold more LIP that cells cultured in low iron media (Núñez et al., 2004). Moreover, cells with higher LIP invariably present higher levels of reactive oxygen species. Thus, the LIP is a marker not only of total cell iron content but also determines the redox state of the cell (Kruszewski, 2003; Núñez et al., 2004).

Over 90% of cell iron is safely stored in ferritin, a multimeric protein that accept up to 4,500 iron atoms in its central core. Since ferritin iron is not redox-active, it is considered "safe" iron. Nevertheless, ferritin iron is not completely safe. Every time ferritin is degraded (microglial ferritin turnover: 3–3.5 h (Mehlhase et al., 2005), its iron will contribute transiently to the LIP. Immunohystochemical studies of ferritin distribution in brain cells show a ubiquitous label for oligodendrocytes and microglia and a weak mark in neurons from cortex, medial habenula, paraventricular nucleus, amygdale and supraoptic nucleus (Connor et al., 1994; Hansen et al., 1999). Thus, we might conjecture that in the majority of neurons, iron uptake and export would be more important than ferritin turnover in determining LIP.

Tf-mediated iron uptake

Tf is present in extracellular fluids either in the apo, monoferric or diferric forms. Under physiological conditions, iron enters the cell by Tf endocytosis. In the acidic pH of the endosome, iron is released from Tf, reduced to Fe^{2+} by a ferric reductase and transported to the cytosol (Núñez et al., 1990). Once in the cytosol, Fe^{2+} becomes part of LIP (Breuer et al., 1997). Plasma Tf saturation in normal individuals is about 35%, which makes monoferric Tf the predominant plasmatic form (Williams and Moreton, 1980). Tf saturation is different in brain cells. Cerebral spinal fluid (CSF) Tf and iron concentrations are about 0.24 and 0.70 μM, respectively (Symons and Gutteridge, 1998). Thus, cerebral spinal fluid Tf is saturated and considerable amounts of non-Tf-bound iron are present. Providing the presence of DMT1 or TfR in the plasma membrane, brain cells will carry out both transferrin-bound and non transferrin-bound iron uptake.

The iron transporter DMT1

DMT1 transports iron into cells by an electrogenic mechanism that involves the co-transport of Fe^{2+} and one proton. In the brain, DMT1 messenger and protein are present mainly in neuronal cells (Gunshin et al., 1997). The highly reductive property of CSF, contributed by ascorbate concentrations of approximately 160 µM (Reiber et al., 1993), determines that Fe^{2+} is the predominant Fe species. Fe^{2+} is readily available for direct incorporation into the cell by the Fe^{2+} transporter DMT1 (Gunshin et al., 1997; Arredondo et al., 2003) in a process known as non-transferrin bound iron uptake. Importantly, non-transferrin bound iron uptake does not have the tight regulation of transferrin-bound iron uptake, exerted by the IRE/IRP system over TfR translation. Thus, neurons with high expression of DMT1 should be particularly susceptible to iron accumulation. In particular, neurons from ventral mesencephalon have one of the highest DMT1/TfR expression ratios (Gunshin et al., 1997; Hill et al., 1985), so these neurons should be prone to iron accumulation.

In searching for DMT1 expression in the rat mesencephalon, we found that co-localization of DMT1 with the dopaminergic marker tyrosine hydroxylase (TH) is higher in the SNpc than in the ventral tegmental area (VTA) (Fig. 2). We hypothesize that he presence of high levels of DMT1 in SNpc might explain its higher susceptibility to neurodegenerative processes.

Four isoforms of DMT1 are generated by alternative splicing of the 5′-end exons (exons 1A or 1B) and of the 3′-end exons (exons 16 (or +IRE) or 16a (or −IRE)) (Hubert and Hentze, 2002). Concordant with the presence of an IRE element in the 3′flanking region, DMT1 expression is down regulated by high cell iron. Nevertheless, there is no agreement about the specific mechanisms causing this regulation. Expression of the 1A/+IRE isoform makes cells particularly sensitive to cell iron levels; expression of the 1A/−IRE isoform yield cells that also responds to iron changes, whereas cells expressing the 1B/+IRE or the 1B/−IRE isoforms do not respond. Thus, it is possible that the regulation of DMT1 expression involves two regulatory regions, one contained in exon 1A and another in exon 16. There is no report on the nature of the DMT1 isoforms present in different brain areas. This information is of primary interest to understand regulation of DMT1 expression.

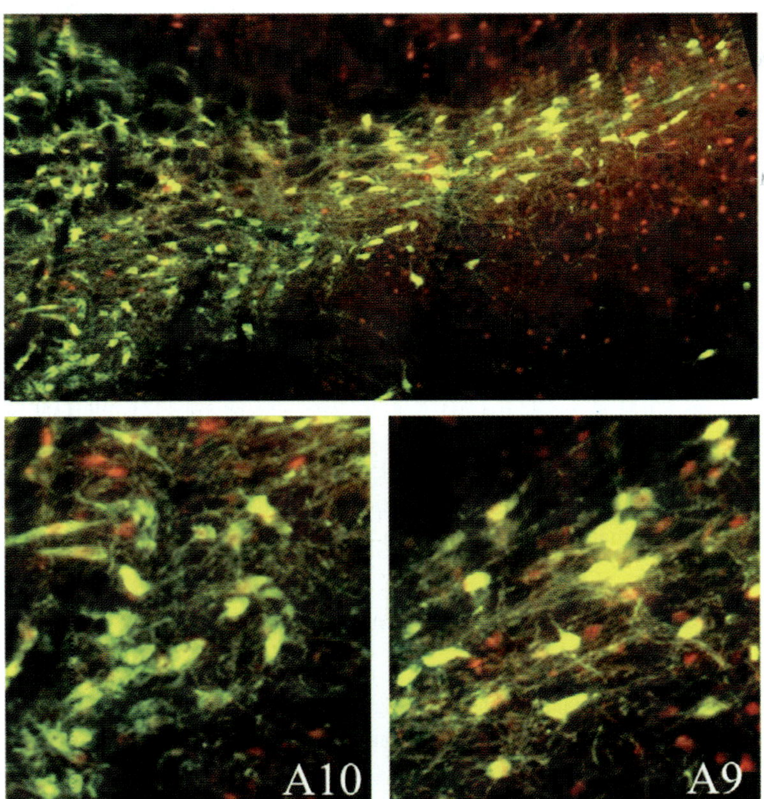

Fig. 2. DMT1 localization in the ventral mesencephalon. Immunohistochemistry against tyrosine hydroxylase (TH, green) and DMT1 IRE+ (red) in a coronal slice of rat mesencephalon. A9, substantia nigra pars compacta. A10, ventral tegmental area. In TH-positive cells, DMT1 immunoreactivity was more intense in A9 than in the A10 area

Iron export

Ireg1 (also called ferroportin 1 and MTP1) is the only member of the SLC40 family of transporters and the first reported protein that mediates the exit of iron from cells (McKie et al., 2000). The protein is expressed mainly in enterocytes and macrophages. In enterocytes, Ireg1 is responsible for iron efflux during the process of intestinal iron absorption, while in Kupffer cells Ireg1 mediates iron export for reutilization by the bone marrow (Devalia et al., 2002). The regulation of Ireg1 expression is unknown. In enterocytes, iron deficiency induces Ireg1 expression (McKie et al., 2000) whereas in macrophages iron deficiency decreases it (Yang et al., 2005). In the brain, we can find Ireg1 messenger and protein in endothelial cells of the blood–brain barrier, in neurons, oligodendrocytes, astrocytes, the choroid plexus and ependymal cells (Wu et al., 2004). In a recent study we reported that SHSY5Y neuroblastoma cells and hippocampal neurons that survive an iron accumulation protocol, evoke an adaptive response consisting of decreased synthesis of DMT1 and increased synthesis of Ireg1 (Aguirre et al., 2005). Thus, the concerted regulation of iron transporters is clearly cell-specific and adjusts to the particular functions of the cells.

The iron reductase Dcytb

Before iron uptake via the membrane transporter DMT1, ferric iron reduction to ferrous iron is attained by the enzyme duodenal cytochrome b (Dcytb) (McKie et al., 2001). Dcytb is also expressed in spleen and probably liver (Latunde-Dada et al., 2004), but no report on the expression of Dcytb in brain cells is available. It is possible that the highly reductive environment of CSF makes redundant Dcytb expression for non-transferrin iron uptake. Nevertheless, Tf-bound iron uptake still should require a Fe^{3+} to Fe^{2+} reduction step before transport into the cytosol (Núñez et al., 1990). Thus, the presence of Dcytb, or a related reductase, in endosomal compartments of brain cells is possible.

The iron oxidases

Two ferroxidases has been described to account for Fe^{2+} oxidation prior to Tf binding, the membrane-bound oxidase hephaestin and serum ceruloplasmin. Hephaestin is a membrane-bound ferrireductase homologous to ceruloplasmin, highly expressed throughout the small intestine, and at low levels in several other tissues (Anderson et al., 2002). No role for hephaestin in human neuronal iron efflux has been demonstrated, thus in the brain, the main ferroxidase involved in iron exit seems to be ceruloplasmin. This member of the multicopper oxidase family exists in the brain predominantly as a glycosylphosphatidylinositol-linked astrocyte protein (Patel and David, 1997). Aceruloplasminemia, a condition characterized by the complete lack of ceruloplasmin ferroxidase activity caused by mutations in the ceruloplasmin gene, results in excessive iron accumulation in the pancreas, retina, and brain (Miyajima et al., 2003). Magnetic resonance imaging of an aceruloplasminemia patient revealed abundant iron deposition in neurons of the putamen, dentate nuclei, substantia nigra, red nuclei, inferior and superior colliculi, and thalamic nuclei (Grisoli et al., 2005). These data can be interpreted as the need of several neuronal areas to discharge iron in order to avoid excessive accumulation.

Iron regulatory proteins: translational regulation

In vertebrates, cellular iron levels are post-transcriptionally controlled by the activity of iron regulatory proteins (IRP1 and IRP2), cytosolic proteins that bind to structural elements called iron-responsive elements (IREs). IREs are found in the untranslated region of the mRNAs of the major proteins that regulate cellular iron homeostasis: the transferrin receptor, involved in plasma-to-cell iron transport, and the iron-storage protein ferritin (reviewed in Eisenstein and Ross, 2003). The activities of both IRP1 and IRP2 respond to changes in cellular Fe through different mechanisms. In iron-replete conditions, IRP1 has a 4S-4Fe cubane structure that renders the protein active as a cytosolic aconitase but inactive for IRE-binding. Low levels of intracellular Fe induce disassembling of the 4S-4Fe cluster, which causes IRP1 to bind and stabilize TfR mRNA. Furthermore, IRP1 binds to ferritin mRNA, thus diminishing its translation. Besides iron, effectors such as nitric oxide (Bouton et al., 1997; Kim and Ponka, 2002), hydrogen peroxide (Martins et al., 1995), hypoxia (Hanson et al., 1999), and phosphorylation (Schalinske and Eisenstein, 1996) also regulate IRP1. In contrast to IRP1, IRP2 activity is down-regulated through iron-induced oxidative damage followed by ubiquitination and proteasome degradation (Guo et al., 1995).

Iron accumulation in neurodegeneration

Transition metals such as iron and copper are frequently associated with neurodegenerative diseases like Alzheimer's disease (AD), Parkinson's disease (PD) and Amyotrophic lateral sclerosis (ALS) (Gerlach et al., 1994; Sayre et al., 2000; Perry et al., 2003).

Iron accumulation in Parkinson's disease

Iron accumulates with age in redox-sensitive tissues such as *substantia nigra pars compacta* (SNpc) (Sofic et al., 1988; Dexter et al., 1989; Riederer et al., 1989). Postmortem studies describe higher levels of iron in normal SNpc than in other brain regions and a further iron accumulation in SNpc of patients with PD (Riederer et al., 1989; Youdim and Riederer, 1993; Shoham and Youdim, 2002; Gotz et al., 2004; Hirsch et al., 1991). This has been confirmed by MRI imaging and ultrasound studies (Gorell et al., 1995; Berg et al., 1999). This increase in iron levels is also present in animal models of PD using the neurotoxins N-methyl-1,2,3,6 tetrahydropyridine (MPTP) or 6-Hydroxydopamine (6-OHDA). In sum, these findings led to the hypothesis that excess iron is the cause of dopaminergic neuronal death in PD (Double et al., 2000). Nevertheless, the position of iron accumulation in the cascade of events that trigger PD has been object of intense debate. Is this accumulation a primary event? PD patients with mild loss of dopaminergic neurons and patients with incidental Lewy body disease (ILBD), postulated as pre-symptomatic PD, present with no significant changes in iron levels in SN (Riederer et al., 1989; Dexter et al., 1994). In addition, in MPTP-treated monkeys, dopaminergic cell death precedes iron elevation (He et al., 2003). However, a causative association cannot be discarded since the status of the LIP in early stages of the disease is not known. However, it seems clear that iron contributes to the disease progression. Recent works report that iron chelation protects against MPTP and 6-OHDA neurotoxicity (Kaur et al., 2003; Youdim et al., 2004), and several pre-clinical trials are already in course to evaluate iron chelators that can cross the haematoencephalic barrier as neuroprotective agents (Youdim et al., 2005).

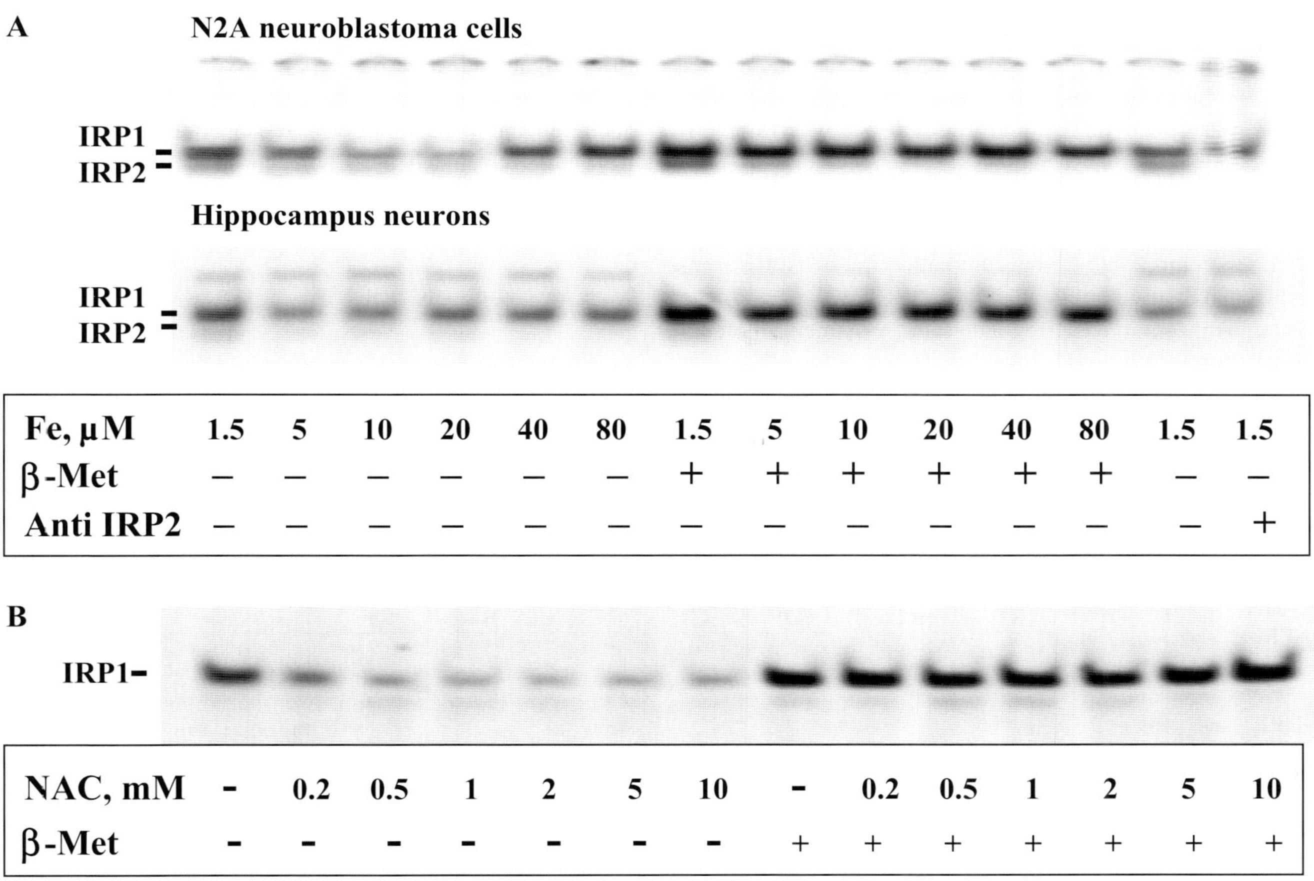

Fig. 3. Effect of iron and antioxidants on IRP activity of neuronal cells. **A** N2A neuroblastoma cells or hippocampal neurons were incubated for 2 days in a media containing 1.5, 5, 10, 20, 40, or 80 µM Fe. Cell extracts were prepared and IRP activity was determined by band-shift assay, using ^{32}P-labeled IRE derived from ferritin cDNA (Núñez-Millacura et al., 2002). The high molecular weight band represents the IRP1-^{32}P-IRE complex, an expression of IRP1 binding activity. Treatment with 2% β-mercaptoethanol (β-Met) maximally activates IRP1, giving a notion of total (active + inactive) IRP1. Following an initial decrease in IRP1 activity as a function of increasing iron, further increases resulted in sustained IRP1 activity. **B** Band-shift assay of IRP activity of N2A cells stimulated for 2 days with 40 µM Fe in the presence of the stated concentrations of the antioxidant N-acetyl-L-cysteine (NAC). It is observed that NAC abolishes the sustained iron-induced IRP1 activity (Fig. adapted from Núñez-Millacura et al. (2001))

We do not know what causes iron accumulation and the factors responsible for overcoming the iron regulatory system. Diferric transferrin binding sites are decreased on melanized neurons of SN (Faucheux et al., 1997). IRP1 activity and the amount of H-Ferritin and L-Ferritin messengers and proteins, present no significant differences between the SNpc of PD patients and control subjects (Faucheux et al., 2002).

An association between ROS/RNS toxicity and PD was found in studies describing: (i) oxidative damage to DNA, lipids and proteins in the SNpc of patients with PD (Alam et al., 1997; Dexter et al., 1989; Floor and Wetzel, 1997); and (ii) NO damage to proteins in Lewis body containing neurons (Good et al., 1998). Thus, considering modulation of IRPs activity by ROS and RNS, it is possible that free radicals in PD impede the expected inactivation of IRP1 at high iron concentrations.

In neuroblastoma cells and cultured neurons, the activity of IRP1 in function of iron concentration shows a biphasic curve: a first component in which iron IRP1 decreases as iron augments, and a second component in which IRP1 increases with further rise in iron concentration (Núñez-Millacura et al., 2002). Interestingly, the upward component is dependent on oxidative stress, since it is reversed by the anti-oxidant N-acetyl cysteine (Fig. 3). These results led us to think that, even when dopaminergic cell might be trying to compensate iron accumulation, globally, the iron-induced oxidative stress maintains IRP1 active, with the consequent failure to up-regulate ferritin (Núñez-Millacura et al., 2002).

A role for inflammation in PD is supported by microglial activation, cell infiltration and augmented cytokines reported in the nigrostriatal system of parkinsonian brains (Hirsch et al., 2003). Conspicuously, studies in monocytic cells, bronchial epithelial cells and endothelial cells showed increased levels of DMT1 and/or decreased level of Ireg1/ferroportin as a consequence of exposition to lipopolysaccharide, TNFα or INFγ (Ludwiczek et al., 2003; Wang et al., 2005; Nanami et al., 2005). Furthermore, NFκB augments the transcription of DMT1 1B (Paradkar and Roth, 2005), and nuclear immunoreactivity of NFκB in PD brains was reported to be over 70-fold that of control subjects (Hunot et al., 1997). To our knowledge, there is no report of the status of DMT1 and Ireg1 expression in SN of PD brains. We hypothesize that dopaminergic cells, which abundantly express TNFα receptors (Boka et al., 1994), will be prone to have increased iron content by the unfavorable expression of iron import and export transporters (Aguirre et al., 2005).

Recent works have revealed that ubiquitin-proteasome system, the main pathway of cellular protein degradation, is specifically impaired in the SN of parkinsonian brains (McNaught and Olanow, 2005). Given that IRP2 is degraded by this system, its impairment could favors IRP2 accretion and increases of iron. Although, band shift assays have failed to find IRP2 activity in human brains, we can search for changes of protein levels.

Iron regulatory proteins and DMT1 in an animal model of Parkinson's disease

In order to test a putative activation of IRP1 and DMT1, we examined IRP activity and protein content of DMT1 in an animal model of PD. We selected the model of partial lesion with striatal injection of 6-OHDA (20 μg/5 μl for

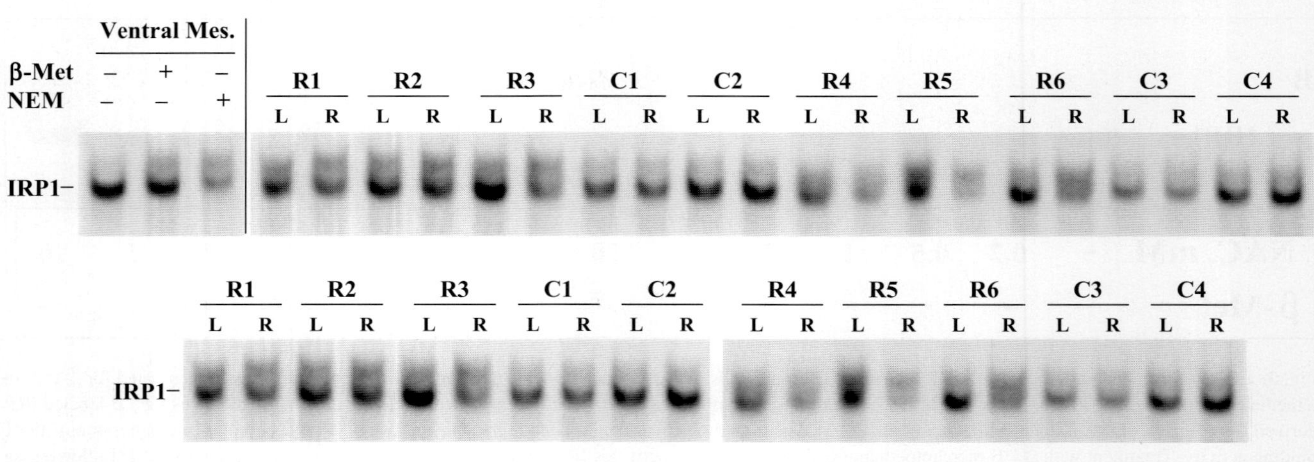

Fig. 4. IRP activity in ventral mesencephalon from 6-OHDA treated rats. IRP activity was determined in cell extracts of ventral mesencephalon It is observed that IRP1 activity is higher in the ventral mesencephalon ipsilateral to the side of 6-OHDA injection (L) in all experimental rats (R1–6). No differences where found between both sides in sham operated rats (C1–4)

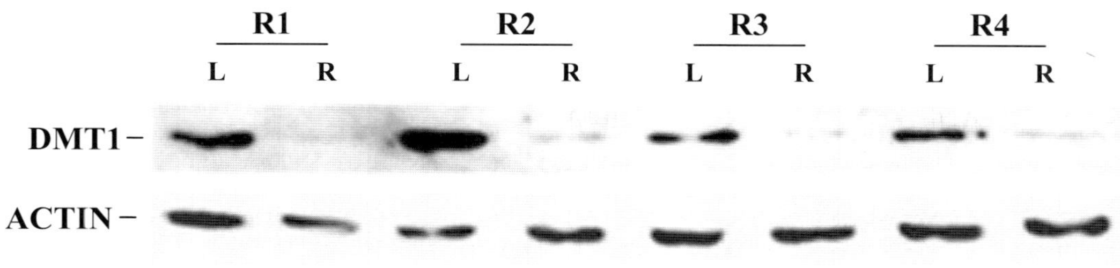

Fig. 5. DMT1 expression in ventral mesencephalon from 6-OHDA treated rats. Ventral mesencephalon from 6-OHDA-treated or control rats was dissected and proteins resolved by SDS-PAGE electrophoresis. DMT1 was recognized by Western immunoblotting using an antibody that recognizes the +IRE isoform of DMT1. To control for gel load, the membranes were acid-stripped after the detection of DMT1 and re-probed with anti-actin (Aguirre et al., 2005). The intensity of the DMT1 band was higher in the ventral mesencephalon ipsilateral to the side of 6-OHDA injection (L) in all experimental rats (R1–4). No differences where found between both sides in sham operated (data not shown)

animal in one injection) because microglial activation and cytokines rise have been reported for this model (Henze et al., 2005; Mogi et al., 1999). In addition, unilateral injections offer the possibility of a control side. At 21 days post-injection, SN of treated rats presented a 40% loss of tyrosine hydroxylase (TH)-positive cells when compared with the control side. Total iron levels were 36% augmented in the SN ipsilateral to the lesion compared with the control side, as measured by mass spectrometry. The ventral mesencephalon (containing the SN) of accurately lesioned rats was dissected and tested in band-shift assays for IRP activity (Fig. 4) and western blot for DMT1 protein levels (Fig. 5). We found an augmentation in both IRP1 activity and in DMT1 protein levels in the SN of all lesioned animals. These finding points to a severe dysregulation of iron homeostasis in 6-OHDA animals. It remains to be determined what is first: unchecked iron accumulation and a positive feedback loop of oxidative stress and IRP1/DMT1 dysregulation or IRP1/DMT1 dysregulation induced by an unknown process resulting in iron accumulation. If increased DMT1 activity is a pathognomonic sign of iron dysregulation, we predict that animals presenting a mutated DMT1 transporter, such as the Belgrade rat and the *mk*-mouse, would present with less susceptibility to neurotoxins causing nigral degeneration.

Concluding remarks

In PD, the iron regulatory mechanisms in neurons of SNpc are surpassed. Recent evidence suggests that IRP1-mediated iron dyshomeostasis and sustained DMT1 presence may underlie iron accumulation in this disease. In this context, an evaluation of DMT1 and Ireg1 expression in parkinsonian brain is capital to understand the cause of iron accumulation and to design neuroprotective and therapeutic strategies to prevent progression of PD.

Acknowledgement

This work was supported by Programme Alban, the European Union Programme of High Level Scholarships for Latin America, scholarship No. E04D044044CL, by project P99-031 from the Millennium Scientific Initiative, Santiago, Chile and by Departamento de Investigación of University of Chile.

References

Aguirre P, Mena N, Tapia V, Arredondo M, Núñez MT (2005) Iron homeostasis in neuronal cells: a role for IREG1. BMC Neurosci 6: 1–3

Alam ZI, Jenner A, Daniel SE, et al. (1997) Oxidative DNA damage in the parkinsonian brain: an apparent selective increase in 8-hydroxyguanine levels in substantia nigra. J Neurochem 69: 1196–1203

Anderson GJ, Frazer DM, McKie AT, Vulpe CD (2002) The ceruloplasmin homolog hephaestin and the control of intestinal iron absorption. Blood Cells Mol Dis 29: 367–375

Arredondo M, Muñoz P, Mura CV, Núñez MT (2003) DMT1, a physiologically relevant apical Cu^{1+} transporter of intestinal cells. Am J Physiol Cell Physiol 284: 1525–1530

Berg D, Grote C, Rausch WD, Maurer M, Wesemann W, Riederer P, Becker G (1999) Iron accumulation in the substantia nigra in rats visualized by ultrasound. Ultrasound Med Biol 25: 901–904

Boka G, Anglade P, Wallach D, Javoy-Agid F, Agid Y, Hirsch EC (1994) Immunocytochemical analysis of tumor necrosis factor and its receptors in Parkinson's disease. Neurosci Lett 172: 151–154

Bouton C, Hirling H, Drapier JC (1997) Redox modulation of iron regulatory proteins by peroxynitrite. J Biol Chem 272: 19969–19975

Breuer W, Greenberg E, Cabantchik ZI (1997) Newly delivered transferrin iron and oxidative cell injury. FEBS Lett 403: 213–219

Connor JR, Boeshore KL, Benkovic SA, Menzies SL (1994) Isoforms of ferritin have a specific cellular distribution in the brain. J Neurosci Res 37: 461–465

Devalia V, Carter K, Walker AP, Perkins SJ, Worwood M, May A, Dooley JS (2002) Autosomal dominant reticuloendothelial iron overload associated with a 3-base pair deletion in the ferroportin 1 gene (SLC11A3). Blood 100: 695–697

Dexter DT, Wells FR, Lees AJ, Agid F, Agid Y, Jenner P, Marsden CD (1989) Increased nigral iron content and alterations in other metal ions occurring in brain in Parkinson's disease. J Neurochem 52: 1830–1836

Dexter DT, Sian J, Rose S, Hindmarsh JG, Mann VM, Cooper JM, Wells FR, Daniel SE, Lees AJ, Schapira AH, et al. (1994) Indices of oxidative stress and mitochondrial function in individuals with incidental Lewy body disease. Ann Neurol 35: 38–44

Double KL, Gerlach M, Youdim MB, Riederer P (2000) Impaired iron homeostasis in Parkinson's disease. J Neural Transm [Suppl 60]: 37–58
Eisenstein RS, Ross KL (2003) Novel roles for iron regulatory proteins in the adaptive response to iron deficiency. J Nutr 133: 1510S–1516S
Epsztejn S, Kakhlon O, Glickstein H, Breuer W, Cabantchik I (1997) Fluorescence analysis of the labile iron pool of mammalian cells. Anal Biochem 248: 31–40
Faucheux BA, Hauw JJ, Agid Y, Hirsch EC (1997) The density of [125I]-transferrin binding sites on perikarya of melanized neurons of the substantia nigra is decreased in Parkinson's disease. Brain Res 749: 170–174
Faucheux BA, Martin ME, Beaumont C, Hunot S, Hauw JJ, Agid Y, Hirsch EC (2002) Lack of up-regulation of ferritin is associated with sustained iron regulatory protein-1 binding activity in the substantia nigra of patients with Parkinson's disease. J Neurochem 83: 320–330
Floor E, Wetzel MG (1997) Increased protein oxidation in human substantia nigra pars compacta in comparison with basal ganglia and prefrontal cortex measured with an improved dinitrophenylhydrazine assay. J Neurochem 70: 268–275
Gerlach M, Ben-Shachar D, Riederer P, Youdim MBH (1994) Altered brain metabolism of iron as a cause of neurodegenerative diseases? J Neurochem 63: 793–807
Good PF, Hsu A, Werner P, Perl DP, Olanow CW (1998) Protein nitration in Parkinson's disease. J Neuropathol Exp Neurol 57: 338–342
Gorell JM, Ordidge RJ, Brown GG, Deniau JC, Buderer NM, Helpern JA (1995) Increased iron-related MRI contrast in the substantia nigra in Parkinson's disease. Neurology 45: 1138–1143
Gotz ME, Double K, Gerlach M, Youdim MB, Riederer P (2004) The relevance of iron in the pathogenesis of Parkinson's disease. Ann NY Acad Sci 1012: 193–208
Grisoli M, Piperno A, Chiapparini L, Mariani R, Savoiardo M (2005) MR imaging of cerebral cortical involvement in aceruloplasminemia. Am J Neuroradiol 26: 657–661
Gunshin H, Mackenzie B, Berger UV, et al. (1997) Cloning and characterization of a proton-coupled mammalian metal ion transporter. Nature 388: 482–488
Guo B, Phillips JD, Yu Y, Leibold EA (1995) Iron regulates the intracellular degradation of iron regulatory protein 2 by the proteasome. J Biol Chem 270: 21645–21651
Gutteridge JM, Halliwell B (2000) Free radicals and antioxidants in the year 2000. A historical look to the future. Ann NY Acad Sci 899: 136–147
Hansen TM, Nielsen H, Bernth N, Moos T (1999) Expression of ferritin protein and subunit mRNAs in normal and iron deficient rat brain. Brain Res Mol Brain Res 65: 186–197
Hanson ES, Foot LM, Leibold EA (1999) Hypoxia post-translationally activates iron-regulatory protein 2. J Biol Chem 274: 5047–5052
Hauptmann N, Cadenas E (1997) The oxygen paradox: Biochemistry of active oxygen. In: Scandalios JG (ed) Oxidative stress and the molecular biology of antioxidant defenses. Cold Spring Harbor Laboratory Press, New York, pp 1–20
He Y, Thong PS, Lee T, Leong SK, Mao BY, Dong F, Watt F (2003) Dopaminergic cell death precedes iron elevation in MPTP-injected monkeys. Free Radic Biol Med 35: 540–547
Hellman NE, Gitlin JD (2002) Ceruloplasmin metabolism and function. Annu Rev Nutr 22: 439–458
Henze C, Earl C, Sautter J, Schmidt N, Themann C, Hartmann A, Oertel WH (2005) Reactive oxidative and nitrogen species in the nigrostriatal system following striatal 6-hydroxydopamine lesion in rats. Brain Res 1052: 97–104
Hill JM, Ruff MR, Weber RJ, Pert CB (1985) Transferrin receptors in rat brain: neuropeptide-like pattern and relationship to iron distribution. Proc Natl Acad Sci USA 82: 4553–4557
Hirsch EC, Brandel JP, Galle P, Javoy-Agid F, Agid Y (1991) Iron and aluminum increase in the substantia nigra of patients with Parkinson's disease: an X-ray microanalysis. J Neurochem 56: 446–451
Hirsch EC, Breidert T, Rousselet E, Hunot S, Hartmann A, Michel PP (2003) The role of glial reaction and inflammation in Parkinson's disease. Ann NY Acad Sci 991: 214–228
Hubert N, Hentze MW (2002) Previously uncharacterized isoforms of divalent metal transporter (DMT)-1: implications for regulation and cellular function. Proc Natl Acad Sci USA 99: 12345–12350
Hunot S, Brugg B, Ricard D, Michel PP, Muriel MP, Ruberg M, Faucheux BA, Agid Y, Hirsch EC (1997) Nuclear translocation of NF-kappaB is increased in dopaminergic neurons of patients with Parkinson disease. Proc Natl Acad Sci USA 94: 7531–7536
Kakhlon O, Cabantchik ZI (2002) The labile iron pool: characterization, measurement, and participation in cellular processes. Free Radic Biol Med 33: 1037–1046
Kaur D, Yantiri F, Rajagopalan S, Kumar J, Mo JQ, Boonplueang R, Viswanath V, Jacobs R, Yang L, Beal MF, DiMonte D, Volitaskis I, Ellerby L, Cherny RA, Bush AI, Andersen JK (2003) Genetic or pharmacological iron chelation prevents MPTP-induced neurotoxicity in vivo: a novel therapy for Parkinson's disease. Neuron 37: 899–909
Kim S, Ponka P (2002) Nitrogen monoxide-mediated control of ferritin synthesis: implications for macrophage iron homeostasis. Proc Natl Acad Sci USA 99: 12214–12219
Kruszewski M (2003) Labile iron pool: the main determinant of cellular response to oxidative stress. Mutat Res 531: 81–92
Latunde-Dada GO, Vulpe CD, Anderson GJ, Simpson RJ, McKie AT (2004) Tissue-specific changes in iron metabolism genes in mice following phenylhydrazine-induced haemolysis. Biochim Biophys Acta 690: 169–176
Ludwiczek S, Aigner E, Theurl I, Weiss G (2003) Cytokine-mediated regulation of iron transport in human monocytic cells. Blood 101: 4148–4154
Martins EA, Robalinho RL, Meneghini R (1995) Oxidative stress induces activation of a cytosolic protein responsible for control of iron uptake. Arch Biochem Biophys 10: 128–134
McKie AT, Marciani P, Rolfs A, Brennan K, Wehr K, Barrow D, Miret S, Bomford A, Peters TJ, Farzaneh F, Hediger MA, Hentze MW, Simpson RJ (2000) A novel duodenal iron-regulated transporter, IREG1, implicated in the basolateral transfer of iron to the circulation. Mol Cell 5: 299–309
McKie AT, Barrow D, Latunde-Dada GO, et al. (2001) An iron-regulated ferric reductase associated with the absorption of dietary iron. Science 291: 1755–1759
McNaught KS, Olanow CW (2005) Protein aggregation in the pathogenesis of familial and sporadic Parkinson's disease. Neurobiol: Epub ahead of print
Mehlhase J, Sandig G, Pantopoulos K, Grune T (2005) Oxidation-induced ferritin turnover in microglial cells: role of proteasome. Free Radic Biol Med 38: 276–285
Miyajima H, Takahashi Y, Kono S (2003) Aceruloplasminemia, an inherited disorder of iron metabolism. Biometals 16: 205–213
Mogi M, Togari A, Tanaka K, Ogawa N, Ichinose H, Nagatsu T (1999) Increase in level of tumor necrosis factor (TNF)-alpha in 6-hydroxydopamine-lesioned striatum in rats without influence of systemic L-DOPA on the TNF-alpha induction. Neurosci Lett 268: 101–104
Nanami M, Ookawara T, Otaki Y, Ito K, Moriguchi R, Miyagawa K, Hasuike Y, Izumi M, Eguchi H, Suzuki K, Nakanishi T (2005) Tumor necrosis factor-alpha-induced iron sequestration and oxidative stress in human endothelial cells. Arterioscler Thromb Vasc Biol 25: 2495–2501
Núñez MT, Gaete V, Watkins JA, Glass J (1990) Mobilization of iron from endocytic vesicles: the effect of acidification and reduction. J Biol Chem 265: 6688–6692
Núñez MT, Gallardo V, Múñoz P, Tapia V, Esparza A, Salazar J, Speisky H (2004) Progressive iron accumulation induces a biphasic change in the glutathione content of neuroblastoma cells. Free Radic Biol Med 37: 953–960

Núñez-Millacura C, Tapia V, Muñoz P, Maccioni RB, Núñez MT (2002) An oxidative stress-mediated positive-feedback iron uptake loop in neuronal cells. J Neurochem 82: 240–248

Paradkar PN, Roth JA (2005) Post-translational and transcriptional regulation of DMT1 during P19 embryonic carcinoma cell differentiation by retinoic acid. Biochem J: Epub ahead of print

Patel BN, David S (1997) A novel glycophosphatidylinositol-anchored form of ceruloplasmin is expressed by mammalian astrocytes. J Biol Chem 272: 20185–20190

Perry G, Taddeo MA, Petersen RB, Castellani RJ, Harris PLR, Siedlak SL, Cash AD, Liu Q, Nunomura A, Atwood CS, Smith MA (2003) Adventiously-bound redox active iron and copper are at the center of oxidative damage in Alzheimer disease. Biometals 16: 77–81

Petrat F, de Groot H, Sustmann R, Rauen U (2002) The chelatable iron pool in living cells: a methodically defined quantity. Biol Chem 383: 489–502

Reiber H, Ruff M, Uhr M (1993) Ascorbate concentration in human cerebrospinal fluid (CSF) and serum. Intrathecal accumulation and CSF flow rate. Clin Chim Acta 217: 163–173

Riederer P, Sofic E, Rausch WD, Schmidt B, Reynolds GP, Jellinger K, Youdim MB (1989) Transition metals, ferritin, glutathione, and ascorbic acid in parkinsonian brains. J Neurochem 52: 515–520

Sayre LM, Perry G, Atwood CS, Smith MA (2000) The role of metals in neurodegenerative diseases. Cell Mol Biol 46: 731–741

Schalinske KL, Eisenstein RS (1996) Phosphorylation and activation of both iron regulatory proteins 1 and 2 in HL-60 cells. J Biol Chem 271: 7168–7176

Shoham S, Youdim MB (2002) The effects of iron deficiency and iron and zinc supplementation on rat hippocampus ferritin. J Neural Transm 109: 1241–1256

Sofic E, Riederer P, Heinsen H, Beckmann H, Reynolds GP, Hebenstreit G, Youdim MB (1988) Increased iron (III) and total iron content in post mortem substantia nigra of parkinsonian brain. J Neural Transm 74: 199–205

Symons MCR, Gutteridge JMC eds (1998) Free radicals and iron: chemistry, biology and medicine. Oxford University Press, New York

Wang X, Garrick MD, Yang F, Dailey LA, Piantadosi CA, Ghio AJ (2005) TNF, IFN-gamma, and endotoxin increase expression of DMT1 in bronchial epithelial cells. Am J Physiol Lung Cell Mol Physiol 289: L24–L33

Williams J, Moreton K (1980) The distribution of iron between the metal-binding sites of transferrin human serum. Biochem J 185: 483–488

Wu LJ, Leenders AG, Cooperman S, Meyron-Holtz E, Smith S, Land W, Tsai RY, Berger UV, Sheng ZH, Rouault TA (2004) Expression of the iron transporter ferroportin in synaptic vesicles and the blood–brain barrier. Brain Res 1001: 108–117

Yang F, Haile DJ, Wang X, Dailey LA, Stonehuerner JG, Ghio AJ (2005) Apical location of ferroportin 1 in airway epithelia and its role in iron detoxification in the lung. Am J Physiol Lung Cell Mol Physiol 289: L14–L23

Youdim MB, Riederer P (1993) The role of iron in senescence of dopaminergic neurons in Parkinson's disease. J Neural Transm [Suppl 40]: 57–67

Youdim MB, Stephenson G, Ben Shachar D (2004) Ironing iron out in Parkinson's disease and other neurodegenerative diseases with iron chelators: a lesson from 6-hydroxydopamine and iron chelators, desferal and VK-28. Ann NY Acad Sci 1012: 306–325

Youdim MB, Fridkin M, Zheng H (2005) Bifunctional drug derivatives of MAO-B inhibitor rasagiline and iron chelator VK-28 as a more effective approach to treatment of brain ageing and ageing neurodegenerative diseases. Mech Ageing Dev 126: 317–326

J Neural Transm (2006) [Suppl] 71: 215–227

Journal of Neural Transmission
Printed in Austria

Cerebral oligemia and iron influence in cerebral structures – element of Morbus Parkinson Models?

T. A. Sontag[1,2,3], **C. Heim** (†), **W. Kolasiewicz**[1,4], **J. Horn**[1,5], **I. Pardowitz**[1,5], **K. H. Sontag**[1,2]

[1] Max-Planck-Institut Experimentelle Medizin, Göttingen, Germany
[2] Veterinary-Biological Laboratory, Veterinary Clinic, Northeim, Germany
[3] Institute of Psychology, University of Regensburg, Regensburg, Germany
[4] Polish Academy of Sciences, Institute of Pharmacology, Krakow, Poland
[5] COGITAT R.N.5, Cognitron GmbH, Göttingen, Germany

Summary The consequences of short phases of restricted cerebral blood flow and iron enrichment of striatal tissues resulted in an animal model that could correspond to the basic features of a model for Parkinson's disease. An automatic and computerized hole-board offers simultaneous data on learning and cognitive memory capabilities, learning of distinct patterns of distributed food pellets found and eaten in a given time, switches between different locations of food in the holes and in different layout patterns. Wistar rats after 60 min of bilateral clamping of the carotid arteries (BCCA) under pentobarbital anesthesia received 1.5 μg $FeCl_3$ injected one week after BCCA unilaterally into the ventrolateral striatum. The experiments showed that reduced cerebral blood flow and increased iron within the striatal tissue had the effect of retarding reactions. Rats after BCCA and iron need 180 s to find pellets deep inside holes that are distributed in a distinct pattern. During only 60 or 30 s BCCA plus iron rats are no longer able to find the same number of pellets as over 180 s. Rats after BCCA plus NaCl do not show such reduced success. These results point to the idea that cerebral oligemia and increased iron in the striatum stimulate the pathological symptoms of Parkinson's disease which need also more time to have reaction and success (see Fig. 5).The data covering abbreviated time-spans show how heavily the BCCA + Fe animals are dependent on longer times.

Introduction

We began a thorough analysis of the capabilities of rats which had received a temporally-limited cerebral shortage of oxygen and cerebral dopamine, a procedure chosen on the basis of the established manifold roles of the neurotransmitter dopamine and of oxygen. Human beings as well and animals need a definite amount of time for perception, decision-making and motor activity. The question then arose whether the model of Parkinson's disease we had developed could reproduce circumstances which are not only significant in themselves but also indicate that definite time periods are required in order to successfully achieve a particular object.

The studies of Jellinger and co-workers (1990) were the first to recognize and demonstrate the cellular localisation of increased iron as well as ferritin levels in parkinsonian substantia nigra. Transient ischemia in rats leads to selective neuronal damage in discrete brain regions such as the CA1 pyramidal cells in the hippocampus and the small-to-medium sized neurons in the striatum (Ginsberg et al., 1985; Pulsinelli et al., 1982). The present work is concerned with the question whether phases of cerebral oligemia have an effect on animals with raised cerebral striatal iron levels. It turned out that rats, following iron supplementation in their ventro-striatal lateral tissue and after additional one-hour occlusion of the carotid arteries, were able to find and to eat hidden pellets over periods of 180 s than animals that had received the same toxic combination of treatment but were tested over a period of 60 or 30 s. However it seemed improbable to us that iron supplementation and phases of oligemia would at the same time have a beneficial effect. We therefore looked for the underlying reasons.

The lack of qualified models was also expressed on the occasion of the 16th International Congress on Parkinson disease and relayed disorders in Berlin by the president of the congress 2005.

The animal models

Rats who underwent a bilateral clamping of carotid arteries (BCCA) plus intrastriatal iron (+Fe), (BCCA + Fe) and

Correspondence: Prof. Dr. K.-H. Sontag, Max Planck Institute for Experimental Medicine, Hermann Rein Strasse 3, 37075 Göttingen, Germany
e-mail: thomas-alexander.sontag@psychologie.uni-regensburg.de

BCCA + buffer, sham + buffer and sham + Fe were tested in the study on a special automatic working hole board system (Heim et al., 2000). The system accumulates all movements and inspections of holes synchronously, filled and not filled with one food pellet, distributed in a definite order. The activities of the animals' spontaneous behaviour are reduced in time sequences of 180 s, 60 s and 30 s. The question whether the used model may indicate some of the early symptoms which characterize Morbus Parkinson is open for discussion.

The influenes of oxygen deficiencies and dopamine lost in the cerebral structures

The striatum and the hippocampus are most vulnerable to oxygen deficiencies (Smith et al., 1984). The striatum is suggested to be responsible for motor performance (Devan and White, 1999; Cools, 1980). Increased levels of dopamin and acethylcholin in the hippocampus are necessary during learning processes. The hippocampus is also importantly involved in processing informations essential to recognition memory (Wittmann et al., 2005). During oxygen deficiencies in the striatum an immediately dopamine release occurred, whereas glutamate and aspartate increased more in the latter perfusion phase (Heim et al., 2000). During bilateral clamping of both carotid arteries (BCCA) in anasthesia the hippocampus and the striatum release glutamate, aspartate and gamma-aminobutyric acid (GABA), followed by hydroxyl free radicals, measured as 2,3-dihydroxybenzoic (2,3-DHBA) (Heim et al., 2000). The hippocampus receives dopaminergic innervations by the ventral tegmental area (VTA), the rubral area (RA) and the substantia nigra (SN) (Scatton, 1980).

Episodes of BCCA initiate lipid peroxidation in the cortex (CRT) and also in the striatum (Melsacka et al., 1994), as well as after BCCA alone and more intensive after BCCA + Fe in the hippocampus, too (Heim et al., 1995).

Defects of the ventrolateral striatum neurones stimulate incorrect substantia nigra pars compacta neurones and dentrites of the pars reticulata ipsilaterally and affected retrorubral area dopaminergic fibres ipsilateral and contralaterally in the striatum and contralateral acting substantia nigra afferents (see Heim et al., 2002).

The VTA and the SN project also to the HPC with a predominance of dopaminergic fibres at the temporal pole and to the caudal and also to the ventral part of the HPC (Verny et al., 1985), which was considered as a part of an interface between limbic and central motor mechanisms (Nauta, 1982).

It is known that the loss of dopamine unilaterally in the ventrolateral striatum leads to a loss of dopamine in the ipsilateral neurones of the substantia nigra compacta, as well as a loss of dendrites in the pars reticulata, loss of neurones in the VTA and in the RA ipsilaterally and contralaterally in the striatum, which should belong to the contralaterally-acting substantia nigra afferents (see Heim et al., 2002). Dopaminergic A9 fibres in the striatum reduce the organisms ability arbitrarily to switch cerebral programmes, whereas a dopamine deficit in the terminal region of dopaminergic A10 fibres in the striatum reduces the organism's ability to switch cerebral programmes (Cools et al., 1980).

Among other effects, the impairment of the performance by the BCCA + Fe treated animals was also referable back to the loss of sufficient dopamine directing activities in the hippocampus. Dopaminergic afferents to the hippocampal formation originate from the A10 and A9 dopaminergic cell groups (Scatton et al., 1980).

Morris et al. (2003) argue that synaptic plasticity is a critical component of the neural mechanisms underlying learning and memory. Morris and colleagues argue that synaptic plasticity would be critical for the encoding and intermediate storage of memory traces that are automatically recorded in the hippocampus.

Methods

In these studies the rats were subjected to a neurotoxically-affecting restriation of cerebral blood flow by clamping of both carotid arteries under anesthesia for one hour together with increased intrastriatal $FeCl_3$, and examined on week later as the earliest. We analysed the animals' behaviour in different environments and during new tasks. The animals were given the opportunity to find food pellets distributed in deep holes in a specially designed hole-board (see Heim et al., 2000).

We used the COGITAT system (Heim et al., 2000). This system records all movements of the experimental animals at fixed times (see Table 1). The system permits detailed and automatic recording of the cognitive and motor behaviour of each animal during the time it is on the board in given time periods. In this study we present 9 out of the 25 parameters measured (Heim et al., 2000).

Pathophysiological data of the model

1. BCCA (bilateral clamping of carotid area) of rats for 60 minutes in pentobarbital anesthesia lead to reduction of cerebral blood flow to oligemic levels. During such experiments the local cerebral blood flow in cortical, hippocampal and striatal tissues did not fall to values lower than to 16 ± 4, 23 ± 6 and 18 ± 8 ml/100 g/min, respectively (see Block et al., 1993).
2. BCCA increased the amount of lipid peroxidation in cortical, striatal (see Melzacka et al., 1994) and hippocampal tissues (Heim et al., Suppl. 1995).

Table 1.

– **1) INSPECTIONS NON-BAITED HOLES** learning **pattern A**, n interruption upper beam
180 s ANOVA
F(3,38) = 5.52, p = 0.0010; BCCA + Fe vs. sham + buffer, sham + Fe;
Gabriel's test for variable: DIST Comparison significant at the 0.05 level are indicated by***
BCCA + Fe; BCCA + buffer; sham + Fe; sham + buffer
180 s BCCA + Fe vs. sham + Fe; BCCA + Fe vs. sham + buffer***

60 s ANOVA
F(3,38) = 7.00, p = 0.0002; BCCA + buffer vs. sham + buffer, sham + Fe, BCCA + buffer ANOVA
Gabriel's test for variable: DIST Comparison significant at the 0.05 level are indicated by***
BCCA + Fe; BCCA + buffer; sham + Fe; sham + buffer
60 s BCCA + buffer vs. BCCA + Fe; BCCA + buffer vs. sham + buffer; BCCA + buffer vs. sham + Fe***

30 s ANOVA
F(3,38) = 30.78, p = 0.0001; BCCA + buffer vs. sham + buffer, sham + Fe, BCCA + Fe ANOVA
Gabriel's test for variable: DIST Comparison significant at the 0.05 level are indicated by***
BCCA – Fe; BCCA + buffer; sham + Fe; sham + buffer
30 s BCCA + buffer vs. BCCA + Fe; BCCA + Fe vs. sham + buffer; BCCA + buffer vs. sham + Fe***

INSPECTIONS NON BAITED HOLES learning **pattern B**, n interruption upper beam
F(3,38) = 9.44, p = 0.0001; BCCA + buffer vs. sham + buffer, sham + Fe; ANOVA
Gabriel's test for variable: DIST Comparison significant at the 0.05 level are indicated by***
BCCA – Fe; BCCA + buffer; sham + Fe; sham + buffer
BCCA + buffer vs. BCCA + Fe; BCCA + buffer vs. sham + Fe; BCCA + buffer vs. sham + buffer***

– **2) INSPECTIONS OF BAITED HOLES** learning **pattern A** n interruption upper beam
180 s ANOVA
n.s.
Gabriel's test for variable: DIST Comparison significant at the 0.05 level are indicated by***
n.s.

60 s ANOVA
n.s.
Gabriel's test for variable: DIST Comparison significant at the 0.05 level are indicated by***
n.s.

30 s ANOVA
F(3,38) = 11.39, p = 0.0001; BCCA + Fe vs. sham + buffer, sham + Fe;
Gabriel's test for variable: DIST Comparison significant at the 0.05 level are indicated by***
BCCA + Fe; BCCA + buffer, sham + Fe, sham + buffer
30 s BCCA + buffer vs. sham + buffer; BCCA + buffer vs. sham + Fe; BCCA + Fe vs. sham + Fe***

INSPECTIONS OF BAITED HOLES pattern B learning n interruption ANOVA
Gabriel's test for variable: DIST Comparison significant at the 0.05 level are indicated by***
BCCA + buffer vs. sham + buffer; BCCA + buffer vs. BCCA + Fe***

– **3) LOWER BEAM pattern A** learning, n of interruption
180 s ANOVA
F(3,38) = 6.72, p = 0.0002; BCCA + Fe vs. sham + buffer, BCCA + buffer;
Gabriel's test for variable: DIST Comparison significant at the 0.05 level are indicated by ***
BCCA + Fe; BCCA + buffer; sham + Fe; sham + buffer
180 s BCCA + Fe vs. sham + buffer; BCCA + Fe vs. BCCA + buffer***

60 s n.s. ANOVA
Gabriel's test for variable: DIST Comparison significant at the 0.05 level are indicated by***
BCCA + Fe; BCCA + buffer; sham + Fe; sham + buffer
60 s n.s.

30 s n.s. **ANOVA**
Gabriel's test for variable: DIST Comparison significant at the 0.05 level are indicated by ***
BCCA + Fe; BCCA + buffer; sham + Fe; sham + buffer
30 s BCCA + Fe vs. sham + Fe ***

LOWER BEAM pattern B learning, n of interruptions ANOVA
n.s.
Gabriel's test for variable: DIST Comparisons significant at the 0.05 level are indicated by ***
n.s.

(*continued*)

Table 1 (*continued*)

– 4) UPPER BEAM pattern A learning, n of interruption
180 s ANOVA
F(3,38) = 6.52, p = 0.0003; BCCA + Fe vs. sham + buffer, BCCA + buffer, sham + Fe;
Gabriel's test for variable: DIST Comparisons significant at the 0.05 level are indicated by***
BCCA + Fe; BCCA + buffer; sham + Fe; sham + buffer
180 s BCCA + Fe vs. sham + buffer, BCCA + Fe vs. BCCA + buffer, BCCA + Fe vs. sham + Fe***

60 s ANOVA
F(3,38) = 4.41, p = 0.0048; BCCA + buffer vs. sham + Fe;
Gabriel's test for variable: DIST Comparisons significant at the 0.05 level are indicated by***,
BCCA + Fe; BCCA + buffer; sham + Fe; sham + buffer
60 s BCCA + buffer vs. sham + Fe***

30 s ANOVA
F(3,38) = 26,68, p = 0.0001; BCCA + learning vs. sham + buffer, sham + Fe; BCCA + Fe vs. sham + Fe;
Gabriel's test for variable: DIST Comparisons significant at the 0.05 level are indicated by***,
BCCA + Fe; BCCA + buffer; sham + Fe; sham + buffer
30 s BCCA + buffer vs. BCCA + Fe, sham + buffer, sham + Fe; BCCA vs. sham + Fe***

UPPER BEAM pattern B learning, n of interruptions ANOVA
F(3,38) = 6.94, p = 0.0001; BCCA + buffer vs. sham + buffer, sham + Fe, BCCA + Fe;
Gabriel's test for variable: DIST Comparisons significant at the 0.05 level are indicated by***
BCCA + buffer vs. sham + buffer, BCCA + sham + Fe***

– 5) INSPECTIONS learning **pattern A** n interruption upper beam
180 s ANOVA
F(3,38) = 3.34, p = 0.0196; BCCA + Fe vs. sham + buffer;
Gabriel's test for variable: DIST Comparison significant at the 0.05 level are indicated by***
BCCA + Fe; BCCA + buffer, sham + Fe, sham + buffer
180 s BCCA + Fe vs. sham + buffer***

60 s ANOVA
F(3,38) = 6.10, p = 0.0005; BCCA + buffer vs. sham + buffer, sham + Fe, BCCA + buffer;
Gabriel's test for variable: DIST Comparison significant at the 0.05 level are indicated by***
BCCA + Fe; BCCA + buffer, sham + Fe, sham + buffer
60 s BCCA + buffer vs. BCCA + Fe, BCCA + buffer vs. sham + buffer; BCCA + sham + Fe***

30 s ANOVA
F(3,38) = 32.38, p = 0.0001; BCCA + buffer vs. sham + buffer, sham + Fe, BCCA + Fe; BCCA + Fe vs. sham + Fe;
Gabriel's test for variable: DIST Comparison significant at the 0.05 level are indicated by***
BCCA + Fe; BCCA + buffer, sham + Fe, sham + buffer
30 s BCCA + buffer vs. BCCA + Fe, BCCA + buffer vs. sham + buffer, BCCA + buffer vs. sham + Fe***

INSPECTIONS pattern B learning, n of interruptions ANOVA
F(3,38) = 10.19, p = 0.0001; BCCA + buffer vs. sham + buffer, sham + Fe, BCCA + Fe; ANOVA
Gabriel's test for variable: DIST Comparison significant at the 0.05 level are indicated by***
BCCA + buffer vs. BCCA + Fe; BCCA + buffer vs. sham + Fe, BCCA + buffer vs. sham + buffer***

– 6) REFERENCE MEMORY ERRORS TOTAL, learning **pattern A**
180 s ANOVA
F(3.38) = 8.09, p = 0.0001; BCCA + buffer vs. sham + buffer, sham + Fe; BCCA + Fe vs. sham + buffer, sham + Fe;
Gabriels's test for variable: DIST Comparison significant at the 0.05 level are indicated by***
BCCA + Fe; BCCA + buffer; sham + Fe; sham + buffer
BCCA + buffer vs. sham + Fe; BCCA + buffer vs. sham + buffer; BCCA + Fe vs. sham + Fe, BCCA + buffer vs. sham + buffer***

60 s ANOVA
Fe(3,38) = 3.36, p = 0.0001; BCCA + buffer vs. sham + buffer, sham + Fe, BCCA + Fe;
Gabriel's test for variable: DIST Comprarison significant at the 0.05 level are indicated by***
BCCA + Fe; BCCA + buffer; sham + Fe; sham + buffer
BCCA + buffer vs. BCCA + Fe; BCCA + buffer vs. sham + buffer; BCCA + buffer vs. sham + Fe***

30 s ANOVA
F(3,38) = 16.67, p = 0.0001; BCCA + buffer vs. sham + buffer, sham + Fe, BCCA + buffer;
Gabriels'test for variable: DIST Comparison significant at the 0.05 level are indicated by***
BCCA + Fe; BCCA + buffer; sham + Fe; sham + buffer
BCCA + buffer vs. BCCA + Fe; BCCA + buffer vs. sham + buffer; BCCA + vuffer vs. sham + Fe***

(*continued*)

Table 1 (*continued*)

REFERENCE MEMORY ERRORS TOTAL, learning **pattern B**
180 s
n.s.
Gabriels'test for variable: DIST Comparison significant at the 0.05 level are indicated by***
BCCA + Fe; BCCA + buffer; sham + Fe; sham + buffer
n.s.

– 7) WORKING MEMORY ERRORS TOTAL (LOWER AND UPPER BEAM, learning **pattern A**
180 s ANOVA
$F(3,38) = 4.88$, $p = 0.0025$; BCCA + buffer vs. BCCA + Fe; sham + Fe
Gabriel's test for variable: DIST Comparison significant at the 0.05 level are indicated by***
BCCA – Fe; BCCA + buffer; sham + Fe; sham + buffer
BCCA – Fe vs. BCCA + buffer; sham + Fe vs. BCCA + buffer***

60 s ANOVA
n.s.
Gabriel's test for variable: DIST Comparison significant at the 0.05 level are indicated by***
BCCA – Fe; BCCA + buffer; sham + Fe; sham + buffer
n.s.

30 s ANOVA
$F(3,38) = 4.82$, $p = 0.0026$; BCCA + buffer vs. sham + buffer, sham + Fe
Gabriel's test for variable: DIST Comparison significant at the 0.05 level are indicated by***
BCCA + Fe; BCCA + buffer; sham + Fe; sham + buffer
BCCA + buffer vs. sham + buffer; BCCA + buffer vs. sham + Fe***

WORKING MEMORY ERRORS TOTAL (LOWER AND UPPER BEAM, learning **pattern B**
n.s. ANOVA
Gabriel's test for variable: DIST Comparison significant at the 0.05 level are indicated by***
BCCA + Fe; BCCA + buffer; sham + Fe; sham + buffer
BCCA + buffer vs. sham + buffer; BCCA + buffer vs. sham + Fe
n.s.

– 8) REINSPECTION BAITED AND/OR UNBAITED HOLES learning **pattern A**
180 s ANOVA
$F(3,38) = 3.04$, $p = 0.0293$; BCCA + Fe vs. sham + buffer;
Gabriel's test for variable: DIST Comparison significant at the 0.05 level are indicated by ***
BCCA + Fe; BCCA + buffer; sham + Fe; sham + buffer
180 s BCCA + Fe vs. sham + buffer***

60 s ANOVA
$F(3,38) = 3.88$, $p = 0.0098$; BCCA + buffer vs. sham + Fe;
Gabriel's test for variable: DIST Comparison significant at the 0.05 level are indicated by ***
BCCA + Fe; BCCA + buffer; sham + Fe; sham + buffer
60 s BCCA + buffer vs. sham + Fe***

30 s ANOVA
$F(3,38) = 11{,}28$, $p = 0.0001$; BCCA + buffer vs. sham + buffer, sham + Fe; ANOVA
Gabriel's test for variable: DIST Comparison significant at the 0.05 level are indicated by***
BCCA + Fe; BCCA + buffer; sham + Fe; sham + buffer
30 s BCCA + buffer vs. sham + buffer; BCCA + buffer vs. sham + Fe; BCCA + Fe vs. sham + Fe***

REINSPECTION BAITED AND/OR UNBAITED HOLES learning **pattern B**, n interruption upper beam
180 s ANOVA
$F(3,38) = 4.50$; $p = 0.0040$; BCCA + buffer vs. sham + buffer, BCCA + Fe; ANOVA
Gabriel's test for variable: DIST Comparison significant at the 0.05 level are indicated by***
BCCA + Fe; BCCA + buffer; sham + Fe; sham + buffer
BCCA + buffer vs. sham + buffer***

– 9) SERIAL COLLECTION learning **pattern A**
180 s ANOVA
$F(3,38) = 3.83$, $p = 0.0101$; BCCA + buffer vs. sham + buffer;
Gabriel's test for variable: DIST Comparison significant at the 0.05 level are indicated by***
BCCA + Fe; BCCA + buffer; sham + Fe; sham + buffer
sham + buffer vs. BCCA + buffer***

(*continued*)

Table 1 (*continued*)

60 s ANOVA
F(3,38) = 6.57, p = 0.0003; BCCA + buffer vs. sham + buffer, sham + Fe, BCCA + Fe;
Gabriel's test for variable: DIST Comparison significant at the 0.05 level are indicated by***
BCCA + Fe; BCCA + buffer; sham + Fe; sham + buffer
sham + buffer vs. BCCA + buffer; sham + Fe vs. BCCA + buffer; BCCA + Fe vs. BCCA + buffer***

30 s ANOVA
F(3,38) = 11.80, p = 0.0001; BCCA + buffer vs. sham + buffer, sham + Fe, BCCA + Fe;
Gabriel's test for variable: DIST Comparison significant at the 0.05 level are indicated by***
BCCA + Fe; BCCA + buffer; sham + Fe; sham + buffer
sham + buffer vs. BCCA + buffer; sham + Fe vs. BCCA + buffer; BCCA + Fe vs. BCCA + buffer***

SERIAL COLLECTION learning **pattern B**
n.s. ANOVA
Gabriel's test for variable: DIST Comparison significant at the 0.05 level are indicated by***
BCCA + Fe; BCCA + buffer; sham + Fe; sham + buffer
n.s.

3. In contrast to the changes consequent on ischemic conditions, staining for light microscopy failed to show overt cell damage in these and other vulnerable brain structures in the rats used in this study (Melzacka et al., 1994; Heim and Sontag, 1994).
4. During long-term survival following surgery, in situ hybridisation showed decreased D1 dopa receptor mRNAs in the dorsal striatum compared with the sham-operated controls as late as 19 months after surgery (Heim et al., 1999).
5. Physiological variables of rats under pentobarbital anaesthesia prior to BCCA showed a pH of 7.368 ± 0.0012 and 55 min during BCCA a pH value of 7.393 ± 0.025. The pO2 blood pressure indicated 67.5 ± 1.7 in the beginning and values of 79.9 ± 6.9 partial blood pressure after 55 min (see Block et al., 1993a).
6. The local temperature in striatum, hippocampus and frontal cortex decreased during BCCA by two degrees. In such rats the arterial blood flow in hippocampus and striatum is not lower than 23 ± 6 or 18 ± 8 ml/100 g.min respectively (Block et al., 1993b). BCCA episodes initiate in striatal dialysates a significant increase of released dopamine and at the end of the BCCA phase a significant increase of DOPAC, HVA, glutamate, aspartate, 2,3-DHBA and GABA (Heim et al., 2000).

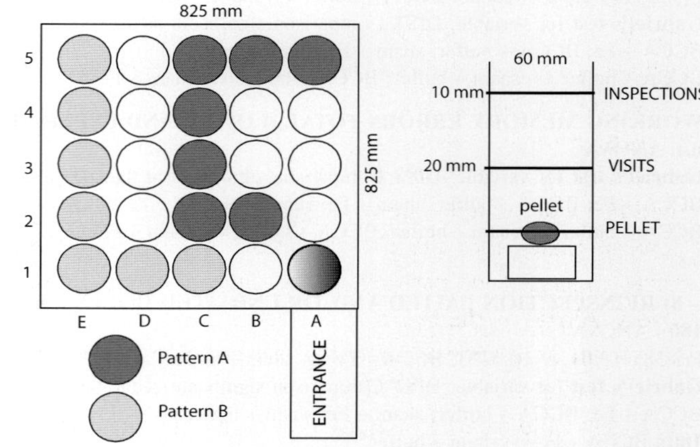

Fig. 1. The COGITRON – System. The hole-board with the pattern for 8 distributed pellets (pattern A, black circles or gray circles pattern B) and the sectional drawing of the holes with the positions of the infrared beams

The test procedure

The automatic hole-board system (COGITAT*) (Heim et al., 2000) makes it possible to measure a variety of parameters associated with learning, memory, re-learning, cognition, and cognitive shifts, inclusive exploratory and sensorimotor performance (Table 1). The surrounding board with transparent Plexiglas had 25 holes (Fig. 1) each consisting of a cylindric tube which is closed off at its lower end by an adjustable feeding plate. The porous base-plate of the system, which the animals cannot see, is covered with the identical food pellets, so that the smell of food is evenly distributed, which prevents the animals from following a path on the basis of olfactory tracking. For a run, 8 out of all the cylinders are baited with one pellet. During a time-limited experimental phase the animals are provided with the opportunity of finding and eating the food pellets. At the same time, however, they also have the opportunity of recognising as well as noting the pattern

*COGITAT R.N.5, Cognitron GmbH, P.O.B. 2121, 37011 Göttingen, Germany.

in which the pellets are presented. The animals should be placed on starvation rations which should cause a weight reduction of not more than circa 10–15%. The system records activities by a set of infrared beams which are situated at different levels in transparent tubes mounted within the holes of the opportunity to find food pellets distributed in deep holes in a specially designed hole-board (see Heim et al., 2000).

We used the COGITAT system (Heim et al., 2000). This system records all movements of the experimental animals at fixed times (see Table 1). The system permits detailed and automatic recording of the cognitive and motor behaviour of each animal during the time it is on the board in given time periods. In this study we present 9 out of the 25 parameters measured.

The software used inter alia also includes a graphical interface to analyse and display information about inspected holes on the surface of the plate.

Before entering the hole-board, the animals remain in their home cage for adaptation to the laboratory for 1 hour and receive some of their daily ration (!). The animals are then tested in a random manner. Eight of the holes are baited in a manner not visible to the animals while walking.

The animals learn the pattern during exploration over several sessions (one per day), using their own individual strategy. A trial on the board is finished either when a fixed time is over or as soon as an animal has collected and eaten all of 8 pellets. Animals with a good knowledge of the pattern are able to collect eight pellets within an average time of 20 sec. As soon as every animal of the corresponding control group had found all of the pellets, the time was switched from 180 to 60 s and later on to 30 s per trial in following period by gradual stages in following days. The learning process was regarded as complete when all of the control animals had succeeded in the collection of all eight pellets during the allotted time period of 30 seconds. Each rat has only one run per day (more information see Heim et al., 2000).

The data obtained in this way allowed evaluation of the individual animals'search-strategies and their learning and memory capabilities.

9 from 23 test parameters (see also the complete Table 1)

(1) Inspections non baited holes. The number of unbaited holes inspected by interruption of the upper beam.
(2) Inspections baited holes. The number of baited holes inspected by interruption of the upper beam.
(3) Lower beam: the interruption of the lower beam.
(4) Upper beam: the number of unbaited holes inspected by interruption of the upper beam.
(5) Inspections: the number of holes inspected by interruption of the upper beam.
(6) Reference memory total (visits and inspections): the percentage of the sum of inspections and visits to unbaited holes in relation to the total number of holes inspected and visited.
(7) Working memory errors, total (lower and upper beam), the percentage of the sum of inspections and visits to previously baited holes in relation to the total number of holes inspected and visits.
(8) Reinspections baited and/or unbaited holes. Inspections of the upper beam.
(9) Serial collection. The number of holes that were baited with pellets that are emptied in a serial order without intermediate inspections or visits in other holes than those in the pattern.

Results

Inspections non baited holes, learning pattern A

During 9 days with one run per day during 180 s BCCA + Fe rats showed the most interruptions of upper beams (Fig. 2). But more interruption of the upper beams during 60 s and 30 s of BCCA + Fe could not be observed. Now the BCCA + buffer rats indicate the most number of interruptions of upper beams (Fig. 2). With learning pattern B also the BCCA + buffer rats showed cognitive capacities (Fig. 2) (ANOVA and Gabriel's test).

BCCA + Fe treated rats found and eath distinct amount pellets only during 180 s and not during 60 or 30 s (Heim et al., 2002) that indicate that such rats need longer times to initiate movements, ideas and/or developable, which can not be seen after BCCA plus iron in the substantia nigra (bcfeSN); see also Figs. 2–4.

BCCA + Fe rats require 180 s to search for pellets on the hole-board successfully (But during a 9-day period BCCA + Fe treated rats found and ate the first pellets on day 4, and 3–4 pellets on day 6, and on day 9, the (last of the test series), only 6–7 pellets out of the 8 distributed (see Fig. 5). (A group of BCCA + Fe rats injected with the same concentration of Fe into the substantia nigra was much quicker in finding and eating pellets distributed in the same pattern, not shown here). It is thus of decisive significance which time interval is allowed to the animals when the animals are obliged to employ their cognitive system. When this is not taken into account one has to discard unusable data. For this reason arbitrary time spans in test-

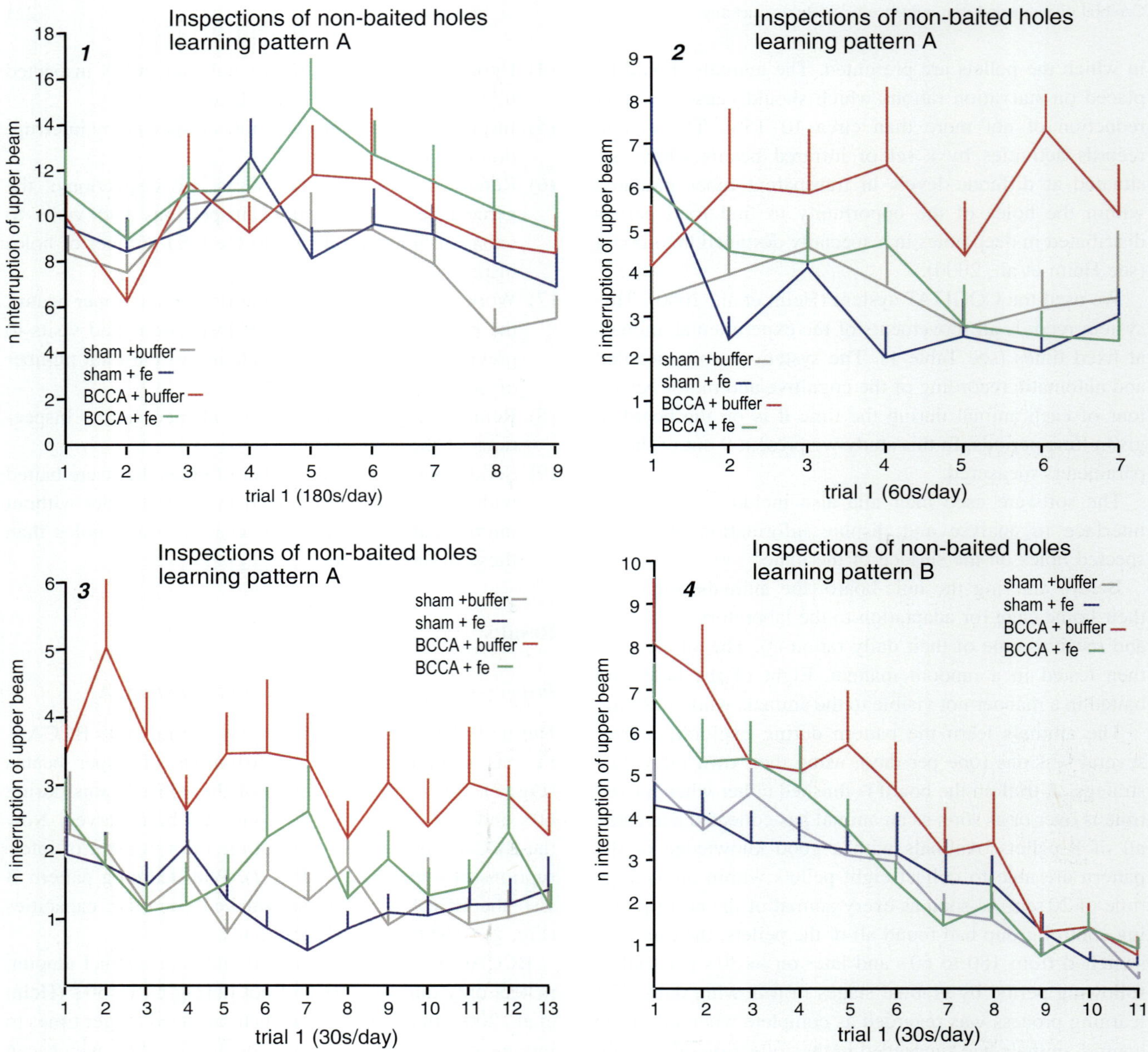

Fig. 2. INSPECTIONS NON-BAITED HOLES learning pattern A, and B n interruption upper beam
180 s
F(3,38) = 5.52, p = 0.0010; BCCA + Fe vs. sham + buffer, sham + Fe; ANOVA
Gabriel's test far variable: DIST Comparison significant at the 0.05 level are indicated by***
BCCA + Fe; BCCA + buffer; sham + Fe; sham + buffer
80 s BCCA + Fe vs. sham + Fe; BCCA + Fe vs. sham + buffer***
60 s F(3,38) = 7.00, p = 0.002; BCCA + buffer vs. sham buffer, sham + Fe, BCCA + buffer ANOVA
Gabriel's test for variable: DIST Comparison significant at the 0.05 level are indicated by ***
BCCA + Fe; BCCA + buffer; sham + Fe; sham + buffer
60 s BCCA + buffer vs. BCCA + Fe; BCCA + buffer vs. sham + buffer; BCCA + buffer vs. sham + Fe***
30 s F(3,38) = 30.78, p = 0.0001; BCCA + buffer vs. sham + buffer, sham + Fe, BCCA + Fe ANOVA
Gabriel's test for variable: DIST Comparison significant at the 0.05 level are indicated by***
BCCA + Fe; BCCA + buffer; sham + Fe; sham + buffer
30 s BCCA + buffer vs. BCCA + Fe; BCCA + Fe vs. sham + buffer; BCCA + buffer vs. sham + Fe***

INSPECTIONS NON BAITED HOLES learning pattern B, n interruption upper beam
F(3,38) = 9.44, p = 0.0001; BCCA + buffer vs. sham + buffer, sham + Fe; ANOVA
Gabriel's test for variable: DIST Comparison significant at the 0.05 level are indicated by***
BCCA + Fe; BCCA + buffer; sham + Fe; sham + buffer
BCCA + buffer vs. BCCA + Fe; BCCA + buffer vs. sham + Fe; BCCA + buffer vs. sham + buffer***

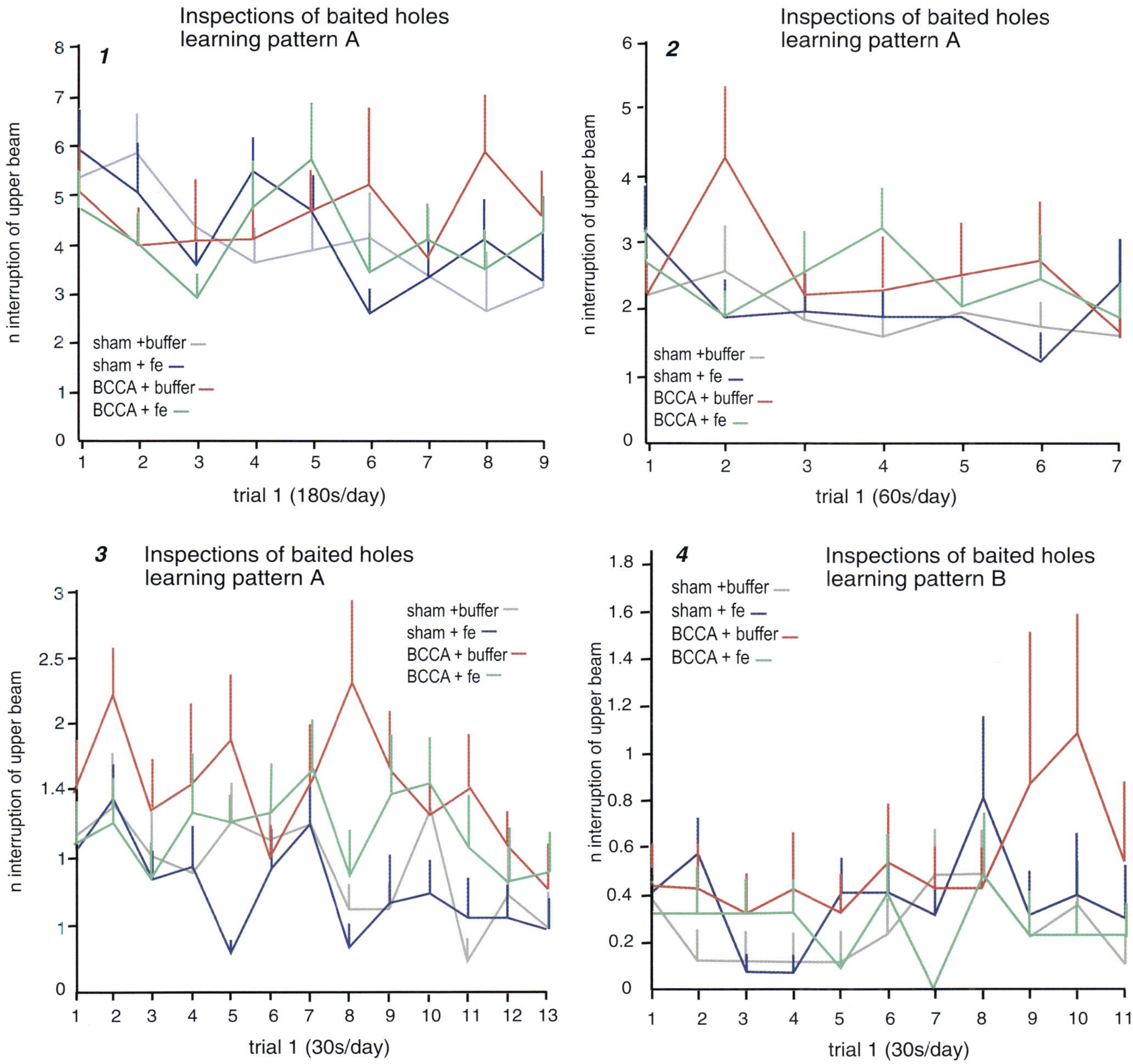

Fig. 3. INSPECTIONS OF BAITED HOLES learning pattern A and B n interruption upper beam
180 s
n.s.
Gabriel's test for variable: DIST Comparison significant at the 0.05 level are indicated by***
n.s.
60 s
n.s.
Gabriel's test for variable: DIST Comparison significant at the 0.05 level are indicated by***
n.s.
30 s
$F(3,38) = 11.39$, $p = 0.0001$; BCCA + Fe vs. sham + buffer, sham + Fe; ANOVA
Gabriel's test for variable: DIST Comparison significant at the 0.05 level are indicated by***
BCCA + buffer vs. sham + buffer; BCCA + buffer vs. sham + Fe; BCCA + Fe vs. sham + Fe***

INSPECTIONS OF BAITED HOLES learning pattern B, n interruption upper beam
Gabriel's test for variable: DIST Comparison significant at the 0.05 level are indicated by***
BCCA + buffer vs. sham + buffer; BCCA + buffer vs. BCCA + Fe***

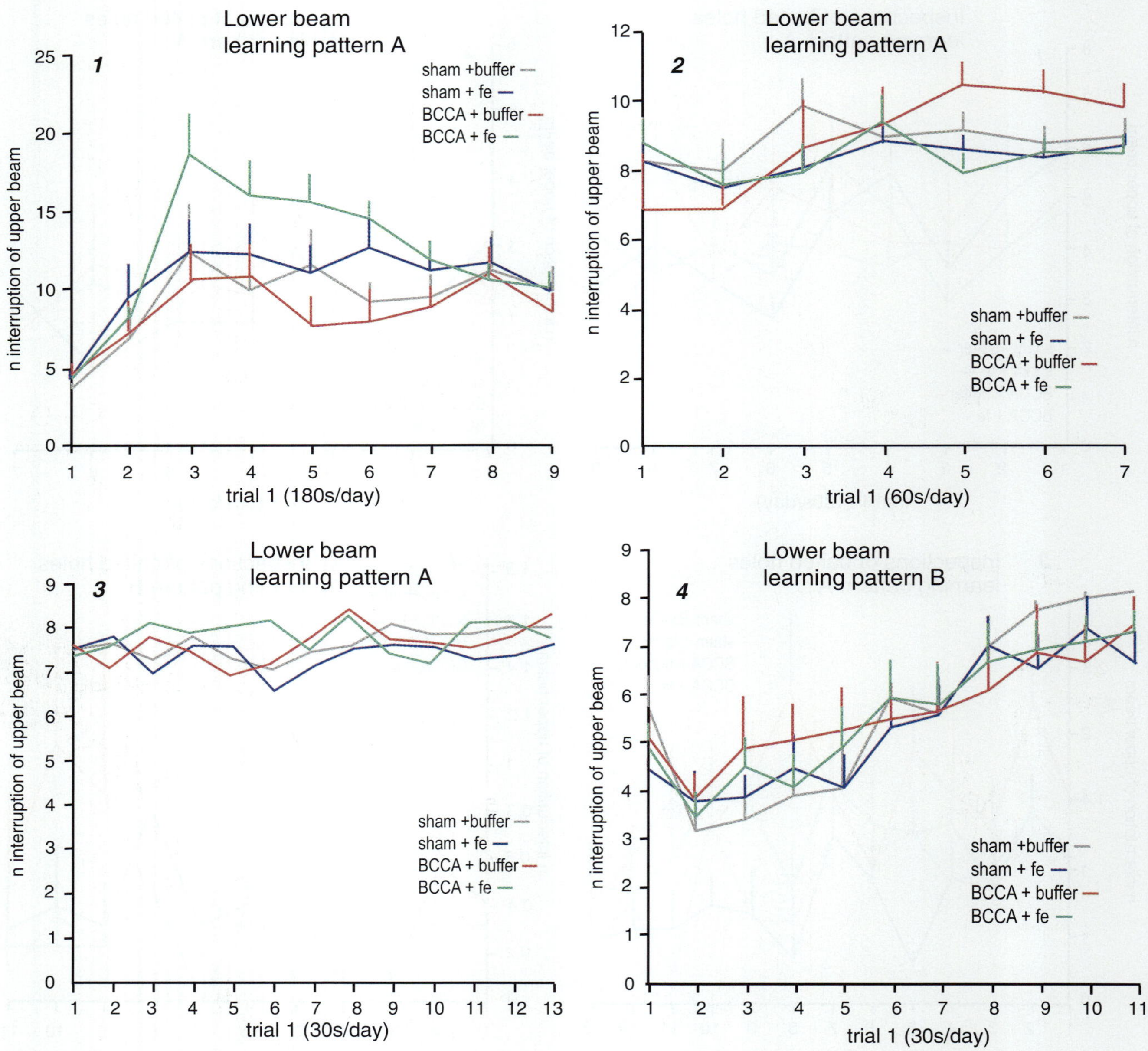

Fig. 4. LOWER BEAM learning pattern A and B, n interruption upper beam
180 s
$F(3,38) = 6.72$, $p = 0.0002$; BCCA + Fe vs. sham + buffer, BCCA + buffer; ANOVA
Gabriel's test for variable: DIST Comparison significant at the 0.05 level are indicated by***
BCCA + Fe; BCCA + buffer; sham + Fe; sham + buffer;
180 s BCCA + Fe vs. sham + buffer; BCCA + Fe vs. BCCA + buffer***
60 s n.s.
Gabriel's test for variable: DIST Comparison significant at the 0.05 level are indicated by***
BCCA + Fe; BCCA + buffer; sham + Fe; sham + buffer;
60 s n.s.
30 s n.s. ANOVA
Gabriel's test for variable: DIST Comparison at the 0.05 level are indicated by***
30 s BCCA + Fe sham + Fe***
LOWER BEAM pattern B learning, n of interruptions pattern B learning
n.s. ANOVA
Gabriel's test for variable: DIST Comparisons significant at the 0.05 level are indicated by***
n.s.

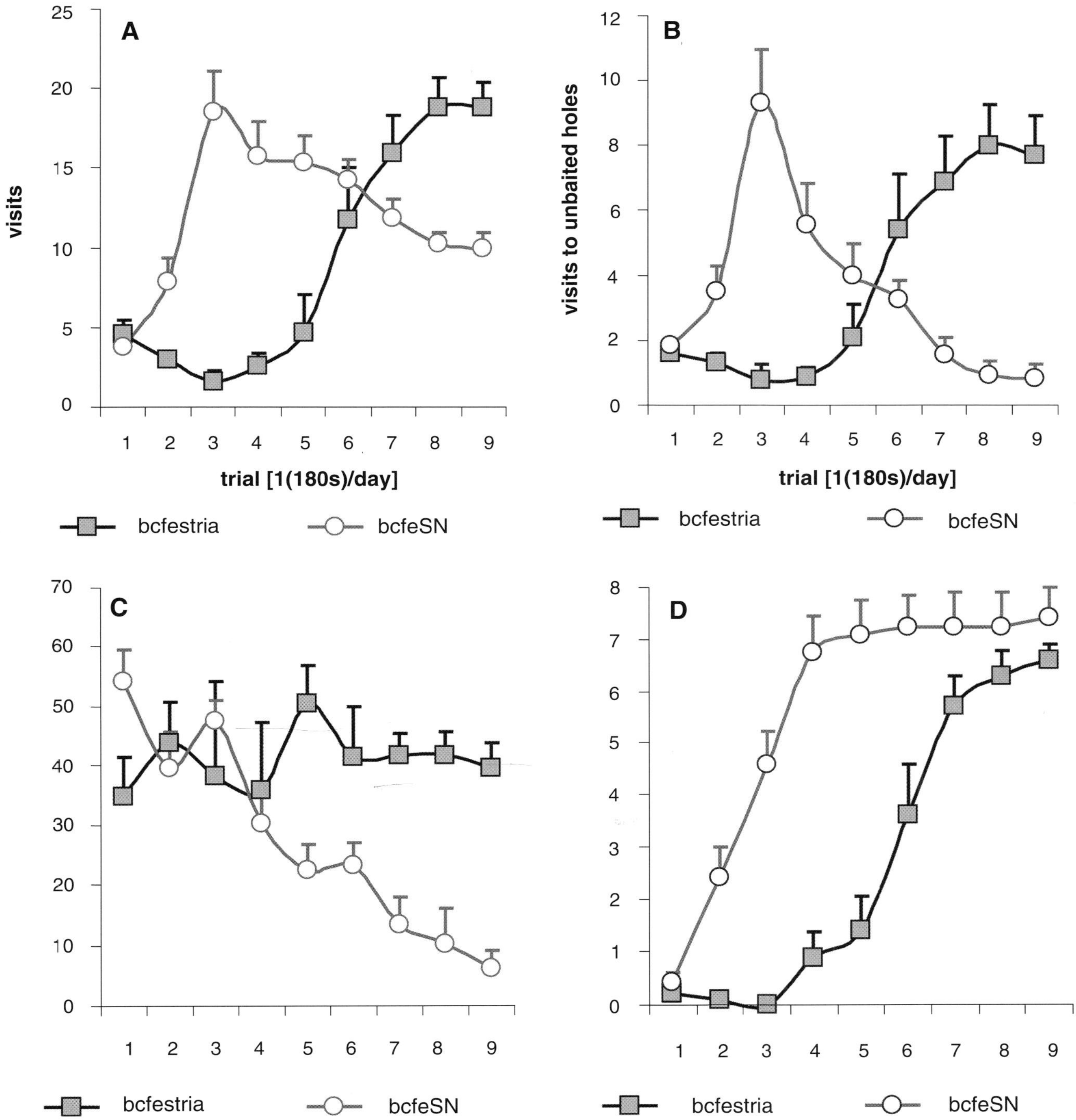

Fig. 5. Rats after BCCA and $FeCl_3$ into the Striatum (bcfestria) and rats after BCCA and $FeCl_3$ into the nigra (bcfeSN) showed different interest to look for pellets and to eat the pellets (A and D). In B, rats with iron in the ventrolateral striatum showed a comparable diminished activity. B shows also that BCCA rats with an injection iron in the subtantia nigra very quickly recognized that visits to unbaited holes are senseless. The cognitive behaviour is also reflected in C

ing of realisation and recognition are not meaningful. This aspect was consistently put into practice in the present test procedure, so that in the material presented here no erroneous interpretations have been made.

Inspections of baited holes, learning pattern A

During 9 and 7 days with one run per day lasting 180 or 60 s BCCA + Fe rats indicated no significances versus the number of interruption of the upper beam (Fig. 3).

Over 30 s the inspections of baited holes by BCCA + Fe showed significant differences compared with sham + buffer and sham + Fe (Fig. 3) ANOVA and in learning pattern B the differences between BCCA + buffer versus sham + buffer and BCCA + buffer versus BCCA + Fe were significant.

Lower beam, learning pattern A

It appears that this can be interpreted as comparable with the early study with inspections of non-baited.

Over a 9 day period at 180 s the activity of BCCA + Fe rats was significantly different compared with sham + buffer and BCCA + buffer (Fig. 4), there was no significant difference over 60 s during 7 days, but over 30 s (during 13 days) there was no difference BCCA + Fe and sham + Fe (during 13 days). No significance could be found in learning pattern B. But with pattern B there appeared an increased number of interruptions of the holes over 11 days, which shows that all groups were employing cognitive performance, i.e. from day to day became more successful (Fig. 4).

But the situation during 180 s reveals a new aspect. While in the situation of 180 s the BCCA + Fe treated rats were most active compared with sham + buffer and BCCA + buffer, it seems that the influence of BCCA + Fe seems to be helpful in finding and to eating pellets, but this is incorrect. As we know (Heim et al., 2000), BCCA + Fe treated rats need a very long time to understand and to start an initiative in a comparable situation when pellets are distributed in the same hole-board like shown in (Fig. 5d) During a 9-day period BCCA + Fe treated rats found and ate at first at day 4 the first pellet, at day 6–4 pellets and at day 9 (the end of the test) 6–7 pellets eaten of 8 distributed pellets (Fig. 5). (A group of rats after BCCA + Fe injected with the same concentration of Fe into the substantia nigra was much faster and more successful in finding and eating pellets distributed in the same pattern).

Table 1 shows the results of two statistic calculations. The ANOVA system indicates which group of animals are most active in fixed times versus other groups; the Gabriel's test ask whether groups are significantly different against other groups in the experiment covering 180 s, 60 s and 30 s or in learning the pattern of distributed pellets. These calculations are very important because animals change it activities mostly in very short time periods. This means that the data of longer periods of 180 s and 60 s are important only if immobile behaviours are of interest.

The analysis showed that over 180 s the BCCA + Fe treated rats were the most active animals during this time-span. However, these rats required the long 180 s period. Figure 5 shows that rats with the BCCA + Fe treatment combination took a long time to realise that food pellets were being presented to be found (Fig. 5, bcfestria). We therefore focused our interest on what the statistical analysis showed (ANOVA) and what can be seen with the help of the Gabriel test: which group is most affected during 30 s and which combination provides the most information about the Parkinson comparable pathology, iron alone, BCCA alone or the combination of both; and furthermore which system is not generally affected and which learning is the best for further studies.

Discussion

It is well-known that there is no satisfactory and no specific test procedure that can be applied to simulate the appearance and development of Parkinson's disease and which might provide understanding and explanation of the causative mechanism. The procedure presented here was developed in the last few years in which all the rats used to exhibit largely normal behaviour. In spite of this some of the animals may in some circumstances exhibit pathological indications.

First of all attention should be focused on the BCCA + Fe animals over 180 s. They exhibited the highest directed meaningful activity in inspections of non-baited holes and inspections of lower beams on the hole-board. But this high capability on the hole-board was no longer evident when the available times were shortened to 60 or 30 s. This indicated that the time available for realisation, initiation and action plays an important part. If in such an experiment all the measurements had been carried out solely after 180 s, one might have concluded that the toxic combination of BCCA with increased iron concentration in the ventrolateral striatum was a combination that might act in a stimulatory fashion. However, as turned out, the circumstances are different when the available times were reduced to 60 or 30 s. The BCCA + $FeCl_3$ animals are now no longer the most active. These rats showed lipid peroxidation in cerebral structures and a loss of dopaminergic neurones and network disaggregation in cerebral structures (Heim et al., 2002; Melzacka et al., 1995).

The region of recognition and reaction is normally limited to few seconds. This was shown by the hole-board when rats had learnt the pattern of provided pellets. They could find and eat the pellets in less than 20 s of directed action, something demanding cognitive and motor activity. The conclusion is that under normal physiologically accepted circumstances recognition referable to the central and motor systems take place within very brief time phases. Figure 2 shows an example of a negative character. This shows that within 180 s an entirely satisfactory performance was achieved which was however almost entirely devoid of value because in normal life such prolonged realisation and translation into action is practically useless. Such a circumstance would be pathological to a large extent.

Since we geared our approach towards a model for Parkinson's disease, it was obvious to compare the experimentally obtained picture with the delays of recognition and motor activities typically suffered by patients with Parkinson's disease. Thus when being suddenly greeted among other reactions it takes them some time to understand and to respond.

The question also arose whether there were any animals that even over 180 s failed to show any significance superiority of BCCA + Fe. Among our nine groups there were only two groups where instead of a BCCA + Fe superiority there was a superiority of BCCA + buffer. These were the animals of the group serial collection and reference memory errors total. Here it must be explained that the hitherto described pathologically-affected structures do not come so much into question. It has up to now proved impossible to create such effects with neurological assignments to the expression of such behaviour. Experimental studies have to be based on limited lessions and their effects have to be followed morphologically, neurochemically and genetically. This can however only be approximately successful if the experimental animals and their inherent system are able to react in a natural way.

Summarising, the example presented is meant to show that after ventrolateral $FeCl_3$ loading and the results of cerebral oligemic stress and their effects on network proliferation, animals'multilateral reactions were investigated in ways that had not been achieved hitherto.

Conclusion

This new method permits us to test already available and also newly-developed substances rapidly and extensively for their effects towards potentially Parkinson-like similarities. The effectiveness of any intervention is dependent on the duration of the exposition.

References

Block F, Sieklucka M, Schmidt-Kasten R, Heim C, Sontag KH (1993a) Metabolic chances during and after transient clamping of carotid arteries in normotensive rats. Brain Res Bull 31: 91–96

Block F, Szabo L, Jaspers RMA, Heim C, Sontag K-H (1993b) Levemopamil reduces spatial learning deficit following transient occlusion of common carotid arteries in normotensive rats. Acta Neurol Scand 88: 33–40

Cools AR (1980) Role of the neostriatal dopaminergic activity in sequencing and selecting behavioural strategies-facilitation of processes involved in selecting the best strategy in a stressful situation. Behav Brain Res 1: 361–378

Devan BD, White NM (1999) Parallel information processing in the dorsal striatum: Relation to hippocampal function. J Neurosci 19: 2789–2798

Ginsberg MD, Graham DI, Busto R (1985) Regional glucose untilization and blood flow following graded forebrain ischemia in the rat: correlation with neuropathology. Ann Neurol 18: 470–481

Heim C, Arzberger T, Sontag T, Xiao A, Herbinger KH, Weindl A, Sontag K-H (1999) Progressive degeneration of dopamine system functions after transient cerebral oligemia in rats. Brain Res 851: 235–246

Heim C, Sontag K-H (1994) Reference memory is affected by transient bilateral clamping of the carotid arteries in rats. J Neural Transm 7: 47–59

Heim C, Melzacka M, Kolasiewicz W, Jaros T, Sieklucka M, Wesemann W, Sontag K-H (1995) Cerebral oligemic hypoxia and iron toxicity in the mesolimbic system of rats. J Neural Transm [Suppl] 46: 165–173

Heim C, Pardowitz I, Sieklucka M, Kolasiewicz W, Sontag T, Sontag K-H (2000) The analysis system CGITAT for the study of cognitive deficiencies in rodents. Behav Res Methods Instrum Comput 32: 140–156

Heim C, Sowa L, Kurz T, Kolasiewicz W, Schwegler H, Sontag K-H (2002) Partial loss of dopaminergic neurons in the substantia nigra, ventrotegmental area and the retrorubral area – model of the early beginning of Parkinson's symptomatology? J Neural Transm 109: 691–709

Jellinger K, Paulus W, Grudke-Iqbal I, Riederer P, Youdim MBH (1990) Brain iron and ferritin in Parkinson's and Alzheimer's diseases. J Neural Transm 2: 327–340

Melzacka M, Weiner N, Heim C, Schmidt-Kastner R, Sieklucka M, Sontag K-H, Wesemann W (1994) Effect of transient reduction of cerebral blood flow on membrane anisotropy and lipid peroxidation in different rat brain areas. Neurochem Int 25: 161–168

Morris RGM, Moser EI, Riedel G, Martin SJ, Sandin J, Day M, O'Carroll C (2003) Elements of a neurobiological theory of the hippocampus – the role of activity-dependent synaptic plasticity in memory. Philos Trans R Soc Lond B Biol Sci 358: 773–786

Nauta HJW, Cuenod M (1982) Perikaryal cell labelling in the subthalamic nucleus following the injection of H-3-labeled gamma-aminobutyric acid into the pallidal complex-an autoradiographic study in cat. Neuroscience 7: 2725–2734

Pulsinelli WA, Brierley JB, Plum F (1982) Temporal profile of neuronal damage in a model of transient forebrain ischemia. Ann Neurol 11: 491–498

Scatton B, Simon H, Le Moal M, Bischoff S (1980) Origin of dopaminergic innervation of the rat hippocampal formation. Neurosci Lett 18: 125–131

Smith ML, Auer RN, Siesjö BK (1984) The density and distribution of ischemic brain injury in the rat following 2–10 min of forebrain ischemia. Acta Neuropathol (Berl) 64: 319–332

Wan F-J, Lin H-C, Kang B-H, Tseng C-J, Tung C-S (1999) D-amphetamine-induced depletion of energy and dopamine in the rat striatum is attenuated by nicotinamide pretreatment source. Brain Res Bull 50: 167–171

Wittmann B, Schott BH, Guderian S, Frey JU, Heinze H-J, Düzel E (2005) Reward-related fMRI activation of dopaminergic midbrain is associated with enhanced hippocampus-dependent long-term memory formation. Neuron 45: 459–467

Youdim MBH, Ben-Shachar D, Riederer P (1994) Iron and Parkinson's Disease Advances in research on neurodegeneration. In: Mizuno Y, Calne DB, Horowski R (eds) Birkhäuser, Boston, pp 63–78

J Neural Transm (2006) [Suppl] 71: 229–236

Journal of
Neural
Transmission
Printed in Austria

Impact of selenium, iron, copper and zinc in on/off Parkinson's patients on L-dopa therapy

G. A. Qureshi[1], A. A. Qureshi[1], S. A. Memon[2], S. H. Parvez[3]

[1] Medical Research Center, Liaquat University of Medical & Health Sciences, Jamshoro, Pakistan
[2] M. A. Kazi Institute of Chemistry, University of Sindh, Jamshoro, Pakistan
[3] Institute Alfred Fessard de Neurosciences, Bat 5, Parc Chateau CNRS, 91190 Gif Yvette, France

Summary We have quantitated CSF and serum levels of Selenium, iron, copper and zinc by Atomic absorption spectrophotometer in 36 patients with parkinson's disease all on L-dopa therapy. Out of these 19 showed on or positive response to L-dopa where as 21 patients showed on and off response. These data were compared with 21 healthy controls. The results showed that serum levels of iron, copper and zinc remained unchanged where as in CSF, significant decrease in zinc was found in both on and on/off PD patients indicating the deficiency of zinc which continues in the worsening clinical condition of off patients. The level of copper remained unchanged in both on and on/off PD patients. Iron and selenium increase in CSF of both patients which is a clear evidence of relationship between increased iron and selenium level in brain which could be correlated with decrease in dopamine levels and oxidative stress in PD Patients.

Introduction

Oxidation and nitration of proteins, DNA, and lipids are markers of neurodegeneration in postmortem tissues. It is impossible to determine with certainty using postmortem analysis, whether oxidative stress has a primary role in neurodegeneration or is a secondary end-stage epiphenomenon. Growing evidence suggests that the generation of oxidants does not result simply from an accidental disruption of aerobic metabolism, but rather from an active process crucial for the nonspecific immune defenses of the brain. And, during the active research in this area during few decades, it is suggested that a possible role of oxidative stress, neuromelanin, mitochondrial dysfunction, calcium-binding protein deficiency, nitric oxide, trophic factors deficiency, and cytokines, in the pathogenesis of Parkinson's disease. The major basic processes inducing neurodegeneration are considered multifactorial ones caused by genetic, environmental, and endogenous factors (Jellinger, 2003; Qureshi et al., 2004a). They include abnormal protein dynamics with defective protein degradation and aggregation, many of them related to the ubiquitin-proteasomal system, oxidative stress and free radical formation, impaired bioenergetics and mitochondrial dysfunctions, and "neuroinflammatory" processes. Oxidative stress, reactive oxygen (ROS), and nitrogen (RNS) species have been known to be involved in a multitude of neurodegenerative disorders such as Parkinson's disease (PD), Alzheimer's disease (AD), and amyotrophic lateral sclerosis (ALS). Both ROS and RNS have very short half-lives, thereby making their identification very difficult as a specific cause of neurodegeneration. These mechanisms that are usually interrelated in complex vitious circles finally leading to programmed cell death cascades (Jellinger, 2003). The formation of extracellular or intracellular deposits of amyloid-like protein fibrils is a prominent pathological feature of many different neurodegenerative diseases, including Alzheimer's disease (AD) and Parkinson's disease (PD).

Accumulation of transition metals has been suggested to be responsible for the deteriorated nigrostriatal dopaminergic system in Parkinson's patients. In addition to this, zinc-induced oxidative stress may result in apoptosis followed by reduced dopaminergic function in the nigrostriatal dopaminergic system (Lin et al., 2003). Abnormalities in the metabolism of the transition metals iron and copper have been demonstrated to play a crucial role in the pathogenesis of various neurodegenerative diseases (Perry et al., 2002). While there is documented evidence for alterations in the

Correspondence: G. A. Qureshi, Medical Research Center, Liaquat University of Medical & Health Sciences, Jamshoro, Pakistan
e-mail: ghulamali48@hotmail.com

homeostasis, redox-activity and localisation of transition metals, it is also important to realise that alterations in specific copper- and iron-containing metalloenzymes appear to play a crucial role in the neurodegenerative process. These changes provide the opportunity to identify pathways where modification of the disease process can occur, potentially offering opportunities for clinical intervention. As understanding of disease aetiology evolves, so do the tools with which diseases are treated. The extracellular microenvironment of the brain contains numerous biological redox agents, including ascorbate, glutathione, cysteine and homocysteine. During ischemia/reperfusion, aging or neurological disease, extracellular levels of reductants can increase dramatically owing to dysregulated homeostasis (Qureshi and Parvez, 1998; Qureshi, et al., 2004b).

Although the aetiology of Parkinson's disease (PD) and related neurodegenerative disorders is still unknown, recent evidence from human and experimental animal models suggests that a misregulation of iron metabolism, iron-induced oxidative stress and free radical formation are major pathogenic factors. These factors trigger a cascade of deleterious events leading to neuronal death and the ensuing biochemical disturbances of clinical relevance.

Besides iron, copper is an essential element for the activity of a number of physiologically important enzymes. Enzyme-related malfunctions may contribute to severe neurological symptoms and neurological diseases: copper is a component of cytochrome c oxidase, which catalyzes the reduction of oxygen to water, the essential step in cellular respiration. Copper is also a cofactor of Cu/Zn-superoxide-dismutase which plays a key role in the cellular response to oxidative stress by scavenging reactive oxygen species. Furthermore, copper is a constituent of dopamine-beta-hydroxylase, a critical enzyme in the catecholamine biosynthetic pathway. Copper binding proteins play important roles in the establishment and maintenance of metal-ion homeostasis, in deficiency disorders with neurological symptoms (Menkes disease, Wilson disease) and in neurodegenerative diseases such as Alzheimer's disease (Strausak et al., 2001).

Zinc on the other hand is an important trace element in biology. An important pool of zinc in the brain is the one present in synaptic vesicles in a subgroup of glutamatergic neurons. In this form it can be released by electrical stimulation and may serve to modulate responses at receptors for a number of different neurotransmitters. These include both excitatory and inhibitory receptors, particularly the NMDA and GABA(A) receptors.

Furthermore, the trace element Selenium is a very important mineral which works as an anti-oxidant substance. It is a constituent of glutathione peroxidase and acts as a cofactor in enzymatic reactions (Levander, 1988). Recently, it is shown that selenium itself is not an antioxidant at all, and even not in general when incorporated into glutathione peroxidases, and a moderate oxidative stress is beneficial rather than detrimental since it can induce defense mechanisms counteracting xenobiotic and oxidative stress (Brigelius-Flohe et al., 2005). Several studies have shown data on these metals suggesting the presence of oxidative stress, however, the significance of these findings is still unclear (Fahn and Cohen, 1992; Kienzl et al., 1995; Jimenez-Jimenez et al., 1998). Nothing is known on the role of selenium, iron, copper and zinc in Parkinson's patient with off and on status kept on L-dopa therapy. This study highlights the levels of selenium, iron, zinc and copper in both serum and cerebrospinal fluid. The results are presented with the view that CSF levels represent its level in brain. By conducting this study, it is of vital importance to understand the role of these metals in PD patients and the influence of L-dopa therapy in on and off status.

Patients and methods

All PD patients fullfilled diagnostic criteria for PD (Hughes et al., 1992) and were evaluated with internationally accepted Staging System (Hochn and Yahr, 1967). All 38 patients were recruited from the department of Neurology, Huddinge University Hospital. 21 healthy controls were also included in this study. Their sex, age, diagnosis and clinical data is summarized in Table 1.

The research ethical commitee of Karolinska Institute, Stockholm approved the study and all patients gave written informed consent to participate. All 38 PD patients were at different stages of illness (Hoehn and Yahr range 2–4) and were on L-dopa therapy containing 200 mg of this drug with or without the DA agonist bromocriptone and MAO-B inhibitor selegiline. 17 PD patients who showed positive response were lebeled as on group where as 19 who have been trated between 6 and 8 years with the similar drug showed severely off response were classified as off PD group. These off PD patients had Hoehn and range of −3 to −4. For control purpose, 21 persons were included who has tension headache without any proven organic ethiology, ischemic cerebrovascular disease and polyneuropathy. All these control group exhibited no signs or symptoms indicating any Daergic dysfunction.

10–12 ml cerebrospinal fluid (CSF) was collected from each patient and healthy control in sitting position at L4–L5 levels by lumbar puncture technique. Blood samples were collected by venipuncture. Both blood

Table 1. *Clinical data on healthy control (HC) and Parkinson patient with on and on/off status on L-dopa*

Patients	*n*	Females	Age	CSF-Albumin	CSF-IgG	IgG-index
HC	21	8	62 ± 11	227 ± 24	29 ± 5	0.45 ± 0.021
PD (on)	17	7	70 ± 15	$335 \pm 35^{*}$	$48 \pm 7^{**}$	0.43 ± 0.015
PD (on/off)	19	6	72 ± 17	$318 \pm 31^{*}$	$46 \pm 6^{**}$	0.42 ± 0.013

$^{*}p < 0.05$, $^{**}p < 0.01$

Table 2. *Levels of iron, copper, zinc and selenium in healthy control (HC) and Parkinson patient with on and on/off status on L-dopa*

Metal	Healthy controls (21)	PD (on) (17)	PD (on/off) (19)
Iron			
(a) Serum (mg/l)	1.16 ± 0.05	1.02 ± 0.11	1.09 ± 0.12
(b) CSF ((μg/l)	237 ± 37	$345 \pm 47^{**}$	$397 \pm 50^{***}$
Copper			
(a) Serum (mg/l)	1.22 ± 0.15	1.16 ± 0.12	1.27 ± 0.16
(b) CSF (μg/l)	132 ± 17	119 ± 18	109 ± 19
Zinc			
(a) Serum (mg/l)	0.89 ± 0.02	0.91 ± 0.07	0.79 ± 0.04
(b) CSF ((μg/l)	161 ± 31	$117 \pm 19^{**}$	$96 \pm 11^{***}$
Selenium			
(a) Serum (μg/l)	20.7 ± 1.5	$28.3 \pm 1.7^{**}$	$30.6 \pm 2.1^{***}$
(b) CSF ((μg/l)	14.2 ± 1.8	$19.7 \pm 1.9^{**}$	$22.7 \pm 2.1^{**}$

$^{*}p<0.05$, $^{**}p<0.01$, $^{***}p<0.001$

and CSF were taken from all individual early in the morning between 7 and 8 A.M. after a night fasting. The basic CSF analyses included cell counting by phase contrast microscopy (Seisjo, 1967), determination of CSF/serum albumin ratio and CSF serum immunoglobuline G (IgG) index (Link and Tibbling, 1977). Serum and CSF albumin and IgG were determined using Hitachi 737 Automatic analyzer (Naka Works, Hitachi Ltd., Tokyo, Japan). Both CSF and serum samples were kept at −80°C and protected from light exposure with aluminium foil until analysis.

An atomic absorption spectrophotometer (AAS, model 3110) equiped with an electrothermal atomizer (modelHGA 400) and an autosampler (all from Perkin- Elmer Beaconfield, Buck, UK) were used for the analysis of iron, copper and zinc in both serum and CSF samples. The analysis of selenium was performed with the same atomic coupled with an hydride generation system. The interday coefficint of variation (CV) was less than 3% for all metals both in CSF and serum samples. All our results are expressed as mean ± standard error of mean (SEM). The statistical analysis was done using ANOVA and two-tailed Student's test.

Results

Table 2 shows CSF and serum levels of iron, copper, selenium and zinc in PD patients both with on and on/off status and both these groups are compared with healthy controls. Serum levels of all metals except selenium remained unchanged whereas in CSF, iron increased significantly where as zinc decreased significantly in both PD groups. Although the level of copper in CSF shows the tendency of decrement but it is not significant. The level of selenium both in serum and CSF of PD patient were found significantly increased.

Discussion

A number of essential trace elements play a major role in various metabolic pathways. Selenium (Se), copper (Cu), zinc (Zn), and iron (Fe) are essential trace elements that have been studied in many diseases, including autoimmune, neurological, and psychiatric disorders. These observations suggest that alterations in essential trace elements Se, Cu, Zn and Fe may play a role in the pathogenesis of Parkinson patients. However, findings from plasma levels of trace element show a variety of results that are difficult to interpret. The extracellular concentrations of transition metals such as copper and iron are substantially elevated during aging and in some neurodegenerative disorders. Increases in the extracellular redox capacity can potentially generate neurotoxic free radicals from reduction of Cu(II) or Fe(III), resulting in neuronal cell death. Anatomical and histological studies have established the existence of selective regional vulnerability to neurodegeneration and cell death. For example, the dopaminergic neurons in the substantia nigra are selectively injured in Parkinson disease, whereas motor neurons in the spinal cord are selectively lost in amyotrophic lateral sclerosis (ALS), and loss of cholinergic neurons frequently occurs in the forebrain of individuals with Alzheimer disease. Despite this regional sensitivity, oxidative processes may represent a specific and selective unifying mechanism for neurodegeneration. Several aspects of this working hypothesis are evident in Parkinson disease and ALS. Parkinson disease may serve as an excellent example to discuss the significance of oxidative processes as a central but not an initiating event for the development of clinical disease (Lee et al., 2002). Environmental toxins (e.g., paraquat, rotenone, and MPTP) that epidemiological studies have shown to be risk factors are capable of generating reactive intermediates, directly alkylating reduced thiols, inhibiting complex I of the mitochondrial transport chain, inducing α-synuclein aggregation, and activating microglia. Possibly, they may also alter iron or other divalent metal homeostasis as well as dopamine metabolism, permitting an increase in nonvesicle-associated dopamine levels. All these events permit formation of reactive oxygen and nitrogen intermediates that propagate cellular dysfunction, leading to cell death (Qureshi et al., 2004a). We have indeed found significant increase in CSF iron levels in both PD groups.

Iron is considered as an essential metal for almost all living organisms due to its involvement in a large number of iron-containing enzymes and proteins, yet it is also toxic. The nervous system, including the brain, spinal cord, and peripheral nerves, is rich in both unsaturated fats (which are prone to oxidation) and iron (Halliwell, 1992). The high lipid content of nervous tissue, coupled with its high metabolic (aerobic) activity, makes it particularly susceptible to oxidant damage (Dawson and Dawson, 1996). The high level of brain iron may be essential, particularly during development, but its presence also means that injury to brain cells may release iron ions that can lead to oxidative stress via the iron-catalyzed formation of reactive oxygen species (Gerlach et al., 1994). This syndrome highly promotes formation of hydrogen peroxide, and hydrogen peroxide thus produced can be a main factor to cause serious damages to DNA and proteins (oxidative stress), yielding a copper(II)- or manganese(II)-peptide complex and its peroxide adduct, which are the serious agents to induce the structural changes from the normal prion protein (PrP(c)) to abnormal disease-causing isoforms (Nishida, 2003), PrP(Sc), or the formation of PrP 27–30 (abnormal cleavage at site 90 of the prion protein). In a recent study (Lan and Jiang, 1997) a chronic cerebral iron-loaded model was established by feeding mice with high iron diet. Data indicated that brain iron concentrations were significantly increased in iron-fed mice compared with those of controls. A significant increase in oxidized glutathione (GSSG), decrease in total glutathione (oxidized and reduced glutathione, GSSG + GSH), and therefore increase in the GSSG/(GSSG + GSH) ratios were observed in iron-loaded mice. Hydroxyl radical (OH) levels in striatum and brainstem were also significantly increased. It is also believed that excessive iron alone did not change either dopamine (DA) or lipid peroxidation (LPO) concentrations in striatum. However, a single injection of 1-methyl-4-phenyl-1,2,3,6-tetrahydropyridine (MPTP, 30 mg/kg, i.p.) into the iron-loaded mice caused a great enhancement in all these biochemical abnormalities. These findings suggest that iron does induce oxidative stress, but not severely injury neurons. Excessive iron accumulation in the brain, however, is a potential risk for neuronal damage, which may promote by triggering factor(s). This supports the hypothesis that excessive cerebral iron may contribute to the aetiology of Parkinson's disease (Bharath et al., 2002; Gupta et al., 2001).

The brain shares with other organs the need for a constant and readily available supply of iron and has a similar array of proteins available to it for iron transport, storage, and regulation. However, unlike other organs, the brain places demands on iron availability that are regional, cellular, and age sensitive. Failure to meet these demands for iron with an adequate supply in a timely manner can result in persistent neurological and cognitive dysfunction (Ponka, 2004; Andersen, 2004). Consequently, the brain has developed mechanisms to maintain a continuous supply of iron. However, in a number of common neurodegenerative disorders, there appears to be an excess accumulation of iron in the brain which suggests a loss of the homeostatic mechanisms responsible for regulating iron in the brain. As a result of a loss in iron homeostasis, the brain becomes vulnerable to iron-induced oxidative stress. Oxidative stress is a confounding variable in understanding the cell death that may result directly from a specific disease and is a contributing factor to the disease process. The underlying pathogenic event in oxidative stress is cellular iron mismanagement (Thompson et al., 2001; Wagner et al., 2002). Here, we propose that iron and iron-induced oxidative stress constitute a common mechanism that is involved in the development of neurodegeneration as we have already shown high levels of NO and homocysteine and low levels of vitamin B12 previously (Qureshi et al., 2003, 2004a). Also, we suggest that, at least in some neurodegenerative disorders, brain iron misregulation is an initial cause of neuronal death and that this misregulation might be the result of either genetic or non-genetic factors as has been suggested by other group (Qian and Shen, 2001). The potential of Fe(II) to catalyse hydroxyl radical formation via the Fenton reaction means that iron is potentially toxic. The toxicity of iron in specific tissues and cell types (liver, macrophages and brain) is illustrated by studies with appropriate cellular and animal models. In liver, the high levels of cyoprotective enzymes and antioxidants, means that to observe toxic effects substantial levels of iron loading are required. In reticuloendothelial cells, such as macrophages, relatively small increases in cellular iron (2–3-fold) can affect cellular signalling, as measured by NO production and activation of the nuclear transcription factor NF kappa B, as well as cellular function, as measured by the capacity of the cells to produce reactive oxygen species when stimulated (Crichton et al., 2002). Iron potentiates the generation of the highly reactive and toxic hydroxyl radical, and, thus, of oxidative damage. Iron deprivation may represent the first really efficient antioxidant, preventing oxidative stress in all subcellular compartments, tissues, and organs. Iron/iron deprivation also modulates programmed cell death (apoptosis), which should be the subject of further studies to better define the mechanisms mediating these complex effects (Polla, 1999). A review of the available data in PD provides the following evidence in support of this hypothesis: (i) an increase of iron in the brain, which in PD selectively involves neuromelanin in substantia nigra (SN) neurons; (ii) decreased availability of glutathione (GSH) and other antioxidant substances; (iii) increase of lipid peroxidation products and reactive oxygen (O_2) species (ROS); and (iv) impaired mitochondrial electron transport mechanisms. Although it is not clear whether iron accumulation and oxidative stress are the initial events causing cell death or consequences of the disease process, therapeutic efforts aimed at preventing or at least delaying disease progression by reducing the overload of iron and generation of ROS may be beneficial in PD and related neurodegenerative disorders. Decreased levels of antioxidant enzyme activity are found in Parkinson's disease patients (Fahn and Cohen, 1992). Current pharmacotherapy of PD (Jellinger, 1999), in addition to symptomatic levodopa treatment, includes 'neuroprotective' strategies with dopamine agonists, monoamine oxidase-B inhibitors (MAO-B), glutamate antagonists, catechol O-methyltransferase inhibitors and other antioxidants or free radical scavengers. In the future, these agents could be used in combination with, or partly replaced by, iron chelators and lazaroids that prevent iron-induced generation of deleterious substances. Changes in central iron homeostasis have been most closely investigated in PD, as this disorder is well characterised both clinically and pathologically. PD is associated with a significant increase in iron in the degenerating substantia nigra (SN) and is measureable in living PD patients and in post-mortem brain. This increase, however, occurs only in the advanced stages of the disease, suggesting that this phenonoma may be a secondary, rather than a primary initiating event, a hypothesis also supported by evidence from animal experiments. The source of the increased iron in off PD patients as we have shown in this study is unknown but a variety of changes in iron homeostasis have been identified in PD, both in the brain and in the periphery. The possibility that an increased amount of iron may be transported into the SN is supported by data demonstrating that one form of the iron-binding glycoprotein transferrin family, lactotransferrin, is increased in surviving neurons in the SN in the PD brain and that this change is associated with increased numbers of lactotransferrin receptors on neurons and microvessels in the parkinsonian SN. These changes could represent one mechanism by which iron might concentrate within the PD SN. Alternatively, the measured increased in iron might result from a redistribution of ferritin iron stores. Ferritin is located in glial cells while the degenerating neurons do not stain positive for ferritin. As free radicals are highly reactive, it is unlikely that glial-derived free radicals diffuse across the intracellular space in sufficent quantities to damage neuronal constituents. If intracellular iron release contributes to neuronal damage it seems more probable that an intraneuronal iron source is responsible for oxidant-mediated damage. Such a iron source is neuromelanin (NM), a dark-coloured pigment found in the dopaminergic neurons of the human SN. In the normal brain, NM has the ability to bind a variety of metals, including iron, and increased NM-bound iron is reported in the parkinsonian SN. The consequences of these phenomena for the cell have not yet been clarified. In the absence of significant quantities of iron NM can act as an antioxidant, in that it can interact with and inactivate free radicals. On the other hand, in the presence of iron NM appears to act as a proxidant, increasing the rate of free radical production and thus the oxidative load within the vulnerable neurons. Given that increased iron is only apparent in the advanced stages of the disease such as in off PD patients, it is unlikely that NM is of importance for the primary aetiology of PD. A localised increase in tissue iron and its interaction with NM may be, however, important as a secondary mechanism by increasing the oxidative load on the cell, thereby driving neurodegeneration (Double et al., 2000). Recently it is hypothesize that increased oxidative stress associated with the disease may result in dysregulation of iron homeostasis in midbrain dopaminergic neurons via alterations in binding of iron regulatory proteins (IRPs). This would mechanistically explain the noted increase in cellular iron levels in the Parkinsonian SN which appear to Contribute to subsequent neurodegeneration (Andersen, 2004).

Ceruloplasmin is a ferroxidase that oxidizes toxic ferrous iron to its nontoxic ferric form. It is previously reported that a glycosylphosphatidylinositol-anchored form of ceruloplasmin is expressed in the mammalian CNS. Therefore, the antioxidant effects of ceruloplasmin could have important implications for various neurodegenerative diseases such as Parkinson's disease and Alzheimer's disease in which iron deposition is known to occur (Patel et al., 2002).

In our results there is no significant decrease in copper CSF levels in both PD patient groups, however, there is significant decrease in zinc CSF levels. We have already shown that in these both PD patients groups, there is increase in CSF homocysteine and free radical nitric oxide and at the same time decrease in dopamine and vitamin B12 levels which could well depend on the accumulation of iron and could be correlated with oxidation stress (Qureshi et al., 2004a, b).

Copper (Cu), a redox active metal, is an essential nutrient for all species studied to date. During the past decade, there has been increasing interest in the concept that marginal deficits of this element can contribute to the development and progression of a number of disease states including cardiovascular disease and diabetes. The essentiality of Cu can be attributed to its role as a cofactor in a number of enzymes that are involved in the defence against oxidative stress. Cu, however, has a second face, that of a toxic compound as it is observed with accumulating evidence in hepatic, neurodegenerative and cardiovascular diseases. Disease progression, assessed through a clinical score, was generally unassociated with toenail trace element levels, with the exception of an inverse relation with zinc and selenium content and a direct correlation with copper concentration (Bergomi et al., 2002). Copper and zinc have significant antiatherogenic effect influencing activity of antioxidant enzymes (glutathione-peroxidase and superoxide-dismutase), mechanism of apoptosis and other mechanisms.

Elevated selenium intake may be associated with reduced cancer risk and may alleviate other pathological conditions including oxidative stress and inflammation. Selenium appears to be a key nutrient in counteracting the development of virulence and inhibiting HIV progression to AIDS. It is required for sperm motility and may reduce the risk of miscarriage. Selenium deficiency has been linked to adverse mood states and some findings suggest that selenium deficiency may be a risk factor in cardiovascular diseases. Selenium is an essential trace element although the level of selenium in food items reflects the soil in which they were grown and thus varies markedly between different parts of the world. The metabolism of selenium by the brain differs from other organs in that at times of deficiency the brain retains selenium to a greater extent. The preferential retention of selenium in the brain suggests that it plays important functions. To date mood is the clearest example of an aspect of psychological functioning that is modified by selenium intake (Benton, 2002). The underlying mechanism of Selenium involvement in oxidative stress is unclear although a response to supplementation was found with doses greater than those needed to produce maximal activity of the selenoprotein glutathione peroxidase. Although the functions of many selenoproteins are unknown some play important roles in anti-oxidant mechanisms (Benton, 2002). Its connection with Glutathione (GSH) is well worked out. GSH is an important antioxidant, and its depletion in neurons has been implicated in several neurodegenerative disorders. The studies demonstrate a critical role for extracellular trace copper in neuronal cell death caused by GSH depletion and may have important implications for the understanding of toxic processes in neurodegenerative diseases (White and Cappai, 2003). Consequently, one of the fundamental molecular mechanisms underlying the pathogenesis of cell death in AD and PD, and possibly other neurodegenerative or amyloid diseases, could be the direct production of hydrogen peroxide during formation of the abnormal protein aggregates (Tabner et al., 2002). A number of in vitro studies have shown that antioxidants, both endogenous and dietary, can protect nervous tissue from damage by oxidative stress. Uric acid, an endogenous antioxidant, was found to prevent neuron damage in rats, both in vitro and in vivo, from the metabolic stresses of ischemia (oxidative stress as well as exposure to the excitatory amino acid glutamate and the toxic compound cyanide) (Yu et al., 1998). Vitamin E was found to prevent cell death (apoptosis) in rat neurons subjected to hypoxia followed by oxygen reperfusion (Tagami et al., 1998). The same study showed that vitamin E prevented neuronal damage from reactive nitrogen species (Tagami et al., 1998). Both vitamin E and beta-carotene were found to protect rat neurons against oxidative stress from exposure to ethanol (Mitchell et al., 1999). In an experimental model of diabetes-caused neurovascular dysfunction, beta-carotene was found to protect cells most effectively, followed by vitamin E and vitamin C (Cotter et al., 1995).

Add to this, from these results, evidence for alterations in the homeostasis, redox-activity and localisation of transition metals, it is also important to realise that alterations in specific zinc-, copper- and iron-containing metalloenzymes appear to play a crucial role in the neurodegenerative process. These changes provide the opportunity to identify pathways where modification of the disease process can occur, potentially offering opportunities for clinical intervention. As understanding of disease aetiology evolves, so do the tools with which diseases are treated. Deficits of zinc or copper can result in rapid changes in cellular redox balance, tissue oxidative stress, inappropriate patterns of cell death, alterations in the migration of neural crest cells and changes in the expression of key patterning genes. In addition to well-recognized malformations, mineral deficiencies during perinatal development can result in behavioral, immunological and biochemical abnormalities that persist into adulthood. Although these persistent defects can in part be attributed to subtle morphological abnormalities, in other cases they may be secondary to epigenetic or developmental changes in DNA methylation patterns. Epigenetic defects combined with subtle morphological abnormalities can influence an individual's risk for certain chronic diseases and thus influence his or her risk for morbidity and mortality later in life (Gaetke and Chow, 2003).

Zinc is an important trace element in biology. An important pool of zinc in the brain is the one present in synaptic vesicles in a subgroup of glutamatergic neurons. In this form it can be released by electrical stimulation and may serve to modulate responses at receptors for a number of different neurotransmitters. Zinc is released in high concentrations from the hippocampus during seizures. Unfortunately, there are contrasting observations as to whether this zinc serves to potentiate or decrease seizure activity. Zinc may have an additional role in causing death in at least some neurons damaged by seizure activity and be involved in the sprouting phenomenon which may give rise to recurrent seizure propagation in the hippocampus. In Alzheimer's disease, zinc has been shown to aggregate beta-amyloid, a form which is potentially neurotoxic. The zinc-dependent transcription factors NF-kappa B and Sp1 bind to the promoter region of the amyloid precursor protein (APP) gene. Zinc also inhibits enzymes which degrade APP to nonamyloidogenic peptides and which degrade the soluble form of beta-amyloid. The changes in zinc metabolism which occur during oxidative stress may be important in neurological diseases where oxidative stress is implicated, such as Alzheimer's disease, Parkinson's disease, and amyotrophic lateral sclerosis (ALS). Zinc is a structural component of superoxide dismutase 1, mutations in which give rise to one form of familiar ALS. After HIV infection, zinc deficiency is found which may be secondary to immune-induced cytokine synthesis. Zinc is involved in the replication of the HIV virus at a number of sites (Cuajungco and Lees, 1997). The levels of zinc in both PD group are significantly decreased in our study. Generally speaking, the metabolism of zinc in the brain is regulated by a number of transport proteins, some of which have been recently characterized by gene cloning techniques. The changes in zinc metabolism which occur during oxidative stress may be important in neurological diseases where oxidative stress is implicated, such as Alzheimer's disease, Parkinson's disease, and amyotrophic lateral sclerosis (ALS). Zinc is a structural component of superoxide dismutase 1, mutations in which give rise to one form of familiar ALS. After HIV infection, zinc deficiency is found which may be secondary to immune-induced cytokine synthesis. Zinc is involved in the replication of the HIV virus at a number of sites (Cuajungco and Lees, 1997).

This study highlights the implication of selenium, iron, copper and zinc in Parkinson disease and provide us with the knowledge how the influence of L-dopa therapy has on their levels showing deficiency of some of these metals in brain and elevation of others so that the proper therapy should be adopted.

References

Andersen JK (2004) Iron dysregulation and Parkinson's disease. J Alzheimers Dis 6 [Suppl 6]: S47–S52

Benton D (2002) Selenium intake, mood and other aspects of psychological functioning. Nutr Neurosci 6: 363–374

Bergomi M, Vinceti M, Nacci G, Pietrini V, Bratter P, Alber D, Ferrari A, Vescovi L, Guidetti D, Sola P, Malagu S, Aramini C, Vivoli G (2002) Environmental exposure to trace elements and risk of amyotrophic lateral sclerosis: a population-based case-control study. Environ Res 89: 116–123

Bharath S, Hsu M, Kaur D, Rajagopalan S, Andersen JK (2002) Glutathione, iron and Parkinson's disease. Biochem Pharmacol 64: 1037–1048

Brigelius-Flohe R, Kluth D, Banning A (2005) Is there a future for antioxidants in atherogenesis? Mol Nutr Food Res 49: 1083–1089

Cotter MA, Love A, Watt MJ, Cameron NE, Dines KC (1995) Effects of natural free radical scavengers on peripheral nerve and neurovascular function in diabetic rats. Diabetologia 38: 1285–1294

Crichton RR, Wilmet S, Legssyer R, Ward RJ (2002) Molecular and cellular mechanisms of iron homeostasis and toxicity in mammalian cells. J Inorg Biochem 91: 9–18

Cuajungco MP, Lees GJ (1997) Zinc metabolism in the brain: relevance to human neurodegenerative disorders. Neurobiol Dis 4: 137–169

Dawson VL, Dawson TM (1996) Nitric oxide neurotoxicity. J Chem Neuroanat 10: 179–190

Double KL, Gerlach M, Youdim MB, Riederer P (2000) Impaired iron homeostasis in Parkinson's disease. J Neural Transm [Suppl 60]: 37–58

Fahn S (1991) An open trial of high-dosage antioxidants in early Parkinson's disease. Am J Clin Nutr 53 [Suppl]: 380S–382S

Fahn S, Cohen G (1992) The oxidant stress hypothesis in Parkinson disease: evidence supporting it. Ann Neuro 32: 804–812

Gaetke LM, Chow CK (2003) Copper toxicity, oxidative stress, and antioxidant nutrients. Toxicology 189: 147–163

Gerlach M, Ben-Shachar D, Riederer P, Youdim MB (1994) Altered brain metabolism of iron as a cause of neurodegenerative diseases? J Neurochem 63: 793–807

Halliwell B (1992) Reactive oxygen species and the central nervous system. J Neurochem 59: 1609–1623

Hoehn MM, Yahr MD (1967) Parkinsonism: onset, progression and mortality. Neurology 17: 427–442

Huges AJ, Ben-Shlomo SE, Daniel ST, Lees AJ (1992) What features improve the accuracy of clinical diagnosis in Parkinson's disease? A clinopathalogical study. Neurology 42: 1142–1146

Jellinger KA (1999) The role of iron in neurodegeneration: prospects for pharmacotherapy of Parkinson's disease. Drugs Aging 14: 115–140

Jellinger KA (2003) General aspects of neurodegeneration. J Neural Transm [Suppl 65]: 101–144

Jimenez-Jimenez FJ, Molina JA, Aguilar MV, et al. (1998) Cerebrospinal fluid levels of transition metals in patients with Parkinson's disease. J Neural Transm 105: 497–505

Kienzl E, Punchingar L, Jellinger K, Linert W, Stachelberger H, Jameson RF (1995) The role of transition metals in the pathogenesis of Parkinson's disease. J Neurol Sci 134: 69–78

Lan J, Jiang DH (1997) Excessive iron accumulation in the brain: a possible potential risk of neurodegeneration in Parkinson's disease. J Neural Transm 104: 649–660

Lee HJ, Shin SY, Choi C, Lee YH, Lee SJ (2002) Formation and removal of alpha-synuclein aggregates in cells exposed to mitochondrial inhibitors. J Biol Chem 277: 5411–5417

Levander OA (1988) Selenium, chromium and manganese. In: Shils ME, Young MR (eds) Modern Nutrition in health and Disease. Lea 7 Febiger, Philadelpia, pp 263–277

Lin AM, Fan SF, Yang DM, Hsu LL, Yang CH (2003) Zinc-induced apoptosis in substantia nigra of rat brain: neuroprotection by vitamin D3. Free Radic Biol Med 34: 1416–1425

Link H, Tibbling G (1977) Principles of Albumin and IgG analyses in neurological disorders III. Evaluation of IgG synthesis within the central nervous system in multiple sclerosis. Scand J Clin Lab Invest 37: 297–301

Mitchell JJ, Paiva M, Heaton MB (1999) Vitamin E and beta-carotene protect against ethanol combined with ischemia in an embryonic rat hippocampal culture model of fetal alcohol syndrome. Neurosci Lett 263: 189–192

Nishida Y (2003) Elucidation of endemic neurodegenerative diseases – a commentary. Z Naturforsch 58: 752–758

Patel BN, Dunn RJ, Jeong SY, Zhu Q, Julien JP, David S (2002) Ceruloplasmin regulates iron levels in the CNS and prevents free radical injury. J Neurosci 22: 6578–6586

Perry G, Sayre LM, Atwood CS, et al. (2002) The role of iron and copper in the aetiology of neurodegenerative disorders: therapeutic implications. CNS Drugs 16: 339–352

Polla BS (1999) Therapy by taking away: the case of iron. Biochem Pharmacol 57: 1345–1349

Ponka P (2004) Hereditary causes of disturbed iron homeostasis in the central nervous system. Ann NY Acad Sci 1012: 267–281

Qian ZM, Shen X (2001) Brain iron transport and neurodegeneration. Trends Mol Med 7: 103–108

Qureshi GA, Parvez SH (1998) The role of aspartic acid, glutamic acid and GABA in neurologic disorders. Biogenic Amines 13: 565–578

Qureshi GA, Memon SA, Qureshi AA, Collin C, Parvez SH (2003) Neurotoxicity and dynamic Parkinson's patients in on-off phenomena. Biogenic Amines 18: 55–78

Qureshi GA, Memon SA, Parvez SH (2004a) Role of cobalamin and its impact on free radical NO homocysteine in Parkinson's on and off patients. Biogenic Amine 19: 26–44

Qureshi GA, Collins C, Memon SA, Parvez H (2004b) Parkinson's Disease and neurotransmitters interplay in on/off phenomena. Biogenic Amines 19: 44–62

Siesjö R (1967) A new method for the cytological examination of cerebrospinal fluid. J Neurol Neurosurg Psych 30: 568–577

Strausak D, Mercer JF, Dieter HH, Stremmel W, Multhaup G (2001) Copper in disorders with neurological symptoms: Alzheimer's, Menkes, and Wilson diseases. Brain Res Bull 55: 175–185

Tabner BJ, Turnbull S, El-Agnaf OM, Allsop D (2002) Formation of hydrogen peroxide and hydroxyl radicals from A(beta) and alpha-synuclein as a possible mechanism of cell death in Alzheimer's disease and Parkinson's disease. Free Radic Biol Med 32: 1076–1083

Tagami M, Yamagata K, Ikeda K, Nara Y, et al. (1998) Vitamin E prevents apoptosis in cortical neurons during hypoxia and oxygen reperfusion. Lab Invest 78: 1415–1429

Thompson KJ, Shoham S, Connor JR (2001) Iron and neurodegenerative disorders. Brain Res Bull 55: 155–164

Wagner KR, Sharp FR, Ardizzone TD, Lu A, Clark JF (2002) Heme and iron metabolism: role in cerebral memorrhage. J Cereb Blood 91: 9–18

White AR, Cappai R (2003) Neurotoxicity from glutathione depletion is dependent on extracellular trace copper. J Neurosci Res 71: 889–897

Yu Z, Bruce-Keller AJ, Goodman Y, Mattson MP (1998) Uric acid protects neurons against excitotoxic and metabolic insults in cell culture, and against focal ischemic brain injury in vivo. J Neurosci Res 53: 613–625

J Neural Transm (2006) [Suppl] 71: 237–247

Journal of Neural Transmission
Printed in Austria

Metal specificity of an iron-responsive element in Alzheimer's APP mRNA 5′untranslated region, tolerance of SH-SY5Y and H4 neural cells to desferrioxamine, clioquinol, VK-28, and a piperazine chelator

S. Bandyopadhyay[1,*], X. Huang[1,*], H. Cho[2], N. H. Greig[2], M. B. Youdim[3], J. T. Rogers[1]

[1] Neurochemistry Laboratory, Department of Psychiatry, Genetics and Aging Research Unit, Massachusetts General Hospital
[2] NIA, Baltimore, MD
[3] Technion, Haifa, Israel

Summary Iron closely regulates the expression of the Alzheimer's Amyloid Precursor Protein (APP) gene at the level of message translation by a pathway similar to iron control of the translation of the ferritin L- and H mRNAs by Iron-responsive Elements in their 5′untranslated regions (5′UTRs). Using transfection based assays in SH-SY5Y neuroblastoma cells we tested the relative efficiency by which iron, copper and zinc up-regulate IRE activity in the APP 5′UTR. Desferrioxamine (high affinity Fe^{3+} chelator), (ii) clioquinol (low affinity Fe/Cu/Zn chelator), (iii) piperazine-1 (oral Fe chelator), (iv) VK-28 (oral Fe chelator), were tested for their relative modulation of APP 5′UTR directed translation of a luciferase reporter gene. Iron chelation based therapeutic strategies for slowing the progression of Alzheimer's disease (and other neurological disorders that manifest iron imbalance) are discussed with regard to the relative neural toxic action of each chelator in SH-SY5Y cells and in H4 glioblastoma cells.

Abbreviations: *IRE* Iron-responsive element, *IRP* iron-regulatory protein, *DFO* desferrioxamine, *CQ* clioquinol, *PIP-1* piperazine-1, *Fe* iron, *Cu* copper, *Zn* zinc, *AD* Alzheimer's disease.

Introduction

Iron and Alzheimer's disease

Recent studies confirmed the central role of iron in the etiology of Alzheimer's disease (AD). For example, the known iron transporter, P97, is a potential early detection biomarker for AD (Jeffries et al., 2001; Ujiie et al., 2002). Also null ferritin heterozygous mutants developed oxidative features in the cortex reminiscent of Parkinson's disease (PD) and AD (Thompson et al., 2003).

Genetic and biochemical evidence have linked the biology of iron to Alzheimer's disease. The genetic discovery that alleles in the hemochromatosis gene accelerate the onset of disease by five years has certainly validated interest in the model wherein metals (iron) accelerate the course of AD (Sampietro et al., 2001). Also another study of 6558 adults from 1971–1992 reported the risk of developing AD was much greater in persons who had both elevated iron and high cholesterol compared to risk from each factor alone (Mainous et al., 2005).

Iron accumulation certainly may not be the direct cause, but a consequence of normal cellular senescence in vitro contributing to the increased oxidative stress and cellular dysfunction seen in senescent cells. Iron accumulates as a function of age and is associated with the pathology of numerous age-related diseases (Killilea et al., 2004). In the case of AD pathology the integral role of iron in disease progression was directly supported from an MRI imaging study of the brains of Alzheimer's patients that revealed elevated levels of iron, particularly in the neurons of the basal ganglia (Bartzokis et al., 2000). Confirming these results, an elegant spectroscopic study demonstrated that amyloid plaques harbor an increase burden of iron copper and zinc (Lovell et al., 1998). Here iron and zinc levels were measured to be present at concentrations as high as the 1 mM level in the vicinity of amyloid plaques.

In support of a model for iron as a pathological risk factor for AD, Atamna and Frey (2004) demonstrated that heme levels were elevated in the brain of AD patients. AD brain demonstrated 2.5-fold more heme-b ($P < 0.01$) and 26% less heme-a ($P = 0.16$) compared with controls, resulting in a highly significant 2.9-fold decrease in heme-a/heme-b ratio ($P < 0.001$) (Atamna and Frey, 2004).

Correspondence: J. T. Rogers, Ph.D, Genetics and Aging Research Unit, MGH, Charlestown MA 02129,
e-mail: Jrogers@partners.org
* These authors contribute equally.

Heme/porphines inhibit prion formation during scrapies infection (Caughey et al., 1998; Priola et al., 2000). In this regard, porhyrins have been suggested as useful in-vivo chelators of AD (Howlett et al., 1997).

A functional iron-responsive element and the translational control of amyloid precursor protein

We previously reported similarities between APP holoprotein and ferritin gene expression, both of which are driven by translational regulatory events in hepatoma, neuronal, and astrocytic cells (Rogers et al., 1999, 2002; Thomson et al., 2005). Here, expression of the APP gene was upregulated at the translational level by iron and IL-1, paralleled by the action of 5′ untranslated region 5′UTR sequences that are similar to the 5′UTR sequences in the mRNAs coding for the L- and H-subunits of ferritin.

Evidently, iron-responsive elements (IREs) are involved in the post-transcriptional regulation of several genes that control intracellular iron homeostasis. The rationale for an IRE stem-loop in any given transcript to be a tag for the involvement of it's encoded protein in iron metabolism was already exemplified by other iron-associated proteins. For example:-

a) The 5′UTRs of both the L- and H- transcripts of the central iron storage multimer, ferritin, encode IRE RNA stem-loops which bind to the Iron Regulatory Proteins (IRP-1 and IRP-2) to cause translational repression. Iron influx releases IRPs to facilitate ferritin translation (Fillebeen et al., 2005). Enhanced ferritin accumulation during inflammation appears to prevent iron catalyzed cellular damage by providing an increased reservoir for the safe storage of toxic iron (Thomson et al., 2005).
b) Transferrin receptor (TfR) is the central iron transporter of iron loaded transferrin into cells, and TfR mRNA stability is increased when IRPs (IRP-1/IRP-2) bind to the 5 canonical IRE stem-loops in the 3′UTR of the transcript (Klausner et al., 1993). An IRE-related RNA stem-loop was also shown to be present in the 5′UTR of the mRNAs coding for the serum iron carrier protein transferrin (Tf) (Cox et al., 1995).
c) An IRE stem-loop is present immediately downstream from the stop codon of the mRNA for DMT-1 (Gunshin et al., 2001). The divalent metal ion transporter, DMT-1 assimilates cellular Cu^{2+}, Zn^{2+}, Fe^{2+} and Mn^{2+}. Expression of DMT-1 is restricted to duodenal enterocytes and reticulocytes where mutations in the DMT-1 gene cause microcytic anemia in mice and the Belgrade rat phenotype, with impaired iron accumulation in red blood cells to diminish hemoglobin synthesis (Gunshin et al., 2005).
d) A functional IRE is present in the 5′UTR of the transcript for IREG-1 which transports iron from enterocytes into the bloodstream (McKie et al., 2000). Human haephestin is the Cu dependent iron oxidase associated with IREG-1 that promotes duodenal iron export prior to loading of Fe^{3+} onto transferrin for circulation in blood (Vulpe et al., 1999).
e) The presence of an IRE in the stem-loop in APP-mRNA suggested that this ubiquitous membrane-associated protein has a significant role in iron metabolism.

The Alzheimer's disease brain harbors dysregulated binding of IRPs to IREs (Pinero et al., 2000), an event that would be predicted to have implications for the expression of any of these iron-related proteins. Certainly the generic IRE RNA stem-loop may be an important site to cause mis-regulation of these key proteins (above) during the course of AD. The absence of IRP-2, which controls iron homeostasis, was associated with a misregulated iron metabolism and ferritin translation and TfR mRNA stability in the gut mucosa and caused central nervous system dysfunction in IRP-2 knockout mice (LaVaute et al., 2001).

Oxidative stress in Alzheimer's disease

Perturbed regulation of iron metabolism appears to promote oxidative stress and is associated with altered ferritin levels in the brains of AD patients (Jellinger et al., 1990; Zecca et al., 2004). Oxidative stress has been strongly associated with the neurotoxicity in AD (Smith et al., 1991, 1994, 1997; Thome et al., 1997). For example, over-expression of superoxide dismutase-1 protected neurons against beta-amyloid peptide (Aβ) toxicity (Celsi et al., 2004). The antioxidant, Co-enzyme Q, has already been tested for efficacy in animal models receiving increased oxidative stress, and is currently being tested for efficacy to AD (Beal, 2003).

In PD, AD and other progressive neurodegenerative diseases neurotoxic events such as oxidative stress, iron accumulation, excitotoxicity, inflammatory processes, nitric oxide, inhibition of mitochondrial complex I, lack of neurotrophic factors and apoptosis have been implicated in their pathogenesis (Youdim et al., 2004). In these disorders, iron accumulation occurs at sites where neurons die. For example, in PD an increase of iron is observed in microglia, astrocytes, oligodendrocytes and melanin containing dopamine neurons of the substantia nigra pars compacta. A similar feature has also been reported to occur in 6-OHDA (6-hydroxydopamine) lesion and MPTP (1-methyl-4-phenyl-1,2,3,6-terahydropyridine) models of PD, as well as in a kainate model of Huntington disease, where iron accumulates in the dentate gyrus and hippocampus CA1 and CA3 regions.

Certainly a new model for amyloid induced neuronal loss in AD (Huang et al., 1999b) can be explained by the binding of Aβ-peptides to copper and iron to catalyze the generation of toxic H_2O_2. Equation 1 shows the standard Fenton reaction by which iron or copper react with hydrogen peroxide and superoxides to generate the toxic and deadly hydroxyl radicals that mediate neuronal loss during AD (Halliwell, 1984). The presence of reduced copper (Cu^{1+}) and iron (Fe^{2+}) also implied that even more damaging hydroxyl radical would be formed by the Fenton and Haber-Weiss chemical reactions (Bush, 2003; Gutteridge, 1994) (Eq. 1).

$$Fe^{-2}(Cu^{2+}) + H_2O_2 \longrightarrow Fe^{+3}(Cu^{1+}) + OH^- + {}^{\bullet}OH$$

An appealing model suggests that the pathologically damaging production of hydrogen peroxide generated by Aβ is the result of a corruption of a beneficial superoxide dismutase activity associated with Aβ In fact, Aβ dimers may form a copper-zinc protein (8 kDa) that has intrinsic superoxide dismutase activity and is capable of converting O_2^- into H_2O_2. (Curtain et al., 2001). This hydrogen peroxide can then be converted into two water molecules by catalase to complete an antioxidant function.

Iron/copper chelators and their clinical efficacy in AD and PD

Because iron participates in redox, with the production of reactive hydroxyl radicals to induce oxidative stress, iron is thought to have a pivotal role in the pathogenesis of PD and other neurodegenerative diseases where iron dysregulation has been reported. However, it is not known whether its role is primary or secondary (Zecca et al., 2004). Intraventricular pretreatment with the prototype iron chelator, desferal, was able to be protective against a 6-OHDA model of PD in rats (Ben-Shachar et al., 1991; Youdim et al., 2004), with confirmation coming also from the MPTP model (Lan and Jiang, 1997). These results have been confirmed pharmacologically with the copper and iron chelator, clioquinol and by genetic over expression of ferritin in mice that results in neuroprotection against MPTP neurotoxicity (Kaur et al., 2003). Furthermore, recent studies employing systemic pretreatment with a brain permeable iron chelators, VK-28 and M30, have shown neuroprotection against 6-OHDA and MPTP, respectively, lesions of striatal dopamine neurons in rats and mice (Shachar et al., 2004) as well as in a kainate model of Huntington (Youdim et al., unpublished results).

There remains considerable controversy as to whether copper or iron actually accelerate the onset of AD. Two studies demonstrated that copper appeared to lower the amyloid burden in the AD brain of APP transgenic mice. In the first study Phinney et al. (2003) demonstrated an in vivo reduction of amyloid-Aβ by a mutant copper transporter. They used a well-known spontaneous mutation of a special strain of mutant toxic-milk mice that accumulate too much copper. Eventually those animals displayed a liver disease, which is a facsimile of a human disorder called Wilson's disease. In direct contrast another study demonstrated that Cu in the water supply dramatically accelerated amyloid plaque formation in APP transgenic mice (Sparks and Schreurs, 2003).

The finding that iron and copper chelation therapy was effective clinically (with desferioxamine and clioquinol treatment) lent more weight to the possibility that mis-regulation of these metals has a role in the etiology of AD and PD. Deferrioxamine has been used clinically for the past four decades to lower the iron burden after red blood cell transfusions to sickle cell patients, and in thalassemia patients. A clinical trial (Toronto, Canada) demonstrated that deferrioxamine was therapeutic in AD patients (Crapper McLachlan et al., 1991). Clioquinol, the copper-zinc-iron antibiotic, was tested with success in late onset patients for use for AD in clinical trial (Phase II) (Ritchie et al., 2003).

Several orally available iron chelators, including deferiprone and deferasirox and also piperazine derivatives, may prove efficacious for therapy to limit amyloid burden in AD patients. Already novel iron chelators have become available for many beneficial therapies associated with iron chelation (transfusion iron overload, protection against myocardiotoxicity) (Wu et al., 2004). One chelator, VK-28 (5-[4-(2-hydroxyethyl) piperazine-1-ylmethyl]-quinoline-8-ol), an orally available iron chelator, completely protected against ICV 6-OHDA (250 μg) induced striatal dopaminergic lesion, as measured by dopamine (DA), dihydroxyphenylacetic acid (DOPAC) and homovanilic acid (HVA) levels (model for PD) (Shachar et al., 2004).

This report sets out to determine the relative capacity of desferrioxamine, clioquinol, a piperazine analog (piperazine-1) and VK-28, respectively to inhibit the APP 5′UTR conferred translation to a stably transfected luciferase gene. We provide data as to the relative neurotoxicity (LD-50 values) of these chelators to neuroblastoma SH-SY5Y cells and H4 glioblastoma cells. We also investigated the relative efficiency of Fe/Cu chelators to suppress APP 5′UTR (Iron-responsive Element) conferred luciferase gene expression in stable transfected cell lines. Finally this report evaluated which of copper, iron or zinc was more effective to change APP 5′UTR driven gene expression.

Materials and methods

Generation of DNA constructs; pIRES (APP mRNA 5′UTR)

The PGAL construct containing the full-length 146-nucleotide APP mRNA 5′UTR upstream from the luciferase gene start codon was prepared as described previously (Rogers et al., 2002). This firefly (Photinus pyralis) luciferase reporter gene is translationally regulated by the APP mRNA 5′UTR that bears the IL-1 responsive element and an additional 55 nucleotides immediately downstream from the 5′-cap site of APP mRNA that had the novel IRE within it.

To generate an APP mRNA 5′UTR driven luciferase reporter gene construct with GFP as an internal specificity control, we excised the APP mRNA 5′UTR-luciferase fragment from the PGAL construct by *Hin*dIII and *Xba*I digestion. The excised fragment was blunt-ended by *klenow DNA polymerase I* treatment. This fragment was then ligated to *SmaI* digested linearized pIRES-EGFP vector (Clontech, Mountain View, CA). The plasmid construct was amplified in bacteria in medium containing kanamycin. This construct was named pIRES(APP mRNA 5′UTR). The colonies were isolated, and the PCR (QIAGEN, Valencia, CA) generated cassette was confirmed from band size after treatment with *Bam*HI restriction enzyme. Bi-directional DNA sequencing confirmed the identity of the clones using GL2 and RV3 primers, the sequencing primers for PGL3[26] (PROMEGA, Madison, WI). The construct obtained permits both the gene of interest, i.e., APP mRNA 5′UTR driven by luciferase, and the EGFP gene to be translated from a single bicistronic mRNA (Fig. 1).

Generation of stable SH-SY5Y transfectants

The SH-SY5Y neuroblastoma cell line was transfected with AMAXA cell line Nucleofactor kit V (AMAXA biosystems, Gaithersburg, MD) following manufacturer's instructions. Briefly, the cells were plated in 100 mm culture dishes and grown to 75–80% confluence, then trypsinized and a total of 1.5×10^6 cells were centrifuged and resuspended in 100 μl of nucleofactor^{TM} solution V (0.5 ml supplement mixed with 2.25 ml nucleofactor^{TM} solution provided with the AMAXA kit). 2–10 μg of plasmid (pIRES APP mRNA 5′UTR) was electroporated using G-04 program of an AMAXA

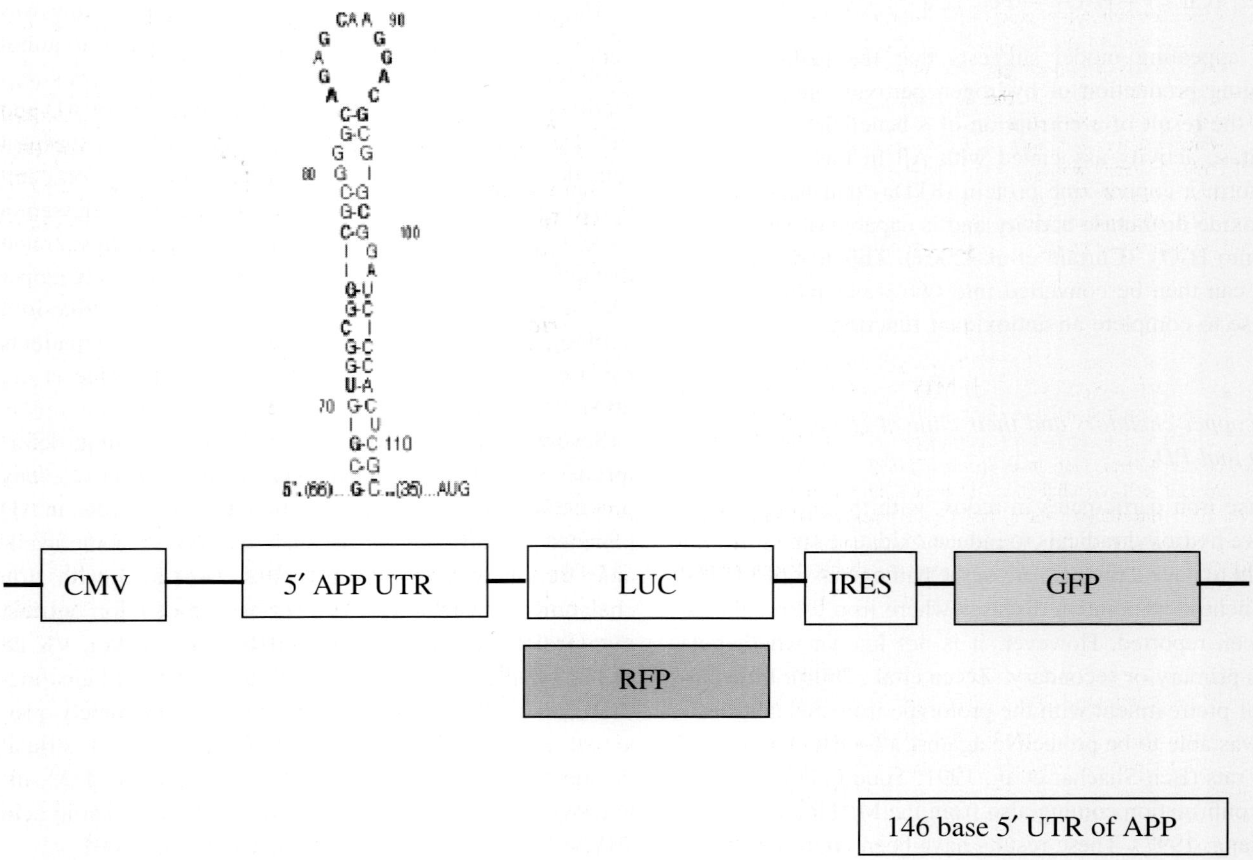

Fig. 1. The Dicistronic pIRES(APP mRNA 5′UTR) Construct. This construct was generated by ligating a DNA cassette encoding the 146 nt APP 5′UTR in front of the luciferase gene (excised from PGAL construct (Rogers et al., 2002)) into the linearized pIRES-EGFP vector. The APP mRNA 5′UTR driven luciferase reporter gene construct incorporated EGFP as an internal specificity control

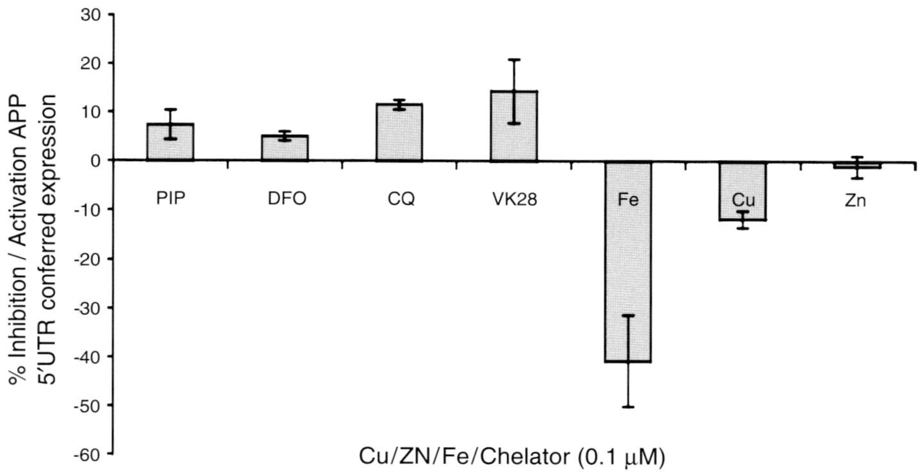

Fig. 2. Relative inhibition/activation of APP 5′untranslated region conferred luciferase expression in response to changed levels of Fe/Cu/Zn in stable pIRES(APP 5′UTR) transfectants. Capacity of four chelators (delivered to SH-SY5Y cells at 0.1 μM for 48 h) to inhibit APP 5′UTR driven luciferase expression in SH-SY5Y cells as (i) desferrioxamine (DFO), (ii) clioquinol (CQ), (iii) piperazine analogue (piperazine-1), and (iv) VK-28 (N = 10). Capacity of Fe, Zn, Cu (delivered to SH-SY5Y cells at 0.1 μM for 48 h) to activate APP 5′UTR driven luciferase expression in SH-SY5Y cells

electroporator according to manufacturer's instructions. 2 μg of pIRES-EGFP plasmid (Clontech) was transfected into the cells as a positive control. The cells were then cultured in complete growth medium. After 48 hours, the medium was removed and replaced with geneticin-supplemented medium for selection of stable clones; the medium was then changed regularly every 4–5 days. Within 10 days, a mixed population with 70% of pIRES (APP mRNA 5′UTR)/pIRES (PrP mRNA 5′UTR) transfected cells was obtained, which was then split and a stock maintained.

Transfection efficiency was determined by counting GFP positive cells observed under a NIKON TE 300 fluorescence microscope with GFP filters (excitation: 465–495 and emission: 515–555). Images were taken under a 20× magnification objective lens.

Viability assay (MTS)

Cell viability was performed by MTS assay (PROMEGA) following manufacturer's instruction. Briefly, 10 μl MTS reagent was added to each well. As negative control, cells in some wells were lysed in 10% Triton X-100. The plate was incubated for 2 hours at 37°C, and the absorbance was recorded at 490 nm read in a Spectra Max plate reader (Molecular Device). Percent cell viability was calculated by the formula: % cell viability = 100× (absorbance − avg. lysis)/(avg. background − avg. lysis); where avg. background is the average absorbance calculated from wells with DMSO alone, and avg. lysis is the average absorbance calculated from lysed cells.

Cell plating to assess the inhibitory action of desferrioxamine, clioquinol, VK-28, piperazine-1

After assay optimization, pIRES(APP mRNA 5′UTR) – transfected stable SH-SY5Y cells were trypsinized, harvested, resuspended in culture medium and strained with a cell strainer (BD Falcon, Bedford, MA) to avoid clogging the multidrop channels with clumped cells. A Multidrop 384 cell dispenser (Thermo Lab systems, NJ) was used to add 40 μl containing 1000 cells to the 23 columns of black 384-well culture plates. Untransfected SH-SY5Y cells were added to the 24th column. The cells were incubated for 2 hours before addition of the chelators at the indicated concentrations as described in Fig. 2).

Results

We previously had identified a functional IRE RNA stem loop in the 5′UTR of the APP transcript (Rogers et al., 2002). Figure 1 shows this APP 5′UTR stem loop, which is known to encode a 76% base homology with the H-ferritin mRNA 5′UTR Iron-responsive Element (IRE-like domain corresponds to APP 5′UTR sequences (+82 to +94). In Fig. 1 the APP 5′UTR IRE is shown in the context of the *pIRES (APP mRNA 5′UTR)* construct.

Desferrioxamine, clioquinol, piperazine-1 and VK-28 confer APP 5′UTR specific inhibition

Desferrioxamine (high affinity Fe^{3+} chelator) and Clioquinol (low affinity chelator of Cu/Zn/Fe) were reported to both inhibit translation conferred to an APP 5′UTR/Luciferase reporter gene in transfection based assays (Rogers et al., 2002). Using the 146 nucleotide APP 5′UTR UTR as a screening target, we identified metal chelators as a significant subclass of the 5 classes leads. For example, the Hg, Pb chelator, dimercaptoporopanol selectively reduced APP holoprotein expression but not APLP-1 expression, in SH-SY5Y cells in a secondary, Western blot assay (Payton et al., 2003).

Since the APP 5′UTR sequences were functionally iron responsive we measured the inhibitory capacity of desferrioxamine, clioquinol, piperazine-1 and VK-28 as chelators to suppress APP IRE driven luciferase reporter gene expression in pIRES(APP mRNA 5′UTR)/stable transfectants (Fig. 2). The average APP 5′UTR inhibitory capacity of DFO, Clioquinol, piperazine-1 and VK-28 was measured at the 0.1 μM concentration of each chelator exposed to SH-SY5Y cells for 48 hours. The histogram in Fig. 2 represents the average data of two separate experiments (N = 5 each) using stable pIRE-S(APP mRNA 5′UTR)/stable transfectants (N = 10, $P < 0.005$). The potency of each chelator to inhibit APP 5′UTR activity was ranked at VK-28 > CQ > PIP-1 > DFO for the 0.1 μM concentration (N = 10). It is noteworthy that desferrioxamine inhibition significantly increased at higher concentrations and/or longer (78 h) incubation times.

Consistent with Fe chelator activity, the same experiment demonstrated that Fe > Cu > Zn activated APP 5′UTR conferred translational expression of a luciferasereporter gene (Fig. 2). These data suggested that the APP 5′UTR was more responsive to iron than copper (0.1 μM concentration for 48 h treatment of SH-SY5Y cells).

Under all conditions of intracellular iron chelation, inhibition of APP synthesis was via a molecular pathway associated with the translational efficiency of APP mRNA. At the same time as iron induced APP 5′UTR driven translation of the luciferase reporter gene, we observed a reduction in RNA binding protein interaction with APP 5′UTR probes (Cho H-Y et al., In Preparation).

Neurotoxicity of desferrioxamine, clioquinol, piperazine-1, and VK-28

In Fig. 3 we compared the dose responsive action of desferrioxamine, clioquinol, piperazine-1 and VK-28 towards neurotoxicity in SH-SY5Y cells (lethal dose at 50% cell viability (LD-50) were established). An MTS viability assay was performed (48 h assay) to determine SH-SY5Y neuroblastoma cell and H4 neuroglioblastoma cell growth in response to increasing concentrations of DFO, CQ, PIP-1, VK-28 (0.01 μM, 0.1 μM, 1 μM, 10 μM, 100 μM).

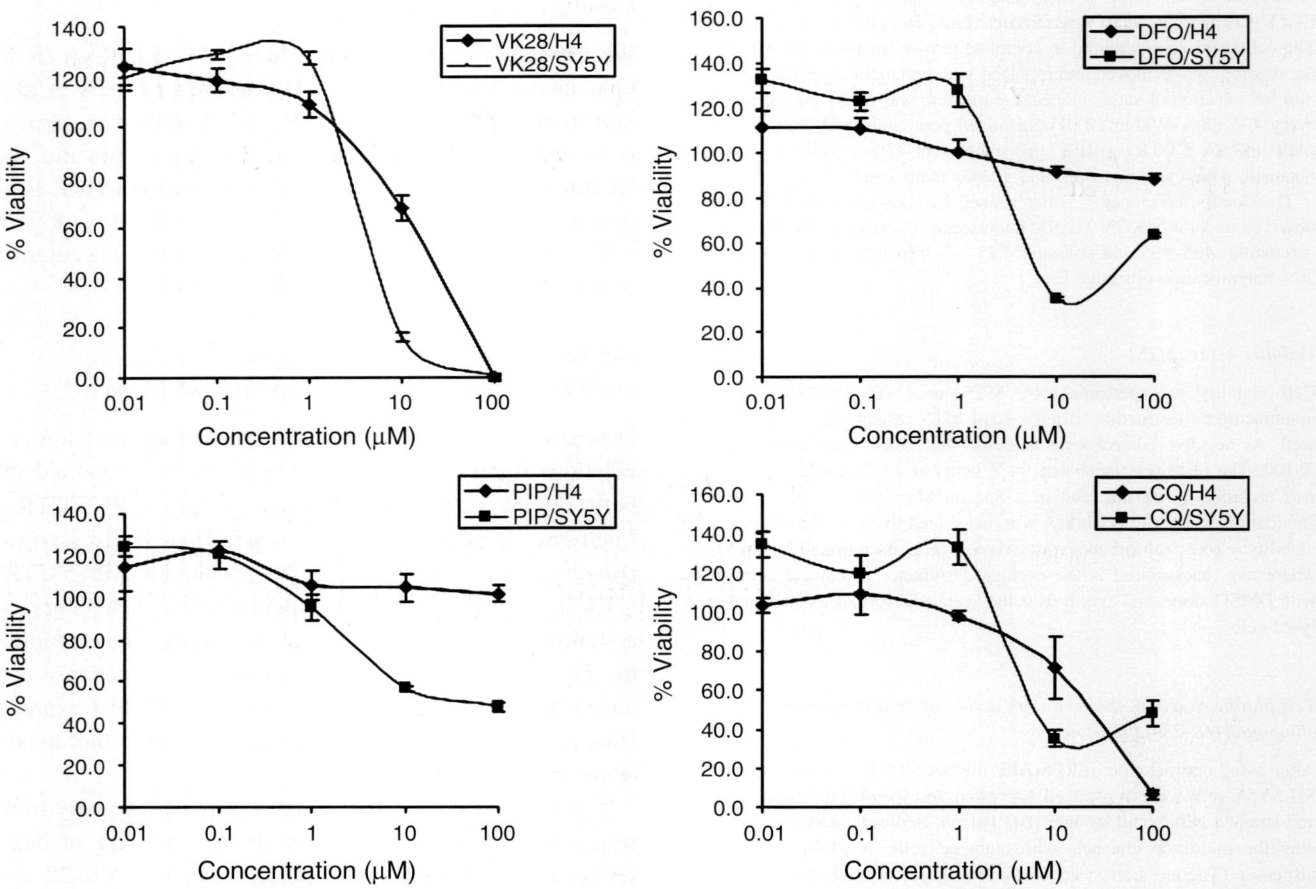

Fig. 3. Dose responsive effect of Desferrioxamine, Clioquinol, Piperazine-1 and VK-28 on cell viability using SH-SY5Y neuroblastoma and H4 neuroglioblastoma models. Cell viability was measured by a standard MTS assay to stain mitochondria. Concentration on the x axis is micromolar chelator for 48 h treatment of SH-SY5Y and H4 cells

Desferrioxamine and clioquinol

Our dose-responsive experiments established that clioquinol was more neurotoxic to H4 cells than desferrioxamine, whereas the two chelators demonstrated similar viability to SH-SY5Y cells. Clioquinol demonstrated and LD-50 of 8 μM in SH-SY5Y cells and 50 μM in H4 cells. Desferrioxamine was toxic to SH-SY5Y cells at a LD-50 of 8 μM. We consistently observed 60% viability for SH-SY5Y cells at 100 μM DFO. DFO was relatively non-toxic to H4 neuroglioblastoma cells (H4 cells were 95% viable at 100 μM DFO).

VK-28 and piperazine-1

Like clioquinol, VK-28 demonstrated and LD-50 of 8 μM in SH-SY5Y cells and 50 μM in H4 neurogliobastoma cells. Piperazine-1 (PIP-1) was far less toxic, and demonstrated an LD-50 value of 100 μM PIP-1 for SH-SY5Y cells. Piperazine-1 was not toxic to H4 cells at the range provided in the assay shown in Fig. 3.

Interestingly all 4 chlelators, piperazine-1, desferriofxamine (Fe^{3+} specific), clioquinol (Cu/Zn/Fe specific) and VK-28 promoted SH-SY5Y growth by 25–30% when delivered to cells at concentrations <1 μM for 48 h. Formally the increased cell viability in response to VK-28, DFO and CQ occurred at the same time that these agents inhibited APP 5′UTR translational activation, although for concentration >1 μM DFO cell viability was reduced at the same time as inhibition of APP 5′UTR directed translation (Rogers, Unpublished Data). In the case of VK-28 and DFO, inhibition of APP 5′UTR directed translation correlates with a therapeutically promising reduction of intracellular APP holoprotein levels, and lowered Aβ peptide secretion from neuroblastoma cells.

Discussion

These experiment confirmed that a potent, functional IRE RNA stem-loop exists in the 146 nucleotide 5′Untranslated region of the Alzheimer's APP transcript (Rogers et al., 2002; Venti et al., 2004). We identified that the APP 5′UTR UTR element was more selective for iron over copper and showed the APP 5′UTR sequence to be unresponsive to zinc (Fig. 2, Fe > Cu > Zn). Chelator dependent APP 5′UTR conferred translation of luciferase reporter was monitored in an internally standardized transfection assay (Fig. 2). These data demonstrated the APP 5′UTR inhibitory capacity of the chelators to be VK-28 > clioquinol > piperazine-1 > desferrioxamine. Desferrioxamine was the most potent chelator at higher concentrations. Each of these chelators exhibit differing specificity towards Fe/Cu/Zn.

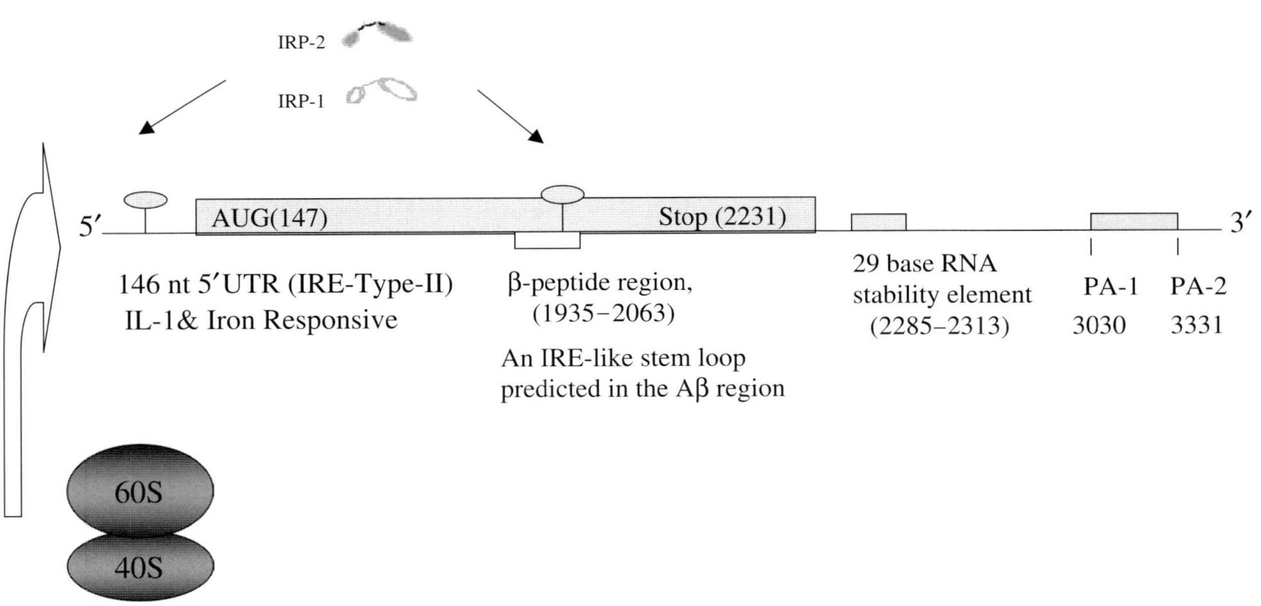

Fig. 4. Regulatory domains mapped to the APP Transcript. The 3 kb APP transcript is controlled at the level of message translation by the action of 5′UTR regulatory domains, conferring translational control by iron (Rogers et al., 2002) and IL-1 (Rogers et al., 1999). The 3′untranslated region is alternatively poly-adenylated, and the longer APP transcript is translated more efficiently than the shorter transcript (Mbella et al., 2000). A 29 nt RNA destabilizing element was mapped to the 1 kb 3′UTR of APP mRNA (Zaidi and Malter, 1994). Ribosome attachment to APP mRNA and translation of APP holoprotein is regulated by both 5′UTR and 3′UTR sequences. IRP-1/IRP-2 interacts *in vitro* and in vivo with APP mRNA

Certainly the expression of the APP is regulated at several levels, including transcription (Lahiri, 1995), RNA stability (Zaidi and Malter, 1994), and message translation (Rogers et al., 1999; Mbella et al., 2000)). The predominance of each of these regulatory levels depends on cell lineage. Iron, IL-1 and TGFβ regulatory elements are present in the 146 nucleotide APP 5′untranslated region (Fig. 4). APP 3′untranslated region sequences (1 kb) control translation of the Aβ-precursor in Chinese hamster ovary cells, whereas APP mRNA stability was shown to be regulated in response to the serum status of endothelial cells (Rajagopalan and Malter, 2000) (Fig. 4).

The APP 5′UTR is a pivotal point for APP production in cells since this 146 nt element harbors both TGFβ transcriptional control sequences (Lahiri et al., 2003), and iron and IL-1 responsive translational sequences (Rogers et al., 1999, 2002). Of recent interest is the report that an APP proximal promoter and APP 5′UTR sequences encode a CAGA sequence (Maloney et al., 2004). This CAGA sequences actually resides within the loop region of the predicted RNA stem-loop specific to the APP 5′UTR, but not within the 5′UTRs of APLP-1 and APLP-2 mRNAs. We are currently investigating whether the CAGA sequence, therefore, may be an IRE specific to amyloid generating genes.

This study characterized the potential of four chelators to limit APP expression via APP 5′UTR sequences. The pharmacological properties of desferrioxamine, clioquinol, VK-28 and a piperazine analogue (Piperazine-1) were compared for their APP 5′UTR inhibitory action in SH-SY5Y cells. Their relative toxicity (LD-50) was established in H4 glioblastoma cells and in SH-SY5Y cells (Fig. 3).

Desferrioxamine

Desferrioxamine (DFO) is a bacterial siderphore that is eliminated from humans in the urine and feces after forming a high affinity hexadentate chelate with Fe^{3+} (26.5 pM affinity for iron) (Rogers and Lahiri, 2004). DFO has already been shown to provide benefit for the treatment of AD (Crapper McLachlan et al., 1991). In a model of PD DFO also protected against proteosome inhibitor-induced nigral degeneration (Zhang et al., 2005). Moreover Youdim and colleagues had reporterd that desferrioxamine was protective to MPTP and 6-OHD treated animal models PD as early as 1975, and 1991 (Ben-Shachar et al., 1991). A major drawback for the clinical use of desferrioxamine is that the chelator does not readily penetrate the blood–brain barrier and has to be administered subcutaneously (Rogers and Lahiri, 2004). These data demonstrated that desferrioxamine selectively inhibited APP 5′UTR conferred translation of a luciferase reporter gene in stable SH-SY5Y transfectants (Fig. 2). Like the Hg/Pb chelator, dimercaptopropanol (Payton et al., 2003), DFO reduced APP holoprotein but also the secretion of Aβ output from SH-SY5Y cells (Cho et al., 2006, in preparation).

Clioquinol

Clioquinol (CQ) binds to metals (Cu, Zn, Fe) at a lower but broader affinity that DFO (Bush, 2002). These current findings showed that this Cu/Zn binding antibiotic selectively inhibited APP 5′UTR conferred translation of a luciferase reporter gene in stable SH-SY5Y transfectants to a greater degree than DFO at the 0.1 μM concentrations, although higher concentrations DFO were more inhibitory than CQ. These transfection-based experiments confirmed that CQ chelated Fe, in addition to Cu and Zn, since the IRE to it in the 5′UTR of the APP transcript was responsive to this antibiotic (Rogers et al., 2002).

CQ inhibited Aβ production *in vivo* by pathways additional to APP 5′UTR directed translation, including dissolution of Aβ amyloid deposits (Cherny et al., 2001), and perhaps inhibition of APP transcription in response to a copper-responsive element in the APP 5′ proximal promoter (Bellingham et al., 2004; Maloney et al., 2004). Clioquinol may have therapeutic benefit to reduce huntingtin protein levels as a therapeutic agent for Huntington's disease (Nguyen et al., 2005).

Certainly clioquinol has been tested in human clinical trials. Ritchie et al. (2004) demonstrated that this broad based low affinity metal chelator was beneficial to AD patients in a limited Phase II clinical trial after CQ (Ritchie et al., 2003). As was the case for desferioxamine (Zhang et al., 2005), CQ provided neuroprotection in the MPP+ mouse model for Parkinson's disease, as has been reported (Kaur et al., 2003). A problem reported for Clioquinol was its neurotoxic effect on murine cortical neurons grown *ex vivo* (Benvenisti-Zarom et al., 2005).

VK-28 and piperazine-1 as novel iron chelators

We show pilot data as to the potential of two new iron chelators, VK-28 and a novel piperazine analog, piperazine-1 (Figs. 2 and 3). Similar to desferrioxamine the high affinity Fe chelators piperazine-1 and VK-28, described in this report, appeared to inhibit translation APP holoprotein expression similar to ferritin translation (Rogers et al., 2002; Thomson et al., 2005). This effect was not targeted to general 5′ cap dependent translation since expression of β-actin and other cellular mRNAs (including APLP-1 and APLP-2) was maintained at high levels when SH-SY5Y cells were treated with all chelators at non-toxic concentrations (MTS assay for cell viability as shown in Fig. 3).

VK-28 was used for PD therapeutics as an iron chelator that protects against dopaminergic lesions in mice (Shachar et al., 2004). VK-28 proved very effective (Fig. 2 showed 15% inhibition of APP 5′UTR driven translation for luciferase reporter expression (at 0.1 μM), although VK-28, like clioquinol, was neurotoxic to SH-SY5Y cells at higher doses >10 μM). Several derivatives of VK-28 are in line from the laboratory of Professor Youdim (Eve Topf and US National Parkinson Foundation Centres of Excellence For Neurodegenerative Diseases, Technion-Rappaport Family Faculty of Medicine) and await further testing as powerful candidates of therapeutic potential for Alzheimer's disease (Gal et al., 2005).

The piperazine derivative, piperazine-1, was a modest inhibitor of APP 5′UTR directed translation. However piperazine-1 was the least neurotoxic of the 4 chelators tested in this report and hence could be dose escalated. Piperazine-based chelators are already effectively employed clinically to diminish cardiotoxicity in cancer patients administered anthracycline antibiotics (Venturini et al., 1996; Wu and Hasinoff, 2005). There remains controversy as to whether piperazine analogs protect cardiac myocytes from doxirubicin toxicity in cancer patients by sequestering iron and limiting the formation of Fe catalysis of OH radical formation by Fenton chemistry (Wu et al., 2004).

The clinical use of desferrioxamine has been hindered by the fact that this Fe chelator is not orally administered and has caused ototthalamic and ophthalamic toxicity (Chiodo et al., 1997). For this reason a new range of orally available iron chelators have been tested for clinical treatment of iron overload associated with blood transfusions. The most commonly used of these agents include deferiprone (Brittenham et al., 2003), Deferasirox (Kontoghiorghes, 2005). Several other novel brain permeable Fe chelators are becoming available. Relevant to this report VK-28 can be administered orally and is brain permeable (Shachar et al., 2004), as was the case for clioquinol (Kaur et al., 2003).

The Alzheimer's APP mRNA 5′untranslated region is a physiologically active element that contributes to set the amount of APP translation in most tissues and cells (Rogers, 2005). We are currently testing how effective the APP 5′UTR acts as a target to discover drugs that inhibit APP holoprotein production and Aβ levels without altering compensatory APLP-1 and APLP-2 levels in the cells. The APP 5′UTR interacts with APP 3′UTR sequences, which may have to be considered in future drug screens for inhibitors of APP translation (Venti et al., 2004).

We have recently screened for potenial anti-amyloid drugs that influence reporter expression translationally driven by both APP 5′UTR/3′UTR sequences. To this end a molecular library of 1200 FDA approved drugs was employed. Indeed, several hits in this FDA library pilot screen were found to be metal chelating agents (i.e., dimercaptopropanol, chloroquine). In progress is a high throughput screen of a molecular library comprising 110,000 compounds (LDDN library) several of which appear to be chelators. These APP 5′UTR directed leads will require further testing of their capacity to limit amyloid Aβ peptide output *in vitro* and *in vivo*.

There is an emerging potential for the use of chelators as therapeutic agents for neurodegenerative disease, including the use of novel Fe chelators as a therapy for AD. This is the case since both DFO (Crapper McClachlan) and clioquinol (Ritchie, 2004) provided useful clinical efficacy in human clinical trials. The efficacy of the APP 5′UTR directed chelators in this report were measured in tissue culture at 0.1 μM concentrations wherein the agents were non-toxic in the SH-SY5Y and H4 cell lines (Fig. 3). It will be necessary to establish the efficacy of each of these chelators (DFO, CQ piperazine-1 and VK-28) to limit amyloid Aβ peptide production.

Acknowledgements

This work was supported by grants from the National Institutes of Health (AG21081) and the Alzheimer's Association (AG18884) to JTR. Dr. Huang is supported by grants from NIMH/NIH (5K01MH002001) and AFAR. The authors would like to thank D. Rudolph Tanzi and Dr. Ashley Bush for continued support, help and scientific discussions concerning this manuscript. Dr. Rogers is particularly grateful to Dr. Lorenzo Refolo and Dr. Howard Fillit (ISOA).

References

Atamna H, Frey WH 2nd (2004) A role for heme in Alzheimer's disease: heme binds amyloid beta and has altered metabolism. Proc Natl Acad Sci USA 101: 11153–11158

Bartzokis G, Sultzer D, Cummings J, Holt LE, Hance DB, Henderson VW, Mintz J (2000) In vivo evaluation of brain iron in Alzheimer disease using magnetic resonance imaging. Arch Gen Psychiatry 57: 47–53

Beal MF (2003) Mitochondria, oxidative damage, and inflammation in Parkinson's disease. Ann N Y Acad Sci 991: 120–131

Bellingham SA, Lahiri DK, Maloney B, La Fontaine S, Multhaup G, Camakaris J (2004) Copper depletion down-regulates expression of the Alzheimer's disease amyloid-beta precursor protein gene. J Biol Chem 279: 20378–20386

Ben-Shachar D, Eshel G, Finberg JP, Youdim MB (1991) The iron chelator desferrioxamine (Desferal) retards 6-hydroxydopamine-induced degeneration of nigrostriatal dopamine neurons. J Neurochem 56: 1441–1444

Benvenisti-Zarom L, Chen J, Regan RF (2005) The oxidative neurotoxicity of clioquinol. Neuropharmacology 49: 687–694

Brittenham G, Nathan D, Oliveieri N, Pippard M, Weatherall D (2003) Deferiprone versus desferrioxamine in thalassaemia, and T2 validation and utility. Lancet 361

Bush A (2002) Metal complexing agents as therapies for Alzheimer's disease. Neurobiol Aging 23: 1031–1038

Bush AI (2003) The Metallobiology of Alzheimer's disease. Trends in Neurosciences 26: 207–214

Caughey WS, Raymond LD, Horiuchi M, Caughey B (1998) Inhibition of protease-resistant prion protein formation by porphyrins and phthalocyanines. Proc Natl Acad Sci USA 95: 12117–12122

Celsi F, Ferri A, D'Amrosi N, Rotliiio G, Costa A, Volonte C, Carri M (2004) Overexpression of superoxide dismutase 1 protects against beta = amyloid peptide toxicity: effect of estrogen and copper chelators. Neurochem Int 44: 25–33

Cherny RA, Atwood CS, Xilinas ME, Gray DN, Jones WD, McLean CA, Barnham KJ, Volitakis I, Fraser FW, Kim Y, et al. (2001) Treatment with a copper-zinc chelator markedly and rapidly inhibits beta-amyloid accumulation in Alzheimer's disease transgenic mice. Neuron 30: 665–676

Chiodo AA, Alberti PW, Sher GD, Francombe WH, Tyler B (1997) Desferrioxamine ototoxicity in an adult transfusion-dependent population. J Otolaryngol 26: 116–122

Cox LA, Kennedy MC, Adrian GS (1995) The 5′-untranslated region of human transferrin mRNA, which contains a putative iron-regulatory element, is bound by purified iron-regulatory protein in a sequence-specific manner. Biochem Biophys Res Commun 212: 925–932

Crapper McLachlan D, Dalton AJ, Kruck TPA, Bell MY, Smith WL, Kalow W, Andrews DF (1991) Intramuscular desferrioxamine in patients with Alzheimer's disease. Lancet 337: 1304–1308

Curtain CC, Ali F, Volitakis I, Cherny RA, Norton RS, Beyreuther K, Barrow CJ, Masters CL, Bush AI, Barnham KJ (2001) Alzheimer's disease amyloid-beta binds copper and zinc to generate an allosterically ordered membrane-penetrating structure containing superoxide dismutase-like subunits. J Biol Chem 276: 20466–20473

Fillebeen C, Caltagirone A, Martelli A, Moulis JM, Pantopoulos K (2005) IRP1 Ser-711 is a phosphorylation site, critical for regulation of RNA-binding and aconitase activities. Biochem J 388: 143–150

Gal S, Zheng H, Fridkin M, Youdim MB (2005) Novel multifunctional neuroprotective iron chelator-monoamine oxidase inhibitor drugs for neurodegenerative diseases. In vivo selective brain monoamine oxidase inhibition and prevention of MPTP-induced striatal dopamine depletion. J Neurochem 95: 79–88

Gunshin H, Allerson CR, Polycarpou-Schwarz M, Rolfs A, Rogers JT, Kishi F, Hentze MW, Rouault TA, Andrews NC, Hediger MA (2001) Iron-dependent regulation of the divalent metal ion transporter. FEBS Letters 509: 309–316

Gunshin H, Fujiwara Y, Custodio AO, Direnzo C, Robine S, Andrews NC (2005) Slc11a2 is required for intestinal iron absorption and erythropoiesis but dispensable in placenta and liver. J Clin Invest 115: 1258–1266

Gutteridge JM (1994) Hydroxyl radicals, iron, oxidative stress, and neurodegeneration. Ann N Y Acad Sci 738: 201–213

Halliwell B, Gutteridge JM (1984) Oxygen toxicity, oxygen radicals, transition metals and disease. Biochem J 219: 1–14

Howlett D, Cutler P, Heales S, Camilleri P (1997) Hemin and related porphyrins inhibit beta-amyloid aggregation. FEBS Lett 417: 249–251

Huang X, Atwood CS, Hartshorn MA, Multhaup G, Goldstein LE, Scarpa RC, Cuajungco MP, Gray DN, Lim J, Moir RD, et al. (1999a) The A beta peptide of Alzheimer's disease directly produces hydrogen peroxide through metal ion reduction. Biochemistry 38: 7609–7616

Huang X, Cuajungco MP, Atwood CS, Hartshorn MA, Tyndall JD, Hanson GR, Stokes KC, Leopold M, Multhaup G, Goldstein LE, et al. (1999b) Cu(II) potentiation of Alzheimer A beta neurotoxicity. Correlation with cell-free hydrogen peroxide production and metal reduction. J Biol Chem 274: 37111–37116

Jeffries W, Dickstein D, Ujiie M (2001) Assessing p97 as an Alzheimer's disease serum biomarker. J Alzheimers Dis 3: 339–344

Jellinger K, Paulus W, Grundke-Iqbal I, Riederer P, Youdim MB (1990) Brain iron and ferritin in Parkinson's and Alzheimer's diseases. J Neural Transm Park Dis Dement Sect 2: 327–340

Kaur D, Yantiri F, Rajagopalan S, Kumar J, Mo JQ, Boonplueang R, Viswanath V, Jacobs R, Yang L, Beal MF, et al. (2003) Genetic or pharmacological iron chelation prevents MPTP-induced neurotoxicity in vivo: a novel therapy for Parkinson's disease. Neuron 37: 899–909

Killilea DW, Wong SL, Cahaya HS, Atamna H, Ames BN (2004) Iron accumulation during cellular senescence. Ann N Y Acad Sci 1019: 365–367

Klausner R, Rouault TA, Harford JB (1993) Regulating the fate of mRNA: the control of cellular iron metabolism. Cell 72: 19–28

Kontoghiorghes GJ (2005) Effects of ICL670 (deferasirox) on cardiac iron concentrations. Lancet 366: 804

Lahiri D, Chen D, Vivien D, Ge Y-W, Greig N, Rogers J (2003) The role of cytokines in the gene expression of amyloid β-protein precursor: identification of a 5′UTR binding nuclear factor and its implications for Alzheimer's disease. JAD 5: 81–90

Lahiri DK, Nall C (1995) Promoter activity of the gene encoding the beta-amyloid precursor protein is up-regulated by growth factors, phorbol ester, retinoic acid and interleukin-1. Brain Res Mol Brain Res 32: 233–240

Lan J, Jiang DH (1997) Desferrioxamine and vitamin E protect against iron and MPTP-induced neurodegeneration in mice. J Neural Transm 104: 469–481

LaVaute T, Smith S, Cooperman S, Iwai K, Land W, Meyron-Holtz E, Drake SK, Miller G, Abu-Asab M, Tsokos M, et al. (2001) Targeted deletion of the gene encoding iron regulatory protein-2 causes misregulation of iron metabolism and neurodegenerative disease in mice. Nat Genet 27: 209–214

Lovell MA, Robertson JD, Teesdale WJ, Campbell JL, Markesbery WR (1998) Copper, iron and zinc in Alzheimer's disease senile plaques. J Neurol Sci 158: 47–52

Mainous AG 3rd, Eschenbach SL, Wells BJ, Everett CJ, Gill JM (2005) Cholesterol, transferrin saturation, and the development of dementia and Alzheimer's disease: results from an 18-year population-based cohort. Fam Med 37: 36–42

Maloney B, Ge YW, Greig N, Lahiri DK (2004) Presence of a "CAGA box" in the APP gene unique to amyloid plaque-forming species and absent in all APLP-1/2 genes: implications in Alzheimer's disease. Faseb J 18: 1288–1290

Mbella EG, Bertrand S, Huez G, Octave JN (2000) A GG nucleotide sequence of the 3′ untranslated region of amyloid precursor protein mRNA plays a key role in the regulation of translation and the binding of proteins. Mol Cell Biol 20: 4572–4579

McKie AT, Marciani P, Rolfs A, Brennan K, Wehr K, Barrow D, Miret S, Bomford A, Peters TJ, Farzaneh F, et al. (2000) A novel duodenal iron-regulated transporter, IREG1, implicated in the basolateral transfer of iron to the circulation. Mol Cell 5: 299–309

Nguyen T, Hamby A, Massa SM (2005) Clioquinol down-regulates mutant huntingtin expression in vitro and mitigates pathology in a Huntington's disease mouse model. Proc Natl Acad Sci USA 102: 11840–11845

Payton S, Cahill CM, Randall JD, Gullans SR, Rogers JT (2003) Drug discovery targeted to the Alzheimer's APP mRNA 5′-untranslated region: the action of paroxetine and dimercaptopropanol. J Mol Neurosci 20: 267–275

Phinney A, Drisaldi B, Schmidt S, Lugowski S, Coronado V, Liang Y, Horne P, Yang J, Sekoulidis J, Coomaraswarmy J, et al. (2003) In vivo reduction of amyloid-β by a mutant copper transporter. PNAS 100: 14193–14198

Pinero DJ, Hu J, Connor JR (2000) Alterations in the interaction between iron regulatory proteins and their iron responsive element in normal and Alzheimer's diseased brains [in process citation]. Cell Mol Biol (Noisy-Le-Grand) 46: 761–776

Priola SA, Raines A, Caughey WS (2000) Porphyrin and phthalocyanine antiscrapie compounds [see comments]. Science 287: 1503–1506

Rajagopalan LE, Malter JS (2000) Growth factor-mediated stabilization of amyloid precursor protein mRNA is mediated by a conserved 29-nucleotide sequence in the 3′- untranslated region. J Neurochem 74: 52–59

Ritchie CW, Bush AI, Mackinnon A, Macfarlane S, Mastwyk M, MacGregor L, Kiers L, Cherny R, Li QX, Tammer A, et al. (2003) Metal-protein attenuation with iodochlorhydroxyquin (clioquinol) targeting Abeta amyloid deposition and toxicity in Alzheimer disease: a pilot phase 2 clinical trial. Arch Neurol 60: 1685–1691

Rogers J (2005) APP and Ferritin Translation, Metals and Alzheimer's disease, in Metals and Medicine, Sessler J, ed. J Am Chem Soc pp 215–251

Rogers JT, Lahiri DK (2004) Metal and inflammatory targets for Alzheimer's disease. Curr Drug Targets 5: 535–551

Rogers JT, Leiter LM, McPhee J, Cahill CM, Zhan SS, Potter H, Nilsson LN (1999) Translation of the Alzheimer amyloid precursor protein mRNA is up-regulated by interleukin-1 through 5′-untranslated region sequences. J Biol Chem 274: 6421–6431

Rogers JT, Randall JD, Cahill CM, Eder PS, Huang X, Gunshin H, Leiter L, McPhee J, Sarang SS, Utsuki T, et al. (2002a) An iron-responsive element type II in the 5′-untranslated region of the Alzheimer's amyloid precursor protein transcript. J Biol Chem 277: 45518–45528

Rogers JT, Randall J, Eder PS, Huang X, Bush AI, Tanzi RE, Venti A, Payton SM, Giordano T, Nagano S, Cahill CM, Moir R, Lahiri DK, Greig N, Sarang SS, Gullans SR (2002b) Alzheimer's disease drug discovery targeted to the APP mRNA 5′untranslated region. J Mol Neurosci 19: 77–82

Sampietro M, Caputo L, Casatta A, Meregalli M, Pellagatti A, Tagliabue J, Annoni G, Vergani C (2001) The hemochromatosis gene affects the age of onset of sporadic Alzheimer's disease. Neurobiol Aging 22: 563–568

Shachar DB, Kahana N, Kampel V, Warshawsky A, Youdim MB (2004) Neuroprotection by a novel brain permeable iron chelator, VK-28, against 6-hydroxydopamine lession in rats. Neuropharmacology 46: 254–263

Smith CD, Carney JM, Starke-Reed PE, Oliver CN, Stadtman ER, Floyd RA, Markesbery WR (1991) Excess brain protein oxidation and enzyme dysfunction in normal aging and in Alzheimer disease. Proc Natl Acad Sci USA 88: 10540–10543

Smith MA, Kutty RK, Richey PL, Yan SD, Stern D, Chader GJ, Wiggert B, Petersen RB, Perry G (1994) Heme oxygenase-1 is associated with the neurofibrillary pathology of Alzheimer's disease. Am J Pathol 145: 42–47

Smith MA, Richey Harris PL, Sayre LM, Beckman JS, Perry G (1997) Widespread peroxynitrite-mediated damage in Alzheimer's disease. J Neurosci 17: 2653–2657

Sparks D, Schreurs B (2003) Trace amounts of copper in water induce beta-amyloid plaques and learning deficits in a rabbit model of Alzheimer's disease. PNAS 100: 11065–11069

Thome J, Gsell W, Rosler M, Kornhuber J, Frolich L, Hashimoto E, Zielke B, Wiesbeck GA, Riederer P (1997) Oxidative-stress associated parameters (lactoferrin, superoxide dismutases) in serum of patients with Alzheimer's disease. Life Sci 60: 13–19

Thompson K, Menzies S, Muckenthaler M, Torti F, Wood T, Torti S, Nentze M, Beard M, Connor J (2003) Mouse brains deficient in H-ferritin have normal iron concentration but protein profile of iron deficiency and increased oxidative stress. J Neurosci Res 71: 46–63

Thomson AM, Cahill CM, Cho HH, Kassachau KD, Epis MR, Bridges KR, Leedman PJ, Rogers JT (2005) The acute box cis-element in human heavy ferritin mRNA 5′-untranslated region is a unique translation enhancer that binds poly(C)-binding proteins. J Biol Chem 280: 30032–30045

Ujiie M, Dickstein D, Jeffires W (2002) p97 as a biomarker for Alzheimer's disease. Front Biosci 7: 42–47

Venti A, Giordano T, Eder P, Lahiri DK, Greig NH, Rogers JT (2004) The integrated role of desferrioxamine and phenserine targeted to an iron-responsive element in the APP-mRNA 5′-untranslated region. Ann N Y Acad Sci 1035: 34–48

Venturini M, Michelotti A, Del Mastro L, Gallo L, Carnino F, Garrone O, Tibaldi C, Molea N, Bellina RC, Pronzato P, et al. (1996) Multicenter randomized controlled clinical trial to evaluate cardioprotection of dexrazoxane versus no cardioprotection in women receiving epirubicin chemotherapy for advanced breast cancer. J Clin Oncol 14: 3112–3120

Vulpe CD, Kuo YM, Murphy TL, Cowley L, Askwith C, Libina N, Gitschier J, Anderson GJ (1999) Hephaestin, a ceruloplasmin homologue implicated in intestinal iron transport, is defective in the sla mouse. Nat Genet 21: 195–199

Wu X, Hasinoff BB (2005) The antitumor anthracyclines doxorubicin and daunorubicin do not inhibit cell growth through the formation of iron-mediated reactive oxygen species. Anticancer Drugs 16: 93–99

Wu X, Patel D, Hasinoff BB (2004) The iron chelating cardioprotective prodrug dexrazoxane does not affect the cell growth inhibitory effects of bleomycin. J Inorg Biochem 98: 1818–1823

Youdim MB, Stephenson G, Ben Shachar D (2004) Ironing iron out in Parkinson's disease and other neurodegenerative diseases with iron chelators: a lesson from 6-hydroxydopamine and iron chelators, desferal and VK-28. Ann N Y Acad Sci 1012: 306–325

Zaidi SH, Malter JS (1994) Amyloid precursor protein mRNA stability is controlled by a 29-base element in the 3′-untranslated region. J Biol Chem 269: 24007–24013

Zecca L, Youdim MB, Riederer P, Connor JR, Crichton RR (2004) Iron, brain ageing and neurodegenerative disorders. Nat Rev Neurosci 5: 863–873

Zhang X, Xie W, Qu S, Pan T, Wang X, Le W (2005) Neuroprotection by iron chelator against proteasome inhibitor-induced nigral degeneration. Biochem Biophys Res Commun 333: 544–549

J Neural Transm (2006) [Suppl] 71: 249–257

Journal of Neural Transmission
Printed in Austria

Green tea catechins as brain-permeable, non toxic iron chelators to "iron out iron" from the brain

S. Mandel, O. Weinreb, L. Reznichenko, L. Kalfon, T. Amit

Eve Topf and US NPF Centers for Neurodegenerative Diseases and Department of Pharmacology, Faculty of Medicine, Technion, Haifa, Israel

Summary Evidence to link abnormal metal (iron, copper and zinc) metabolism and handling with Parkinson's and Alzheimer's diseases pathology has frequently been reported. The capacity of free iron to enhance and promote the generation of toxic reactive oxygen radicals has been discussed numerous times. Metal chelation has the potential to prevent iron-induced oxidative stress and aggregation of alpha-synuclein and beta-amyloid peptides. The efficacy of iron chelators depends on their ability to penetrate the subcellular compartments and cellular membranes where iron dependent free radicals are generated. Thus, natural, non-toxic, brain permeable neuroprotective drugs, are preferentially advocated for "ironing out iron" from those brain areas where it preferentially accumulates in neurodegenerative diseases. This review will discuss the most recent findings from *in vivo* and *in vitro* studies concerning the transitional metal (iron and copper) chelating property of green tea and its major polyphenol, (−)-epigallocatechin-3-gallate with respect to their potential for the treatment of neurodegenerative diseases.

Abbreviations: *AD* Alzheimer's disease; *Aβ* amyloid beta peptide; *APP* amyloid precursor protein; *DA* dopamine; *DFO* desferrioxamine; *EGCG* (−)-epigallocatechin-3-gallate; *HIF-1* hypoxia inducible factor-1; *IRE* iron responsive element; *IRP* iron regulatory protein; *MPTP* N-methyl-4-phenyl-1,2,3,6-tetrahydropyridine; *6-OHDA* 6-hydroxydopamine; *OS* oxidative stress; *PD* Parkinson's disease; *PKC* protein kinase C; *sAPP-α* soluble APP-alpha; *SN* substantia nigra; *Tf* transferrin; *TfR* transferrin receptor; *ROS* reactive oxygen species.

Introduction

The consumption of tea is believed to have been initiated five thousands years ago in China and India (Gutman, 1996). In general, tea is consumed in the form of green tea, oolong tea or black tea, which are all derived from *Camellia sinensis*, a small plant grown mainly in China, Japan and Southeast Asia. Green and black teas are differently manufactured. Preservation of the intact green leaf is of highest importance in the preparation of green tea. The freshly harvested leaves are steamed to prevent fermentation, rolled and then dried. This process yields a chemical composition in green tea similar to the fresh tea leaf. The preparation of black tea involves a "fermentation" process in which fresh leaves are withered, rolled and crushed, initiating a chain of oxidative reactions of the catechin polyphenols contained in them. This results in polymerization of the catechins converting them into higher molecular weight theaflavins and thearubigins, conferring tea its strong dark color and special flavor. A less extensive, partial fermentation leads to a lighter flavored tea, known as oolong tea (Cooper et al., 2005).

Nowadays, tea is considered as a source of dietary constituents endowed with biological and pharmacological activities with potential benefits to human health. The increasing interest in the health properties of tea extract and its main catechin polyphenols have led to a significant rise in scientific investigation for prevention and therapeutics in several diseases. Several of these are subject, in the last few years, of intensive investigation in diverse medical disciplines, such as cardiology, oncology (Wiseman et al., 2001; Higdon and Frei, 2003; Galati and O'Brien, 2004), inflammatory diseases and neurology. The favorable properties of green tea extract had been ascribed to their high content of polyphenolic flavonoids. Fresh tea leaves, contains a high amount of catechins, a group of flavonoids or flavanols, known to constitute 30–45% of the solid green tea extract (Yang and Wang, 1993; Wang et al., 1994). Among the tea catechins, (−)-epigallocatechin-3-gallate (EGCG) is the major constituent, accounting for more than 10% of the extract dry weight followed by (−)-epigallocatechin, (EGC) > (−)-epicatechin and (EC) ≥ (−)-epicatechin-3-gallate (ECG). Ingested tea catechins are absorbed mainly in the small intestine and metabolized by enzymatic reactions of glucuronidation, sulfation and *O*-methylation.

Correspondence: Dr. S. Mandel, Efron St., P.O.B. 9697, Haifa 31096, Israel
e-mail: mandel@tx.technion.ac.il

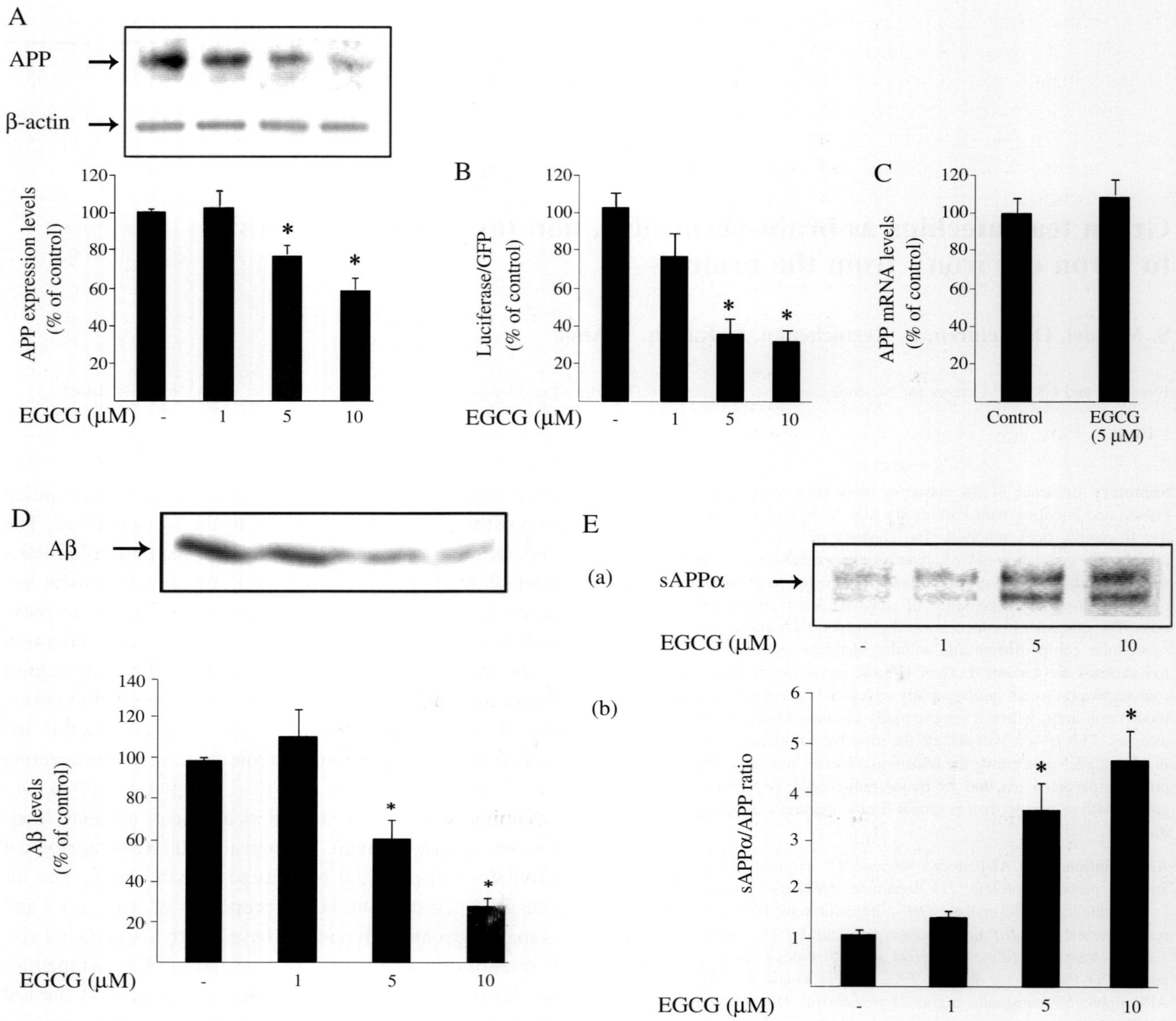

Fig. 1. Effect of EGCG on holo-APP protein and mRNA expression levels, sAPPα secretion and Aβ generation (adapted from Reznichenko et al., 2006). **A**, **B** Human neuroblastoma SH-SY5Y cells were treated without (control) or with increasing concentrations of EGCG (1–10 μM) for 48 h. **A** EGCG dose-dependently reduced holo-APP protein levels (43.1 ± 5.7% at 10 μM), as assessed by Western blot analysis, using antibody 22C11. The histogram under the gel micrograph summarizes the values from three independent experiments normalized to β-actin and expressed as percentage of control. $^{*}p < 0.01$ vs control. **B** The efficacy of EGCG as an iron chelator, to modulate the translation of a luciferase reporter gene driven by the APP 5′-UTR sequences was tested in U-87-MG glioma cells, co-transfected with 10 μg of DNA from pGALA plasmid (APP 5′-UTR + APP 3′-UTR sequences) and 5 μg of DNA from a construct that expresses GFP, to standardize for transfection efficiency. Cell plates were grown in the absence (control) or presence of increasing concentrations of EGCG (1–10 μM) for 48 h. Values represent luciferase activity normalized to GFP (mean ± SEM, from four independent experiments, each conducted in six replicates). $^{*}p < 0.01$, vs untreated control. EGCG gradually suppressed APP 5′-UTR reporter gene expression in a concentration-dependent manner (maximal inhibition of 68.4 ± 5.0% at 10 μM EGCG vs. the untreated control). **C** APP gene expression was measured by quantitative real-time RT-PCR. The amount of the products was normalized to the housekeeping gene 18S-rRNA and expressed as percentage of control. EGCG did not affect APP mRNA levels, indicating a post-transcriptional regulatory mechanism. **D** The regulatory effect of EGCG on the amyloidogenic Aβ peptides was analyzed in CHO/ΔNL cells, stably transfected with the "Swedish" APP mutation, since Aβ levels in the medium of SH-SY5Y are undetectable. EGCG treatment for 48 h markedly reduced Aβ levels in the medium of CHO/ΔNL cells, achieving a maximal decrease (72.8 ± 4.7%) with 10 μM EGCG. **E** The effect of EGCG on secreted soluble APP-alpha. sAPPα was assessed in SH-SY5Y cells under long-term, 48 h culture conditions. (a) EGCG significantly induced sAPPα release into the medium (at 10 μM, 241 ± 19% of control) and (b) progressively increased the ratio sAPPα/holo-APP along the EGCG concentration range (at 10 μM, 460% of control), indicating that the compound favors the non-amyloidogenic pathway of APP processing

These forms are detected in plasma and excreted in bile and urine (for review see Bravo, 1998). There is evidence that polyphenol metabolites and their parent compounds have access to the brain. Studies with radioactively labeled EGCG in mouse or chemiluminescence-based detection of EGCG in rats, demonstrated its incorporation into brain, as well as in various organs including kidney, heart, liver, spleen and pancreas (Nakagawa and Miyazawa, 1997; Suganuma et al., 1998).

Catechin polyphenols have been demonstrated to act directly as radical scavengers of oxygen and nitrogen species and exert indirect antioxidant effects through activation of transcription factors and antioxidant enzymes such as catalase and superoxide dismutase, thus modulating the cellular redox state (see reviews: Wiseman et al., 1997; Rice-Evans, 2001; Higdon and Frei, 2003). In addition to their radical scavenging action, green tea catechins possess well established metal chelating properties. Structurally important features defining their chelating potential are the 3′,4′-dihydroxyl group in the B ring (Hider et al., 2001), as well as the gallate group (Guo et al., 1996; Kumamoto et al., 2001), which may neutralize ferric iron to form redox-inactive iron, thereby protecting cells against oxidative damage (Grinberg et al., 1997). In fact, the ability of green tea catechins to act as antioxidants *in vitro* is based on their metal chelating capacity and on the potent quenching of singlet oxygen (Tournaire et al., 1993).

This review aims to shed light on the relevance of the divalent metal chelating properties of green tea polyphenols to neurodegeneration, where increased amounts of ionic, redox-active toxic metals trigger a cascade of neurotoxic events and cause aggregation of proteins such as alpha-synuclein (α-synuclein) and amyloid-β peptide (Aβ).

Iron and neurodegeneration

Various metals have been implicated in the pathophysiology of certain neuropsychiatric diseases. Thus, iron is present in substantia nigra, globus pallidus, and dentate gyrus at a concentration equal to or greater than that found in the liver. These three brain regions are known to be associated with neurodegenerative diseases (Youdim and Riederer, 2004). Specifically, redox-active iron has been observed in the rim of Lewy body, the morphological hallmark of Parkinson's disease (PD), composed also of lipids, aggregated α-synuclein (concentrating in its peripheral halo) and ubiquitinated, hyperphosphorylated neurofilament proteins (Jellinger, 2003). Altered iron homeostasis has also been reported in Alzheimer's disease (AD), as indicated by changes in the levels of iron, ferritin and transferrin receptor (TfR) in the hippocampus and cerebral cortex (Beard et al., 1993; Sipe et al., 2002; Honda et al., 2005). Iron promotes both deposition of Aβ and induction of oxidative stress (OS), which is associated with the plaques. Indeed, it has been demonstrated that amyloid deposits are enriched with zinc, iron and copper (Atwood et al., 2003).

Conventional neurochemical studies as well as genomic and proteomic profiling of brain autopsy material from PD patients and more recently from AD, have provided evidence for the involvement of supplementary processes, including glutamatergic neurotoxicity, nitric oxide elevation, dysfunction of ubiquitin-proteasome system and mitochondria, which may lead to breakdown of energy metabolism and consecutive intraneuronal calcium overload, increased expression of apoptotic proteins and loss of tissue reduced glutathione (GSH; an essential factor for removal of hydrogen peroxide) (Riederer et al., 1989; Blum et al., 2001; Linazasoro, 2002; McNaught et al., 2002; Blalock et al., 2004; Grunblatt et al., 2004; Poon et al., 2005; Zhang et al., 2005). These series of neurotoxic events may act independently or cooperatively, leading eventually to the demise of the neurons. Thus, considering the multifactorial nature of neurodegenerative disorders, drugs directed against single functional components of the different disease pathologies, such as cognition or movement disorder will be limited in efficacy. It is likely that strategies considering the application of multi-site directed drugs (polypharmacology) or combining drugs with different therapeutic targets may be more suitable to address the varied pathological aspects of the disease.

Neuroprotection by metal chelation with EGCG

One innovative therapeutic approach could be the use of non-toxic, brain-permeable natural plant polyphenols, reported to possess multifunctional activities (Guo et al., 1996; Morel et al., 1999; Hider et al., 2001; Rice-Evans, 2001; Joseph et al., 2005) and as recently reviewed (Mandel et al., 2004b, 2005). Of particular importance to neurodegenerative diseases, such as PD, AD and amyotrophic lateral sclerosis (ALS), is the ability of catechins to act as antioxidants, to inhibit peroxynitrite-mediated oxidation of dopamine (DA), to inhibit nitration of tyrosine residues (Pannala et al., 1998; Kerry and Rice-Evans, 1999) and to chelate divalent metals (Guo et al., 1996; Kumamoto et al., 2001). Research from our laboratory has demonstrated that the antioxidant-iron chelating activity of the major green tea polyphenol EGCG plays a major role in the prevention of neurodegeneration in a variety of cellular and animal models of neurodegenerative diseases (Mandel et al., 2004a; Mandel and Youdim, 2004). Thus, EGCG was reported to protect human neuroblastoma cells from damage induced by 6-hydroxydopamine (6-OHDA) and 1-methyl-4-phenylpyridinium (MPP^+) (Levites et al., 2002); to protect primary hippocampal neurons (Choi et al., 2001) and rescue rat pheochromocytoma (PC12) cells from Aβ-induced toxicity, presumably through the scavenging of ROS (Levites et al., 2003). More recently, EGCG was shown to exert a neurorescue activity in long-term serum-deprived PC12 cells and to promote neurite outgrowth (Reznichenko et al., 2005). This could have important implications with regard to aging, PD and AD, suggesting a potential therapeutic use of EGCG in regenerating injured neuronal cells.

Accumulating studies indicate that the neuroprotective/neurorescue activity of catechin flavonoids are likely the result of activation of an array of different signaling pathways involved in cellular survival, growth and differentiation as protein kinase C (PKC) and extracellular mitogen-activated protein kinase (MAPK) (Schroeter et al., 2002; Mandel et al., 2005). In the context of cell survival, EGCG was shown to down-regulate pro-apoptotic genes, such as bad, bax, mdm2, caspase-1, cyclin dependent kinase inhibitor p21 and TNF-related apoptosis-inducing ligand (TRAIL) (Levites et al., 2002; Weinreb et al., 2003) and to regulate transcriptional activation (Wiseman et al., 1997; Higdon and Frei, 2003; Townsend et al., 2004; Zhou et al., 2004; Thomas and Kim, 2005). These findings and the well acknowledged antioxidant/iron chelating attributes of tea catechins, suggest that green tea extract may be a source of neuroprotectants, with particular relevance to neurodegenerative diseases where OS has also been implicated.

Reduction of amyloid precursor protein (APP) and toxic Aβ by EGCG: implication of iron chelation

Whether iron has a primary or a secondary role in neurodegeneration is unknown. The limited number of neuroprotective studies that have been carried out so far, indicate that iron-chelation therapy could be a viable neuroprotective approach for neurodegenerative disorders (Rogers and Lahiri, 2004; Zecca et al., 2004; Youdim and Buccafusco, 2005). Treatment with desferal/desferrioxamine (DFO) as an iron chelator or with the antibiotic iron and copper chelator, 5-chloro-7-iodo-8-hydroxyquinoline (clioquinol) was shown to be neuroprotective against the neurotoxins 6-hydroxydopamine (6-OHDA) and N-methyl-4-phenyl-1,2,3,6-tetrahydropyridine (MPTP)-induced neurotoxicity in rats and mice, respectively (Ben-Shachar et al., 1991; Kaur et al., 2003). Furthermore, treatment with clioquinol inhibited Aβ accumulation in AD transgenic mouse model (Cherny et al., 2001). However, DFO is a very poor brain penetrating agent and clioquinol is highly toxic (Meade, 1975). More recently, the multifunctional iron chelator/monoamine oxidase (MAO)-A and -B inhibitor, brain-permeable compound, M-30 (Youdim et al., 2004; Youdim and Buccafusco, 2005), showed neuroprotective activities in neuronal rat PC12 and P19 cell cultures against serum deprivation and 6-OHDA (Zheng et al., 2005a, b) and in MPTP-induced parkinsonism (Gal et al., 2005).

In AD pathology, iron may regulate APP translation, via a mechanism involving the iron responsive element-type II (IRE-type II) located in the 5′UTR region of APP mRNA (Rogers et al., 2002). This is consistent with biochemical evidence pointing to APP as a redox-active metalloprotein (Huang et al., 2004). APP was found to be post-transcriptionally regulated by iron regulatory proteins (IRPs), which are labile iron pool-sensitive cytosolic RNA proteins binding specifically to the IRE located in the 5′ or 3′ untranslated regions of iron metabolism-associated mRNAs. Changes in the iron status (iron overload or depletion) lead to compensating changes in the IRP/IRE system of translational control of iron homeostasis. For example, the APP 5′-UTR-conferred translation was selectively down-regulated upon intracellular iron chelation, in a similar manner as the iron-storage protein ferritin, which also possesses an IRE in its 5′UTR mRNA (Rogers et al., 2002).

The evidence that tea catechins, including EGCG, are well established metal ion chelators and the involvement of metal chelation in APP/Aβ regulation raised the question whether EGCG could affect APP processing. This possibility was recently investigated by our group, demonstrating a dual regulatory effect of EGCG on Alzheimer's APP: EGCG reduces holo-APP, presumably through iron chelation, and induces non-amyloidogenic soluble APP-alpha (sAPPα) release via PKC activation, resulting ultimately in inhibition of Aβ peptide generation (Reznichenko et al., 2006) (Fig. 1A). The observed reduction in APP protein levels was linked to the chelation of intracellular free-iron labile pool by EGCG, as this polyphenol was shown to suppress the translation of a luciferase reporter gene driven by the APP 5′-UTR sequences (Fig. 1B), as has been recently described for other metal chelators, such as DFO, clioquinol and dimercaptopropanol (Rogers et al., 2002; Payton et al., 2003). Since EGCG did not alter APP mRNA levels (Fig. 1C), the decrease in the levels of APP protein was attributed to the suppression of APP translation. The finding that exogenous iron supplementation reversed EGCG action on APP, reinforces the likelihood that these effects are mediated through modulation of the intracellular iron pool. The *in vitro* findings are supported by a previous *in vivo* study, which demonstrated that prolonged administration of EGCG to mice induced a significant reduction in membrane-associated APP levels in mice hippocampus (Levites et al., 2003). Furthermore, different experimental strategies have shown that EGCG markedly reduced secreted Aβ levels in the conditioned medium of Chinese hamster ovarian cells, overexpressing "Swedish" mutated APP (CHO/ΔNL) (Reznichenko et al., 2006) (Fig. 1D) and in primary neuronal cells derived from transgenic mice bearing the APP "Swedish" mutation (Rezai-Zadeh et al., 2005). Other lines of research focusing on Aβ stability and toxicity reported that green tea or wine polyphenols (e.g. resveratrol) are able to inhibit formation, extension and destabilization of Aβ fibrils *in vitro* (Ono et al., 2003, 2004), to lower the levels of secreted and intracellular Aβ in various cell lines (Marambaud et al., 2005) and to protect against Aβ-induced neurotoxicity (Levites et al., 2003). Thus, attenuation of both APP synthesis and Aβ production by EGCG could be of therapeutic value for AD therapy, as increased generation of β-amyloid peptides plays a central role in AD plaque formation (Cuajungco et al., 2005).

The other important pharmacological action of EGCG is related to recent reports demonstrating that either short- or long-term incubation with EGCG promotes the generation of the soluble N-terminal fragment, sAPPα, via PKC-dependent activation of α-secretase (Reznichenko et al., 2006; Levites et al., 2003) (Fig. 1E). In this context, EGCG has been shown to up-regulate PKCα and PKCε isoforms in mice striatum and hippocampus (Levites et al., 2003; Mandel et al., 2004a). New supportive data came from a study conducted in Alzheimer transgenic mice, showing that EGCG promotes sAPPα generation through activation of α-secretase cleavage (Rezai-Zadeh et al., 2005). This was accompanied by a significant reduction in cerebral Aβ levels and β-amyloid plaques. Since sAPPα and Aβ are formed by two mutually exclusive mechanisms, stimulation of the secretory processing of sAPPα might prevent the formation of the amyloidogenic Aβ. Thus, EGCG may influence Aβ levels, either via translational inhibition of APP or by stimulating sAPPα secretion. Cleavage of APP within the Aβ domain by α-secretases is of physiological interest, not only because it precludes the formation of Aβ, but also because it promotes the generation of sAPPα that exhibits neuroprotective properties (Mattson, 1997; De Strooper and Annaert, 2000). Moreover, shedding of the ectodomain is a prerequisite for the cleavage of the intracellular domain of γ-secretases, a process that liberates a C-terminal fragment with transcriptional activity (Cao and Sudhof, 2001; Gao and Pimplikar, 2001; Leissring et al., 2002). Thus, promotion of α-secretase-mediated APP processing, rather than down-regulation of Aβ production, may offer a novel approach to AD treatment (Esler and Wolfe, 2001).

Induction of iron/hypoxia-responsive genes by green tea catechins

The interplay of iron and oxygen is most interesting in hypoxic condition where they interact causing brain damage. The link between hypoxia and iron is reflected by the hypoxic-mediated regulation of proteins that modulate iron homeostasis like IRPs (IRP1 and IRP2), ferritin and TfR. Indeed, all the major genes of iron metabolism respond to hypoxia (Sorond and Ratan, 2000). Substantial amounts of chelatable iron are released from storage during hypoxia and ischemia (Bralet et al., 1992). One of the adaptive responses employed by hypoxic mammalian cells is the induction of hypoxia-inducible factor-1 (HIF-1), considered as the master regulator of the "hypoxic world", being responsible for the concerted expression of a myriad of genes which participate in the processes of angiogenesis, cell proliferation/survival and glucose/iron metabolism (Lee et al., 2004; Sharp and Bernaudin, 2004). Thus, the reduction in the small, chelatable iron pool by iron chelation will affect not only the post-transcriptional regulation of iron homeostasis-related mRNAs (e.g. TfR, ferritin) but also the induction of a wide array of genes tightly regulated by HIF-1 (Fig. 2).

Iron was recently shown to block HIF-1 activation induced by the green tea catechins, EGCG and epicatechin-3-gallate (ECG), as well as by DFO (Zhou et al., 2004; Thomas and Kim, 2005). In fact, both HIF-1 and IRP2 share a common iron-dependent proteasomal degradation pathway, by the activation of key iron and oxygen sensors prolyl hydroxylases, which become inactivated by iron chelation (Hanson et al., 2003; Wang et al., 2004). Thus, the reduction in the free-iron pool by EGCG chelation may result in the inhibition of prolyl hydroxylases and consequently, in the concerted activation of both HIF and IRP2. As IRPs and HIF-1 coordinate the expression of a wide array of regulators involved in cellular iron homeostasis, survival and proliferation (Templeton and Liu, 2003; Sharp and Bernaudin, 2004), their activation could be of major importance in neurodegenerative diseases (Fig. 2).

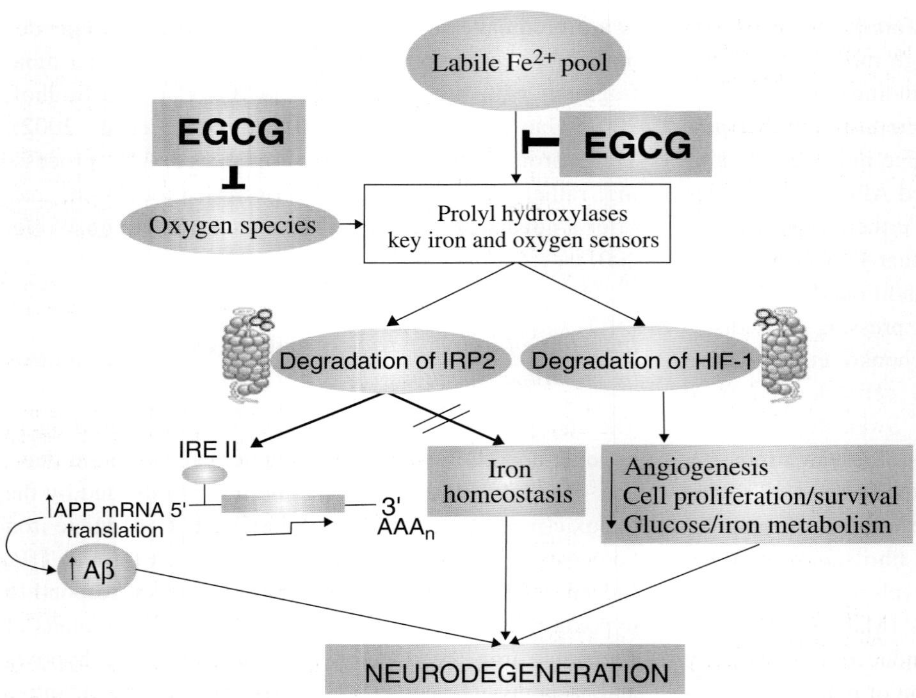

Fig. 2. Iron-induced neurodegeneration in AD via transcriptional activation of APP mRNA and suppression of hypoxia-inducible genes. Increase in labile Fe^{2+} pool can elevate the production of APP via proteasomal-mediated inactivation of IRP2, thereby promoting the translation of APP mRNA from its 5′UTR-typeII). Increased iron and oxygen species may activate the prolyl hydroxylase enzymes, which are key iron and oxygen sensors, leading to proteasomal-mediated degradation of the transcription factor HIF-1, a master regulator orchestrating the coordinated induction of a wide array of survival genes. It has been suggested that IRP2, similar to HIF-1, can be enzymatically modified by a prolyl hydroxylase, routing it to proteasomal degradation. Both iron chelation and oxygen species scavenging by EGCG may prevent the degradation of IRP2 and HIF-1, resulting in the promotion of cell survival processes such as angiogenesis, glucose metabolism and maintenance of iron homeostasis. EGCG, (−)-epigallocatechin-3-gallate; IRP, iron regulatory protein; HIF-1, hypoxia inducible factor-1. Sharp arrows indicate positive inputs, whereas blunt arrows are for inhibitory inputs. For a more detailed explanation read text

Conclusion

Although the precise mechanism of neuroprotection/neurorescue exerted by green tea catechins is not fully established, accumulating evidence indicates the participation of multiple pathways, including the pro-survival PKC and extracellular mitogen-activated protein kinase (MAPK) signaling (Mandel et al., 2005); promotion of neurite outgrowth (Reznichenko et al., 2005); down-regulation of pro-apoptotic genes (Levites et al., 2002; Weinreb et al., 2003) and promotion of secreted soluble, non-toxic, non-amyloidogenic form of APP, reputed to have neurotrophic and neuroprotective properties against excitotoxic and oxidative insults (Levites et al., 2003). Recently, a new dimension was added to these actions, associated with the iron chelating property of green tea catechins and the impact on neurodegenerative processes, as inhibitors of OS-mediated protein aggregation, APP synthesis and Aβ plaque formation. Considering the pathological role iron plays in a number of neurological conditions, the use of EGCG as a natural, non-toxic, lipophilic brain permeable neuroprotective drug, could offer potential therapeutic benefits for "iron out iron" from those brain areas where it preferentially accumulates (Youdim and Buccafusco, 2005).

Acknowledgment

The authors of this review would like to honour Moussa Youdim for his outstanding and significant contribution to the field of neuroscience. He was among the pioneers who envisaged the pivotal role iron takes in the "neurodegeneration arena". His high intellect, together with his innovative research on Parkinson's disease and multifunctional drug design, place him among the handful of people who make one feel that the "sky is the limit".

Thank you, Moussa for your unconditional support, for always being there when needed, for the stimulating experience and pleasure of being part of your selected research team, bust most of all, for being a "MENTCH".

References

Atwood CS, Obrenovich ME, Liu T, Chan H, Perry G, Smith MA, Martins RN (2003) Amyloid-beta: a chameleon walking in two worlds: a review of the trophic and toxic properties of amyloid-beta. Brain Res Brain Res Rev 43: 1–16

Beard JL, Connor JR, Jones BC (1993) Iron in the brain. Nutr Rev 51: 157–170

Ben-Shachar D, Eshel G, Finberg JP, Youdim MB (1991) The iron chelator desferrioxamine (Desferal) retards 6-hydroxydopamine-induced degeneration of nigrostriatal dopamine neurons. J Neurochem 56: 1441–1444

Blalock EM, Geddes JW, Chen KC, Porter NM, Markesbery WR, Landfield PW (2004) Incipient Alzheimer's disease: microarray correlation analyses reveal major transcriptional and tumor suppressor responses. Proc Natl Acad Sci USA 101: 2173–2178

Blum D, Torch S, Lambeng N, Nissou M, Benabid AL, Sadoul R, Verna JM (2001) Molecular pathways involved in the neurotoxicity of 6-OHDA, dopamine and MPTP: contribution to the apoptotic theory in Parkinson's disease. Prog Neurobiol 65: 135–172

Bravo L (1998) Polyphenols: chemistry, dietary sources, metabolism, and nutritional significance. Nutr Rev 56: 317–333

Cao X, Sudhof TC (2001) A transcriptionally [correction of transcriptively] active complex of APP with Fe65 and histone acetyltransferase Tip60. Science 293: 115–120

Cherny RA, Atwood CS, Xilinas ME, Gray DN, Jones WD, McLean CA, Barnham KJ, Volitakis I, Fraser FW, Kim Y, Huang X, Goldstein LE, Moir RD, Lim JT, Beyreuther K, Zheng H, Tanzi RE, Masters CL, Bush AI (2001) Treatment with a copper–zinc chelator markedly and rapidly inhibits beta-amyloid accumulation in Alzheimer's disease transgenic mice. Neuron 30: 665–676

Choi YT, Jung CH, Lee SR, Bae JH, Baek WK, Suh MH, Park J, Park CW, Suh SI (2001) The green tea polyphenol (−)-epigallocatechin gallate attenuates beta- amyloid-induced neurotoxicity in cultured hippocampal neurons. Life Sci 70: 603–614

Cooper R, Morre DJ, Morre DM (2005) Medicinal benefits of green tea: Part I. Review of noncancer health benefits. J Altern Complem Med 11: 521–528

Cuajungco MP, Frederickson CJ, Bush AI (2005) Amyloid-beta metal interaction and metal chelation. Subcell Biochem 38: 235–254

De Strooper B, Annaert W (2000) Proteolytic processing and cell biological functions of the amyloid precursor protein. J Cell Sci 113: 1857–1870

Esler WP, Wolfe MS (2001) A portrait of Alzheimer secretases – new features and familiar faces. Science 293: 1449–1454

Gal S, Zheng H, Fridkin M, Youdim MBH (2005) Novel multifunctional neuroprotective iron chelator-monoamine oxidase inhibitor drugs for neurodegenerative diseases. In vivo selective brain monoamine oxidase inhibition and prevention of MPTP-induced striatal dopamine depletion. J Neurochem 95: 79–88

Galati G, O'Brien PJ (2004) Potential toxicity of flavonoids and other dietary phenolics: significance for their chemopreventive and anticancer properties. Free Radic Biol Med 37: 287–303

Gao Y, Pimplikar SW (2001) The gamma -secretase-cleaved C-terminal fragment of amyloid precursor protein mediates signaling to the nucleus. Proc Natl Acad Sci USA 98: 14979–14984

Grinberg LN, Newmark H, Kitrossky N, Rahamim E, Chevion M, Rachmilewitz EA (1997) Protective effects of tea polyphenols against oxidative damage to red blood cells. Biochem Pharmacol 54: 973–978

Grunblatt E, Mandel S, Jacob-Hirsch J, Zeligson S, Amariglo N, Rechavi G, Li J, Ravid R, Roggendorf W, Riederer P, Youdim MBH (2004) Gene expression profiling of parkinsonian substantia nigra pars compacta; alterations in ubiquitin-proteasome, heat shock protein, iron and oxidative stress regulated proteins, cell adhesion/cellular matrix and vesicle trafficking genes. J Neural Transm 111: 1543–1573

Guo Q, Zhao B, Li M, Shen S, Xin W (1996) Studies on protective mechanisms of four components of green tea polyphenols against lipid peroxidation in synaptosomes. Biochim Biophys Acta 1304: 210–222

Gutman RL, Ryu RH (1996) Rediscovering tea: an exploration of the scientific literature. Herbal Gram 37: 33–48

Hanson ES, Rawlins ML, Leibold EA (2003) Oxygen and iron regulation of iron regulatory protein 2. J Biol Chem 278: 40337–40342

Hider RC, Liu ZD, Khodr HH (2001) Metal chelation of polyphenols. Methods Enzymol 335: 190–203

Higdon JV, Frei B (2003) Tea catechins and polyphenols: health effects, metabolism, and antioxidant functions. Crit Rev Food Sci Nutr 43: 89–143

Honda K, Smith MA, Zhu X, Baus D, Merrick WC, Tartakoff AM, Hattier T, Harris PL, Siedlak SL, Fujioka H, Liu Q, Moreira PI, Miller FP, Nunomura A, Shimohama S, Perry G (2005) Ribosomal RNA in Alzheimer disease is oxidized by bound redox-active iron. J Biol Chem 280: 20978–20986

Huang X, Moir RD, Tanzi RE, Bush AI, Rogers JT (2004) Redox-active metals, oxidative stress, and Alzheimer's disease pathology. Ann N Y Acad Sci 1012: 153–163

Jellinger KA (2003) Neuropathological spectrum of synucleinopathies. Mov Disord 18 [Suppl 6]: S2–S12

Joseph JA, Shukitt-Hale B, Casadesus G (2005) Reversing the deleterious effects of aging on neuronal communication and behavior: beneficial properties of fruit polyphenolic compounds. Am J Clin Nutr 81 [Suppl 1]: 313S–316S

Kaur D, Yantiri F, Rajagopalan S, Kumar J, Mo JQ, Boonplueang R, Viswanath V, Jacobs R, Yang L, Beal MF, DiMonte D, Volitaskis I, Ellerby L, Cherny RA, Bush AI, Andersen JK (2003) Genetic or pharmacological iron chelation prevents MPTP-induced neurotoxicity in vivo: a novel therapy for Parkinson's disease. Neuron 37: 899–909

Kerry N, Rice-Evans C (1999) Inhibition of peroxynitrite-mediated oxidation of dopamine by flavonoid and phenolic antioxidants and their structural relationships. J Neurochem 73: 247–253

Kumamoto M, Sonda T, Nagayama K, Tabata M (2001) Effects of pH and metal ions on antioxidative activities of catechins. Biosci Biotechnol Biochem 65: 126–132

Lee JW, Bae SH, Jeong JW, Kim SH, Kim KW (2004) Hypoxia-inducible factor (HIF-1)alpha: its protein stability and biological functions. Exp Mol Med 36: 1–12

Leissring MA, Murphy MP, Mead TR, Akbari Y, Sugarman MC, Jannatipour M, Anliker B, Muller U, Saftig P, De Strooper B, Wolfe MS, Golde TE, LaFerla FM (2002) A physiologic signaling role for the gamma -secretase-derived intracellular fragment of APP. Proc Natl Acad Sci USA 99: 4697–4702

Levites Y, Amit T, Youdim MBH, Mandel S (2002) Involvement of protein kinase C activation and cell survival/cell cycle genes in green tea polyphenol (−)-epigallocatechin-3-gallate neuroprotective action. J Biol Chem 277: 30574–30580

Levites Y, Amit T, Mandel S, Youdim MBH (2003) Neuroprotection and neurorescue against amyloid beta toxicity and PKC-dependent release of non-amyloidogenic soluble precusor protein by green tea polyphenol (−)-epigallocatechin-3-gallate. Faseb J 17: 952–954

Linazasoro G (2002) Neuroprotection in Parkinson's disease: love story or mission impossible? Expert Rev Neurotherapeutics 2: 403–416

Mandel S, Youdim MBH (2004) Catechin polyphenols: neurodegeneration and neuroprotection in neurodegenerative diseases. Free Radical Bio Med 37: 304–317

Mandel S, Maor G, Youdim MBH (2004a) Iron and alpha-synuclein in the substantia nigra of MPTP-treated mice: effect of neuroprotective drugs R-apomorphine and green tea polyphenol (−)-epigallocatechin-3-gallate. J Mol Neurosci 24: 401–416

Mandel S, Weinreb O, Amit T, Youdim MBH (2004b) Cell Signaling Pathways in the Neuroprotective Actions of the Green Tea Polyphenol (−)-Epigallocatechin-3-Gallate: Implications for Neurodegenerative Diseases. J Neurochem 88: 1555–1569

Mandel SA, Avramovich-Tirosh Y, Reznichenko L, Zheng H, Weinreb O, Amit T, Youdim MBH (2005) Multifunctional activities of green tea catechins in neuroprotection. Neurosignals 14: 46–60

Marambaud P, Zhao H, Davies P (2005) Resveratrol promotes clearance of Alzheimer's disease amyloid-beta peptides. J Biol Chem 280: 37377–37382

Mattson MP (1997) Cellular actions of beta-amyloid precursor protein and its soluble and fibrillogenic derivatives. Physiol Rev 77: 1081–1132

McNaught KS, Belizaire R, Jenner P, Olanow CW, Isacson O (2002) Selective loss of 20S proteasome alpha-subunits in the substantia nigra pars compacta in Parkinson's disease. Neurosci Lett 326: 155–158

Meade TW (1975) Subacute myelo-optic neuropathy and clioquinol. An epidemiological case-history for diagnosis. Br J Prev Soc Med 29: 157–169

Morel I, Lescoat G, Cogrel P, Sergent O, Pasdeloup N, Brissot P, Cillard P, Cillard J (1999) Antioxidant and iron-chelating activities of the flavonoids catechin, quercetin and diosmetin on iron-loaded rat hepatocyte cultures. Biochem Pharmacol 45: 13–19

Nakagawa K, Miyazawa T (1997) Absorption and distribution of tea catechin, (−)-epigallocatechin-3-gallate, in the rat. J Nutr Sci Vitaminol (Tokyo) 43: 679–684

Ono K, Hasegawa K, Naiki H, Yamada M (2004) Anti-amyloidogenic activity of tannic acid and its activity to destabilize Alzheimer's beta-amyloid fibrils in vitro. Biochim Biophys Acta 1690: 193–202

Ono K, Yoshiike Y, Takashima A, Hasegawa K, Naiki H, Yamada M (2003) Potent anti-amyloidogenic and fibril-destabilizing effects of polyphenols in vitro: implications for the prevention and therapeutics of Alzheimer's disease. J Neurochem 87: 172–181

Pannala AS, Razaq R, Halliwell B, Singh S, Rice-Evans CA (1998) Inhibition of peroxynitrite dependent tyrosine nitration by hydroxycinnamates: nitration or electron donation? Free Radical Bio Med 24: 594–606

Payton S, Cahill CM, Randall JD, Gullans SR, Rogers JT (2003) Drug discovery targeted to the Alzheimer's APP mRNA 5′-untranslated region: the action of paroxetine and dimercaptopropanol. J Mol Neurosci 20: 267–275

Poon HF, Shepherd HM, Reed TT, Calabrese V, Stella AM, Pennisi G, Cai J, Pierce WM, Klein JB, Butterfield DA (2005) Proteomics analysis provides insight into caloric restriction mediated oxidation and expression of brain proteins associated with age-related impaired cellular processes: Mitochondrial dysfunction, glutamate dysregulation and impaired protein synthesis. Neurobiol Ageing: Epub ahead of print

Rezai-Zadeh K, Shytle D, Sun N, Mori T, Hou H, Jeanniton D, Ehrhart J, Townsend K, Zeng J, Morgan D, Hardy J, Town T, Tan J (2005) Green tea epigallocatechin-3-gallate (EGCG) modulates amyloid precursor protein cleavage and reduces cerebral amyloidosis in Alzheimer transgenic mice. J Neurosci 25: 8807–8814

Reznichenko L, Amit T, Youdim MBH, Mandel S (2005) Green tea polyphenol (−)-epigallocatechin-3-gallate induces neurorescue of long-term serum-deprived PC12 cells and promotes neurite outgrowth. J Neurochem 93: 1157–1167

Reznichenko L, Amit T, Zheng H, Weinreb O, Avramovich-Tirosh Y, Youdim MBH, Mandel S (2006) Reduction of the iron-regulated beta-amyloid precursor protein and toxic beta-amyloid peptides expression by green tea polyphenol (−)-epigallocatechin-3-gallate: implication of iron chelation in Alzheimer's disease. J Neurochem 97: 27–36

Rice-Evans C (2001) Flavonoid antioxidants. Curr Med Chem 8: 797–807

Riederer P, Sofic E, Rausch WD, Schmidt B, Reynolds GP, Jellinger K, Youdim MBH (1989) Transition metals, ferritin, glutathione, and ascorbic acid in parkinsonian brains. J Neurochem 52: 515–520

Rogers JT, Lahiri DK (2004) Metal and inflammatory targets for Alzheimer's disease. Curr Drug Targets 5: 535–551

Rogers JT, Randall JD, Cahill CM, Eder PS, Huang X, Gunshin H, Leiter L, McPhee J, Sarang SS, Utsuki T, Greig NH, Lahiri DK, Tanzi RE, Bush AI, Giordano T, Gullans SR (2002) An iron-responsive element type II in the 5′-untranslated region of the Alzheimer's amyloid precursor protein transcript. J Biol Chem 277: 45518–45528

Schroeter H, Boyd C, Spencer JP, Williams RJ, Cadenas E, Rice-Evans C (2002) MAPK signaling in neurodegeneration: influences of flavonoids and of nitric oxide. Neurobiol Ageing 23: 861–880

Sharp FR, Bernaudin M (2004) HIF1 and oxygen sensing in the brain. Nat Rev Neurosci 5: 437–448

Sipe JC, Lee P, Beutler E (2002) Brain iron metabolism and neurodegenerative disorders. Dev Neurosci 24: 188–196

Sorond FA, Ratan RR (2000) Ironing-out mechanisms of neuronal injury under hypoxic-ischemic conditions and potential role of iron chelators as neuroprotective agents. Antioxidants and Redox Signaling 2: 421–436

Suganuma M, Okabe S, Oniyama M, Tada Y, Ito H, Fujiki H (1998) Wide distribution of [3H](−)-epigallocatechin gallate, a cancer preventive tea polyphenol, in mouse tissue. Carcinogenesis 19: 1771–1776.

Templeton DM, Liu Y (2003) Genetic regulation of cell function in response to iron overload or chelation. Biochim Biophys Acta 1619: 113–124

Thomas R, Kim MH (2005) Epigallocatechin gallate inhibits HIF-1alpha degradation in prostate cancer cells. Biochem Biophys Res Commun 334: 543–548

Tournaire C, Croux S, Maurette MT, Beck I, Hocquaux M, Braun AM, Oliveros E (1993) Antioxidant activity of flavonoids: efficiency of singlet oxygen (1 delta g) quenching. Journal of Photochemistry and Photobiology B 19: 205–215

Townsend PA, Scarabelli TM, Davidson SM, Knight RA, Latchman DS, Stephanou A (2004) STAT-1 interacts with p53 to enhance DNA damage-induced apoptosis. J Biol Chem 279: 5811–5820

Wang J, Chen G, Muckenthaler M, Galy B, Hentze MW, Pantopoulos K (2004) Iron-mediated degradation of IRP2, an unexpected pathway involving a 2-oxoglutarate-dependent oxygenase activity. Mol Cell Biol 24: 954–965

Wang ZY, Huang MT, Lou YR, Xie JG, Reuhl KR, Newmark HL, Ho CT, Yang CS, Conney AH (1994) Inhibitory effects of black tea, green tea, decaffeinated black tea, and decaffeinated green tea on ultraviolet B light-induced skin carcinogenesis in 7,12-dimethylbenz[a]anthracene-initiated SKH-1 mice. Cancer Res 54: 3428–3455

Weinreb O, Mandel S, Youdim MBH (2003) cDNA gene expression profile homology of antioxidants and their anti-apoptotic and pro-apoptotic activities in human neuroblastoma cells. Faseb J 17: 935–937

Wiseman S, Mulder T, Rietveld A (2001) Tea flavonoids: bioavailability in vivo and effects on cell signaling pathways in vitro. Antioxid Redox Signal 3: 1009–1021

Wiseman SA, Balentine DA, Frei B (1997) Antioxidants in tea. Crit Rev Food Sci Nutr 37: 705–718

Yang CS, Wang ZY (1993) Tea and cancer. J Natl Cancer Inst 85: 1038–1049.

Youdim MBH, Riederer P (2004) Iron in the brain, normal and pathological, In: Adelman G, Smith B (eds) Encyclopedia of Neuroscience, Elsevier

Youdim MBH, Buccafusco JJ (2005) Multi-functional Drugs for Various CNS Targets in the Treatment of Neurodegenerative Disorders. Trends Pharmacol Sci 26: 27–35

Youdim MBH, Fridkin M, Zheng H (2004) Novel bifunctional drugs targeting monoamine oxidase inhibition and iron chelation as an approach to neuroprotection in Parkinson's disease and other neurodegenerative diseases. J Neural Transm 111: 1455–1471

Zecca L, Youdim MBH, Riederer P, Connor JR, Crichton RR (2004) Iron, brain ageing and neurodegenerative disorders. Nat Rev Neurosci 5: 863–873

Zhang Y, James M, Middleton FA, Davis RL (2005) Transcriptional analysis of multiple brain regions in Parkinson's disease supports the involvement of specific protein processing, energy metabolism, and signaling pathways, and suggests novel disease mechanisms. Am J Med Genet B Neuropsychiatr Genet 137: 5–16

Zheng H, Gal S, Weiner LM, Bar-Am O, Warshawsky A, Fridkin M, Youdim MBH (2005a) Novel multifunctional neuroprotective iron chelator-monoamine oxidase inhibitor drugs for neurodegenerative diseases: in vitro studies on antioxidant activity, prevention of lipid peroxide formation and monoamine oxidase inhibition. J Neurochem 95: 68–78

Zheng H, Weiner LM, Bar-Am O, Epsztejn S, Cabantchik ZI, Warshawsky A, Youdim MBH, Fridkin M (2005b) Design, synthesis, and evaluation of novel bifunctional iron-chelators as potential agents for neuroprotection in Alzheimer's, Parkinson's, and other neurodegenerative diseases. Bioorg Med Chem 13: 773–783

Zhou YD, Kim YP, Li XC, Baerson SR, Agarwal AK, Hodges TW, Ferreira D, Nagle DG (2004) Hypoxia-inducible factor-1 activation by (−)-epicatechin gallate: potential adverse effects of cancer chemoprevention with high-dose green tea extracts. J Nat Prod 67: 2063–2069

Index

Springer and the Environment

WE AT SPRINGER FIRMLY BELIEVE THAT AN INTERnational science publisher has a special obligation to the environment, and our corporate policies consistently reflect this conviction.

WE ALSO EXPECT OUR BUSINESS PARTNERS – PRINTERS, paper mills, packaging manufacturers, etc. – to commit themselves to using environmentally friendly materials and production processes.

THE PAPER IN THIS BOOK IS MADE FROM NO-CHLORINE pulp and is acid free, in conformance with international standards for paper permanency.